HAND BOOK
ON
HERBAL PRODUCTS

(Cosmetics, Toiletries , Medicines & Perfumes)
in 2 Volumes

Vol. I

IMPORTANT STEPS FOR SELECTION OF AN INDUSTRY

- If you are not in a position to decide an appropriate industry within your range of investment then read this book thoroughly. You will find a number of industries of your interest in the book.

- Select few products and keep them in mind for discussion with your friends and family members.

- For the selection you may seek the services of your consultant who can provide you more informations and guidance on the ins and out of all the products which you have selected and help in the final selection of one or two of the products which suits you.

- Although this book provides you basic information, yet before going in for implementation you are advised to assess the latest prices of plant, machinery and raw materials, market position through your own sources.

- For detailed information on manufacturing process, market survey, selection of appropriate plant and machinery, procurement of loan from financial institutions, and other assistance, you must obtain Practical Project Execution Know-How Report which can be availabe from "National Institute of Industrial Research",106 - E, Kamla Nagar, Delhi - 110 007.

HAND BOOK
ON
HERBAL PRODUCTS
(Cosmetics, Toiletries, Medicines & Perfumes)
in 2 Volumes

Vol. I

by

NIIR Board of Technologists

Publicaton Division
नेशनल इंस्टीट्यूट ऑफ इन्डस्ट्रियल रिसर्च
National Institute of Industrial Research
Regd.Office: 106-E, Kamla Nagar, Delhi-110 007(INDIA)

Published by :

National Institute of Industrial Research

Regd. Office: 106-E, Kamla Nagar, P.B. No.2162, Delhi - 110007 (INDIA)
Ph. : 91-11-23843955, 23845654, 23845886, 9811043595
Fax : 91-11-23841561 **E-Mail** : niir @ vsnl.com
Website : www.niir.org

I.S.B.N. : 81-86623-48-5 (Set)

Price Rs. 1500/- (For 2 Volumes)
Us$ 220/-

Printed & Published by **Ajay Kr. Gupta** for "**National Institute of Industrial Research**", Delhi-110007 & Printed at New Gian Offset Printers, Shahzada Bagh, Delhi-35.

Ist(BJJJBAFAA)
IInd(CAAEBCFAA)

CONTENTS

VOL I

1

Herbel Cosmetics

Cosmetic

Any substance, preparation, or treatment, applied to the person (*a*) to cleanse, (*b*) to alter the appearance, (*c*) to promote the attractiveness of the person. The term thus includes all creams, powders, lotions, and coloring agents applied to the face, scalp, hair, and hands, and many borderline products, such as deodorants, depilatories, and oral and suntan preparations.

According to the broad definitions in the preceding section, the various kinds, of cosmetic products are best grouped in three principal classes: (1) for the skin, (2) for the hair, and (3) for the nails. In form they may be dry powders, pastes, solid or liquid emulsions, or aqueous, alcoholic, or oily solutions. The methods of manufacturing are essentially those employed for the manufacture of other commercial products of similar form. In the following pages, therefore, specific information will be given only for those products that require special techniques, or notes on other points of special interest.

Cosmetology

A branch of applied science that deals with the external embellishment of the person through the use of cosmetic products and treatments. As specified in most state laws, the regions of the body that may be treated in cosmetology are the head, neck, upper chest and back, arms, and hands (now extended to include lower legs and feet). The permitted treatments are hairdressing, haircutting, temporary and permanent waving, hair bleaching and coloring, and corrective and preventive care, by massage or otherwise, of scalp and skin on face, chest, back, arms, and hands. Related branches are body massage, electrolysis, and chiropody.

INGREDIENTS OF HERBEL COSMETICS

Both organic and inorganic natural materials are used in the manufacture of herbel cosmetic products; the former have undergone a gradual shifting from natural vegetable and animal substances, through metallic compounds, to the synthetic organic. As only certain substances of a class may have the properties desired for a certain cosmetic product, the range of possible ingredients is usually limited.

Among the types of organic substances used in cosmetics are: natural and synthetic oils, fats, and waxes; liquid, semisolid, and solid hydrocarbons; soaps and synthetic surface-active agents; starches, gums, and resins; dyes and pigments; acids, alcohols, and esters; alkyl- and alkanolamines; and many others. The inorganic substances include water and hydrogen peroxide; metallic salts and oxides; acids, ammonia, fixed alkalies; and many others.

Cosmetic Emulsions

Cosmetic lotions and creams are emulsions of water-based and oil-based phases. An emulsion is a two-phase system consisting of two incompletely miscible liquids, the internal, or discontinuous, phase dispersed as finite globules in the other. Special designations have been devised for oil and water emulsions to indicate which is the dispersed and which the continuous phase. Oil-in-water (o/w) emulsions have oil as the dispersed phase in water as the continuous phase. In water-in-oil (w/o) emulsions, water is dispersed in oil, which is the external (continuous) phase (8-9) (see Emulsions).

Properties of Emulsions

The properties that are most apparent, and thus are usually most important, are: case of dilution, viscosity, color, and stability. For a given type of emulsification equipment, these properties depend upon: (1) the properties of the continuous phase, (2) the ratio of the external to the internal phase, (3) the particle size of the emulsion, (4) the relationship of the continuous phase to the particles (including ionic charges), and (5) the properties of the discontinuous phase. In any given emulsion, the properties depend upon which liquid constitutes the external phase, ie, whether the emulsion is o/w or w/o. The resulting emulsion type is controlled by: (1) the emulsifier: type, and amount, (2) the ratio of ingredients, and (3) the order of addition of ingredients during mixing.

The dispersibility (solubility) of an emulsion is determined by the continuous phase; thus if the continuous phase is water-soluble; the emulsion can be diluted with water; conversely, if the continuous phase is oil-soluble, the emulsion can be diluted with oil.

The ease with which an emulsion can be diluted, increased by decreasing the viscosity of the emulsion. The viscosity of an emulsion when the continuous phase is in excess is essentially the viscosity of the continuous phase. As the proportion of internal phase increases, the viscosity of the emulsion increases to the point that the emulsion is no longer fluid. When the volume of the internal phase exceeds the volume of the external phase, the emulsion particles become crowded and the apparent viscosity is partially structural viscosity

An emulsion is stable as long as the particles of the internal phase do not coalesce. The stability of emulsion depends upon: (1) the particle size; (2) the difference in density of the two phase; (3) the viscosity of the continuous phase and of the completed emulsion; (4) the charges on the particles; (5) the nature, effectiveness, and amount of the emulsifier used; and (6) conditions of storage, including temperature variation, agitation and vibration, and dilution or evaporation during storage or use. The stability of an emulsion is affected by almost all factors involved in its formulation and preparation. In· formulas containing sizable amounts of emulsifier, stability is predominantly a function of the type and concentration of emulsifier.

Emulsifiers

Emulsifiers can be classified as ionic or nonionic according to their behaviour. An ionic emulsifier is composed of an organic lipophilic group (L) and a hydrophilic group (H). The hydrophilic- lipophilic balance (HLB) is often used to characterize emulsifiers and related surfactant materials. The ionic types may be further divided into anionic and cationic, depending upon the nature of the ion-active group. The lipophilic portion of the molecule is usually considered to be the surface-active portion.

Nonionic emulsifiers are completely covalent and show no apparent tendency to ionize. They can, therefore, be combined with other nonionic surface-active agents and with either anionic or cationic agents as well. The nonionic emulsifiers are likewise less susceptible to the action of electrolytes than the anionic surface-active agents. The solubility of an emulsifier is of the greatest importance in the preparation of emulsifiable concentrates.

Emulsifiers, being surface-active agents, lower surface and interfacial tensions and increase the tendency of their solution to spread.

O/w emulsifying agents produce emulsions in which the continuous phase is hydrophilic; hence, such emulsions are generally dispersible in water and will conduct electricity. The surfactants that are capable of producing such emulsions usually have an HLB of more than 6.0 (preferably 7), the hydrophilic portion of their molecules being predominant. (Between HLB 5 and 7 many surfactants will function as either w/o or o/w emulsifiers, depending on how they are used).

O/w emulsifiers		HLB
P.E.G. 300 distearate	nonionic	7.3
sorbitan monolaurate	nonionic	8.6
P.E.G. 400 distearate	nonionic	9.3
triethanolamine stearate	anionic	12.0
P.E.G. 6000 monolaurate	nonionic	19.2

W/o emulsifiers produce emulsions in which the continuous phase is lipophilic in character (oil, wax, fat, etc). Such emulsions are not generally dispersible in water and do not conduct electricity. The surfactants capable of producing such emulsions usually have an HLB of less than 6.0 and preferably below 5. The lipophilic portion of their molecules is predominant.

W/o emulsifiers		HLB
lanolin alcohols	nonionic	ca 1.0
ethylene glycol monostearate S/E	nonionic	2.0
propylene glycol monostearate S/E	anionic	3.2
sorbitan monooleate	nonionic	4.3
P.E.G. 200 dilaurate	nonionic	6.0

COSMETICS FOR THE SKIN

Under cosmetics for the skin may be included all preparations used for conditioning or embellishment—creams, lotions, masks, powders, colorings and products used for personal hygiene—toilet soaps, accessories for the bath, deodorants, and hair removers.

CREAMS

Creams constitute the largest class of cosmetic preparations used on the skin. Although the variety may seem bewildering, every true cream consists basically of an emulsion of oily and watery substances in solid or liquid form. According to their function, creams fall into three principal groups: cleansers, emollients, and finishers. Most cleansing creams and all emollient creams are water-in-oil emulsions; most of the finishing creams are oil-in-water emulsions. The Toilet Goods Association has published standards for most of the raw materials used in the making of cosmetic creams.

Cleansing creams are of three types: cold creams, "quick-liquefying" creams, and liquid cleaners. A satisfactory cleansing cream is a water-in-oil emulsion that melts at the temperature of the body and spreads readily over the skin. The oily ingredients should be light enough to penetrate a little to clear the skin of impurities, and flow away. It should not contain any appreciable amounts of substances that might be retained by the skin. The product should not be sticky; after it is removed, the skin should feel smooth, clean but not greasy, and relaxed.

The product known as *cold cream* is of historical interest because the original recipe for a cream of this kind dates from the *Ceratum refrigerans Galeni*, introduced by Galen, a physician of ancient Rome (A.D. 130-200). It consisted of almond oil, bees-wax, and rose water; the designation *cold* was undoubtedly applied to it because of the sensation produced on the skin as the water evaporated. An early modification of the recipe, long official in some pharmacopeias, contained spermaceti and a small amount of borax as an auxiliary emulsifying agent; still later, varying amounts of mineral oil, paraffin, and other related substances were included. This type of cleanser is satisfactory for the normal skin as well as for a skin that tends to dryness. Some typical compositions for cold cream are given in Table I (3, 4, 6 9, 13). Among other fatty and waxy materials occasionally incorporated in cold creams are: carnauba wax, castor oil, ceresin, cocoabutter, olive oil, oleic acid, peanut oil, sesame oil, stearic acid (triple pressed, XXX), and certain synthetic fats and waxes. Among many newer emulsifying agents are: aminoglycol, alkanolamines, and esters of polyhydric alcohols. Distilled or de-ionized water is now used instead of rose water: practically all cleansing creams are delicately perfumed.

Table I. Compositions of Cleansing Creams.

	Typical recipe, % by wt. in					
Ingredient	1	2	3	4	5	6
Almond oil	34	50	35	–	–	–
Beeswax	16	12	12	8	13	5
Lanolin	–	–	15	–	–	20
Mineral oil	–	–	–	50	45	–
Paraffin wax	–	–	–	–	–	35
Spermaceti	–	12	8	12	6	55
Borax	1	1	–	1	1	–
Distilled water	–	–	–	–	35	35
Stronger rose water	49	25	28	29	–	–
Total	100	100	100	100	100	100

The so-called *quick-liquefying creams* as originally prepared were not really creams, that is, emulsions, but simply mixtures of liquid and solid hydrocarbons, melted together and perfumed. The principal purpose of this type of product is to melt and spread rapidly, but it is not equally effective in removing all kinds of dirt. As the long continued use of petroleum hydrocarbons is admittedly drying, cleansers of this type are more satisfactory for skins that tend toward oiliness. To meet this criticism, some compositions have ben modified to contain animal and vegetable fats and waxes, and even to produce them as emulsions. For some typical compositions, see Table II.

Table II. Compositions of Quick-Liquefying Creams.

	Typical recipe, % by wt. in:				
Ingredient	1	2	3	4	5
Beeswax	16	–	9	–	7
Ceresin	–	12	–	–	12
Mineral oil	74	88	50	50	43
Ozokerite	5	–	–	–	–
Paraffin wax	5	–	18	30	–
Petrolatum	–	–	23	20	38
Total	100	100	100	100	100

Emollient creams are those intended for the special purpose of softening the skin, and are usually employed as lubricants or while resting. They were formerly designated "skin foods," "rejuvenating creams," "nourishing creams," etc., and are now recognizable as "night creams," or "massage creams," etc.

In physical properties, emollient creams often are of a heavier consistency than cleansing creams; because of the presence of lanolin, they are often yellowish and appreciably tacky. As lanolin, itself, is entirely too viscous to permit free motion over the skin, emollient creams contain varying percentages of vegetable and mineral oils. To avoid the yellowish tinge, mixtures of sterols with inert hydrocarbons—the so-called absorption bases—are often substituted for lanolin.

Other ingredients of emollient creams may be: benzoinated land, cocoa butter, beeswax, spermaceti; almond, corn, castor, and olive oils; hydrogenated vegetable oils; cetyl and stearyl alcohols, glycerol, glycol, and derivatives; lecithin, vitamins and estrogenic substances. Because of the relative case with which lanolin creams seem to penetrate the skin, they serve as vehicles for products with specifically intended properties; that is, bleaching, astringent, and medicated creams. The effectiveness of organotherapeutic agents, as applied externally in cosmetic creams, has been the subject of intensive research and is still a subject of controversy despite steadily encouraging reports on research. Some typical compositions for emollient creams are given in Table III.

Table III. Compositions of Emollient Creams.

	Typical recipe, % wt. in:				
Ingredient	1	2	3	4	5
Almond oil	–	–	10	10	–
Beeswax	20	8	4	10	–
Borax	1	–	–	0.5	–
Cetyl alcohol	2	2	–	–	–
Cholesterol	2.5	2	–	–	3
Cocoa butter	7	6	–	10	–
Lanolin (anhydrous)	–	10	10	5	50
Olive oil	–	50	10	–	–
Lecithin	–	1	–	–	–
Petrolatum (solid or liquid)	45.5	–	20	40	–

Stearic acid (XXX)	–	–	–	–	10
Spermaceti	–	–	4.5	5	–
Triethanolamine	–	–	–	–	8
Perfume	1	1	0.5	0.5	1
Preservative	0.5	1	0.2	0.5	1
Water, to make	100.0	100.0	100.0	100.0	100.0

Products that are high in lanolin content are specifically good as lubricants for massage of a dry skin. For the oily skin, a composition containing little or no lanolin is more satisfactory; many operators find a cleansing cream satisfactory for this purpose.

Finishing creams are those used after the skin is cleansed (and in facial treatments, after the massage) as a foundation for make-up. They are of two types: vanishing creams and pigmented foundations.

Vanishing creams is essentially an oil-in-water emulsion of stearic acid and water in which a small amount of a suitable emulsifier serves as the binder. The latter may be formed *in situ* by first mixing a portion of the stearic acid with sodium or potassium hydroxide, triethanolamine, aminoglycol, etc. This type of product is readily recognizable by its pearly luster. Sodium stearate produces a relatively harder, and potassium stearate a relatively softer, cream; the latter is usually preferable.

The so-called vanishing creams do not actually disappear into the skin, but simply spread a thin smooth film over it, which temporarily conceals roughness and enhances the effect of face powder. Because some skins are appreciably dry, modifying substances are usually added to the basic emulsion; glycerol is often present as a humectant. Among the substances used to vary the properties of vanishing creams are: cocoa butter, lanolin, cetyl alcohol, benzoinated lard, mineral oil (for superficial oiliness), and certain synthetic waxes.

The proportion of glycerol present is a most important factor. Many of the objections to vanishing creams in the early days were due to an inadequate understanding of the properties and effects of glycerol. As it can combine with water in all proportions, it may serve as a humectant and be beneficial to the skin; if used in excess, it may extract water from the tissues causing a drying or burning sensation. In humid weather it also absorbs moisture from the atmosphere, causing stickiness and spotting in face powder. In the past, certain imported creams of this type were found to contain as high as 50% of glycerol; American products are uniformly lower in content. Some typical compositions for vanishing creams are given in Table IV.

Table IV. Compositions of Vanishing Foundation Creams

Ingredient	Typical recipe, % by wt.in: 1	2	3	4	5
Cetyl alcohol	–	–	0.5	0.5	–
Glycerol	10	10	5	8	6
Lanolin	–	1	5	–	4
Mineral oil	–	2	5	–	–
Potassium hydroxide	1	0.5	–	–	2
Sodium hydroxide	–	0.5	–	0.4	–
Stearic acid (XXX)	25	22	20	20	15
Triethanolanine	–	–	2	1.2	–
Perfume	0.5	1	0.5	–	–
Water, to make	100.0	100.0	100.0	100.0	100.0

Pigmented foundations are modifications of the heavy creams used as theatrical make-up. Any good recipe for vanishing cream can serve as the base, the opacity being supplied by incorporating a good powder composition in appropriate shades. Some of these products are applied like vanishing cream, directly from the tube or jar, and are carefully spread over the skin a little at a time. Others, in the form of a compressed cake of cream or paste, are applied with water and a sponge, and allowed to dry. Depending upon the composition, the effect of one of these foundations may or may not be satisfactory without the application of face powder over it.

If properly compounded, these pigmented foundations (also called *cake make-up* and *powder base*) may be used on any type of skin. They are especially effective on skin that tends to oiliness because they give a smooth finish and effectively conceal the conspicuous pores and other blemishes commonly found in oily skin.

Special creams comprise all those whose composition is modified to effect some definite purpose, such as bleaching or tightening the skin, or clearing it of minor lesions.

A stringent creams are used during facial treatments for the massage of an oily skin, and for overnight use at home. Almost any good emollient cream can serve as a basis; substances added for the astringent effect are alum, zine phenolsulfonate, zinc sulfate, and the like. The exact nature of the mechanism by which an astringent cream functions is not definitely understood (see *Astringents*). As the so-called pores (actually the pilosebaceous openings) cannot be reduced in size, it is believed that the appearance of reduction results from varying degrees of swelling in the tissue surrounding the lumen of the pore. In practice the use of an astringent cream is usually supplemented by application of an astringent lotion.

Bleaching creams contain a variety of ingredients, selected either for lightening the color of the skin or for covering it with an opaque white film. Any good composition for emollient cream can serve as the basis, and the product is used both in beauty shops and at home, either as a step in a facial treament or overnight. Stronger bleaching agents incorporated in these creams are mercury compounds (chiefly ammoniated mercury, permissible to 5%); among the milder compounds commonly used are peroxides of hydrogen, magnesium, and zinc, and mild (weak) acids, such as dilute acetic, citric, and lactic. As they act slowly, these creams are supplemented by the use of bleaching lotions. The whitening creams contain titanium dioxide or zinc oxide (occasionally bismuth "subnitrate") and simply spread white pigment over the face. Older products of this type appear as thick pastes, compounded with water instead of in a cream base, or as powders, to be mixed with water.

Acne creams, intended to help in clearing the complexion of pustules and other minor lesions, are more properly classed as drugs than as cosmetics. A good emollient cream should serve as the base, preferably one very soft in consistency so that the product can be spread easily without irritating the skin. Among the active ingredients commonly employed for treatment of acne are: benzoin, β-naphthol, cade oil, camphor, boric and salicylic acids, phenol, sulfur, zinc carbonate (calamine), and zinc oxide. The composition of such a cream should be based on sound dermatological principles.

"All-purpose" creams are actually misnamed. From the foregoing discussion of the desired properties and the functions of various standard types of cosmetic creams, it should be clear that no single product can serve the purpose of all of them equally well. A cleansing cream, for example, which is intended to act superficially and leave the

skin relaxed and receptive, cannot also carry effective substances into the skin, constringe it, and serve as a basis for make-up. The composition that most nearly meets multiple demands could be a well-compounded cold cream containing additional lanolin, which both softens the skin and leaves sufficient residue to serve as a foundation for powder and makeup.

Miscellaneous special creams (for example, *eye creams* or *throat creams*) are generally emollients with a base of lanolin, stiffened with natural or synthetic waxes, and containing compounds intended specifically to make wrinkles and fine lines less conspicuous.

Estrogenic Creams, The possibility of improving the condition and appearance of the skin by the external application of estrogenic substances has been for several years a subject of controversy between medical authorities and scientific investigators. Intensive research, however, undertaken independently by several reputable manufacturers, has yielded results that substantiate the claims made for estrogenic creams. According to one published report (3a), topical application of a well-compounded estrogenic cream causes considerable improvement in the skin of older women (deficient in estrogenic substance), without evidence of systemic effects or any indication of malignancy (see also *Hormones*).

Protective creams, also called *industrial creams*, came into long-delayed recognition during World War II through the need for protecting the hands from injury—or merely soiling—in the prosecution of many industrial processes. The widespread adoption of these products and their admitted success should insure for them a permanent place in industrial plants.

The wide diversity of chemical irritants might seem to call for almost as many protective agents. The ideal product must spread easily and if possible penetrate into the hair folicles; it must remain stable in contact with most chemical agents, providing an oily film of low surface tension; it must not dehydrate the skin; and it must be readily removable with any good soap.

Protective creams are of four types: mixtures of fats and oils; jellies containing physical barriers; emulsions; and soap bases. Each type offers certain advantages and disadvantages, but the best all-around product seems to be an emulsion of fats and waxes with water, made with triethanolamine, and incorporating magnesium stearate or talc as the physical and chemical barrier (13).

The advantages of these protective creams in preventing industrial dermatoses are inestimable. The success of similar products, applied by women to protect their hands while doing their daily household chores, should stimulate research for better protectin of the hands in chemical and other industrial plants.

Liquid Creams

Practically any of the creams described here can be made in fluid form. Some manufacturers offer an entire line of liquid cleansing, emollient, and finishing creams (occasionally called "milks"); for advantages and disadvantages, these must be tested and judged on individual properties and personal preference. The compositions may contain up to 90% of water.

The most popular use of liquid creams is as so--called *hand lotions*, of which the long established "honey-and-almond cream" is typical. They are usually oil in-water emulsions, much improved in recent years by the use of the newer emulsifying agents, notably triethanolamine, polyhydric alcohol fatty acid esters, etc. As the stability of such emulsions is of paramount importance, the methods of manufacture frequently depend upon the nature of the emulsifying agents used, and are usually more complicated than those suitable for solid creams.

Manufacture of Creams

For the manufacture of most *creams in emulsion, form,* the following equipment should be available: mixing kettle, with thermometer (or thermostat) and agitator; source of heat—steam or water in jacket of kettle (direct heating is usually not advisable); melting container for fats, or immersion heater for removing small amounts of solid fats from drums. For fatty mixtures, pastes, and ointments, a colloid mill or some form of homogenizer is also required. The actual pieces to be used depend upon the nature of the ingredients, occasionally upon the type of emulsifying agent employed. For makig small batches of cream, some items of household equipment, such as a double boiler, an egg beater, a meat chopper, and many of the modern mechanical mixing and emulsifying devices have proved satisfactory.

The oils, waxes, emulsifiers, and other oilsoluble components are heated to 75°C in a steam-jacketed kettle. The water-soluble components (alkalis, alkanolamines, polyhydric alcohols, and preservatives) are dissolved in the aqueous phase and heated to 75°C in another steam-jacketed kettle. To allow for evaporation of water during the heating and emulsification, about 3-5% excess water (based on formula weight) is added.

The procedure for preparing o/w and w/o emulsions is to add the warmed inner phase very slowly to the outer phase (also at 75°C), stirring constantly and homogenizing to assure efficient emulsification. Finely dispersed o/w emulsions can also be prepared by adding the aqueous phase to the oils. Initially the low concentration of water forms a w/o emulsion according to the phase-volume relationship. The slow addition and emulsification of the water increases theviscosity of the system while the oil phase expands to a maximum. At this point, the continuous oil phase breaks up into minute droplets as emulsion inversion occurs, characterized by a sudden decrease in viscosity. This emulsification technique proceeds smoothly at the critical inversion point in a well-balanced, low oilwax system, but it frequently causes coagulation in high oilwax emulsions. The conventional procedure of adding the iner phase to the outer is preferable for creams and lotions.

The rates of addition and mechanical agitation of the dispersed phase are critically important in determining the efficiency of emulsification. The product formed may vary from a completely dispersed inner phase in a well emulsified system, to a mixed emulsion in a poorly emulsified system, the latter owing to excessive rate of addition of inner phase and to inadequate stirring. This in turn affects the consistency, viscosity, and stability of creams and lotions.

Total stirring times and cooling rates are important to lotion viscosity, cream consistency, and emulsion stability. Experimental formulas are often developed in vessels that are not equipped with a heating and cooling jacket. Under these air-cooled conditions, longer stirring times are necessary. The transition to full scale production in jacketed equipment introduces a variable in the physical factors contributing to emulsion preparation. If cooling is started too soon after emulsification is complete, crystallization of the higher melting waxes may occur.

The temperature at which the perfume oils are added to the cream or lotion is another factor contributing to emulsion instability. The addition of perfume to a w/o amulsion proceeds smoothly owing to its solubility in the external phase. In o/w systems, the oils must break through the continuous aqueous phase to the emulsified.

If the cream is to be hot-poured, it is stirred to 5°C above the congealing point, any required color solutions are added, and the cream held at that temperature with occasional stirring during the filling procedcure. If cold-filling is preferred, the cream is stirred to 35°C, any color solutions are added, and filling proceeds at room temperature.

In the packaging of creams they are transferred to containers either while they are still warm enough to be fluid, or after they are cooled. Most cold creams, cleansing creams, and emollient creams are filled warm; vanishing creams, pastes, and ointments are usually filled while cold. Apparatus includes gravity-and vacuum-operated devices. Precautions to be observed are the avoidance of air pockets in the tubes or jars, effecting of a neat smooth surface onthe cream, and complete cooling of the jars before capping.

In any modern, well-equipped factory, manufacturing proceeds in an efficient manner through continuous successive operations from the mixing kettles to filling, labeling, packing in boxes or cartons, and optional steps such as the enclosing of inserts, outer wrapping, and sealing. Equipment is available, or can be devised, to meet the needs of the most exacting packaging problem.

The manufacture of *liquid creams* is more complicated because of the possibility of breaking the emulsion. As stated earlier, the method of manufacture may vary considerably with the nature of the emulsifying agent, but the proportions and purity of ingredients, the manner and speed of mixing, and other factors are highly important. All creams should be perfected in small batches before any attempt is made to make them on a large scale.

Liquid creams may be filled by gravity from large tanks, handfilled with multiple nozzles, or filled entirely automatically by vacuum apparatus. The manner of closing the bottles varies depending upon whether the closure is a cork with a decorative top, a glass stopper, a threaded metal or plastic cap, etc.

All jars, bottles, and closures must be perfectly clean before they are filled, and kept free from all contamination during the entire manufacturing process.

Cosmetic Lotions

The oils and waxes in lotions are identical to those of an emollient cream but they are present in lower concentration. An o/w emollient lotion usually contains more water than the corresponding cream; a w/o type may thave the same water content, with oily components replacing part of the waxlike materials. These lotions are preferred for use during the day because they produce a lighter or less oily emollient film. However, they can be formulated to contain the same concentration of oil phase ordinarily used in creams. The sales appeal of emollient lotions dervies partly from their convenience and partly from the greater variety of package design possible for liquid emulsions.

The formulation of lotions of all emulsifier and emulsion types is similar to that of emollient creams. The emulsion must be stable at elevated temperatures (45-50°C) for whaterver period is deemed necesary and at room tempertures for a minimum of one year. In the freeze-thaw test of emulsion sability, the lotion is subjected to a temperature of–5°C for 24 h and is then allowed to return to room temperature, at which time it should be stable and pourable.

An example of an all-purpose hand, face, and body lotion prepared with an anionic emulsifier is: 4.00% stearic and (triple-pressed), 1.50% lanolin anhydrous, 1.50% mineral oil, 1.00% cetyl alcohol, 0.80% triethanolamine, 0.25% preservative [methyl and propyl paraben (5:1)], 90.60% distilled or deionized water, and 0.35% perfume.

A representative all-purpose hand, face, and body lotion, prepared with cationic emulsifiers is: 1.00% cetyl alcohol, 0.50% stearyl alcohol, 1.00% lanolin anhydrous, 4.00% mineral oil, 0.10% *N*-(colaminoformylmethyl) pyridinium chloride, 0.80% *N*-(colaminoformylmethyl) pyridinium chloride stearate, 0.25% preservative [methyl and propyl paraben (5:1)], 6.00% propylene glycol, 64.80% distilled or deionized water, 0.125% sodium chloride, 0.125% sodium benzoate, 11.00% distilled or deionized water, 0.30% perfume, and 10.00% denatured alcohol no. 40.

In composition, the lotions used in cosmetic treatments vary according to the purpose for which they are intended; that is, they may be astringent, bleaching, cleansing, emollient, medicated, or refreshing lotins; still others are especially compounded for the eyes and for after shaving.

Table V. Compositions of Astringent Lotions

Ingredient	Typical recipe, % by wt. in: 1	2	3	4
Alcohol	10	16	50	10
Alum	1.5	4	–	1
Boric acid	3	–	–	–
Glycerol	5	2	–	10
Zinc phenolsulfonate	–	2	2	–
Zinc sulfate	–	–	–	1
Water, to make	100.0	100	100	100

Astringent lotions are generally used inthe treatment of oily skin and conspicuous pores. For an immediate degreasing effect, some recipes contain as much as 50% of alchol (ethyl or isopropyl), but results seem to be more satisfactory with less alcohol and a good selection of salts or other compounds of aluminum, magnesium, and zinc. Mild acids, for example, acetic, boric, citric, and salicylic, extract of witch hazel, b-naphthol, and resoreinol, are also used. In planning an astringent lotion it must be remembered that many compounds that might seem suitable because of their property of coagulating proteins will be incompatible with certain other substances and compounds in solution. The properties of all proposed ingredients should be studied before any decision is made.

Bleaching lotions are not so much in demand now as they were formerly, undoubtedly because of the vogue for tanning. At best the merits of such preparations are questionable. As the pigment-forming mechanism of the skin is situated at the base of the epidermis, any true bleaching agent strong enought to penetrate to the site of pigment and actually lighten the color of it could readily harm the epidermis itself.

Melanin, the pigment in skin and hair, can be bleached to a lighter color by hydrogen peroxide (at least 5%, 17-volume). A clear bleaching solution may be made of hydrogen peroxide and rose water or orange-flower water. Other suggestions are for mild acids (acetic, citric, lactic, tartaric) in scented water, with or without the addition of glycerol (to 10%). Potassium chlorate, sodium perborate, and other oxidizing chemicals are also included occasionally in bleaching lotins.

Cloudy lotions or those containing a sediment, which are to be shaken before application, may contain bismuth subnitrate, ammoniated mercury (maximum allowed, 5%), or metallic peroxides (zinc, magnesium). Lotions recommended especially for lightening freekles usually contain ammoniated mercury, which causes exfoliation of the pigment and may irritate the epidermis.

Another type of so-called bleaching lotion actually masks, rather than lightens, the color of the skin. Like the whitening creams, these lotins usually contain zinc oxide or titanium dioxide with various proportions of alcohol, glycerol, and water. As delicate flesh tints may also be added, such products often serve more properly as liquid powders.

In cosmetic treatments, as given professionally in the beauty shop, bleaching lotions are applied to supplement the usually stronger action of bleaching creams and pastes; at home they are generally used instead of these products.

Cleansing lotions are used to supplement the action of cleansing creams, and at any time for quick cleansing or for more thorough cleansing than is afforded by soap and water; they are of several types.

Lotions intended for cleansing the *dry skin* should contain relatively little alcohol or mineral oil, and only small percentages of alkaline salts or synthetic surface-active agents because all of these ingredients can only aggravate a tendency toward dryness. Borax and triethanolamine may be present to the extent of 1%; glycerol (or glycol compounds) to 5-10%; ethyl or isopropyl alcohol to 5-10%. Tincture of benzion is occasionally included; magnesium carbonate is also added to some mixtures to serve as a mechanical aid to cleansing. Such lotions must bewell shaken before they are applied, because the white powder settles on standing.

Cleansing lotions for *oily skin* many contain up to 50% of alcohol. Although the primary purpose of these lotions is to remove oil and shine from the face, many of them are so compounded that continual use may have an astringent effect and thus counter act the oily condition. Among the compounds included are synthetic detergents, mild acids (boric, salicylic), acetone, camphor, and witch hazel.

Freshening lotions (formerly called *skin toning lotions*) are used for mild stimulation of the skin, and for the complete removal of creams before the application of make--up. Alcohol may or may not be present; rose water or orange-flower water is often used as the base. Preservatives are usually required. Menthol, when used for cooling effect, must be kept to the minimum, as its secondary reaction is an occasionally unpleasant overstimulation of the skin. Glycerol is included for its humectant properties. Other common ingredients of skin fresheners are alum, camphor, witch hazel, and mild organic acids (3, 6, 9, 10, 13).

Medicated lotions, although used for their cosmetic effect in certain treatments, are on the borderline, if not actually over the line, into the category of drugs. It is not permissible to recommend any true cosmetic lotion for the cure of any lesion or eruption in the skin. All such claims require proof of accomplishment, and a declaration of the active ingredients of the product on the label.

Lotions commonly used for the alleviation of minor blemishes may contain antiseptics, such as alcohol, phenol, hexylresorcinol; also camphor, sulfur, resorcinol; and various zinc compounds (phenolsulfonate, carbonate, sulfate, oxide). For indirect alleviation of minor conditions by thorough cleansing of the skin, triethanolamine, either alone or in compounds with fatty acids, is used; certain synthetic detergents of the class of fatty acid sulfonates or alkyl sulfates are also used in some of the newer .products.

Shaving lotions are offered for either before or after shaving. *Before-sharing preparations* may be of two types: (*1*) Those intended primarily to soften the beard usually have as active ingredient a wetting agent, in a base of water and glycerol, perfumed and tinted. Those to be applied before using an electic razor act like strong astringents, contracting the skin to make the hair stand up more straight. *After-shaving lotions* are usually similar in composition to astringent lotions, with a higher percentage of alcohol, which serves to cool, the skin and to counteract any irritation. The alcohol also acts as a mild antiseptic to aid against infection of any abrasions. As many of the suggested ingredients may deteriorate, lotions of this type should contain preservatives.

Special Lotions

In addition to the various types of lotions used as washes for the skin of the face, at least two other types have become popular and have been the subjects of considerable sound research.

Eye lotions, used to cleanse, soothe, and brighten the eyes, should be so compounded that in pH and osmotic pressure they approxmiate the natural fluid, tears. Many older, compendia gave recipes for eye-washes, based on herbal extracts (camphor, cherry laurel, eupharasia or "eyebright," fennel, fleabane, snakewort, witch hazel), which could well serve the same purpose in modern preparations. In practice, herbal extracts are usually combined with boric acid, ammonium, potassium, or sodium chloride, sodium borate or salicylate, zinc salts or other suitable compounds. If any natural organic substances are used, a preservative must be added; for obvious reasons this should be selected with great care. Claims for eye lotions should be most conservative. Nothing of this kind should be recommended for the treatment of abnormal or pathological conditions; otherwise the product falls automatically into the class of drugs.

Hand lotions are of two principal types; (*1*) creamy fluids ("honey and-almond" type). (*2*) thin mucilages. They deserve to be even more widely used than they are at present because of the protection they afford to the skin of hands and arms (and legs) in cold weather, and, at any time, to hands that are exposed to soap and water or any other cause of defatting.

About the oldest of the preparations still in use is a mixture of glycerol and rose water. It was made formerly with 50% of glycerol, but the quantity has been cut to an average of 25%; in commercial production, a perservative should be added. Sorbitol is also used in place of some of the glycerol.

The familiar translucent, gelatinous or mucilaginous hand lotions consist of one or more gums (acacia, chondrus, karaya, tragacanth) with varying percentages of alcohol, glycerol (or glycols), boric acid, camphor, or benzoin; benzoic acid or one of the newer benzoic acid esters to used as the preservative.The gums are occasionally also added to the emulsion type of hand cream. Other thickening agents used in hand lotions are agar, marsh-mallow root, starch, pectin, and the extracts from seeds of flax, psyllium, and quince.

Manufacture of Lotions

To have the proper esthetic appeal, a lotion that is intended to be clear should have the brilliance and clarity of a jewel, whether water-white or colored. Clouding can be prevented by careful study of all the ingredients of the product, in relation to their mutual interactions and compatibility. Stability at various temperatures is also important; otherwise, certain ingredients may precipitate out of the solution under varying climatic conditions. Time should always be allowed for possible changes during storage; "shelf tests" should preferably be of the full duration, rather than accelerated.

Most solutions of these types improve if they are allowed to stand for a while before they are filtered and bottled. Whenever possible, filtration by gravity is preferable to the application of vacuum or pressure. As a mechanical aid in clarification, fuller's earth, asbestos, magnesia, talc, or other substances that are inert to the solution may be distributed over the filtering medium.

As insurance against deterioration, all bottles, caps, and filing apparatus should be cleaned, and the atmosphere of the room should be kept as free as possible from all sources of contamination. The filling and capping of bottles by available standard equipment presents no difficulties.

For mucilaginous lotions, the gum-producing substances must be soaked in water, and some must be forced through sieves or fabrics to prepare them for combination with the other ingredients. General information cannot be given for all conditions; successful preparation of any product requires carefull attention to all steps in the manufacturing process outlined for it.

Deodorants and Antiperspirants

Deodorant and antiperspirant products are marketed as aerosols, creams, gels, lotions, powders, soaps,and sticks.

The FDA product and ingredient review panel for over-the-counter antiperspirants (OTC panel) has assigned three classifications to antiperspirants: category 1, safe to use; category 2, does not meet requirements, remove offending materials; category 3, may be marketed while testing continues.

The initial proposal states that color and fragrance apparently have no effect on safety; buffers do not apparently make a product more effective; a product, to remain on the market, must be at least 20% effective on at least one half of the persons tested. With a confidence rate of 95%, special tests will be set up to evaluate claims of extra effectiveness (30% or more); products aimed at combatting problem and emotional perspiration will require special tests; if a new ingredient is used tests are required for skin irritation and compatibility with normal flora.

Active Ingredients

Aluminum chloride, once commonly used in deodorants and antiperspirants, may cause fabric damage and skin irritation because of its low pH. This has led to the development of various basic aluminum compounds. The most widely used compound is aluminum chlorhydroxide (ACH) . Other compounds that have been or are now used are: basic aluminum bromide, iodide, and nitrate, and basic aluminum hydroxychloride–zirconyl hydroxy oxychloride, with the without glycine. Zirconium salts, formerly used in antiperspirants, were banned for use in aerosol in 1977.

An example of an antiperspirant rollon is: 33.60–40.60% methyl cellulose 65 HG (high gain), 400 mPa.s (=cP), 3% solution [96.9% distilled or deionized water, 3.0% methyl cellulose 65 HG, 400 mPa.s (=cP), 0.1% methyl paraben]; 30.00–36.0% aluminum chlorhydroxide complex, 50% solution; 16.25–29.25% alcohol SDA no. 40; 4.65% propylene glycol; and 2.50% solubilized perfume [solubilizer and perfume oil (4:1)].

Deodorant–Antiperspirant Sticks

Sodium stearate, the primary gelling agent for deodorant sticks, constitutes about 7-9 wt% of these products. The grade employed depends on the fatty acid used in making the stearate. Derivatives such as acetylated sucrose distearates also can be used but are more common in antiperspirant sticks to gel cetyl alcohol-based formulations (typical use level, 28%).

There are three main types of stick formulations for antiperspirants: hydroxyethyl stearamide, which produces clear-melting, homogeneous sticks; stearamides and cetyl alcohol dry-powder dispersions of ACH; and stearamides coupled with propoxylated alcohol. The stearamide wax content is 26-29%; the active concentration, 20-25%.

Volatile silicones, the siloxanes, are employed in the newer antiperspirant sticks at levels as high as 40-50%. They function as a processing aid, reducing cracking and crumbling of the stick. The tetrameric and pentameric cyclic silicones are preferred because of their volatility (see Silicon compounds). When the stick is applied to the skin, the silicones evaporate, leaving the ingredients on the skin in a nonsticky film. The silicones are useful in pump antiperspirants, acting as a lubricant for valves and a suspending agent for the active material. The compounds also act as skin lubricants and emollients.

A typical deodorant stick formula is: 75.35 wt % alcohol SDA no. 40; 17.00 wt % propylene glycol; 6.00 wt % sodium stearate, purified USP; 1.50 wt % perfume; and 0.15 wt % trichlorocarbanilide.

A typical antiperspirant stick formula is: 27.5 wt % stearic acid monoethanolamide; 240 wt % poly (dimethylsiloxane) (low viscosity, volatile); 20.0 wt % rehydrol powder: 15.0 wt % propoxylted myristyl alcohol; 9.0 wt % propylene glycol; 3.0 wt % distilled or deionized water; 1.0 wt % perfume; and 0.5 wt % myristyl lactate.

A typical dry compressed antiperspirant stick formula is: 65.75 wt % microcys talline cellulose; 25.00 wt % ultrafine powdered aluminum chlorohydrate; 9.00 wt % talc; and 0.25 wt % magnesium stearate.

Deodorizers merely prevent the emanation of an odor from the sweat, or substitute a pleasant odor for an unpleasant one. These products pass as true cosmetics and therefore require no statement of ingredients on the label. They may be prepared as powders, creams, or liquids; as used under the arms, on palms or soles, and on sanitary napkins, the first two types predominate. Common ingredients are: boric, benzoic, and salicylic acids; zinc oxide and peroxide; magnesium carbonate, talc and hydroxyquinoline sulfate. A few typical recipes are given in Table VI.

Table VI. Compositions of Deodorizers.

	Typical recipe, % by wt. in:								
	Powders			Creams			Liquids		
Ingredient	1	2	3	1	2	3	1	2	3
Alcohol	–	–	–	–	–	–	50	–	–
Boric acid	30	–	40	10	10	15	3	–	–
Colloodial clay	–	–	–	4	–	–	–	–	–
Glycerol	–	–	–	16	–	–	15	–	–
Hydroxyquinoline sulfate	–	10	–	–	–	–	–	2	–
Petrolatum	–	–	–	–	65	62	–	–	–
Salicylic acid	–	–	2	–	–	3	4	–	–
Talc	38	90	48	8	–	–	–	–	–
Water	–	–	–	40	25	15	28	98	95
Zinc peroxide	32	–	–	–	–	–	–	–	–
Zinc phenolsulfonate	–	–	–	2	–	5	–	–	5
Zinc stearate	–	–	10	20	–	–	–	–	–
Total	100	100	100	100	100	100	100	100	100

Antiperspiratns are strong astringents that are believed to coagulate and precipitate proteins in the skin at the site of application; the sweat is thus deflected to other regions. Products that thus "affect a function of the body" are considered drugs rather than cosmetics, and all active ingredients must be listed on the label.

Antiperspirants are usually prepared as liquids, creams, and paste in sticks. The active ingredients of first choice are salts of aluminum and zinc, of which many organic and inorganic salts are available; those most commonly used are the chloride, sulfate, chlorohydroxide complex, and acetate of aluminum (also potassium alum), and the chloride, sulfate, and phenolsulfonate of zinc. Other ingredients are formalin, hexamethylenetetramine, tannic acid and tannin, and hydroxyquinoline sulfate.

The compounding of these products calls for considerable care to keep within limits of solubility of the salts, but especially to avoid irritation of the skin and damage to clothing. The liquid preparations have most commonly been the more serious offenders on the last point.

The simplest antiperspirant is a 16-20% solution of aluminum chloride in distilled water; this may be modified by adding alum, hydroxyquinoline sulfate, glycerol, and other organic compounds. As a base for the creams, the vanishing type seems to be the most generally satisfactory, using glycerol monostearate as the principal ingredient. A few typical recipes are given in Table VII.

Table VII. Compositions of Antiperspirants.

	Typical recipe, % by wt. in:						
	Liquid		Cream			Stick	
Ingredient	1	2	1	2	3	1	2
Alcohol	–	6	–	10	–	–	–
Alum	8	22	–	–	10	5	–
Aluminum chloride	10	10	–	5	–	–	–
Beeswax	–	–	–	–	–	25	–
Boric acid	10	–	–	–	–	–	–
Formalin	–	–	–	1	–	–	–

Glycerol monostearate	–	–	25	15	25	–	20
Glycerol	–	–	–	–	–	–	10
Hexamethylenetetramine	–	–	–	–	–	–	3
Lanolin	–	–	–	–	–	6	–
Hydroxyquinoline sulfate	–	22	2	3	–	2	–
Petrolatium	–	–	8	4	–	30	–
Mineral oil	–	–	–	–	–	10	–
Titanium dioxide	–	–	4	–	2	2	–
Talc	–	–	–	–	–	15	–
Water	72	80	61	62	58	–	67
Zinc phenolsulfonate	–	–	–	–	5	5	–
Total	100	100	100	100	100	100	100

Manufacture of Deodorants. A few points should be observed in the making of various deodorants. Perfumes should be selected with care in order to avoid any that may be incompatible with the ingredients of the products, or that may be irritating. Hydroxyquinoline sulfate is readily contaminated and discolored by contact with iron or other metals; therefore, if it is not handled properly it may impart color to the finished product after it has stood for some time.

Deodorizers and antiperspirants are packaged in many ways: the powders, in carton, plastic, or metal containers with a sifter top; the liquids (*1*) in small bottles with a glass or plastic applicator and a small rubber sponge, (*2*) on saturated pads, packed closely in air-tight jars, and (*3*) most recently in flexible plastic bottles, which can be squeezed to spray the fluid through an atomizer. The creams must be in jars of convenient size with good closures; sticks are mounted in holders of wood, plastic, or coated metal.

Definitions : A sunscreen *sunburn preventive agent* is an active ingredient that absorbs 95% or more of light in the uv range of 290-320 nm. A sunscreen *suntanning agent* is an active ingredient that absorbs up to 85% of light in the uv range of 290-320 nm but transmits light at wavelengths longer than 320 nm. A sunscreen *opaque sunblock agent* is an opaque agent that reflects or scatters light in the uv and visible range at wavelengths of 290-777 nm.

Recommendations

The panel recommended the product designations based on SPF factors in Table VIII.

Table VIII. Sunscreen Product Designations Bases on SPF Factors

Skin type	Sunburn and tanning history	Recommended SPF factor product category designation
1	burns easily, never tans	8 or more (max)
2	burns easily, minimal tan	6-7 (extra)
3	bunrs moderately, normal tan	4-5 (moderate)
4	burns minimally, tans well	23 (min)
5	burns rarely, tans profusely	2 (min)
6	never burns, deep pigment	none indicated

Safe and effective sunscreen ingredients are listed in Table IX.

For significant residual protection, PABA must be applied at least two hours prior.

Table IX. Safe and Effective Sunscreen Ingredients

Ingredient	Trade or generic name
aminobenzoic acid	
2-ethoxyethyl *p*-methoxycinnamate	Cinoxate
hydroxyethylaminoethyl *p*-methoxycinnamate	
digalloyl trioleate	
2, 2'--dihydroxy--4-methoxybenzophenone	dioxybenzone
ethyl4 [bis(2-hydroxypropyl) amino] benzoate	
2-ethylhexyl 2-cyano--3, 3-diphenylacrylate	
2ethylhexyl *p*-methoxycinnamate	
2-ethylhexyl salicylate	
3,3,5-trimethylcyclohexyl salicylate	Homosalate
glyceryl aminobenzoate	
2-hydroxy, 4-naphthoquinone	Lawsone
methyl anthranilate	
2-hydroxy-4-methoxybenzophenone	oxybenzone
pentyl 4-dimethylaminobenzoate	Padimate A
2-ethylhexyl 4-dimethylaminobenzoate	Padimate O
2-phenylbenzimidazole-5-sulfonic acid	

red petrolatum	
2-hydroxy-4-methoxybenzophenone-5-sulfonic acid	sulisobenzone
titanium dioxide	
2- [bis (2-hydroxyethyl) amino] ethyl salicylate	

Sunscreens

The sun emits energy in a continuous band throughout the electomagnetic spectrum. The shorter wavelengths are absorbed in the upper atmosphere so that at sea level the radiation extends from a cutoff near 290 nm through the near ultraviolet to the conventional end of the ultraviolet range, which is near 400 nm. The intensity of the radiation varies nonlinearly throughout this range.

The production of erythema and the subsequent production of melanin pigment are both maximum with 296.7 nm radiation. As the wavelength increases, both responses fall rapidly, so that $10\ \mu\ W/cm^2$ of 307 nm radiation, $100\ \mu\ W/cm^2$ of 314 nm. $1000\ \mu$ W of 330 nm, and $10{,}000\ \mu W$ of 340 nm radiation are required to equal the effect of $1\ \mu\ W/cm^2$ of 296.7 nm radiation in the production of erythema.

A unit of erythemal flux, the E-viton, is equivalent to the erythema induced by $10\ \mu\ W/cm^2$ of 296.7 nm radiation. The response of the skin to an E-viton (or viton) is constant: irradiation by 10 vitons for one hour produces the same erythemal response as 5 vitons for two hours. The effects owing to irradiation by different wavelengths are additive. About twenty minutes exposure to midsummer sunlight (or 40 viton min) ae needed to produce a minimum perceptible erythema (MPE) on normal Caucasian skin. Thus 1 E-viton acting for 40 min produces an MPE. 10 E-vitons acting 4 min or 40 E-vitons acting for 1 min will produce the same MPE.

With the realization that prolonged exposure to sunlight produces most of the ageing effects on skin and the clear implication of exposure in at least three types of skin cancer (basal cell cancer, squamous cell cancer, melanoma), use of products that protect the skin from excessive exposure has become increasingly widespread.

Sunscreens are of two types: physical and chemical. Physical screening agents, such as titanium dioxide and zinc oxide, are opaque materials that block and scatter light, and thus act as mechanical barriers. Their action is nonselective over all wavelengths. Chemical screening agents, which act by absorbing uv light, offer selective protection against certain uv wave bands, depending on their absorption spectrum. Anthranilates, cinnamates, benzyl and homomenthyl salicylate, and *p*-aminobenzoic acid (PABA) and its ester derivatives belong in this category and have maximal absorption in the sunburn region. A useful sunscreen resists wash-off from swimming or sweating and does not come off during exercise or rubbing. Maintenance of significant protection following swimming or sweating would suggest that the chemical is substantive or can diffuse into the horny skin layer. PABA and its esters are moderately substantive and give appreciable protection after intensive sweating and brief periods of immersion in water (5 to 10 min).

OTC Report

Sunscreen products for over-the-counter (OTC) human use are reviewed in a report on recommendations to the FDA by the OTC panel on Topical Analgesics. Definitions and recommendations made by the panel are reviewed below.

Sun Protection Factor (SPF)

The panel defined the ratio of the amount of energy required to produce a minimum erythemal dose (MED) to the amount of energy to produce the same MED without any treatment by the SPF. Examples given are: SPF to immersion. This probably reflects the time required for penetration into the stratum corneum. It is highly important, especially during the first few days of exposure to the sun, to reapply PABA-type sunscreens after swimming. With repeated daily applications increased protection.

Sunscreens with much greater resistance to swimming can be formulated with acrylate polymers, which leave flexible films on the surface. A chemical sunscreen incorporated in the formulation will tend to be bound in the film and remain in place despite sweating and bathing.

Table X lists some effective physical and chemical sunscreens; information on various sunscreens is included in patents (17-18).

Table X. Sunscreens

Chemical sunscreens	*Trade name*
2 ethoxyethyl *p*-methoxycinnamate	Giv-tan F (Givaudan)
menthyl anthranilate	

homomenthyl salicylate	
glyceryl *p*-aminobenzoate	Escalol 106 (Van Dyk)
isobutyl *p*-aminobenzoate	Cycloform (RSA Corp.)
isoamyl-*p*-dimethylaminobenzoate	Escalol 506 (Van Dyk)
2-hydroxy-4-methyxybenzophenone-5 sulfonic acid	Uvinul MS-40 (GAF)
2,2'-dihydroxy-4methoxybenzophenone	Uvinul D-49 (GAF)
2-hydroxy-4methoxybenzophenone	Uvinul M-40 (GAF)
p-aminobenzoic acid	
4-mono-and 4-bis (3-hydroxypropyl) aminoisomers of ethyl benzoate	Amerscreen P (Amerchol)
2-ethylhexyl *p*-dimethylaminobenzoate	Escalol 507 (Van Dyk)

Natural oils (in order of effectiveness)

(1) mink oil
(2) avocado oil
(3) sweet almond oil
(4) sesame oil
(5) persic oil
(6) safflower oil
(7) peanut oil
(8) jojoba oil
(9) coconut oil
(10) olive oil

Physical sunscreens (opaque)

titanum dioxide

zinc oxide

Examples of sunscreen formulations are the following:

Clear Sunscreen Lotion: 74.50 wt % poly (alkylene glycol) (Ucon LB-625, Union Carbide); 20.00 wt % alcohol denatured no. 40; 5.00 wt % PABA (sunscreen); and 0.50 wt % perfume.

Opaque Sunscreen Lotion: 67.60 wt % distilled or deionized water; 10.00 wt % sesame oil (preserved, contains antioxidant); 10.00 wt % mineral oil (Saybolt viscosity at 37.8°C is 65/75); 5.00 wt % PABA (sunscreen); 3.00 wt % stearic acid, triple pressed; 2.90 wt % propylene glycol; 0.50 wt % cetyl alcohol; 0.50 wt % triethanolamine, 98 wt % solution; 0.25 wt % preservative [methyl and propyl paraben (5:1)]; and 0.25 wt % perfume.

Because of the extent of sunscreen application to skin, any perfume used must be chosen with attention to its potential to irritate. Careful testing of its stability to heat and sunlight are also required.

Aerosols

Such cosmetic products as having creams, hair sprays, deodorants and anti-perspirants, colognes, and sunscreens are now commonly packaged as aerosol sprays. In a bulletin released in 1966 the Aerosol Scientific Committee of the Chemical Specialities Manufacturers Association defined an aerosol product as a liquid, solid, gas, or a mixture that is discharged by a propellant force of liquified and/or nonliquified compressed gas, usually from a disposable-type container and through a valve.

The three main components of aerosol products are the propellants, solvents and the active ingredients. Previously, the liquified gas propellants have primarily been the chloroflurocarbons (eg, Freons by DuPont) but these were banned in 1978 for use in all personal and household aerosol products, except for pharmaceuticals such as asthma spray.

Compressed gases (N_2, Co_2) and liquified hydrocarbons have become the primary propellants in revised formulations.

Make-up

The term *make-up*, originally applied to cosmetics used in the theater, now comprises products used by anyone to enhance the coloring of the face or to accentuate facial features. It thus includes face powder, rouge for cheeks and lips, and colorings for use around the eyes.

Color

Straight colorants are referred to in the trade as primary colors, primary dyes, and primaries. The principal primary colors are red, blue and yellow. Practically every hue can be produced by blending red, yellow and blue in proper proportions. Hue, in color, is a quality whereby one color differs from another. Brightness is a measure of the reflectance value of a dye. Strength is a measure of the tinting or coloring value of a dye.

Straight colorants include both primaries and lakes of such primary colorants made by extending the primary colorant on a substratum such as aluminum hydroxide, barium sulfate, a mixture of aluminum hydroxide and barium sulfate, aluminum benzoate, or zinc oxide. These lakes vary in pure dye content strength from 2-80%. The primaries contain over 80% pure dye. Primary colorants are frequently used in diluted forms. Mixtures of two or more primary colorants are sometimes referred to as primary mixtures. Mixtures of two primary colorants are referred to as secondary colorants, and mixtures of three primary colorants, as tertiary colorants.

The initials, FD&C, D&C, and external D&C, which are part of the name of straight colorants, indicate for what use the colorant has been certified. Colorants designated FD&C may be used for foods, drugs, and cosmetics. The name of a mixture usually tells nothing of its permitted use, but if there is a restriction in the use of the colorant, a statement to that effect is required on the product lable (see Colorants for foods, drugs and cosmetics).

For safety, colorants that have been certified for cosmetic use must contain not more than 0.002% of lead, not more than 0.0002% of arsenic, and not more than 0.003% of heavy metals other than lead and arsenic.

Most cosmetic colorants are certified coal-tar colorants. However, a few natural dyes are used in limited amounts to color foods, drugs, and cosmetics. The more important are alkanet, annatto, carotene, chlorophyll, cochineal, saffron, and henna.

Inorganic Colorants

Except for the white pigments, such as titanium dioxide, zinc oxide and talcum, the inorganic colorants are used in a number of cosmetic products. They usually have excellent light fastness and complete insolubility in solvents and aqueous solutions.

The naturally occurring colored minerals that depend for their color upon the presence of oxide of iron are known by such names as ochre, umber, sienna, etc. Because they are naturally occurring products, they possess certain inherent disadvantages. They show greater variation in color and tinting power than do manufactured pigments. The nature and amount of impurities they contain varies and may, form time to time, exclude their use in a domestic product.

The most important inorganic colorants or pigments are the iron oxides, chrome oxide greens, ultramarine pigment blues and pinks, and the carbon blacks. Iron oxide is sold in the form of yellow hydrated iron oxide, or ochre; brown iron oxide, red iron oxide, and black iron oxide. The yellow iron oxide is made by an alkaline precipitation from a ferrous salt, followed by an oxidation the product is ca 85% Fe_2O_3, and is supplied in shades from light lemon yellow to a deep orange.

The brown iron oxides, umber, are made by treating a mixture of red, yellow and black iron salt with alkali and partially oxidizing the precipitate. The brown oxide is a mixture of Fe_2O_3 and Fe_3O_4. The red iron oxides, sienna, are usually made by heating the precipitated yellow iron oxides. Light to dark red can be obtained depending on heating conditions, and the product is 96-98% Fe_2O_3.

The black iron oxide is formed by precipitation of Fe_3O_4 under carefully controlled conditions. The chromium oxide green is pure Cr_2O_3. The anhydrous pigment has a dull green shade; the hydrated pigment shows a bluish tint. This type of pigment is used in eye makeup.

Carbon blacks are of vegetable or natural gas origin. These blacks find wide cosmetic application, particularly in eye makeup.

The ultramarine blues and pinks are made from a mixture containing sulfur, sodium carbonate, charcoal, pitch or rosin, and several other ingredients carefully heated for a lengthy period. The finely pulverized pigment gives shades of ultramarine blue from the pink to the green, depending on its silica content.

Dye Stability

It is well known that many dyes are pH indicators. Such dyes change in hue with pH variations. Those that do not change much in hue can be affected in other important properties. It is, therefore, important to consider the pH conditions in a cosmetic product. In general, the inorganic colors are not as much affected by pH conditions as are the coal-tar dyes.

The hue of some dyes varies with the percentage of moisture present. The term bleeding is used to refer to the strengthening of the hue of a color in the presence of moisture, particularly in moist powders that are stored for a long period of time.

All water or organo-soluble dyes and most insoluble dyes and pigments are destroyed or chemically changed by the photochemical action of ultraviolet, visual light, infrared, and other short wavelength radiations. The degree of sensitivity varies with the dye and with the conditions.

The dyes change in tinctorial strength and hue, becoming progressive weaker, and usually duller, as the destruction of the dyestuff progresses. This is considered normal fading. The ability of the certified dyes to resist this chemical change owing to photochemical action has been charted for a number of the dyes and is available in tabular form.

The absence of moisture greatly retards photolytic effects. Absence of air, oxygen, hydrogen, and other oxidizing or reducing reagents also retards fading. The presence of titanium dioxide greatly accelerates it.

Judging Color Effects

Many factors affect the judgment of color, including the nature of the light source, the degree of transparency or opacity of the color, and eye strain or color memory.

Face Powders

Formulation

Face powders, both the loose the now - popular cake or pressed, is a blend of white pigments, tinted and perfumed . The function of a face powder is to impart a smooth, matte finish to the skin by masking any shine owing to the secretions of the sebaceous and sweat glands. To obtain this effect, the powder must be neither too transparent to mask the shine, nor too opaque, lest it give a masklike appearance. In addition, it must posses reasonable lasting properties; it must adhere to the skin and be reasonably resistant to the mixed secretions of the skin. Finally, through intimate contact of its perfume - laden particles over a warm and relatively large area, it should disseminate a pleasing odor, the psychological value of which is often underestimated.

No single substance possesses all the desired properties; covering power, slip, absorbency, adhesiveness, and bloom. Therefore; a modern face powder is a blend of several constituents, each one chosen for some specific quality. The materials most commonly used can be grouped in the following manner.

Covering power. To cover skin defects, such as enlarged pores and skin shine. Examples: Titanium dioxide, zinc oxide, kaolin, and magnesium oxide.

Slip. To assist in spreading and to give the characteristic smooth feeling. Examples: talc, zinc satearate, magnesium streate, and starch.

Absorbency. To absorb sebaceous or oily secretions and perspiration, and thus reduce shine. Examples: precipitated chalk, magnesium carbonate, starch, and kaolin.

Adherence. To improve clinging to the face. Examples: Metallic Soaps, such as magnesium and zinc stearates, and small quantities of oil or fatty materials in the powder base.

Bloom. To give a smooth, velvetlike appearance to the skin. A matte effect, Examples: chalk and starch.

Representative formulas for loose and pressed powders are:

Loose face powder	*Wt %*	
kaolin	3.0	
talc (Italian)	64.0	
talc (Sierra)		
magnesium stearate	1.5	base
magnesium carbonate	0.5	
zinc oxide	15.0	
corn starch	10.0	
D&C red # 2 (lake) 20% in talc		
D&C red # 3 (lake) 10% in talc		
D&C orange # 4 (lake) 10% in talc	5.0	colorant dilutions
yellow iron oxide 20% in talc		
brown iron oxide 20% in talc		
perfume	1.0	

Cake or pressed powder	Wt %	
kaolin	10.0	
zinc stearate	5.0	
zinc oxide	10.0	base
magnesium stearate	5.0	
talc (French)	61.4	
mineral oil light	2.0	
cetyl alcohol	1.0	binding agent
lanolin	0.3	
D&C orange # 4 (lake) 10% in talc	2.7	
D&C red # 2 (lake) 20% in talc	0.8	colorant dilutions
brown iron oxide 20% in talc	1.0	
perfume	0.8	

The function of face powder is to conceal shine and endow the skin with a new and better looking color or tint. The finer the particle size of face powder, the greater the diffusion of light and the better the bloom, with correspondingly less shine. The reason for this is that the light is reflected in many different angles, somewhat like reflection from the frosted surface of glass. Within certain limits, the smaller the powder particles, the higher the covering power and the better the tinting. Titanium dioxide, with its extremely fine particle size, provides especially good covering power. The percentage used is generally in the range of 5–8%. A common method of determining fineness of particles is the bite test, which consists of grating the ingredients between the teeth. The gritty threshold on grating chalk powder between the teeth has been placed at ca 12 μm. The materials used in a face powder should, therefore, be passed through at least a 50μm (300-mesh) sieve, or, more properly, through a micronizing or micropulverizing machine.

The designation, light, medium, heavy, applied to a face powder denotes not weight, but covering power. A dry skin requires, in the absence of exceptional skin defects, a light powder; but since such a skin is lacking in grease, either the powder must possess increased powders of adherence, or a powder base must be used. A greasy skin, on the other hand, requires a powder of high opacity and grease resistance. Adherence is supplied by the skin itself, and in this case a powder containing sufficient grease-resistant constituents such as kaolin, together with a drying agent such as zinc oxide, may be used. The latter powder would be termed a heavy powder. Most women prefer a light to medium weight powder, since both are suitable to dry or normal skin.

Manufacture

The following is a procedure commonly used in manufacturing loose face powder: (*1*) All basic materials are screened into a Day spiral (ribbon) mixer, and blended. (*2*) The inorganic colorants and lakes or toners are diluted with either some of the mixed base material or with a portion of the talcum and screened. These diluted colorants are then added to the base. (*3*) The perfume, diuted and thoroughly mixed with a portion of the mixed base material or the talcum and screened, is added to the mixer. (*4*) The mixture is well blended and then transferred to a 50-μm (300-mesh) silk or stainless steel screen where it is screened several times and checked for color. An efficient and rapid method of screening consists of passing the material through a micronizer, using a suitable screen. (*5*) If the color check indicates that adjustments are necessary, the estimated amount of colorant dilutions are added and extra base and perfume to compensate for the additions are blended in. (*6*) When the color corresponds closely with the standard, the batch should again be thoroughly mixed in the spiral mixer and the entire batch passed through the 50μm (300-mesh) screen or the Fitzpatrick comminuter or a micronizer. (7) The screened material can now be stored in a cool, dry place, or can be sent to the packaging room.

The manufacturing procedure for compact powder closely parallels that for loose powder, except that the moistening agent must be added slowly and mixed well in the base materials. If water is used to moisten the base materials, the water content of the mixed powder should be reduced by drying to ca 2.5-3%. Few manufacturers use water to moisten the powder because drying lengthens the process considerably and because water may cause some bleeding. The finished powder, having been passed by the control laboratory for shade, can be stored in the same way that the loose powder is stored.

Before the powder is placed in the pans for pressing it must be agitated because the inclusion of air, introducting during the mixing and screening process, may cause breakage of the compact powder unless it is vibrated before pressing.

Because vibration does not necessarily remove all included air, the process known as prepress is a part of the manufacturing procedure for compact powder. Prepress consists of applying moderate pressure to the material placed in the pans, and then releasing the pressure before passing the cakes on to the hydraulic press. At the hydraulic press sufficient pressure is applied to make a hard, compact powder cake.

Breakage of the compact cake is a very important factor for rejection. One firm tests the cake of compressed powder by dropping it from a height of ca 0.3 m onto a thin metal plate, cushioned by a few sheets of paper. The cake of compressed powder has to withstand more than ten drops from this height to pass the control test.

Product Stability

The most common reason that loose face powder loses its saleability is loss of perfume. The stability of the perfume in a particular face powder can be readily checked by using the method of minimum quantity to discover whether perfume and powder are reacting with each other. For this test one uses not more than 0.1% of perfume. A good perfume and suitable powder should maintain a slight but agreeable perfumed note for at least two days in a vessel open to the air. The usual failure is the disappearance of all of the perfume, or the appearance of a phenolic or medicated odor.

The stability of the pigment used is of great concern to every manufacturer of face powder.Not all shades can be produced with earth colors exclusively, and it is necessary to use some organic lakes and toners. These should be used sparingly, because they are not light stable for any length of time. A simple check of light stability is to place a puff on the smoothened surface of loose face powder and then put the sample into bright sunlight for about thirty minutes. Any appreciable bleaching of the unprotected area indicates possible trouble.

Zinc stearate may develop an odor on ageing, and it is necessary to use a good grade of zinc stearate for face powder. Kaolin may develop a clalike odor when moistened, and magnesium carbonate may have a deleterious effect on the perfume. All materials used in the preparation of face powders must be carefully tested to prevent the inclusion of impurties. The same precautionary measures taken in preparing loose face powder must be observed in the manufacture of compact or pressed face powder. Additional care must be taken in the choice of ingredients since the compact face powders usually contain moistening ingredients. Off odors may also be introduced by the glues used in powder boxes, puffs or in gluing compressed powder to the metal pan.

Lipstick

Lipstick is a solid fatty-base product containing dissolved and suspended colorant materials. A good lipstick must possess a certain maximum and minimum of thixotropy; ie, it must soften enough a yield a smooth, even application with the minimum of pressure. It should not be necessary to apply a lipstick more often than every 4 to 6 hours. The applied film, no matter how thin, should to some extent be impervious to the mild abrasion encountered during eating, drinking, or smoking. The lipstick should be of such composition as to color only that portion of the lip to which it is applied, and not to bleed, streak or feather into the surrounding tissue of the mouth. It should be of a consistency that can be quickly and easily applied, and the perfume (usually present at 12%) should be carefully compounded so that it does not have an unpleasant taste. The colorants used in lipsticks are either insoluble lakes or oil-soluble dyes of the Eosin group, or both.

The bromo acids, bromo derivatives of fluoroescein, are used to produce indelibility in the applied film. Two are most generally used, dibromo and tetrabromofluorescein. Dibromofluorescein produces a yellow-red color; the tetra compound gives a more purple stain. Usually the two are used in combination, as neither produces desired results separately. From 1-5% of these dyes are used in lipsticks; but ordinarily, 2 or 3% is adequate. Other pigments are used in concentrations of 5-15%, 10% is an average.

A highly refined grade of castor oil (qv) is one of the most common ingredients in lipstick. It is used primarily to impart viscosity to the molded stick and, secondly, because it has a small solvent action on the bromo acids. Castor oil dissolves less than 0.3% of the bromo acids. Its solvent action is owing to the presence of free hydroxyl groups in the glycerides of ricinoleic acid, which make up a large percentage of castor oil.

In the so-called high-stain sticks, a solvent such as polyethylene glycol 400 is used. The polyethylene glycol is not soluble in castor oil. A mutual solvent or coupling agent is, therefore, necessary; propylene glycol monoricinoleate is used for this purpose. Isopropyl myristate, isopropyl palmitate, butyl stearate, and some of the higher esters of the mono-and dihydric alcohols are commonly used in lipsticks, both for their solvent action on the bromo acids, and to reduce the thickness of the castor oil film.

Lanolin and various derivatives are used for their emollient properties and for a degree of tackiness and drag. Acetylated lanolinis more soluble in castor oil than lanolin itself. Lanolin oils, solvent extractions of lanolin, eliminate much of the tack of lanolin. Lanolin helps hold the lipstick mass in a uniform homogenous mi ture. Lanolin, used in the proper ratio, helps to prevent sweating of the solvent oils and confers some protection against abrupt temperature changes.

Various waxes are used to impact different characteristics, such as hardness, thixotropy, melting point, and ease of application. These waxes are used in amounts regulated by the nature of the other components making up the finished stick.

Carnauba wax is responsible for stiffening the stick. If used in the proper proportions, it imparts to the stick exactly the right degree of thixotropy. Its melting point is very high, much higher than any of the other natural waxes. Candelilla wax is used for the same reason, but to a lesser extent. Too much carnauba will cause a granular texture in the finished lipstick, and it is best to keep its concentration as low as possible, usually less than 5%.

Ceresin and ozokerite are both also good stiffening agents, with ceresin exhibiting the greater stiffening action. Since ceresin is merely a mixture of ozokerite and paraffihn, the same effect can be obtained by using these two waxes in combination. Ceresin can have a variety of melting points, depending upon the ratio of ozokerite to paraffin, thus affecting the melting point of the lipstic. Ozokerite is used more often to raise the melting point. A combination of ozokerite and carnauba is most efficient.

Beeswax can be used to raise the melting point. It is a good binder, helping to produce a homogenous mass. In large amounts it causes granulation and a dulling effect. A typical lipstick base formulation is: 49.6 wt % castor oil; 26.3 wt % hydro-genated vegetable oil, a cocoa butter substitute; 11.6 wt % ozokerite 160; 5.0 wt % lanolin anhydrous; 4.5 wt % carnauba wax; 1.7 wt % cetyl alcohol; 1.0 wt % perfume; 0.2 qt % antioxidant; 0.1 wt % preservative, plus the necessary pigment pastes.

Manufacture

In manufacturing lipsticks, the colorants are mixed with part of the oil, usually in a Day Pony mixer, then passed through a 3 roll mill. The color and oil are ground a sufficient number of times to achieve a colorant distribution or better on a grind gage.

Gas that is absorbed on the surface of pigment particles diffuses slowly into the surrounding lipstick mass. A marked improvement is noticed in a pigment dispersion that is placed under vacuum. Dispersion of pigment involves a complicated combination of surface phenomena, eg, absorption, wetting, surface tension, interfacial tension, and formation of phase boundaries. Electrical charges must also be considered. Mechanical force alone cannot produce a satisfactory dispersion.

The base material is heated in a steam-jacketed kettle to 90°C and the ground colorants are added to the base material in the kettle. The batch is stirred with a high speed mixer for several hours. Any adjustment in shade is made by using the ground colorants. Base material is added in proportion to the amount of colorant used in the correction to keep the consistency approximately equal to that in the original formulation.

When the color match is satisfactory, the lipstick mass is drawn from the kettle and passed through a 74-µm (200-mesh) stainless steel screen. It is collected in a molding pan and slabbed for future molding. Prior to molding, the mass is melted with slow agitation in a melting kettle to remove entrapped air.

Temperature control is important throughout processing, with care being taken to avoid excessive temperature in the kettle. The warmed lipstick mass is poured into warm molds, and the molds are passed through a cooling chamber. When cool, the lipsticks are removed from the molds, inserted in the lipstick holders, and flamed by passing them rapidly through a bunsen gas flame. They are then ready for packaging and distribution.

Control Methods

Manufacturing control begins with a thorough check of raw materials. A test of heat resistance of the finished product is made by holding it for 24 h in a constant temperature box at a temperature of 55°C, to determine any tendency to droop or distort. Hardness may be tested using a penetrometer.

The tendency for the stick to sweat or bleed can be checked by putting filled lipstick containers in a desiccator containing water and kept at a constant temperature of 45°C.

Shade and intensity of stain are best judged on the skin by comparison with the standard. Skin tone and undertone are also checked on the skin. Mass tone is judged by comparison with a standard.

Lipsticks

Dow corning describes lipsticks containing alkylmethylsiloxanes, in addition to castor oil, as an emollient, a wax, a suspending agent, a coloring agent and an organsilicone compound (Formula 1).

Shiseido describes a water-in-oil lipstick formulation containing a swellable clay mineral treated with a quaternary ammonium cationic surfactant. The product covers the lips smoothly and provides a long-lasting moisturizing effect as well as long-lasting color. A modified clay dispersion is first prepared by treating magnesium aluminium silicate with benzyl-dimethylstearyl ammonium chloride and adding hydrogenated lecithin, water (aqua) and glycerin. This mixture is then added to a typical lipstick mass to form a w/o emulsion stick (Formula 2).

Improved transfer resistance: A European patent application assigned to Revlon Consumer Products discloses a method of preparing makeup products with improved transfer resistance. The compositions comprise 1-70% of a volatile solvent, 0.1-15% of a silicone resin, 10-45% wax, 5-50% powder and 1-30% oil. The compositions show better transfer resistance than previous cosmetics, which have a tendency to blot or transfer from the skin onto other surfaces, such as glassware or clothing. The compositions are prepared by grinding some of the dry components with the solvent and resin, then adding the wax and oil, followed by the remainder of the dry components.

When filled into suitable receptacles, the compositions may be used as a concealer, blush, eye shadow, foundation, lipstick or the like. An example of a transfer-resistant lipstick composition is shown in Formula 3.

Unilever discloses lipsticks containing polymeric thickening agents. Formula 4 shows a lipstick containing about 10% water (aqua) that uses polybutene and gelatin.

Lipstick overcoat: Nippon Shikizai Kogyo Kenkyush describes a simple lipstick overcoat composition containing perfluoro compounds and powders with a particle size of 0.1-20.0 um. In an example, a lipstick overcoat contains 73% perfluoropoly-methylisopropyl ether, 25% poly (methyl methacrylate) and 2% glycerin. "I presume the poly (methyl methacrylate) represents the dispersed, small-particulate solid the patent specifies. Applying the composition after lipstick application prevents the lipsticks from coming off".

Smooth-spreading lipsticks: A Shiseido patent discloses another lipstick formulated as a w/o emulsion (Formula 12). The emulsion uses alkyl-ether-based emulsifying agents and contains 0.1-10% of a water-soluble polymer, such as polyvinyl alcohol. The resulting lipsticks are said to show smooth-spreading properties and to have long-lasting wearability.

Another Shiseido lipstick patent uses oil-soluble polymers, such as Escorez 1291 (an aliphatic hydrocarbon polymer from Exxon, Japan) to improve spreading and lasting properties.

Sansho Kaken discloses a hydrogel sheet consisting of polyvinyl alcohol, water (aqua) and sodium chloride for removing lipstick color marks left on the skin after being kissed. The sheet, which is pressed against the lipstick marks to remove the stain, may also contain an antibacterial agent/preservative, urea and abrasive powders.

Formula 1. Lipsticks

Octyldodecanol	10.00%
Candelilla (Euphorbia cerifera) wax	7.00
Ozokerite	4.00

Carnauba (Copernicia cerifera) wax	2.50
Acetulan	2.50
Bentone	0.60
Propylparaben	0.10
BHA	0.05
Castor (ricincus communis) oil	28.25
Pigment concentrate 7% pigment, 23% castor oil	30.00
Alkyldimethyl siloxane	15.00
	100.00

Formula 2. Water-in-oil lipstick emulsion

Polyethylene wax	7.00 Parts
Ceresin wax	4.00
Candelilla (Euphorbia cerifera) wax	7.00
Carnauba (Copernicia cerifera) wax	1.00
Castor (ricincus communis) oil	1.00
Mineral oil (paraffinum liquidum)	20.00
Glycerin bis (2-heptylundecanoate)	20.00
Pigments	9.20
Magnesium aluminum silicate (Veegum, RT Vanderbilt)	0.15
Benzyldimethylstearylammonium chloride	0.05
Hydrogenated lecithin	0.05
Water (aqua)	3.00
Glycerin	2.00

Formula 3. Transfer-Resistant Lipstick

Synthetic wax	6.00%
Ceresin	4.00
Paraffin	3.00
Isododecane	10.00
Cetyl stearate/acetylated lanolin, 90:10	5.00
Methylparaben	0.30
Propylparaben	0.10
BHA	0.10

Cyclomethicone	41.50
Isostearyltrimethylolpropane siloxysilicate	5.00
Colors	qs 100.00

Formula 4. Lipstick with polymeric Thickener

Candelilla (Euphorbia cerifera) wax	6.40 parts
Ozokerite wax	3.20
Carnauba (Copernicia cerifera) wax	0.40
Lanolin	4.80
Caprylic/capric triglyceride	6.00
Propylene glycol myristyl ether acetate	6.00
Lanolin oil	2.40
Polybutene	0.80
bis-Diglyceryl caprylate/caprate/ Isostearate/hydroxystearate adipate (Softisan 649, Huls)	9.20
Isopropyl palmitate	12.00
Soy lecithin	1.00
Sunflower oil monoglyceride	4.00
Gelatin, 270 bloom strength	0.36
Water (aqua)	9.64

Formula 5. Oil-in Water Lipstick Emulsion

Microcrystallin wax (cera microcristallina)	3.00%
Ceresin	10.00
Carnauba (Copernicia cerifera) wax	2.00
Lanolin oil	5.00
Jojoba (Buxus chinensis) oil	20.00
Castor (Ricinus communis) oil	10.00
Glyceryl tri-2-ethylhexanoate	31.80
Alkyl-ether-based surfactants	2.00
Pigments	10.00
Water (aqua)	5.00
Glycerin	1.00
Polyvinyl alcohol	0.20
	100.00

Foundations

Procter & Gamble describes an invisible foundation composition containing spherical inorganic components. The foundation, which is invisible on the skin, contains a light-scattering agent, such as silica, having a spherical shape and diameter of up to 30m. Coloring agents are purposely not included to accent the invisibility of the preparation.

Pola Kasei Kogyo described translucent makeup-base cosmetics with fine-pore-covering properties. Cosmetics such as the product shown in Formula 13 resist water and sebum, are translucent and cover fine pores.

Kanebo describes w/o makeup foundations containing 10-35% cyclosiloxanes, 0.5-3% sorbitan monoisostearate and/or diglycerin monoisostearate, and 0.5-3% silicon copolyols (Formula 8). The emulsions have excellent stability, do not discolor and spread easily on the skin.

Procter & Gamble discloses cosmetic tinted gels containing polymer-treated pigments and a hydrophilic gelling agent (Formula 9). This looks like a way of dispersing iron oxide pigments in a carbomer gel. The pigments are treated with water-dispersible polyester or polyester-amide polymers. The gellants may be a cellulose ether, PVP, PVA or carbomers.

Nippon Shikizai Kenkyusho discusses o/w emulsion as foundation bases. Formula 10 may interest makeup formulators.

There appears to be a continuing trend toward the development and use of hollow microspheres for makeup products, perhaps for a feeling of lightness on application, L'Oreal provides the latest example in a patent disclosing a non-compacted powder makeup containing hollow microspheres of a synthetic-thermoplastic material with a specific mass less than 0.1 g/cm^3 (Formula 11).

Elizabeth Arden describes cosmetic compositions, such as facial foundations, said to help minimize fine lines and wrinkles without irritating the skin. The compositions contain C_2-C_{28} a-hydroxy carboxylic acids and rosmarinic acid as well as their salts. A liquid eyeliner containing these materials is shown in Formula 12.

Mascara

Because of the proximity of these products to the eye, the law imposes strict limitations on the ingredients they may contain. The colorants are limited to natural dyes and inorganic and carbon pigments. The commercially available pigments used are the varying shades of the iron oxides, carbon blacks, and ultramarine blues.

Mascara, used to emphasize lashes, makes them appear longer since the ends of the lashes tend to be rather blondish, as compared to the rest of the hair length. The film applied should show good resistance to moisture and to gentle abrasion.

Cream Mascaras

In cream mascara the water has already been incorporated to provide a mascara ready for use without previous trituration. There are some advantates in this type of preparation since a much higher concentration of pigment can be incorporated than in possible in a cake. In addition, the optimum amount of water may be added rather than leaving this to the discretion of the consumer.

A typical cream mascara base is: 46.50 wt % hydrocarbon solvent (Soltrol no. 130); 33.25 wt% distilled or deionized water; 8.25 wt% caranuba wax no.1 refined; 7.50 wt % beeswax, white; 4.00 wt % glyceryl monostearate S.E. (Arlacel C); 0.40 wt % poly-oxyethlene (20) sorbitan stearate (Tween 60); 0.40 wt % borax.5H_2O; 0.10 wt % propyl *p*-hydroxybenzoate; and 0.05 wt % methyl *p*-hydroxybenzoate.

The pigments used in cream mascara are ground into the base material, and the fine grind is then mixed with the necessary water and humectants to form the cream.

Eye Shadows

The colors used in eye shadows are carbon blacks, ultramarine blue, and the various yellows, browns, and reds of the iron oxide pigments. There is usually a higher concentration of pigments in eye shadows than mascaras, sometimes as high as 25%. The base into which the colorants are ground usually consists of beeswax, ozokerite, mineral oil, lanolin, and petrolatum. The method of manufacture consists of melting the waxes and oils together, adding the colorants and titanium dioxide used to impart the desired opacity, and grinding in a three-roll mill.

Eye shadows that have a metallic luster are made by incorporating finely ground aluminum, bronze, silver, or gold powders. The completed formula is heated and stirred slowly to remove occluded air and is then poured into the container.

From time to time power-shadow products, called Kohl, have appeared on the market. These are principally talcum-based with various inorganic colorants.

A prototype formula for an eye shadow is: 40.0 wt % mineral oil 65/75; 24.0 wt % ozokerite 80°C; 20.0 wt % chromic oxide hydrated (40% in petrolatum) 14.0 wt % petrolatum 45-50°C; 1.7 wt % paraffin; and 0.3 wt % propyl para-hydroxybenzoate.

Eye Makeup

L'Oreal describes eye makeup compositions containing a fine wax microdispersion. The waxes, dispersed in water (aqua) using ethoxylated glyceryl monostearate as the dispersing agent, have an average particle size of 184 nm (Formula 13).

Anhydrous eye-makeup compositions having excellent water, perspiration, sebum and oil-resistance are prepared with an oil-soluble resin. An example from a Shiseido patent uses polyisobutylene (Formula 14).

Kao dscribes makeup containing anionic-polymer emulsion with high film-forming ability for waterproof qualities. The anionic-polymer emulsions can also add gloss and help keep sunscreens in place. Formula 15 is an example of a cream eye shadow containing a 30% acrylic acid/butyl acrylate/methyl methacrylate copolymer emulsion in water (aqua).

L'Oreal discloses a surfactant-free eyelash and/or eyebrow makeup consisting of a wax dispersion in an aqueous phase containing water-soluble polymers (Formula 16).

Kanebo describes an emulsion-type mascara that contains a water soluble fibroin peptide (molecular-weight range of 300-3,500), an oily base having a melting point range of 60-110°C, water, a surfactant and, optionally, a hair-setting vinyl polymer. The mascara curls fine eyelashes, impart water resistance and durability, and enhance eyelash luster (Formula 17).

L'Oreal discloses a water-resistant mascara for coating the eyelashes (Formula 18).

Kanebo describes eye-makeup removers containing low-boiling (160-180°C) isoparaffins and polyoxyalkylene alkyl ether surfactants (Formula 19). The resultant products remove both oily, film-forming eye-makeup products and powdery eye shadows.

Formula 6. Eyebrow Cake

Silicone-treated talc	50.00%
Silicone-treated sericite	20.00
Magnesium stearate	2.00
Amino-acid-treated sericite	2.00
Titanium dioxide	1.20
Spherical poly (methyl methacrylate) powder	9.00
Titanium-coated mica	2.00
Titanium carbide/Titanium nitride (30:70) nano powder	8.00
Dimethylsiloxane	3.00
Octyldodecyl dimethyloctanoate	1.40
Octyldodecyl myristate	1.40
	100.00

Formula 7. Pore-covering Makeup

Stearic acid	1.00%
Mocrocrystalline (Cera Microcristallina) wax	1.00
Beeswax (cera alba)	2.00
Sucrose fatty acid ester	3.00
Squalane	2.00
Cyclomethicone	8.00
Glyceryl monostearate	3.00
Polyethyleneglycol monostearate	2.00
Titanium dioxide	3.00
Xanthan gum	0.10
Methylparaben	0.10
Triethanolamine	0.30
1, 3-Butylene glycol	6.00
Water (aqua)	qs 100.00

Formula 8. Water-in-oil Makeup Foundation

Octamethylcyclotetrasiloxane	20.00%
Sorbitan monoisostearate	1.00
Silicone copolyol	1.00

Mineral oil (paraffinum liquidum)	5.00
Petrolatum	1.00
Titanium dioxide	10.00
Iron oxide	0.50
Talc	4.50
Water (aqua)	qs 100.00

Formula 9. Tinted Makeup Gel

Glycerin	5.00%
Carbomer (Carbopol, 950, Goodrich)	0.50
Sodium hydroxide	0.25
Methylparaben	0.20
Methyldibromoglutaronitrile (and) phenoxyethanol (Euxyl K400, S&M)	0.10
Polymer-treated red iron oxide	0.20
Polymer-treated yellow iron oxide	0.40
Polymer-treated black iron oxide	0.05
Water (aqua)	qs 100.00

Formula 10. Foundation Makeup Base

Dimethylsiloxane, 10 cSt	32.90%
Mineral oil (paraffinum liquidum)	10.00
Polybutene	2.00
Paraffin	2.00
1, 3--Butylene glycol	5.00
Neopentyl glycol dioctanoate, HLB 1,3	1.00
Polyether-modified silicones, HLB 4.5	2.00
Diglyceryl disostearate, HLB 6.0	2.00
Methylparaben	0.10
Silicone-treated titanium dioxide	8.00
Silicone-treated talc	5.00
Silicone-treated sericite	3.00
Silicone-treated iron oxides	2.00
Water (aqua)	qs 100.00

Formula 11. Non-compacted Makeup Powder

Mica	23.42%
Kaolin	0.84%
Zinc stearate	0.84
Yellow iron oxide	0.12
Brown iron oxide	0.08
Nylon powder	14.70
Mineral oil (paraffinum liquidum)	49.20
Aroma	0.80
Hollow microspheres based on vinylidene chloride-acrylonitrile polymer (Expancel 551 DE, supplier)	10.0
	100.00

Formula 12. Liquid Eye-liner

Sodium lactate	2.00%
Rosmarinic acid	1.00
Sodium CMC	1.50
Hectorite	0.50
Propylene glycol	5.00
Triethanolamine shellac	5.00
Iron oxide	4.00
Methylparaben	0.10
Diazolidinyl urea (Germall II, Sutton)	0.25
Water (aqua)	qs 100.00

Formula 13. Eye-liner

Carnauba (Copernica cerifera) wax	37.500%
Ethoxylated glyceryl monostearate	9.375
Methylparben	0.200
Black iron oxide	6.000
Hydroxyethyl cellulose	0.250
Water (aqua)	qs 100.000

Formula 14. Water and Oil-resistant Mascara

Carnauba (Copernica cerifera) wax	7.00%
Beeswax (Cera alba)	2.00

Microcrystalline wax (cera microscristallina)	20.00
Lanolin	0.40
Polyisobutylene	57.60
Bentonite	3.00
Pigment	10.00
	100.00

Formula 15. Waterproof Cream Eye Shadow

Microcrystalline wax (cera microcristallina)	3.00%
Stearic acid	3.00
Mineral oil (paraffinum liquidum)	8.50
Lanolin	1.00
Sorbitan monostearate	1.50
Glycerin	5.50
Triethanolamine	1.50
Methyl hydroxypropyl cellulose	0.50
Acrylic acid/butyl acrylate/methyl methacrylate copolymer, 30% emulsion	10.00
Pearl colorant	10.00
Ultramarine blue	2.00
Aroma, preservative	qs
Water (aqua)	qs 100. 00

Formula 16. Eyelash Makeup

Paraffin wax	10.00%
Starch	5.00
Polyethylene	5.00
Black iron oxide	7.00
Carbomer (Carbopol, BF Goodrich)	0.50
Hydroxyethylcellulose	0.50
Panthenol	2.00
Water (aqua)	qs 100.00

Formula 17. Mascara Emulsion

Beeswax (cera alba)	5.00%
Ceresin	4.00
Stearic acid	8.00

Dipropylene glycol	16.00
Tert-Butanol amine	0.80
Fibroin peptide, 7% aq. sol	20.00
Acrylic polymer emulsion	16.00
Alcohol	2.00
Methylparaben	0.10
Butylparaben	0.10
Black iron oxide	12.00
Water (aqua)	qs 100.00

Formula 18. Water-Resistant Mascara

Paraffin wax	12.00%
Lanolin alcohol	15.00
Starch	2.00
Iron oxide	5.00
Isoparaffin	45.00
Montmorillonite clay	8.00
Panthenol	3.00
Chitosan Pyrrolidonecarboxylate (Kytamer PC/Amerchol)	3.00
Water (aqua)	7.00
	100.00

Formula 19. Eye-Makeup Remover

Isoparaffin, b.p. 200-280°C	70.00%
Polyoxyethylene cetyl ether	2.50
Polyoxyethylene behenyl ether	1.00
Polyoxyethlene sorbitan tristearate	1.00
Methylparaben	0.30
Propylene glycol	3.00
Water (aqua)	qs 100.00

Nail Lacquers

Advanced Genetic Technologies describes nail-polish compositions with increased adhesiveness and durability. The products contain protein-adherent polymers with hydroxyl-substituted aromatic groups, such as poly (4-hydroxystyrene). In an example, 150 mg poly (4-hyseozyaryrene). In an example, 150 mg poly (4-hydroxystyrene) was dissolved in ethyl alcohol containing 0.01 M magnesium chloride and coated onto the finger-nails. The resulting finish dried within 2 minutes to a clear, hard, glossy film that could not be scraped or peeled off the nails. The nails could be trimmed clipped or filed without cracking or chipping the finish.

Shinetsu Chem Ind discloses nail lacquers containing polyacetylenes, for products that do not discolor the nails (Formula 20).

International Beauty Design discloses nail-polish compositions that produce hard and durable coatings. A method for strengthening finger nails or toenails comprises three steps:

- Cleaning the nail surface.
- Applying one or more layers of a nail-polish composition consisting of aliphatic urethane acrylate, tripropylene glycol diacrylate, trimethylpropane ethoxylate triacrylate, methacrylic acid, I-hydroxycyclohexylphenyl ketone, butyl acetate and colorants.
- Subjecting the layers to UV treatment for curing.

Pola Chemical Industries describes nail lacquers containing selenium compounds that prevent yellow discoloration of the nails. Formula 21 is an example of a nail lacquer containing 0.01% sodium selenite. No yellow discoloration was noted after using this formula for three months, whereas, severe nail yellowing occurred using products without the sodium selenite.

Unilever discloses nail-polish remover compositions containing gelatin suspension stabilized glycerin and diglycerin. In one example a nail-polish remover contained 85% acetone, 1.0% glycerin, 1.0% diglycerin, 0.2% color, 0.2% aroma, 0.0001% gelating and water (aqua) to 100%. No explanation is given for including gelatin.

NAIL PRODUCTS

Nail Lacquer

Nail lacquer or nail polish usually consists of a resin, plasticizer, solvents, and pigment (30-32). The resins can be nitrocellulose or dinitrocellulose, also known as pyroxylin. Nitrocellulsoe films tend to shrink, so that their surface adhesion may be only moderate. Other resins are, therefore, added to impart adhesion. Gloss and plasticizers are added to reduce shrinkage and make the film flexible.

The solvents used influence the ease of application of the licquer, its rate of drying and hardening and the final characteristics of the film. The preferred solvents for nail lacquers are mixtures of low and medium boiling point alcohols, aromatic hydrocarbons, and aliphantci hydrocarbons.

Plasticizers may be added singly or in combinations of two or more, depending on the formulation. High molecular weight esters are used as well as castor oil. The esters can be dibutyl and dioctyl phthalate, triethyl citrate, and acetyl tributyl citrate.

The pigments used in nail lacquer formulations are carbon black, iron oxides, chromium oxides, ultramarines, metallic powders (gold, bronze, aluminum, copper), titanium dioxide. Transparent systems require the use of solvent-soluble colorants such as D&C red, green, yellow, and violet.

Pearl pigment in nail lacquer may be the natural pearl essence, guanine (2-amino-6-hydroxy purine), or a synthetic pearl that is usually a bismuth salt.

A typical nail lacquer formulation is: 30.5% wt % toluence; 12.8 wt % *n*-butyl acetate; 11.1 wt % *n*-amyl acetate; 11.1 wt % ethyl acetate; 10.0 wt % nitrocellulose; 10.0 wt % aryl sulfonamide–formaldehyde resin; 5.0 wt % isopropanol; 3.0 wt % bentonite; 2.5 wt % camphor (plasticizer); 2.5 wt % dibutyl phthalate; and 1.5 wt % ethanol.

Formula 20. Non-discoloring Nail Lacquer

Poly (1-trimethylsilylpropylene)	0.30%
Nitrocellulose	12.00
Alkyd resin	10.00
Dibutyl phthalate	4.00
Camphor	2.00
Butyl acetate	49.70
Toluene	20.00
Pigment	1.00
Quaternary bentonite	1.00
	100.00

Formula 21. Non-yellowing Nail Lacquer

Sodium selenite	0.01%
Ethyl acetate	20.00
Isobutyl acetate	26.99
Isopropyl alcohol	2.00

Toluene	20.00
Nitrocellulose	17.00
Sucrose acetate isobutyrate	8.00
Di butyl phthalate	3.80
1, 3-Butylene glycol	0.20
Colorant	1.00
Stearalkonium hectorite	1.00
	100.00

Lacquer Removers

Lacquer removers may be made from any of a number of solvents. In most cases, any of the solvents used in the formulation of the enamels can be used as removers. The fastest acting seems to be acetone, but because of its high volatility, ethyl acetate has come into favor as well. Many of the lacquer removers contain an additive designed to leave a film on the nail, since the solvent itself hs so high a degreasing tendency. Various oils and emollient compounds are added to the lacquer removers such as castor oil, lanolins, and lanolin derivatives.

A typical nail polish remover formula is: 40.0 wt % ethyl acetate; 30.0 wt % acetone; 19.0 wt % carbitol; 10.0 wt % dibutyl phthalate; 1.0 wt % sesame oil; and *qs* perfume

Cuticle Removers and Softeners

Cuticle removers and cuticle softeners usually consist of a dilute solution of alkali in water with some glycerol or other humectant added to keep the water from evaporating too easily. Potassium hydroxide, the alkali most often used, results in a somewhat harsh preparation but is effective. Trisodium phosphate, triethanolamine, and some of the quaternary ammonium salts have been used as replacements for potassium hydroxides. These are not as effective as the alkali but do a fair job of softening the cuticle.

Rouge

The term rouge (literally, red), although it properly includes all products intended to impart a glow to cheeks and lips, has gradually become limited to colorings applied to the cheeks. Rouge for the lips (except in theatrical cosmetics) originally was dispensed in little jars or pots, but it is now made in the form of crayons or sticks, and it will be considers here under a separate heading.

Rouge is available in several forms: (*1*) creams, (*2*) pastes, (*3*) compact powder, and (*4*) liquid. Choice is related to the condition of the skin and should be associated with the choice of face powder.

(*1*) *Cream rouge* is recommended for skin that tends toward dryness, because it can be rubbed well over the skin and blended well into the surrounding areas. To enhance the natural effect, light weight powder should be applied over it.

In cream rouge the pigment is dispersed in an emulsion that conforms in type to any of several of the creams described in the earlier section—cold cream, emollient, or vanishing cream. The ingredients are selected from those used in various types of creams, combined to insure case of application, lasting effect, good body, and consistency during changes in temperature. White petrolatum (short fiber), white mineral oil, white beeswax, spermaceti, absorption bases, stearic acid, and cocoa butter are among the oily components used; borax and triethanolamine are used as emulsifying agents; glycerol and glycols are included as humectants.

Table XI. Compositions of Cream and Paste Rouges.

	Typical recipe, % by wt. in:					
Ingredient	Cold creams		Emollient	Vanishing Cream	Pastes	
Beeswax	20	10	10	–	4	
Borax	2	1	1	1	–	–
Ceresin	–	–	–	–	–	21
Cetyl alcohol	–	–	–	4	4	–
Cocoa butter	–	–	–	–	4	–
Glycerol	–	2	–	10	–	–
Lanolin	–	–	5	–	–	–
Mineral oil	–	35	24	–	23	53
Oleic acid	15	–	–	–	–	–
Petrolatum	25	25	40	–	60	23
Spermaceti	–	–	12	–	5	3
Stearic acid	–	2	–	25	–	–
Triethanolamine	4	1	–	–	–	–
Water	34	24	8	60	–	–
Total	100	100	100	100	100	100

The colors of preference for cream rouge are insoluble lakes, although some oil-soluble dyes are occasionally used. Dyes soluble in one or the other of the two phases of the emulsion would cause mottling; darkening due to evaporation of water might also cause unevenness in the product itself and in the effect of it.

(2) *Paste rouge* is made from various fats and waxes, incorporating appropriate colors and perfume, but no water. It is used in the same manner as cream rouge; therefore, the ease of spreading, melting point, and stability are important factors. Recipes for several types of cream and paste rouges are suggested in Table XI (4, 5, 9, 13). The compositions suggested are best prepared as white bases, to be used in proportional amounts with the chosen colors. Perfume, and also a preservative, are also to be added.

(3) *Powder rouge* is usually recommended for the skin that tends toward oiliness, though many women who use the cream or paste also apply a touch of powdered rouge for repairing their make-up at odd times. For regular use on an oily skin, the powdered rouge should be applied over a heavy weight of face powder.

Because of the delicate effect desired, the composition of powder rouge resembles that of lighter-weight face powders. Talc may be present to 80%; starch, stearin, and gums may be used as the binding agent; the remaining ingredients are zinc oxide, zinc stearate, kaolin, precipitated chalk, and titanium dioxide. Many manufacturers use their prepared powder bases, adding what may be required to insure the formation of a good compact product.

(4) *Liquid rouge* is not so popular now as it was formerly, but it still appears occasionally as a novelty. It is usually a dilute solution of appropriate and approved water-soluble colors in a mixture of water, alcohol, and glycerol. Good lasting effect can be obtained by careful adjustment of the amount of cosin present; the addition of a small amount of a wetting agent assists spreading. Recipes for liquid rouge are given in various handbooks.

As *novelties*, rouge also has been offered on leaves of tissue paper in small books or envelopes, and as a white product containing alloxan, which turns red as it is rubbed over the skin.

Colors for rouge are limited by the range of tints and shades that would be normal for the natural tones in the skin, and the color of the blood as seen through it. Many manufactures offer three basic variations—clear red, orange-red, and bluish or purplishred. The merchandising of these products takes advantages of seasonal changes in the basic tone of the skin, and also of the need for slightly different shades of make-up in daylight and under certain types of artificial lighting.

Manufacture of Rouge and Lipstick. Many manufacturers in the field consider the making of rouge and lipstick so difficult and complicated that they consign their recipes to others who specialize in the production of these items. It is true that with older equipment it was inevitable that entire rooms soom became covered with various shades of red deposit; but with the newer equipment and reasonable care this waste can be almost entirely avoided.

For *paste rouge* the fats are melted and well mixed; the finely divided certified colors are added; and the mass is allowed to cool under continuous agitation. When it is about 20°F. above the solidification point, the mass is run through an ointment mill and poured into the containers.

For *cream rouge* the colors are first mixed with a portion of the petrolatum or mineral oil. Water-in oil emulsions are prepared as described under "Creams". After emulsification is complete the colored portion (and perfume) is added, and the whole mass is run through an ointment mill, if necessary, to insure thorough mixing. Oil-in-water emulsions are completely prepared without color; this is added after the mixture is cool, and the whole mass is milled before filling.

Compact powder rouge is prepared as described under face powders; the method of dry compression is preferred.

In the making of *lipsticks* that contain bromo acid this dye is incorporated in the castor oil, *n*-butyl stearate, or other solvent warmed in a jacketed kettle, while the fats, waxes and lakes are melted and thoroughly mixed in another vessel. The second mixture is then added to the first; the whole mass in kept under continuous agitation, and finally run through a steam-jacketed mill to insure uniform dispersion of the colors. The mixture is allowed to cool, and when it is 5-10° above the solidification point it is poured into molds and chilled quickly. The sticks are at once placed in their holders, passed through a gas flame or under an infrared lamp to smooth the surface, and covered for packaging.

Skin Pigmentation

Henkel discloses the use of indolines as tanning agents for human skin. These compounds are applied to the skin as o/w emulsions to impart a brown color to the skin without exposure to the sun (Formula 22).

Shiseido discloses the use of chaulmoogra (Taraktogenos kurzii) oil for the treatment of hypopigmentation (Formula 23). Chaulmoogra (Taraktogenos kurii) oil and its salts and esters induced pigmentation in hypomelanotic spots on the skin by causing an expansion of already pigmented areas.

A patent assigned to Estee Lauder described self-tanning cosmetic compositions dispensed as a spray. The compositions are alchol-and-oil-free and dry quickly on the skin (Formula 24).

Richardson-Vicks (now part of Procter & Gamble) has patented stabilized compositions for imparting an artificial tan to human skin. The improved stability emulsions comprise 0.120% dihydroxyacetone, 0.15% of an alkyl phosphate, such as diethanolamine cetyl phosphate, and 0.025-2.5% of a carboxylic acid copolymer, such as acrylates $C_{10}C_{30}$ alkyl acrylate crosspolymer (Formula 25).

Stiefel Laboratories describes suntanning agents containing a pseudocatalase. Suntanning is enhanced by

L'Oreal describes the use of 4-thiroesorcin derivatives in skin-whitening cosmetics. In an example, 0.01 M 4-mthyl thiroesorcin inhibited tyrosinase activity by 90% (Formula 26).

Kanebo discloses skin-lightening preparations containing cinnamic acid derivatives, which prevent melanin formation and are not irritating to the skin (Formula 27). One of the preferred compounds is 3-[2-(b-glucopyranosyloxy) phenyl]-2-cinnamic acid. At 0.1%, this compound inhibited 97.2% tyrosinase activity.

Kao discloses skin-lightening compositions containing a combination of ascorbic acid and tea-leaf extracts (Formula 28).

Sansei Seiyaku described skin preparations contaiuning oligopeptides for inhibiting melanin formation. A cream containing anserine as the oligopeptide is shown in Formula 29.

Unilever describes topical, retinol-containing cosmetic compositions used to promote the repair of photo-damaged skin and/or to reduce or prevent the damaging effects of UV light on skin and/or to lighten the skin (Formula 30).

A Japanese patent assigned to Nonogawa Shoji YK discloses skin-lightening cosmetics containing proteogylcans and ascorbates. The proteoglycans are extracted from animal tissue. The lotion shown in Formula 31 inhibited malanin formation in vitro tests.

A Mikimoto Seiyaku patent describes cosmetics containing cholesteric liquid crystals and licorice extracts. The licorice extract is used in Japan to lighten skin; the liquid crystals, which may have a skin-moisturizing effect, also enhance the product's appearance (Formula 32).

Kojic acid has been used for many years as a skin-lightening compound in Japan. In the past few years, the use of glabridin, licorice extract, as a skin lightener has increased. Kanebo discloses the latest (Formula 33).

A patent assigned to Kose discloses the use of superoxide dismutase to enhance the effectiveness of skin-lightening agents (Formula 34).

Formula 22. Skin-Coloring Formulation

Zinc stearate	2.00%
Aluminium stearate	0.50
Isopropyl isostearate	13.00
Wheat germ (Triticum vulgare) oil	3.00
Methylglucose dioleate	2.00
PEG-45/dodecyl glycol copolymer	2.00
Beeswax (Cera alba)	3.00
1, 2-Dodecanediol	1.00
Propylparaben	0.20
Lactic acid	0.50
Sodium hydroxide	0.15
Methylparaben	0.20
Magnesium sulfate 7 H_2O	0.70
Glycerin	2.00
5, 6-Dihydroxyindole hydrobromide	0.9 mmole
Water (aqua)	qs 100.00

Formula 23. Treatment Cream for Hypopigmentation

Carbomer 940 (Carbopol 940, BF Goodrich)	0.20%
Triethanolamine	0.25
Butylene glycol	4.00
Glyceryl stearate	3.00
Chaulmoogra (Takaktogenos kurzii) oil	2.00
Myristyl myristate	2.50

Acetylated lanolin	3.00
PEG-20 Stearate	3.00
Cetostearyl octanoate	2.00
Mineral oil (paraffinum liquidum)	1.00
Lanolin alcohol	0.50
Octyl methoxycinnamate	3.00
Methychloroisothiazolinone (and) methylisothiazolinone (Kathon CG, Rohm & Hass)	0.10
Allantion	0.10
Water (aqua)	qs 100.00

Formula 24. Self-Tanning Spray

Dihydroxyacetone	5.00%
1, 3-Butylene glycol	3.00
PPG-12-buteth-16 (Ucon 50 HB660, Union Carbide)	0.50
Hydrolyzed wheat protein (and) hydrolyzed wheat starch (Cropeptide W, Croda)	0.20
Dimethyl isosorbide (Arlasolve DMI, ICI)	10.00
PEG-10 laurate (Protomate 600-ML, Protameen)	1.50
Methyldibromoglutaronitrile (and) phenoxyethanol (Euxyl K-400, Calgon)	0.20
Ethoxydiglycol (Transcutol, Gattefosee)	10.00
Glycereth-7 triacetate (Dermol GL-7A, Alzo)	5.00
PEG-40 castor oil (Surfactol 365, Cas Chem)	1.00
Water (aqua), deionized	qs 100.00

Formula 25. Artificial Tanning Lotion

Carbomer 934	0.20%
Carbomer 980	0.15
Acrylates C_{10}-C_{30} alkyl acrylate crosspolymer (Pemulin TR1, BE Goodrich)	0.15
PPG-20 Methyl glucose ether distearate	2.00

Tocopheryl acetate	1.20
Mineral Oil (paraffinum liquidum)	2.00
Stearyl alcohol	1.00
Shea (Butyrosermum perkii) butter	1.00
Cetyl alcohol	1.00
Ceteareth20	1.00
Ceteth-2	1.00
Ceteth 10	1.00
Diethanolamine cetyl phosphate	0.75
Dihydroxyacetone	3.00
DMDM hydantoin (and) iodopropylbutylcarbamate	0.25
Aroma	1.00
Cyclomethicone	2.0
Water (aqua)	qs 100.00

Formula 26. Skin-whitening Composition

4-Methyl thioresorcin	2.80%
Ethyl alcohol	50.00
PEG-40	30.00
Ethoxydiglycol	5.00
Glycerin	5.00
Water (aqua)	qs 100.00

Formula 27. Skin-lightening Composition

3-[2-(b-glucopyranosyloxy) phenyl]-2-cinnamic acid	0.10%
Olive (Olea europaea) oil	15.00
Isopropyl myristate	5.00
Polyoxyethylene nonyl phenyl ether	0.50
Glycerin	5.00
Methylparaben	0.10
Alcohol	7.00
Water (aqua)	qs 100.00

Formula 28. Skin-lightening Composition

Glyceryl stearate	5.00%

Polyethyleneglycol monostearate	2.00
Squalane	8.00
Glyceryl trioctanoate	8.00
Stearyl alcohol	5.50
Dimethylpolysiloxane	0.20
Propylene glycol	5.00
Disodium edetate	0.10
L-Ascorbic acid phosphate magnesium salt	3.00
Tea leaf (Camillia sinensis) extract	3.00
Citric acid	0.50
Sodium citrate	0.50
Preservatives, aroma, color	qs
Water (aqua)	qs 100. 00

Formula 29. Skin-lightening Cream

PEG-40 stearate	2.00%
Glyceryl stearate SE	5.00
Stearic acid	5.00
Behenyl alcohol	1.00
Mineral oil (paraffinum liquidum)	10.00
Glyceryl trioctanoate	10.00
Glycerin	5.00
Ethylparaben	0.10
Anserine	4.00
Water (aqua)	qs 100.00

Formula 30. Photodamaged skin/lightening Treatment Oil

Retinol	0.20%
Cysteaminophenol	1.00
Isopropanol	10.00
Volatile silicone	80.00
Ethylhexyl palmitate	8.70
Antioxidant	0.10
	100.00

Formula 31. Skin-lightening Lotion

Alcohol	8.00%
PEG hydrogenated castor oil	0.40
Glycerin	5.00

1, 3-Butylene glycol	3.00
Proteoglycan extracts	10.00
L-Ascorbic acid phosphoric acid magnesium salt	3.00
Citric acid	0.50
Sodium citrate	1.00
Aroma	qs
Water (aqua)	qs 100.00

Formula 32. Skin Lightener

Cholesteryl 12-hydroxystearate	3.00%
Cholesteryl heptanoate	3.00
Cholesteryl oleate	2.00
Cholesteryl butyrate	1.00
Licorice (Glycyrrhiza glabra) extract	1.00
Neutralized carboxyvinyl polymer	0.30
Water (aqua)	qs 100.00

Formula 33. Skin Lightener

Alcohol	10.00%
Polysorbate 20	0.50
BHT	0.01
Aroma	0.05
Potassium 2-phenylbenzimidazole 5-sulfonate	0.50
Glabridin	0.10
Glycerin	5.00
Xanthan gum	0.10
Water (aqua)	qs 100.00

Formula 34. Skin-lightening Preparation

Superoxide dismutase	3.12×10^{-5} nM
Kojic acid	1.00%
1, 3-Butylene glycol	20.00
Polyoxyethylene hydrogenated castor oil monoisostearate	1.00
Lactic acid	0.05
Sodium lactate	0.03
Water (aqua)	qs 100.00

Hair

Glycolipids and siloxanes: Kao describes hair dyes containing glycolipids and siloxanes, to provide long lasting colours without damaging the hair. The siloxanes are selected from dinethyl siloxanes, methyl phenyl siloxanes, amino-modified silicones, fatty-acid-modified silicones, alcohol-modified silicones, cyclic silicones, polyether-modified silicones, fluorine-modified silicones and alkyl-modified silicones (Formula 1). Of course, this is the first step; and oxidize must be added to develop the colour in the hair.

Tyroisinase activators and pantothenic acid: A patent assigned to Lion discloses the use of tyrosinase activators and pantothenic acid (and derivaties) to prevent hair from graying. Culturing human melanocytes with both 0.025% of the 2-amino-2-methyl-1, 3-propanediol salt of 8-methyxy-c AMP and 0.05% calcium pantothenate increase tyrosinase activity 240%, compared to a 193% increase without the pantothenate salt. However, Lion's patent gives to date for hair treated with this combination.

Dopa: Unilever cosmetic describes compositions containing dihydroxyphenylalanine (DOPA) derivatives for darkening hair. An analog of DOPA, dihydroxyphenyl serine, can be absorbed by skin or by hair follicles and metabolized in vivo. This leads to melanin formation in skin or the growth of melanin-pigmented hair. Consequently, the composition gives controlled skin darkening that mimics sun-induced tanning or brings about the growth of dark hair in place of gray or white hair (Formula 2). After two days in the presence of 0.1 mm dihydroxyphenylserine, cultured hair follicles were observed to darken. The hair shaft that grew from the follicles showed dark color.

Permanent dyes: Shiseido discloses a unique non-oxidative permanent-dye formulation for hair and synthetic fibres. By mixing a gelling agent, water (aqua), a mercaptan-based reducing agent and a certified FD&C or D&C dye, Shiseido produces a highly effective, easily employed permanent-dye gel composition that imparts a desired color into both natural and synthetic fibres. In the preferred compositions, the user adds the mercaptan-based reducing agent to the composition immediately before applying the gel composition to the fibres. Merely rubbing the gel onto the fibres permanently embeds the desired color into the fibers.

Temporary dyes: Bristol-Myers Squibb discloses compositions and methods for temporarily coloring hair using chemically synthesized or biosynthetic water-soluble melanins. The compositions comprise, in addition to the melanin compound, water-dispersible cationic compounds. The cationic material, which forms a complex with most of the water-soluble melanin, can be a surfactant, such as dicetyldimmonium chloride, or a cationic polymer, such as polyquaternium-6, 11 or -39. The patent procedure dissolves 40 mg solubilized melanin in 5 ml water (aqua) for solution 1 and adds 40 mg dicetyldimmonium chloride to 5 ml water (aqua) to make solution 2. A mixture of solutions 1 and 2 at pH 7.1 is used to treat hair.

Non-oxidative dyes: A recent European patent application discloses an interesting two-step, non-oxidative hair-dye system. The user first applies a composition containing 2--hydroxyl-1, 4-naphthoquinone to the hair. This remain in place for about 30 minutes. In the second step, the user applies a preparation containing 5, 6-dihydroxyindole, which remains on the hair for an additional 10 minutes before being rinsed off. The treatment gives the processed hair a blond color (Formula 3).

Shampoo dyes: Kao describes shampoo containing direct hair dyes that have excellent dyeing and cleansing properties (Formula 4).

Henkel discloses a one-step product for simultaneously washing and coloring the hair that uses a coupler-developer oxidation coloring agent, a cationic polymer, an anionic surfactant and an amphoteric surfactant. Formula 5 gives a medium-blond hair dye.

Clairol discloses direct hair dyes having a quaternary center with a long aliphatic chain. The dyes have a high affinity for hair, are shampoo-stable and impart uniform dyeing. A hair dye comprises 0.2% dimethylhexadecyl--2 (2-nitroanilion) ethyl ammonium iodide, 65% ethyl alcohol and water (aqua) to 100%.

Bleaching agents: Hoyu describes bleaching agents containing sulfite salts, benzyl alcohol and cationic surfactants (pH 7-9) to bleach dyed hair without damaging the hair or changing the native hair color. A gel-type composition containing 4% sodium sulfite, 5% benzyl alcohol and 3% cetyltrimethylammonium chloride effectively bleaching the dyed hair colour without bleaching the native, black color. This almost sounds like a stripping agent for previously used non-oxidative hair dyes.

A Takara Belmont patent describes hair bleaches containing bicarbonates, hydrogen peroxide and persulfates at pH 5-8. These are said to show less damage to hair and a low incidence of irritation to the skin. The product formula describes three mixtures, apparently mixed before use. The first mixture is a 3% water (aqua) solution of ammonium bicarbonate; the second mixture is a 17% water (aqua) solution of 35% hydrogen peroxide. To produce the bleach, Takara Belmont mixes 60 g each of solutions 1 and 2 with 1 g of ammonium persulfate powder. A bundle of hair coated with this mixture, kept at 50°C for 15 minutes. washed and dried, and bleached brightly showed to damage.

A Poly Chemical Industries patent describes hair preparations containing 0.0001% sodium selenite that prevent UV-induced yellowing of hair.

Natural pigments: Kashiwa Chemical discloses hair dyes containing natural pigments extracted from Dactylspius coccus, Monascus purpureus, Coccus lacca and Polygonus tinctrium, including capsaicin, ceraminic acid and laccaic acid (Formula 6).

A German patent describes the enhancement of cosmetic hair coloration via exposure to light. The chemical coloration of hair is enhanced, yielding brighter and stronger colors, by subsequent exposure of the hair to light, especially coherent light in the wavelength range 600-1, 200 nm, preferably 780 nm. This treatment alters the a-helical structure of the hair macrofibrils, particularly the enzyme coordination and redox potential. Researchers irradiated hair by placing a hood with laser diodes set into the inner surface over the head.

E.C. DeWitt and Co. disclose hair-darkening compositions containing thiosulfates and bismuth acetate derivatives. A hair dye was prepared using bismuth citrate, disodium EDTA, glycerine, alcohol, sodium thiosulfate, polysorbate 80 and aroma in an aqueous base.

Bristol-Myers Squibb discloses other melanin-forming hair dyes. A hair-dying kit comprises three items:

- An aqueous solution of DOPA compound
- A water-soluble oxidant
- A buffering agent to maintain a pH of 6-10.

When the DOPA compound reacts with the oxidant in an aqueous environment, it provides a high concentration of a nitrogenous phenolic melanin precursor, which converts to melanin while in the hair. Combining a DOPA (0.15 g DOPA, 7.5 ml 0.1 M HCl) and an oxidant (0.9 g $K_3Fe(CN)_6$, 1.15 g disodium phosphate, 0.3 g hydrated trisodium phosphate and 7.5 ml water (qua) solution provides the aqueous reaction medium, with an initial pH of 7.2. Exposing a swatch of virgin gray hair to the aqueous reaction medium for 30 minutes, rinsing with water (aqua), shampooing and drying leaves the hair several shades darker.

Chlorotrichosis: An article by M. Sticherling et al briefly reviews why hair turns green. The problem of green discoloration, sometimes referred to as chlorotrichosis, often results from deposition of exogenous copper through both occupational and vacation activities.

These days, a common source of exogenous copper is tap water or swimming-pool water. The metal is released from copper fittings by the acidic pH of the water and, according to one report, after flurodiation of drinking water. It is also released after the addition of copper-based algaechides to, or chlorination of, swimming-pool water. In most cases, the problem affects patients with light-blond hair.

Predisposing factors that must be present as well for green discoloration to occur include previous hair damage (either mechanically, by sun or by peroxide bleaching), dyeing, frequent contant with chlorinated water or use of an alkaline shampoo. However, reported causes of green hair other than exogenous copper deposition include use of tar shampoo and industrial exposures to cobalt, chromium and nickel. You may wish to obtain a reprint of this short but through review for your files because it contains almost 40 valuable references on this subject.

Formula 1. Hair Dye

p-Phenylenediamine	1.00%
Oleic acid	10.00
Oleic acid diethanolamide	8.00
Oleyl alcohol	2.00
Polyoxyethylene octyldodecyl ether	10.00
Ethyl alcohol	15.00
Propylene glycol	10.00
Polyether modifies silicone	1.00
Glycolipid hydroxypropyl either	1.00
Ammonia to pH 10.00	qs

Formula 2. Anhydrous Hair Darkener

Dihydroxyphenylserine	5.00%
Isopropyl alcohol	10.00
Ethylhexylpalmitate	8.70
Antioxidant	0.10
Volatile silicone	qs 100.00

Formula 3. Two-step Non-oxidative Hair Dye

First Application

2-Hydroxyl-1, 4-naphthoquinone	0.50%
Carob gum	3.00
Citric acid	4.00
Milk powder	qs 100.00

Dilute with 3 times its weight of water (aqua) and apply to hair for 30 minutes.

Second Application

5, 6-Dihyrdoxyindole	0.50%
Alcohol	10.00
Hydroxypropyl cellulose	1.00
Capryl caprylglucosides (Triton CG 110, Rohm & Haas)	2.00
Triethanolamine	0.75
Tartaric acid	0.30
Preservative	qs
Water (aqua)	qs 100.00

Apply for 10 minutes and rinse from the hair.

Formula 4. Direct Hair-Dye Shampoo

Disodium lauryl ether sulsosuccinate, 30%	27.00%
Sodium lauryl sarcosinate, (30%)	7.50
C_{9-11} Alkylpolyglucoside, (35%)	19.00
Dimenthyllaurylamine oxide, (35%)	6.00
Laurylhydroxysulfobetaine, 30%	3.50
PEG160- sorbitan stearate	1.00
Polysorbate 60	1.00
Preservative	0.30
EDTA	0.50
Polydimethyldiallylammonium chloride	0.50
Citric acid	1.00
Henna (Lawsonia inermis) extract	0.10
Basic yellow no. 57	0.01

Basic red no. 76	0.08
Basic blue no. 99	0.01
Water (aqua)	qs 100.00

Formula 5. Hair-coloring/conditioning Shampoo

C_{12-18} Fatty alcohol	10.50%
Sodium laureth sulfate	5.00
Cocoalkyldimethylammonium betaine	3.00
Polyquaternium-10 (Polymer JR 400, Amerchol)	1.00
a-Naphthol	0.40
1, 3-*bis* (2, 4-diaminophenoxy) proper	0.10
Resorcinol	0.15
p-Toluylene-diamine sulfate	0.21
EDTA	0.20
Sodium sulfate	1.00
Ammonia solution, 25%	6.00
Water (aqua)	qs 100.00

Formula 6. Hair Dye Containing Natural Pigments

Glyceryl monolinoleate	1.80%
Polyoxyethylene polyoxypropylene glycol	1.20
Polyethylene glycol	4.00
Berberine chloride	0.80
Copper/sodium chlorophyll	0.70
Hematin	0.50
Cochineal	1.50
Citric acid	0.20
Aroma	0.30
Water (aqua)	qs 100.00

Hair Preparations

Shampoos

Present day shampoos usually contain a primary detergent which can be a fatty alcohol sulfate, ether sulfate, sarcosinate, or one of many other anionics (see Hair preparations; Surfactants). The primary detergent can also be amphoteric or nonionic. The secondary, or auxiliary, detergent is usually an alkanolamide, which controls the viscosity of the product and increases the quality and volume of the foam (33-39).

Soap Shampoo

Soap shampoos do not cleanse well in hard water areas. They are primarily aqueous solutions of soft soap combined with preservatives, sequestrants, color, and perfume.

Soapless Shampoo

Soapless shampoos are primarily based on aqueous solutions of sulfonated oils such as sulfonated castor oil and sulfonated olive oil combined with preservatives, color, and perfume.

Low pH Shampoos

Unlike many of the propertiees ascribed to shampoos, such as foaming, cleansing, luster, and manageability, pH is an intangible in that it cannot be observed or demonstrated during product usage, and the effects of low pH are not obvious to the user. It has been reported that mild aqueous acids cause antiswelling action on the cuticle scales of the hair. As the cuticle tightens, the hair gains luster because light is more efficiently reflected from the surface of the hair shaft. In the absence of external charges hair shows its highest strength and resiliency at pH 4.0-6.0. Some surfactants do not perform will in an acid medium. Fatty alcohol sulfates hydrolyze rapidly and decompose below pH 4.0. Alkanolamides generally react in a similar manner. However, combinations of triethanolamine, and sodium and ammonium lauryl sulfates with amine oxides can be adjusted to low pH with good stability. Examples of clear, stable shampoo formulations adjusts to pH 4.0 are: 54.0 wt % water; 40.0 wt % ammonium lauryl sulfate (30% solution); 6.0 wt % cocamidoopropylamine oxide (30% solution); and *qs* (as needed) preservative, color, perfume, acid, etc.

Amphoteric Shampoos

Amphoteric surfactants are generally assumed to be less irritating to the eyes than other detergent or soap preprations. They are usually low foam materials, and it is customary to combine them with anionic surfactants. Amphoteric shampoos are based on the use of imidazoline, betaine, and sulfobetaine surfactants. Amphoteric-base shampoos are difficult to thicken and difficult to opacify. Amphoterics can be blended with equal parts of either high foaming anionic lauryl sulfates or the sulfo-succinate half esters. Amine oxides can also be used instead of the more irritating alkanolamides. The keratin substantivity of the betaine amphoterics is greatest at pH 5.5-6.5. The following shampoo formula, which has been adjusted to a pH of 5.8, illustrates the use of amphoterics: 17.0 wt % ammonium lauryl sulfate; 6.0 wt % Monomate CPA-40 (sulfo-sauccinate half ester); 2.0 wt % Monateric ISA-35 (isostearic imidazoline); and *qs* perfume, preservative, color, and water.

Dandruff Shampoos

Dandruff is the product of hyperkeratinization. The rate of keratinization has increased to the point that the scales become more visible. There are not known differences in the incidence of dandruff in men and women or among races. Dandruff shampoos contain ingredients that effectively control dandruff by allowing a normal turnover rate of epidermal cells. Ingredients used in some anti-dandruff shampoos are coal tar, quaternary ammonium compounds, resorcinol, salicylic acid, selenium sulfide, sulfur, undecylenic acid and derivatives and zinc pyrithoine (zinc 2-mercaptopyridine 1-oxide; zinc moadine). Selenium sulfide and zinc pyrithione are cytostatic (reduce epidermal cell turnover rate). Zinc pyrithione is strongly absorbed by the hair, with absorption related to concentration, pH, temperature, product formulation, and time of exposure. Since these are medicated shampoos, formulations should be nonirritating and nonsensitizing.

A typical lotion cream shampoo is: 47.0 wt % distilled or deionized water; 42.1 wt % sodium lauryl sulfate, 28% active; 4.0 wt % ethylene glycol monostearate; 3.0 wt % coconut fatty acid diethanolamide; 3.0 wt % propylene glycol; 0.5 wt % perfume; and 0.4 wt % preservative.

A typical clear liquid shampoo is: 50.0 wt % triethanolamine lauryl sulfate, 65% active; 27.6% wt % distilled or deionized water; 10.0 wt % propylene glycol; 5.0 wt % lauric acid diethanolamide; 4.0 wt % myristic acid; 2.0 wt % oleyl alcohol; 0.8 wt % perfume; 0.4 wt % preservative; 0.1 wt % citric acid; and 0.1 qt % sequesterant Na_2.

A typical viscous liquid shampoo is: 60.0 wt % triethanolamine lauryl sulfate, 38% active; 21.1. wt % distilled or deionized water; 3.0 wt % myristicacid; 2.0 wt % oleyl alcohol; 2.0 wt % propylene glycol; 1.0 wt % perfume; o.5 wt % poly (vinylpyrroliddionone) K-30; and 0.4 wt % preservative.

A typical antidandruff shampoo is: 65.3 wt % water; 25.5 wt % sodium aluryl sulfate; 5.0 wt % stearic acid; 2.1 wt % lauramine oxide; 1.0 wt % zinc pyrithione powder; 0.7 wt % sodium hydroxide pellets; 0.4 wt % sodium chloride; plus preservative, color, and perfume.

Shampoo Additives

Foam builders are principally fatty acid alkanolamides. Conditioning agents are amine oxides, fatty alcohols, lanolin derivatives, esters of fatty acids, silicones, cationic materials, and polyacrylamides. Opacifying agents are higher fatty alcohols, such as stearyl and cetyl, and glycol and glycerol esters of fatty acids. Sequestering agents prevent formation of insoluble calcium and magnesium soaps and prevent discoloration owing to iron contamination. Citric acid, tartaric acid and salts of EDTA are commonly used sequestrants. Viscosity builders are cellulose derivatives, alkanolamides, and carboxy-vinyl polymers. Preservatives are usually the hydroxybenzoates, formaldehyde, imidazolidinyl-urea compounds (Germall), sorbates, and 1 (3-chloroallyl) 3, 5, 7--triazo-1 azoniaadamantane chloride (Dowicil).

Hair Straighteners

Though the thioglycolate straighteners are essentially the same as products used for hair waving, they differ in that the straighteners are appreciably more viscous to help keep the hair straight while it is being softened (see Hair preparations). After application, the hair is repeatedly combed, which may be a factor in scalp irritation. Since curly hair is quite resistant, the softening process takes a rather long time and the danger of hair damage and scalp irritation proportionately increases. When it reaches the desired straightness, the hair is rinsed and treated with a conventional neutralizer such as sodium bromate. A typical formula for a thioglycolate straightener is: 52.00-53.00 wt % distilled or deionized water; 22.00 wt % glyceryl monostearate, pure; 17.50 wt % ammonium thioglycolate (50% solution, 8.75% thio acid); ca 4.50 wt % ammonium hydroxide (28% solution, sufficient to product pH 9.2-9.4); 1.75 wt % Brij 35; 1.00 wt % mineral oil; 0.50-1.00 wt % perfume; and 0.15 wt % preservative [methyl *p*-hydroxybenzoate and propyl *p*-hydroxybenzoate (3:1)].

The Gant and Hersh patent relates to compositions and methods for straightening kinky hair or for curling straight hair.

Depilatories

Products used for the removal of unwanted hair by chemical agents are commonly called depilatories. The requirements of a depilatory are that is should be (*1*) nonirritaring and innocuous, (*2*) efficient in action, removing hair within a 10 min period, and (*3*) be without odor or have the pleasant odor of the perfume.

The activity of the depilatory substance depends upon (*1*) the nature of the depilating or denaturing agent, (*2*) the duration of the action, (*3*) the pH of the cosmetic medium, and (*4*) the temperature of the reaction.

The depilatory most widely used today is based on calcium thioglycolate in a strongly alkaline medium, pH ca 12.3. It also contains a small amount of a wetting agent, a filler, enough slaked lime to attain the required pH, and alkali stable perfume. The commercial products are sold either as thin or very thick pastes, packaged in a jar or collapsible tube.

A typical formula for a depilatory is: 69.0 wt % base cream [60.10 wt % distilled water (solvent); 32.00 wt % calcium carbonate (filler); 6.15 wt % cetyl alcohol (bodying agent for cream); and 1.75 wt % product G--2135 (wetting agent and emulsifier)]; 15.0 wt % distilled water; 6.8 wt % calcium hydroxide (pH control); 5.4 wt % calcium thio-glycolate (depilating agent); 3.4 wt % strontium hydroxide (pH control); and 0.4 wt % perfumePerfumes used for depilatories have to be specially formulated to overcome the intense product sulfide odor and be stable in the high pH medium of 12.3.

In manufacture the following precautions must be observed: (*1*) avoidance of metal contamination from iron or copper or other heavy metals, pure stainless steel is satisfactory; (*2*) avoidance of unnecessary exposure to air as oxidation reduces product strength; (*3*) pH control at ca 12.3, which should be checked before packaging; (*4*) choice of proper packaging, pure tin is best, wax-lined lead tubes, glass, and polyethylene packaging are satisfactory.

Waxing

A very old method for removal of hair makes use of a material known as epilating wax. This wax is a mixture of rosin and beeswax, which is melted, applied to the area to be treated, and allowed to solidify, after which the wax mixture is peeled from the skin. During this peeling action, the hair is actually pulled out and removed from the skin along with the wax mixture.

BATH PRODUCTS

When bathing, dirt, perspiration, and microorganisms are initially removed from the surface of the skin by the water and soap. The water also causes the outermost layers of the epidermis to swell slightly so that they are shed more rapidly. If the bath contains suitable additives, it also can show effects that extend beyond the hygienic aim and contribute cosmetically.

Bath Oils

The subjective response to the use of any bath oil is generally favorable. This is to be expected since bathing itself imparts a feeling of softness to the stratum corneum, and even the slightest deposition of an emollient adds to this effect The addition of fragrances and fragant oils to baths was recorded as early as the Roman era.

Bath oils fall into one of two major categoreis: (*1*) spreading or floating bath oils and (*2*) dispersible bath oils. Spreading bath oil is usually an anhydrous system that is oleaginous. The hydrophobic system floats on the surface of the bath water. The spreading action is facilitated by inclusion of small amounts (usually ca 5%) of an oil soluble surfactant. The lowering of the surface tension of bath water by the surfactant permits the oil to form a continuous film, rather than existing as individual droplets. Ideal surfactatns should demonstrate a reasonably high hydrophilic-lipophilic balance (HLB) (ca 9) yet remain soluble in the oleaginous composition.

From a functional standpoint the floating layer of perfumed oil affords a pleasant fragrance and a desirable feel to the skin. The oleaginous film adheres to the body surface and imparts a hydrophobic barrier to the keratin.

The oleaginous composition may consist of one or more of the commonly accepted hydrophobic components; natural vegetable oils, animal-derived lipids, such as lanolin and mink oil, low melting fatty alcohols, such as oleyl and hexadecyl, low melting synthetic glycerides, such as glyceryl mono-oleate and glyceryl monolaurate, and mineral oils.

Dispersible bath oils contain a sufficient concentration of surface active agents to sulobilize the oleaginous components through micellar solubilization, or to disperse them as the internal phase of an oil-in-water emuslion. The addition of either system to the bath water disperses oil throughout the bath water. Unlike the spreading bath oil, which maintains its oleaginous character in water, the dispersible bath oil loses some of its oleaginous character as the result of oil-in-water dispersibility. Dispersible bath oils leave a layer of dilute oil in a water dispersion on the skin. As the water evaporates from this, a hydrophobic residue remains, providing a moisture barrier on the skin surface.

The nature (HLB) and concentration of the surfactant component also dictates whether the dispersible bath oil turns milky on addition to water (blooming bath oil), whether it remains clear on dispersing in water, or whether the bath oil generates any foam (foaming bath oil). Surfactants with lower HLBs, such as polyoxyethylene oleyl ether (HLB 4.9), are oil soluble and yield oils that produce the characteristic blooming. Perfume is generally employed in a concentration of 3-20%, obviously depending on the nature and quantity of surfactant.

The dispersible bath oils are usually preferred by the consumer over the floating type because they are water dispersible (washable) whereas the latter may leave an oil slick in the tub and may create drain clogging problems.

Foaming Bath Oils and Foam Baths

These are based on suitable surfactants, either liquid or powder, which are blended with color, perfume, and foam stabilizers. Addition of warm or hot running water produces a fragrant foam.

Bath Salts

Two types of bath salts are available. The first is formulated with crystalline salts such as rock salt and epsom salt to which color and perfume are added. These are not water softeners. The second type is the water softening type based on sesquicarbonates, phosphates, and borates. Color and perfume are added and in some products, small percentages of fatty acid ester are included for nondrying effects.

Bubble baths contain sulfated fatty alcohols or their derivatives, sometimes mixed with saponin, water-softening agents, and sodium alginate, which helps to preserve the foam. These products may be made in powdered (granulated) or liquid form. To be most effective in producing bubbles, The material should be added directly to a vigorous steam of water as it flows from the faueet. They serve to disperse perfume, remove curd from hard water, and insure thorough cleansing of the skin. Some of them, however, are sometimes incompatible with soap, and the wetting agents employed may be drying to the skin.

Bath powders, usually designated as *talcum, after-bath, body, or dusting powders,* may consist entirely of talc, but they usually contain also some variable percentage of precipitated chalk, colloidal clay, and magnesium or zinc stearate. The first two additives serve as absorbents for any moisture that may remain on the skin after drying with a towel; the third makes the powder adhere better. Titanium dioxide or zinc oxide may be added to lighten the color of the mixture.

With the exception of the powders used by men after shaving, most powders of this class are not tinted. The perfume should be prefixed, to insure that the earthy odor of talc is well covered.

Baby powders are usually only lightly perfumed, and they may contain a small proportion of boric acid. The so-called antiseptic baby powders usually contain hydroxyquinoline ("oxyquinoline") sulfate.

Manufature of Bath Products. Bath salts serve just as well without either color or perfume, though for esthetic appeal they are usually both tinted and scented. The appropriate color is dissolved in a saturated solution of the compound used (for example, sodium sesquicarbonate). If alcohol soluble dyes are used, a small amount of a gum or resin should be added as a fixative. The solution of dye is then sprayed over the mass of salt, which is under constant agitation in order to distribute the tint evenly and prevent the crystals from clumping.

The perfume for bath salts must be stable to alkalies; it is first combined with a resinous fixative and sprayed over the salts.

For efferverscent bath salts, all the ingredients except the acids must be dried separately and then carefully mixed until thoroughly blended. Bath salts may be prepared in several delicate tints, using the appropriate certified colors, and in many different scents, of which pine seems to be preferred.

Two products, formerly used for the bath but now practically superseded by bath salts, are *violet ammonia,* a strongly perfumed, 30% solution of ammonia, with or without green soap, which effectively softens bath water; and *toilet vinegar,* a solution of various aromatic oils with acetic acid or ethyl acetate and 75-90% of alcohol, which served only to perfume the bath.

Bath oils, for perfuming the bath, are usually mixtures of sulfonated castor or olive oil, or other liquid dispersing agents, and some form of natural or synthetic perfume oil. They disperse quickly throughout the water and are compatible with soap, but they are extremely drying to the skin. The principal advantage offered by these products is that they combine with any hard-water elements and prevent the formation of a ring of curd around the tub. Other subtances suggested for bath oils that do not disperse in water contain solvents such as diethyleneglycol monoethyl ether as perfume vehicle. Creamy bath oils, sometimes called *bath milks*, are liquid emulsions of stearic acid or stearates, with glycerol or glycols, and mineral oil, usually emulsified with organic amines.

SOAPS

Although soaps as a class are not included among the products that come within the purview of the Federal Food, Drug and Cosmetic Act, toilet soaps, in so far as they cleanse, alter the appearance, or promote the attractiveness of the person, may be considered as cosmetics.

It is generally conceded that the best soaps for the skin are those made substantially from olive oil. For various economic reasons, and an unwarranted belief in the merits of copious lathering, coconut oil has been used in increasing amount. Coconut oil soap furnishes abundant lather, but it is admitted to be harsh and irritating to the skin; according, it is commonly used as an addition to soaps made of tallow and palm oil. Good bases for toilet soaps are available in flakes or chips, either as mechanical mixtures of different soaps or combinations made from mixtures of olive, coconut, and other vegetable oils with tallow.

All that should be claimed for a toilet soap is that it cleanse efficiently. In the choice of soap as a cosmetic cleanser, it must be remembered that purity of the ingredients is not so important as the nature of the ingredients. Soap-and-water cleansing is specifically recommended for the oily skin, but not just any soap should be used. A favorite product may actually be 100% a chemically pure soap in itself, but if it is made entirely or largely from coconut oil it may be quite unsatisfactory or unsuitable for cosmetic purposes.

Equal in importance to the oils, fats, and fatty acids used in the making of soap are the alkalies, and the water that assists in cleansing. Sodium and potassium hydroxides and carbonates hae been commonly employed, and more recently several of the organic amino compounds, for example, triethanolamine, have come into use. The prevalence of hard water presents a complication in the satisfactory use of soap because it causes the precipitation of an insoluble soap as an interfering and unsightly curd or secum on whatever is being washed. It is recognized that this can be circumvented by using sufficient soap to insure complete precipitation and then continuing with more. This practice is easier on the skin than the use of soaps that include harsh water softeners, but it is not always practical.

Special Soaps. Practically all good toilet soaps are milled (often designated "French milled", see section on "Manufacture"). They are delicately scented, if not similarly to other products in a manufacturer's line, at least with an odor that does not interfere with that of other cosmetics. Cakes are available in all sizes from 1-1b. pieces for the bath to dainty "guest size" tablets, and still smaller pellets or wafers used for individual manicures.

(1) "*Castile soap*", a term used for centuries (and still commonly believed) to designate a soap made exclusively from olive oil, has been applied to "any nice white soap" since a ruling of the Federal Trade Commission in 1926. Many soaps so designated now consist wholly or largely of coconut oil, with or without other fats and oils.

(2) *Floating soaps*, popular for the bath, result from beating air into the product during manufacturing.

(3) *Green soap* (officially soap mollis, or soft soap), formerly made of linseed oil, now of olive oil, and potash, is the basis of the following tincture.

(4) *Tincture of green soap* (35% alcohol) is often recommended in cosmetology for the treatment of excessively oily skin (and hair), and as an aid in the removal of comedones (balckheads). It is too drying for continued use on normal or dry skin.

(5) *Hard-water soaps* for toilet and bath are usually made of coconut oil, and contain some percentage of sodium carbonate, trisodium phosphate, or other compound that precipitates the calcuim and magnesium salts before they can interfere with the soap. They may be used for the bath, but preferably not on the face.

(6) *Transparent glycerin soaps*, which vary in popularity, are made from tallow, castor oil, and coconut oil, with about 10% of glycerol, 10% of sugar, and usually some alcohol. They seem to have a strong esthetic appeal, but are often found to be drying to the average skin.

(7) *Superfatted soaps*, designed to counteract the drying effect of alkali or other ingredients in plain soap, are supposed to leave an emollient film on the skin after washing. Many of these are practically useless with hard water. If the superfatting principle is wholly or largely lanolin (similar to sebum in the skin), the lathering of the soap is not inhibited to the same extent as it is with the so-called cold-cream soaps, which contain an excess of mineral oil. Moreover, the addition of lanolin seems to benefit the skin, whereas the mineral oil merely leaves it greasy without correcting the drying action of the plain soap.

(8) *Medicated soaps* may contain sulfur, phenol, iodine, or other antiseptic compounds, which may have some effect on certain conditions in the skin. Often the actual effect is more psychological than physical, although some modern antiseptic soaps display a demonstrable capacity of reducing the bacterial flora of the skin.

Although they are used more in shampoos (*q.v.*), so-called "soapless" compounds (synthetic surface-active agents with various properties) have been added also to some toilet soaps. Some of these substances do improve the action of soaps in hard water but, because many of them are extremely drying to the skin, the indiscriminate addition of these compounds to formerly acceptable recipes for toilet soap is not to be recommended without further research.

Specifications for all kinds of toilet soaps have been published by the National Bureau of Standards, the American Society for Testing Materials (1), and other organizations dedicated to protecting both the public and the industry.

Manufacture

Soap manufacture is generally by one of three methods. In the boilded process, the fats, oils, and alkalies are all boiled together until saponification is complete. The soap is salted out with or without varying percentages of glycerol left in the soap. This is the most widely used process. In the semiboiled process, exact chemical amounts of the fats, oils, and alkalis are mixed and heated to start the saponification, after which the reaction is allowed to complete itself. In the cold process, the fats,oils, and a calculated quantity (less than needed for complete saponification) of alkali are placed in a crutcher and gently heated and mixed. When saponification is underway the material is poured into soap frames where the reaction completes itself spontaneously. The glycerol which is the by-product is left in the soap.

Transparent soaps are prepared with sugar, alcohol and glycerol or a combination of these materials in the approximate proportions: sugar, 10-15 wt % of the soap; alcohol, 50% of the fatty acid present in the soap; glycerol, 50% of the fatty acid present in the soap.

Detergency or cleaning ability is usually determined by soiling cloth with a standard smudge or soiling mixture made according to the following formula: lamp or carbon black, 2.0 g; heavy mineral oil, 5.0 g; tallow, 3.0 g; carbon tetrachloride, 2000.0 ml.

It is well known that soaps and detergents remove the natural oil secretions (sebaceous matter) as well as the dirt. This drying effect can be partially overcome by superfatting the soap or detergent bar. The presence of superfatting agents reduces the cleansing efficiency thereby preventing complete degreasing of the skin surface. From a dermatological aspect, the superfatting of soaps should be advantageous. Apart from the dermatological aspect, the addition of superfatting agents to soap also makes the process of milling and plodding easier because the soap is rendered more plastic. it contributes to the quality of the final product by reducing the tendency of the soap cake to split or crack in use. Superfatted soaps have a superior velvety feel and produce an especially smooth lather.

Superfatting agents are: lecithin (qv) (softens and mositurizes skin); amine oxides and fatty acid amides (improve soap texture and lathering properties); lanolin (improves texture of soap); casein (improves lather and skin feel); and cocoa butter (emollient and moisturizer).

Deodorant Soaps

About half the soap market is claimed for deodorant soaps. These are usually quality soap bars containing either Irgasan DP-300 (Triclosan) or 3, 4, 4'-trichlorocarbanilide (Triclocar4ban). A patent was issued in 1972 for a germicidal detergent bar that contains poly (vinylpyrrolidinone)-iodine complex.

Shaving Preparations

Dry hair in the beard is usually quite compact and is resistant to cutting by a razor blade. Preliminary treatment with hot water and soap removes the sebum, a complex mixture of lipids secreted by the sebaceous glands, and absorbed by the beard, that presents a barrier to water and impedes hair softening. The use of a shaving soap or shaving cream provides a wet, lubricatig blanket of water that reduces friction between the razor blade and the skin.

Shave Soap

Shaving soaps or shaving sticks are hard soaps, sodium salts of primarily saturate fatty acids, that are usually applied with a shaving brush.

Lather Shave Cream

Shave creams are formulated as lather shave and brushless shave. Lather shave creams are soft soaps formulated with potassium hydroxide salts of saturated and unsaturated fatty acids, and containing a small percentage of sodium hydroxide to regulate viscosity, body and consistency. Added to the basic product are humerctants such as glycerol and propylene glycol, emollients such as lanolin and lanolin derivatives, boric acid in small percentage to neutralize any excess alkali, and menthol for its cooling effect. The water content of a lather shave is about 35 to 40%, and the pH of the lather is about 10.

A typical formula for shaving cream is: 41.52 wt % water: 30.8 wt % setaric acid; 10.0 wt % glyceol; 7.7 wt % coconut fatty acids; 7.0 wt % potassium hydroxide; 1.0 wt % lonolin; 1.0 wt % boric acid; 0.57 wt % sodium hydroxide; 0.5 wt % sodium silicate; and *qs* perfume.

Brushless Shave Cream

Brushless shave creams are similar to vanishing creams, with an excess of free fatty acid, usually stearic, emulsified into a nonalkaline base of suitable viscosity or consistency. Its softening effect is not so rapid as that obtained with a lather shave.Brushless shave creams have a water content higher than that of lather shaves, and a pH of 6.0-6.5. Additives are similar to those used in lather shave formulations. A typical formulation is: 70.8 wt % water; 17.0 wt % stearic acid; 4.0 wt % glycerol; 4.0 wt % glyceryl monostearate; 2.0 wt % mineral oil; 1.2 wt % triethanolamne; 1.0 wt % lanolin; *qs* preservative; and *qs* perfume. All formulations contain preservatives and usually fragrance to cover the base odor of the soap and additives.

Aerosol Shave Creams

Aerosol shave creams in pressurized containers are convenient to use because the lather is easily obtained in a ready to use form from the can and is easily rinsed off the face. Formulations are either aqueous soap solutions or soap emulsions that are pressurized with a mixture of propane and isobutane. The product is expelled from the container through a valve. The expelled liquid expands to a foam as the propellant is released. Aerosol shave creams contain additives similar to those used in lather shave formulas.

Self-Heating Shave Creams

Self-heating shave creams are formed from an exothermic reaction that occurs when two components, one containing an oxidizing agent and the other a reductant, are expelled together from a dual compartment container.

Gel Shave Creams

Gel Shave creams are emollient aqueous gels that are soap based and contain a volatile solvent such as pentane. Expelled as a soft gel from a pressure container, the shave cream is rubbed on the face, and the solvent is released. The released solvent expands as it volatilizes, and the gel becomes a foam.

ORAL PRODUCTS

Toothpastes

Toothpastes are suspensions of polishing agents and detergents in a suitable binder, generally packaged in a collapsible tube. The Council on Dental Therapeutics of the American Dental Association has established definte criteria for approval of dentifrices. Some of the requirements are based on the degree of hardness, degree of abrasiveness, and particle size of the polishing agent. The use of medicinals or of drugs that should be used only under the supervision of a dentist are not approved by the Council for over-the-counter purchase by the consumer.

The principal ingredients in toothpastes or powders are: polishing agents (calcium carbonate, magensium carbonate, di-or tricalcium phosphate, talc etc); detergents (soap, anionic surface active agents); binders (ecipients) and humectants (glycerol, propylene glycol, sorbitol, mucilages or gums, etc); sweeteners (saccharin, sorbitol); preservatives (benzoic acid, hydroxybenzoates); flavors (essential oils, etc.) and water.

Cellulose derivatives, such as methyl cellulose, are sometimes used to maintain satisfactory consistency and stannous fluoride or sodium monoflurophosphate may be added as anticaries agents.

A prototype formula of toothpase is: 32.200 wt % glycerol; 27.00 wt % calcium phosphate, dibasic 36.675 wt % water; 2.000 wt % sodium N-lauroyl sarcosinate; 1.00 wt % carrageenan TP-4; 0.500-1.000 wt % flavor; 0.400 wt % sodium monofluro-phosphate; 0.125 wt % saccharin sodium USP; 0.100 wt % sodium benzoate USP.

A recently developed dentifrice contains synthetic, amorphous, porous silica xerogel as the polishing and cleansing ingredient. A formula example is: 39.0 wt % water; 34.76 wt % glycerol; 12.0 wt % silica Xerogel V; 6.0 wt % sodium lauryl sulfate (21% in glycerol); 5.0 wt % silica Aerogel 1; 1.5 wt % hydroxyethyl cellulose; 1.1 wt % flavour; 0.41 wt % stannous fluoride; 0.2 wt % saccharin; and 0.03 wt % FD&C Blue no. 1 (1% solution).

Preservatives

Changes and deterioration in cosmetic products can be brought about by changes in acidity or alkalinity, or as a result of hydrolysis, oxidation, heat and light, and bacterial or fungal contamination. The source of bacterial or fungal contamination of cosmetic products can be the raw materials, water from dirty ion exchangers, contaminated equipment, or dirty bottles and cap liners. Even cosmetic products that are properly prepared require addition of preservatives to ensure adequate shelf life. In addition to all other quality assurance tests run by the laboratory, suitable microbiological tests should also be run on the finished product.

Characteristics of the ideal preservative or mixture of preservatives are: (*1*) activity of low concentration; (*2*) physical and chemical compatibility and effectiveness over a wide range of pH; (*3*) effectiveness against a wide range of microorganisms; (*4*) ready solubility and stability to heat and storage, and limited tendency to migrate into the nonaqueous phase; (*5*) lack of odor, color, toxicity, and irritation in the concentrations used.

Preservatives frequently used in cosmetic products are: *p*-hydroxybenzoats (parabens) (most effective in acid pH); dehydroacetic acid (active against fungi); sorbic acid and sorbates (active against fungi, pH-dependent); imidazolidinylurae (Germall (115) (synergistic with other preservatives); 2-bromo-2-nitro-1, 3-propanediol (broopol) (active against gram-negative bacteria, releases formalydehyde): formaldehyde (strong antibacterial); and 1-(3-chloroallyl)-3, 5, 7-triaza-1-azoniaadamantane chloride (Dowicil 200 as cosmetic preservative) (formaldehyde donor).

Cosmetic formulations and packaging may interact with some preservatives. The nonionic emulsifiers commonly used in cosmetic formulations do not significantly interfere with preservative action when used in a concentration below 1%. In higher concentrations the emulsifier can form aggregates that extract preservatives from the oil-water phases, leaving a low concentration of preservative; Lipid-soluble preservatives may migrate into plastic container walls and into plastic cap liners. Some components of a cosmetic formulation can enhance preservative action. The ingredients of many perfume oils, eg, have antimicrobial properties. Synergisms of preservative mixtures are also possible. Mixtures of parabens are more effective than individual parabens, and mixtures of parabens and imidazolidinylurea and significantly more active and widen the range of microorganisms against which the cosmetic product is protected. Whatever preservative system is chosen should undergo microbial challenge testing in the final product.

Antioxidants

An antiodixant is a substance capable of slowing the rate of oxidation of autoxidizable materials (see Antioxidants). It should be soluble in both water and oil; be odorless, nontoxic, nonallergenic, and effective in low concentration; and be stable under conditions of use. Phenolic antioxidants are usually soluble in oil and generally insoluble in water. Propyl gallate has a solubility of about 1.8% in water. The addition of propyl gallate requires a chelating agent to prevent reactions with iron contaminants which will cause color changes. Calcium disodium EDTA is slightly soluble in oil. The most widely used antioxidants are butylated hydroxyanisole (BHA), butylated hydroxytoluene (BHT), PG and nordihydroguaiaretic acid (NDGA). A widely used antioxidant mixture contains 20% BHA, 6% PG, 4% citric acid, and 70% propylene glycol.

Toxicity and Test Methods

Animal Studies

Even though true sensitization does not occur equally in animals and humans, the animal test provides some measure of protection by serving as a screen. Sensitization of animals makes a material suspect, and so great caution is exercised before using the material on humans. On the other hand, a negative sensitizing result on animals indicates that the material is probably not a strong sensitizer and further tests on humans offers little risk. The final tests must, however, be clinical trials on human subjects.

Preliminary animal tests are performed to determine whether the material has an acute or chronic toxicity, and, if so, the MLD_{50}. These tests involve feeding the material to the animals which are subsequently sacrificed for close examination of the organs, glands, and brain.

Percutaneous toxicity is determined by the application of the material to cleanly shaven necks and backs of animals over a regularly scheduled period. The condition of the skin is carefully checked and the animals are observed for any signs of systemic toxicity and their tissues are examined for pathological changes. The final tests must, however, be clinical trials on human subjects.

Human Safety Testing

Irrespective of the completeness of the program carried out with the animals, initial trails on humans must be on a limited number of individuals. Evaluation of sensitizing potential should begin with 10 or 12 panelists. Full-scale tests must then be carried out before the product is released to market. Although 60 panelists are generally adequate as precursors to large-scale studies, forthcoming regulations are expected to require tests on 200.

In human safety trials of topically applied materials the principal concern in most cases is induced cutaneous reactions. If, however, animal studies indicate significant absorption of components of the formulaion, clinical trials must also monitor such absorption by testing blood and urine which may reflect subclinical systemic toxic effects.

The cutaneous reactions that may result from application of cosmetics are of three types: primary irritation, contact, sensitization, and reactions that develop following exposure to the sun. The potential of topically-applied materials to induce these reactions is evaluated by means of patch tests.

Sensitization Potential

One of the most critical evaluations is the determination of sensitizing potential. Two basic procedures have been most frequently employed, and numerous variatios of these have been used. One of the basic procedures has limited value since it detects only very strong sensitizers. Present consideration of the human patch test will primarily be limited to the repeated insult procedure and its various modifications. Two variations were originally developed—one by Shelanski and Shelanski and the other by Draize. Both of these procedures employ repeated applications made over a period of four or five weeks. They differ in that ten sensitizing applications are made in the Draize procedure and fifteen are made in the Shelanski procedure. They differ also in that challenge applications are made only to the original tests sites in the Draize procedure, but are made to previously unpatched sites as well as the original test site in the Shelanski procedure.

A short review of these and other procedures involving human panelists has been presented by Kligman, who suggested the maximization procedure as an alternative. Various methods for achieving the objective of Kligman's maximization procedure have been employed, an interesting one being a Hill Top Research procedure in which the skin is abraded prior to sample application. The test materials are applied to abraded sites on the upper arm under patches. Reactions top the test applications are scored on Wednesday, Friday, and Monday following applications on the preceding Monday, Wednesday, and Friday. The patches are removed by the panelists 24 h after application. Nine applications are made in three successive weeks, and the challenge application is made on Monday of the sixth week. The challenge applications are made to previously unpatched sites. Abrasions of the test sites are made just prior to sample applications on test days, 1, 4, 7, and 11, or preferably, prior to each application. This more frequent scheduling of abrading can be done when up to four materials are evaluated on abraded skin only. The abrasions, in the form of two concentric circles with diameters of 1.25 cm and 1 cm, are inficted by a specially constructed apparatus. The skin areas are cleansed with isopropyl alcohol just prior to abrading. A separate sterile abrader is used for each panelist. All adhesive patches and absorbent pads applied over abraded areas are sterilized by exposure to ethylen oxide prior to use. The usual grading scale is utilized.

Patch test reaction scoring scale

0	no evidence of irritation
1	slight erythema
2	marked erythema

3 erythema and papules
4 edema, erythema may or may not be present
5 erythema, edema, and papules
6 vesicular eruption
7 strong reaction spreading beyond test site min reaction meets minimal requirements for grade assigned

Effect on superficial layers of skin

A slight glazed appearance
B marked glazing
C glazing with peeling and cracking
F glazing with fissures
G film of dried serious exudate covering all or portions of the patch site
H small petechial erosions and/or scabs

Another procedure employed is to strip the skin by repeated application and removal of adhesive tape from the test sites prior to sample applications.

Regardless of the procedure employed in tests on human panelists, mimimal reactions, frequently evoked during the serial applications and at challenge, require expert judgment as to whether the material is a sensitizer or not. It is frequently necessary to conduct rechallenges in order to assess the significance of the observed reactions.

When properly applied, the repeated insult test is a severe test for the sensitizing potential of products. Many products that induce sensitization in a low percentate of panelists tests by this procedure can be used without untoward reactions. The proposed use must be considered. For example, a product that shows minimal sensitization potential and is to be used on the feet should not be marketed. On the other hand, a product that would be used infrequently under nonconclusive conditions could probably be safely marketed.

In addition to its value as predictor of sensitizing potential, the repeated insult patch test furnishes valuable information on the primary irritant characteristics and cumulative primary irritant properties of test materials. The latter property is descriptively referred to frequently as skin fatigue.

Some assurance that products found to be minimal sensitizers can be safely marketed may be obtained by conducting product-use challenges of panelists who have been sensitized in the patch test procedure. If these reactive individuals do not respond to use applications, it is most unlikely that senitization would be induced by normal use of the product. However, this reasoning cannot be applied to products used for whole-body applications. Whole-body exposures by senitized panelists cannot be safely done, and limited area applications may be misleading.

2

Flower Perfumes

Not so long ago it was fashionable in some circles to decry flower perfumes. Why, it was asked, should a women want to smell of flowers? The exclusion of flower perfumes from perfumery has been taking place over a long period. The flower perfume is dead, Authors subsequent observations, however, tended to modify this initial impression, because he went on to praise some forgotten garden scents, gave suggestion for their formulation, and recommended their potential use as background odours in more sophisticated fantasy perfumes.

Despite any extravagant statements to the contrary, flowers and their perfumes are still of very considerable and even basic importance to the perfumer. In the first place they a stimulus, a point reference, and a sources of pleasure and invaluable information. In the second, some of them are still irreplaceable raw materials, despite and any disadvantage that may attach to them in respect of scarcity or cost. And ,in the third place, many flower noted or floral accords form of the essential structure of even the most advanced and up to date fantasy perfumes. The fashionable woman may not wish to smell like a flower, but neither is she improved by smelling like a crude mixture of synthetic chemicals or like a civet cat, a musk deer or a dish of overripe odorants, and in it the floral note still plays a vital and even a dominant part.

We shall be giving in this chapter, for each flower mentioned, a list of constituents used in its reproduction, including, some that may be thought of as tricks- of the -trade, although the main object will always be to approach the true note of each flower. Secondly, we shall give one, two or more complete formulae, by way of illustration. Here it is necessary to point out that such formulae can only be considered as the sum of the actual materials used in preparing them in the first place; and that subsequent reproduction must involve olfactory adjustment in give the desired result.

We shall start with the more familiar perfumes based on flower noted.

Rose

Rose notes vary considerably one from another. In addition to the basic components mentioned below under red rose, Damascene rose and Centifolia Rose, we find some important auxiliary notes in the naturally occurring esters, as well as in a few aldehydes and acetals. Many other odorants also enter, in relatively small amount but with significant effect, into the composition of specialised rose notes, e.g. those of the tea rose.

Red Rose

This is usually considered to be the truest and finest type of rose odour. Its main constituents are rhodinol, phenylethyl alcohol, alpha-ionone and the very useful nerol. A more flowery effect is obtained by the addition of rose absolute and Bulgarian otto. Bulgarian geranium oil can, when obtainable, impart a much - appreciated green note.

Rose Damascena

Among natural essential oils this is represented by Bulgarian rose. The basis of this odour is given by rhodinol phenylethyl alcohol, geraniol expalmarosa oil, and cinnamic alcohol; always in association with certain natural essential oils and esters.

Rose Centifolia

The main constituents here are citronellol, geraniol, phenylethyl alcohol and rhodinol together with smaller amounts of adjuncts which give it a slightly sharp note, such as C_9 aldehyde, citral, etc.

Tea Rose

The basic components are citronellol, phenylethyl alcohol and geraniol. The accessories that impart its special character include guaiyl acetate, menthone and tuberose absolute.

Rose Marechal Niel

In nature this is a yellow rose with a very special perfume. Basically one uses geraniol ex palmarosa oil, citronellol and synthetic geraniol, in association with isoeugenol, benzoin and sandalwood oil etc.

White Rose

Here the base is rhodinol, phenylethyl alcohol, benzyl alcohol and linalool (to give it the slightly acidulated note by which it is identified). The blend is rounded off with a little bergamot, phenylethyl acetate, etc.

In all matters relating to rose perfumes one has to take into consideration the part played by Bulgarian Rose. This notes is often required but unfortunately the widespread use of bulgarian oil of rose in its pure state is limited by considerations of cost. This necessitates research into compositions diluents or extenders, and these must be the best possible for the purpose. By using certain raw materials judiciously one can in fact arrive at some very interesting extenders which will blend well with the natural oil, giving an excellent quality of end product at a reasonable price, The raw materials in question are relatively few in number. One thinks of phenylethyl alcohol, oil of geranium- such as the geranium incolore de grasse, geraniol, rhodinol, 1- citronellol; and very small quantities of nerol and farnesol.

A formula is given below. This is a convenient point to emphasise that no formula can be better than the type and quality of this individual constituents. It is therefore essential for perfumers to make their own trials and adjust their final formulae accordingly. Some readers may be surprised to note the recurrence in certain of these formulae of branded specialities, usually made by some of the leading supply houses. We make no apologies for these inclusion, because they are in fact not obtainable on the market in the pure state, while others are the result of difficult and time- consuming to copy.

Rose Extender 1

Geraniol ex palmarose	1.50
Oil of Grasse Geranium	0.50
Phenylethyl alcohol	2.50
Linalool ex bois de rose, Brazilian	1.20
Rhodinol ex geranium oil	1.20
1- Citronellol,	3.00
Nerol, pure	0.07
Farnesol, pure	0.03
	10.00

Parts by weight . All constituents of the finest available quality. With the aid of this extender, such blends may be made as the following:

Rose No . 1

Rose Bulgarian	75
Rose Extender 1	25

Rose No. 2

Rose Bulgarian	50
Bulgarian absolute	
Oil of rose	4
Rose Extender 1	46

Rose No. 3

rose Bulgarian	25
Bulgarian rose absolute	3
Rose Extender 1	72

In this way one has at hand three different rose formulae, all of a totality approaching that of the Bulgarian Rose but each at a different price level. Formulation over a reasonably wide price range is thus facilitated.

Some formulae of actual rose perfumes follow. The first, called simply F because that happens to be its reference in one's notebooks, is simple and straight forward but has great strength and marked diffusive properties.

Rose F

Rhodinol	40
Ionone alpha	23
Rose No. 2 (as above	6
Phenylethyl alcohol	12
Bois de rose Brazil	12
Rose de Grasse absolute	6.5
Jasmin absolute	0.5
Menthone	trace
	100

Rose H

Rhodionl, 1st quality	10
Phenylethyl alocohol	20
Cinnamic alcohol	6
Geraniol	20
Citronellol	10
Linalool	6
Hydroxycitronellal	5
Linalys acetate	4
Eugenol	4
Rose de Grasse absolute	4
Geranium (African) oil	10
Phenylethyl acetate	1
	100

Rose Rouge

ViletonneA	18

Rose No. 1	4.5
Rose de Grasse absolute	13
Phenylacetic acid	0.4
Lorena (Firmenich)	4.5
Phenylethyl alcohol	9.6
Rhodinol	50
	100

Rose Blanche

Rose No. 1	13.50
Sandalwood oil	6.30
Patchouli oil	6.30
Tuberose NO. 1	5.50
Tubereuse (Synarome)	5
Orris resinoid	5
Jasmonis (Givaudan)	3.50
Benzyl acetate	2
Geraniol synth pure	12
Lorena (Firmenich)	9
Phenylethyl alcohol	11
Iraldeine 100% (de Laire)	9
Rhodiunol P (Rhone-Poulenc)	11.50
Aldehyde C9	0.10
Aldehyde C10	0.15
Aldehyde C.12 (lauric)	0.15
	100.00

Rose M S

Rose H	390
Rhodinol P (Rhone-Poulenc)	110
Geraniol synth., chem. pure	16
Rhodinol (with traces of menthone)	45
Phenylethyl alcohol	150
Geranium Bourbon	5
Hydroxycitrounellal	15
Cinnamic alcohol	7.50
Iraldeine 100% (de Laire)	26.50
Iralia B	3.50
Sandalwood oil	9
Lorena (nerol)	100

Bois de Rhodes (UOP)	1
Diphenyl oxide	5
Aromel (Givaudan)	1
Guaiac wood oil	14.50
Geranyl acetate	2
Phenylethyl acetate	2
Rhodinol acetate	9
Citronellyl formate	14.50
Geranyl formate	5
Rhodinyl formate	4.50
Phenylacetic aldehyde 50%	10
Verbenol	15
Musk ketone	39
	1000.00

Where specialties are cited under the names of specific firms, this simply means that no one firm makes and offers exactly the same end product as the others. In each case one must take into account the fact that chemicals includes in a process as trace impurities are not likely to be present in exactly the same pattern or proportions in a competitive product.

Examples of special shades of odour even among standard chemicals are provided, for examle, by Givaudan's Laurine, which is a hydroxycitronellal with a note of its own-often in great demand-and Lorena of firmenich, which though a nerol, is yet distinguishable from other nerols.

A footnote rose compounding: modern perfumery now also makes use, with restraint, of rose oxide.

JASMIN

Rose and jasmin are still the most important flower notes used in perfumery. Singly or together, they provide a conventional floral background for a great diversity of perfumes. Oil of jasmin has been the subject of much analytical research and, on this basis, it is possible to devise a wide range of formulae for 'jasmin artificial'. Among the basic components one may note benzyl acetate, amyl and hexyl cinnamic aldehydes; benzyl alcohol, formate, salicylate and other ester; indoble and derivatives; phenylethyl alcohol, dimethyl benzyl carbinyl acetate, hydroxycitronellal, linalool, linalyl acetate; esters of propionic acnd butyric acids; Peru balsam etc., To sweeten formulae for artificial jasmins that may be somewhat crude and synthetic, use can be made of jasmin absolute chassis, which is the asbolute obtained by petroleum ether or benzene extraction from jasmin flowers that have previously been treated by the enfleurage process but which have nevertheless retained some of their perfume. This must not be confused with the actual absolute of jasmine d'enfleurage.

It is a principle in fine perfumery that natural materials should be used to sweeten and soften the odours of syntehtic blends. When costing considerations prevent the more liberal use of 'natural', the result of judiciously incorporating even small quantities will usually prove conclusive.

Jasmin No. 1

Benzyl acetate, pure	28
a-Amyl cinnamic aldehyde Prima (Descollonges)	20
Jasmin chassis absolute ex benzene (Schmoller & Bompard), 10% in benzyl benzoate	10
Benzyl propionate	4
Paracresyl isobutyrate	3.2
Dimethyl benzyl carbinyl acetate	1.6
Benzyl alcohol	9.2
Linalyl acetate	2
Mehyl anthranilate	0.4
Isojasmone (Descollonges)	0.05
Bois de rose oil, Brazil	6
Geraniol (synth., chem. pure, (Firmenich)	1.6
Iradeine 100% (de Laire)	2
Allofloral (Allondon-Firmenich)	6.75
Ylang-Yland oil	2.4
Indole, 10%	2.8
	100.00

Jasmin No. 2

Benzyl alcohol	11

Linalyl acetate ex bois de rose	11
Benzyl acetate	129
Benzyl benzoate	6
Ethyl phthalate	3
Jasmin chassis absolute, ex benzens (Schmoller & Bompard)	6
Laurine (Givaudan)	10
Phenylethyl alcohol	8
Linalool	9
Bergamot oil, sesqui terpeneless	4
Peru balsam	5
Yland-ylang oil	3
Benzyl salicylate	5
	100

Jasmin Fantasy No. 3

Phenylethyl alcohol	22
Benzyl acetate	45.5
Cinnamic alcohol	3.5
Methyl anthranilate	2
Diethyl phthalate	5.5
Citronelol	3.5
Geraniol (synth. chem. pure, (Firmenich)	5.8
Ylang-ylang oil	2
Canange oil	1
Isoeugenol	0.5
Benzyl salicylate	2.5
Ethyl salicylate	0.2
Cedrenol (ex cedarwood oil)	3
Virginia cedarwood oil	3
	100.0

Jasmonone No. 4

Benzyl alcohol extra	19
Phenylethyl alcohol	1
Jasmin absolute	2

Benzyl acetate, chem. pure (BBA)	10
Castoreum absolute (Descollonges) 10%	3.5
Narcissus absolute (Charabot)	1
a-Amyl cinnamic aldehyde	20
Jasmin de Provence (Desccollonges)	30
Indole 10%	2
Linalys acetate ex bois de rose	6
Linalool	3.65
Paracresol 10%	0.7
Isojasmone 10%	0.65
Bitter almond oil 10%	0.5
	100

Jasmonone No. 4A

Benzyl acetate	30
Benzyl alcohol	30
Benzyl propionate	5
Methyl anthranilate	2.5
Indole 10%	2.5
Linalyl acetate	5
Linalool	7.5
Buxine (Givaudan)	7.5
Ylang-ylang oil	10
	100.00

This composition has a rather fresh note that facilitates its use in numerous combinations, both with other jasmin components and in perfumes where a sharp and fresh jasmin note contributes to the overall odour.

Jasmin Base No. 5

Cinnamyl acetate	0.8
p. Cresyl isobutyrate	1.1
Methyl anthranilate	0.3
Benzyl alcohol	18
Benzyl acetate	18
Linalool	4.6

Benzyl propionate	3.1
Terpineol, pure	3.1
Amyl cinnamic aldehyde	15.3
Methyl eugenol	1.5
Linalyl acetate	7.5
Raldeine D (Givaudan)	3.8
Hydroxycitronellal	3.11
p. Methyl methylsalicylate	1.5
p. Cresyl phenylacetate	0.7
phenylpropyl aldehyde	2
Aldehyde C. 10	0.15
Indole	0.45
Tolu tincture	15
	100

This base may be improved, as in the following formula (5a).

Jasmin Base No. 5a

Jasmin Base No. 5	70
Jasmin d'Espagne (Givaudan)	13
Jasmin Frutal (Polak's Frutal (Works)	
Jasmin chassis absolute ex benzen (Schmoller & Bompard)	4
	100

Orangeflower and Neroli

Perfumers will be well aware of the differences that exist between these two closely related odours. Both are frequently used, and its could even be said that there are relatively few compositions into which the orangeflower note does not enter. Neroli is particularly valuable in eau de cologne and related notes. Here are some examples.

Orangeflower A

Linalyl acetate	7.1
Petitgrain oil, terpeneless	33.4
Flonol 160 (de Laire)	14.3
Indole 10%	4.7
Eugenol	2.2

Geraniol synthetic	5.6
Geranyl acetate	3.7
Brouts absolute (Robertet)	19
Ylang-ylang oil	1.2
Phenylethyl alcohol	4.7
Lentisque (Mastic) oil	0.8
Methyl anthranilate	2.4
Citral	0.9
	100.0

Neroli A

Petitgrain oil pays (Grasse)	31.5
Methyl anthranilate	25
Eugenol	18.5
Geraniol	6
Phenylethyl alcohol	4.25
Linalyl acetate	7.3
Indole 10%	4.7
Aldehyde C.8 10%	2.75
	100.00

This is a useful type of formula for belending with natural neroli, in certain applications, as a diluent. A suggested proportion is 1 part of natural neroli oil to 2 parts of Neroli A.

In flower perfumes closely associated with the organge blossom note, e.g., hoyneysuckle, syringa (Philadelphus coronarius), gardenia and narcissus, the fruity note of Apricot is often present and should always be borne in mind.

VIOLET

The classic note of violet was adored by ladies at the turn of the century. Two species of the flower should be distinguished. The simple Violet (Nice or Toulouse) may be based on a blend of methyl ionone, alpha ionone, orris absolute or resinoid, violet leaf absolute and phenylethyl alcohol. A floral note, projected as it were by a trace of MNA aldehyde, is imparted by jasmin or cassie. The double or Parma violetis based on varying proportions of beta ionone, alphas ionone and methyl ionone, together with orris resionoid or concrete, a little phenylethyl alcohol, methyl octin carbonate, a trace of vetiver, and a small quantity of hydroxycitronellal and even sometimes, bergamot. Very small amounts of violet leaf absolute may be included, but the green leafy note of Parma violets is much less accentuated. For imparting the necessary sweetness to the base of Parma violet, use may be made of a plum or mirabelle note.

It is difficult to give a violet perfume the 'thrust' required by modern perfumes. An interesting result has been obtained, however, with a very fresh lily-of-the valley composition, used in just sufficient quantity to impart an exuberant freshness but note enough to impair the basic violet note.

Wood violets, with their rather earthy background, may be simulated by the inclusion of very small quantities of a pure grade of amyl acetate, which helps to provide the odour of damp earth and humus. Other humus noted may be similarly employed.

Violet No. 1

Ionone alpha	10
Iralia (Firmenich)	10
Irisone extra (Givaudan)	10
Jasmin No. 2	20
Ysminia (Firmenich)	5
Jasmonis (Givaudan0	2
Violet leaf absoute	2
Orris absolute or Irophore (Firmenich)	1.1
Ylang ylang oil	1
Ylang ylang absolute	0.6
Cassie absolute	0.55
Rose No. 1	0.1
Neroli oil	0.06
Phenylethyl alcohol	1
Bitter orange oil	0.6
Oakmoss absolute (Robertet)	0.16
Folione (Givaudan)	0.03
Linalool	0.5
Bois de rose Brazil	43
Cinnamylal (Givaudan)	4.5
Heliotropin	2
Musk ambrette	0.1
Musk ketone	0.5

Vanillin	0.2
Civet tincture	16.5
Peru balsam tincture	8.5
	100.00

Violet No. 2

Violet No.1	60
Irisone Beta (Givaudan)	6
Iralia (Firmenich)	10
Cetone V (Allyl ionone, (Givaudan)	9
Ylang ylang absolute	4
Irophore (Firmenich)	1.6
Violet leaf absolute	2.6
Cassie absolute	0.8
Mimosa absolute	1.3
Jasmin absolute	1.2
Mirabelle (Firmenich) 1%	3.5
	100.0

The absolute oil of Parma violets, which had a delightful odour, is no longer an item of commerce. The following formula yields a product of fine odour which may be utilised as a 'reconstituted' absolute oil of Parma violets.

Parma Violets Absolute, Art

Violet leaf absolute (Schmoller & Bompard)	1.8
Irophore (Firmenich)	4
Violettone B extra fine 100% (Firmenich)	4
Parmanthene (Firmenich)	0.2
Benzyle benzoate	90
	100.0

The basic formula that follows gives a product of fine quality, which can be used in a multitude of different combinations is order to give effects approaching those of a little violet bouquest. The delicate odour of earth and humus that is so often found in a bunch of violets can be given by Des-colonges' Humuscol or by a mixture of amyl salicylate and pure amyl acetate, etc.

Violet Base

Paracetone (Givaudan)	24
Beta--iso Methyl Ionone	32

Irisone extra incolore (Givaudan)	24
Betá methyl ionone	3
Boronia absolute	1
Ionone alpha	16
Violet leaf absolute	10
Orris absolute (Robertet)	10
	120

The concrete and absolute oils of Boronia, which contain ionone beta in its natural state, are much sought after in violet compositions, where they soften any harshness and add a tendency towards the Parma violet note.

Many other formulae for violet perfumes could be given but we feel that the foregoing should suffice as a general indication to the practising perfumer.

Lilac, Lily-of-the-Valley, Carnation and Tuberrose are also, lie the fore going flower perfumes, widely used to 'floralize' sophisticated perfume blends. It is convenient, however, to arrange them in alphabetical order rather than attempt to do so on the basis of their relative importance.

Acacia

This is not is fact a ture acacia, although the latter species is well represented in perfumery as cassie. The acacia perfume, which finds acceptance chiefly in warmer climates, represents the fragrant and somewhat orangeflower-like dour of the tree, Robinia pseudacacia. The basic odorants entering into its composition are: phenylethyl alcohol cinnamic alcohol, benzyl acetate, hydroxyci tronellal, methyl naphthyl ketone, methyl anthranilite, linallol, terpineol, anisic aldehyde ex anethole and just at touch of apricot.

Broom

Broom, genista or genet is a shrub very popular in the south of France and in Spain; particularly in Catalonia, where the hills of Barcelona and the Tibidabo are covered with retama (the Catalan name for broom) at the approach of summer. Fragrant varieties of broom are also found in the U.K. and elsewhere. From the perfumery point of view, the base is one of orange blossom: methyl anthranialate, fleur d'oranger, etc., associated with methyl paracresol, methyl acetophenone, anisaldehyde and Grasse absolute of gene. Other constituents include alpha ionone, terpineol, linallol, phenylethyl alcohol, heliotropin, systhetic musck and olibaum.

Carnation

From the perfumer's point of view there are three main types of carnation. The carnation of Nice has a rather rosy, honeyed odour. The garden pink has a spicy odour recalling cloves and pepper. The so-called sea pink (not to be confused with Armoria maritima) has the basic odour of carnation plus a note suggesting oilbanum and labdanum: hence the use of such ole oresins as fixatives.

Oeillet de Nice. Here the basis is a blend of eugenol isoeugenol and methyl eugenol, in varying proportions, accompanied by phenylethyl alcohol, benzyl salicylate, and sometimes amyl salicylate, vanilla, vanillin or ethyl vanillin. This base is sweetened with rose notes from rhodinol or rose de Mai absolute, carnation absolute or concrete and, above all, tuberrose absolute. Unfortunately, as the latter has become very expensive, it must usually be replacedas by a blend of synthetic tuberose with the natural material, or by a good ylang-ylang oil or ylang-ylang absolute. As aids to fixation there are benzyl isoeugenol, helitropin and so-caled heliotropin amorphous (a mixture of helitropin, vanillin, anisic and benzoic acids).

Garden Pink, known as Oeillet mignardise, has a slightly more clove-like odour. Hence the use of more eugenol and less isoeugenol in the base, together with a trace of clove oil. The vanilla base will preferably contain methyl vanillin (veratraldehyde). The characteristic note is given by oils of pimento, bay or black pepper.

Sea Pink. This small pink, which has a simple flower whose colour is actually mauve, is found growing wile on dunes by the sea. Its strong odour may be imitated by adding to a garden pink formula amyl salicylate, phenylacetic adlehyde and, if desired, a trace of hyacinth absolute.

Carnation noted have a major role in all kinds of perfumery. Even so, they could probably be exploited yet more fully in the field of masculine perfumes. A straight forward carnation not could be used, in this way, instead of the all too familiar spiced-cologne complexes. Some formulae follow.

Base Claveline No. 1

Eugenol	51.35
Cananga oil	25.7
Ylang-ylang oil	2.55
Rose No. 2	5.6
Benzyl acetate	2.55
Orris absolute	4.25
Ceylon cinnamon oil	0.5
Nutmeg concrete	1.5
Nutmeg oil	1
Benzyl benzoate	3.45
Heliotropin	1.55
	100.00

Base Claveline No. 2

Eugenol	61.5
Ylang-ylang oil	4.16
Canaga oil	4
Rose No. 2	4.6
Cinnamic alcohol	16.7
Banzyl acetate	2.5
Vetiver oil, Java type	1.25
Nutmeg oil	0.65
Labdanum absolute (Lautier)	0.20
Heliotropin	4
	100.00

Oeillet de Nice No. 3

Base Claveline No.	55.9
Isoeugenol	13.9
Rhodinol	1.2
Pimento oil	1.3
Phenylethyl alcohol	0.65
Ionone alpha	0.35
Tuberose absolute synth. (Synarome)	2.5
Carnation absolute (Charabot)	5.9
Vanillin	13.9
Coumarin	3
Musk ketone	1
Musk ambrette	0.4
	100.00

Carnation Flowers No. 4

Base Claveline No. 2	18.3
Oeillet de Nice No. 3	3
Eugenol	6
Isoeugenol	31
Rose No. 3	4.5
Bulgarian rose oil	4.5
Phenylethyl alcohol	9.5
Jasmoide 215 (Synarome)	0.6
Jonquil synth. (Roure-Dupont)	0.6
Terpenelless petitgrain oil	3
Methyl ionone	6
Bois de rose oil, Brazil	3.8
Jasmonis (Givaudan)	0.6
Amyl salicylate	0.4
Hydroxycitronellal	0.5
Phenylpropyl aldehyde	0.4
Benzyl benzoate	1
Ylang-ylang oil	1.5
Peru Balsam Clair (Laujtier)	0.5
Vanillin	3.6
Musk ketone	0.5
Musk ambrette	0.2
	100.0

Oeillet des Dunes No. 5

Eugenol	15
Base calveline No.2	15
Isoeugenol	10.0
Methyl ionone	6.7
Amyl salicylate	5
Jonquil synth (Roure Dupont)	0.65
Tuberose absolute synth. (Synarome)	0.35
Ylang-ylang oil	6.7
Bois de rose oil, Brazil	3.3

Phenylethyl alcohol	13.3
Rose No. 3	3.3
Neroli A	3.3
Wardia (Firmenich)	4
Phenylacetic aldehyde	3.3
Jasmonis (Givaudan)	0.65
Jasmin chassis absolute	0.65
Vanillin	0.6
Musk ketone	1.6
Anisic aldehyde	0.35
Benzyl benzoate	5
Heliotropin	0.35
	100.00

CYCLAMEN

Many species of cyclamen are secnted, notably C. persicum and C. europaeum. The odour of the original small mauve flowers from the mountainous districts of Tamil Nadu is quite mild and may typically be given be cyclamen aldehyde. The basic elements of cyclamen perfumes as a class are hydroxycitronellal, linalool, phenylethyl alcohol, terpineol, cinnamic alcohol, amyl cinnamic aldehyde, styrallyl acetate, rhodinol, phenylacetic aldehyde, ionone, Lilial, Lyral and, finally, the essentail cyclamen aldehyde and some of the classic 'freshness' components.

This perfume theme could, we feel, be subjected to some interesting variations and thus result in novel and interesting compositions. Think, for example of its association with a group containing cyclopentadecanolide, aldehyde MNA, incense and vanilla. This type of association might well provide a very attractive ensemble. The cyclamine odour and its possible derivatives have not yet, in our view, been fully exploited-especially if the cumin note is one of the elements used in its formation.

Fougere (Fern)

The fern or fougere may be one of several thougsand specie, but in any case it will rarely have an odour other than a mild and vague effluvium of humus, greenery and earth. The perfumes known aas fern or foughere are entirely the creations of imaginative perfumers. Most of them have a more or less pronounced note of verdure and moss. The honour of creating the first Fougere went to Paul Parquet circa 1880. Fern perfumes are nowadays divisible into two main groups: (a) one based on the triad bergamot. Tonka bean tincture of coumarin, and a product of musky odour; and (b) the other, in which linaly, terpinyl, geranyl and above all bornyl and isobornyl acetates give a compound of more or less rustic or woodland character.

Fougers No. 1

Tree moss absolute	2
Bergamot oil	10.1
Lavender oil	10.1
Rhodinol	10.1
Roase M.S.	6.1
Patchouli oil	3.1
Geranium absolute incolore (Grasse)	
Methyl ionone	12.15
Cyclopentadecanolide	1
Petitgrain oil, Paraguay	2
Coumarin	14.3
Musk ketone	6.1
Heliotropin	6.1
Phenylethyl salicylate	3.1
Methyl salicylate	1
Eugenol	1
Jasmin No. 1	3.1
Clary sage oil	1.35
Amyl salicylate	2
Musk tincutre	1
Tobacco (I.F.E.)	0.2
	100.00

This is a formula of the category (a) type. See note above the following belongs to category (b).

Fouger No.2

Musk ketone	0.4
patchouli oil	1
Vetiver oil, Java	1
Lavender oil, Mitcham type	6.5

Lavender absolute	1.6
Bergamot oil	35
Linalyl ecetate	2.2
Terpinyl acetate	2
Coumarin	31.4
Cyclopentadecanolide	0.2
Tobacco (I.F.F.)	0.2
Oakmoss absolute, Yugoslav	0.8
Mousse de Chene 1026 (Foure-Dupont)	0.2
Alliantone (Givaudan	1.3
Allofloral (Firmenich) 10%	0.2
Roes No. 3	4.3
Palmarose oil	1.1
Geranium oil	4.7
Neroli A	4.7
Myrtle oil	0.2
Cuir 1073 (Firmenich)	0.8
Bornyl acetate	0.2
	100.0

When it is desired to impart a fruity note other than the classic peach, apricot, prune or mirabelle, one such note that can be extremely successful is strawberry, and this has in fact been incorporated in the above formula.

GARDENIA

In the reproduction of the gardenia odour one uses several of the components of tuberose, but gives more emphasis to the rose-like tonalities. Thus in the first place consideration is given to ylang, jasmin, beyzyl salicylate, phenylethyl alchol, an orange blossom note, etc. Secondly, one turns to dimethyl benzyl carbinol, acetyl isoeugenol, hydroxycitronellal, rose de mai absolute, benzyl acetate, terpineol, etc., And, above all, there is styreallyl acetate, which provides the peculiarly green and fruity note of gardenia, and gamma nonyl lactone.

Apart from its general acceptance as a flower, gardenia has an important role in perfumery. It contributes fragrance to such perfumes as Millot's Crepe de Chine. Absolute oil of a gardenia has been produced and is, when available, a remarkable and attractive product. Among the gardenia compounds introduced by the synthetic chemical houses, one of the best and a contributory, factor in some celebrated perfumes is Givaudan's Gardenia 9058.

Gardenia No. 1

Dimethyl benzyl carbinol	4
Styrallyl (methyl phenyl carbinyl) acetate	9.5
Neroli B	2.5
Isoeugenol	4
Rose de Mai absolute	1
Ylang-ylang oil	7
Benzyl acetate	4
Jasmin absolute	1
Lilol (Givaudan)	6
Ionone alpha	10
Hydroxycitronellal	20
Phenylethyl alcohol	8
Phenylacetic aldehyde 50%	1.5
Citronellol	4.5
Cinnamic alchol ex styrex	7
Coumarin	2.5
Helitiopin	7.5
	100.0

Gardenia No. 2

Musk Ketone	2.5
Musk ambrette	1
Jasmin de Provence B (Descollonges)	1
Jasmin absolute	1
Rose de Mai absolute	3.5
Jonquil absolute	1
Tuberose absolute	3
Opopanax L.G. (Givaudan)	16.9
Muguet No. 2	10.2
Styrallyl acetate	12
Hydroxycitronellal	15
Ylang-ylang oil	5

Cinnamic alcohol ex styrac	2
Phenylethyl alcohol	2
Gardenia 9058 (Givaudan)	23.9
	100.0

At current raw material prices it would obvisouly be essential to replace most of the natural absolutes with the best 'artificials' available within costing limits. In the case of tuberose we suggest the use of one of the compounds given under that name elsewhere in this chapter, or a selected speciality such as Synarome's Tubereuse S, for example.

Gardenia FS

Benzyl acetate	3.00
bergamot oil	3.00
Jasmin absolute, artificial	6.00
Rose de mai, art	2.00
Absolu Rose, Lot 1, Robertet	2.00
Amuguet 33 (de Laire)	3.50
Amyl salicyalte	3.50
Hydroxycironellal	4.50
Ionone alpha	3.,00
Diamthine (Firmenich)	1.50
Ylang-ylang oil	5.00
Methyl ionone	4.50
Styrallyl acetate	3.50
Wardia (Firmentich)	2.00
Aurantiol	1.00
Iris Liquide (de Laire)	1.50
Lianlool	6.00
Vetiver oil	0.75
Patchouli oil	0.25
Civetone	0.15
Castoreum Anhydrol (Givaudan)	0.25
Musk ketone	4.10
Musk ambrette	5.50
Coumarin	6.50
Ethyl vanillin	1.50
Liquidambar II	2.50
Aldehyde C12 (lauric) 10%	2.00

C11 (undecylenic) 10%	2.00
C10	2.00
Diethyl phthalate	17.00
	100.00

HAWTHORN

The base of hawthorn perfumes is anishic aldehyde, in association with anisic alcohol and methyl acetophenone. For middle notes one uses hydroxycitronellal, cinamic alcohol, citronellol, linalool and terpineol. The lower notes are provided by heliotropin and coumarin.

The noted English horticulturist, Graham Thomas, listed 'Crataegus, all species' (including of course the common may or hawthorn, C. oxyacantha) among thirty or so flower scents that he considered 'unsuitable for sensitive noses'. The perfumer may here and in similar cases improve on nature by ignoring the methylamine or other off-notes present in the actual flowers and create, as it were, an idealised version of the natural floral odour.

Heliotrope

The heady, delightful and characteristic perfume of ths helitrope (Heliotropium Peruvianum and other spp.) is duplicated chiefly with heliotropin and helitropin amorphous; the latter being a mixture of helitopin with vanillin etc. With these are associated benzoic and anisic acids, phenylethyl alcohol, ylang-ylang oil, rhodinol, cinnamic alcohol, anisic aldehyde, benzal-dehyde (traces) and benzoin resinod. A synthetic of hazel nut odour, used discreetly will help to give a impression of the real flower. The slight note of greenery is obtainable with an oakmoss or, better still, a mignonette absolute or base. Another useful constitutent is paramethyl hydrocinnamic aldehyde.

Honeysuckle

The honeysuckles, Lonicera fragrantissima, L. brachypoda, L. caprifolium and other species, familiar also in the perfumery literature by their French name, chevrefeuille, are among the most fragrant of flowers. Their general odour, sweet and diffusive but only slightly honeyed, can be simulated with such basic constituents as : muguet, orange blossom, rose and jasmin odorants; cinnamic alcohol, phenylethyl alcohl, terpineol, citronellol, linalool, hydroxycitronoelll, paracresyl phenylacetate and anisic aldehyde. Small quantities of methyl cinnamate, methyl naphythyl ketone, phenylethyl acetate, isoeugenol, and ylang-ylang, enter into consideration. To ensure the correct emphasis on the fruitiness of the natural flower odour, use may be made of an apricot note. A trace of Firmenich's Abricot base 4512, for example, will serve this purpose quite well.

Chevrefeuille No. 1

Petitgrain oil, Paraguay	5
Neroli B	6.55
Brouts absolute (Robertet)	1
Ionone alpha	4.85
Anisic aldehyde	2.5
Linalool	3
Terpineol	10
Geraniol	5.1
Hydroxycitronellal	3.8
Lilac No. 3	5.1
Phenylacetic acid	1
Bergamot oil	5
Benzyl acetate	5.1
jasmonone No. 4	5
Cherefeuille 2035 (Firmenich)	10
Chevrefeuille L.G. (Givaudan)	25
Musk ketone	1.25
Musk ambrette	0.75
	100.00

Hyacinth

The odour of the hyacinth flower is often rather harsh and strident. Variants biased towards the rose or orange blossom are more acceptable. The basic odorants are pheynylacetic aldehyde, hydroxycitronellal, cinnamic and phenylethyl alcohols, terpineol and phenylethyl acetate. And, as products contributing towards the piquant note of hyacinth, which is more or less green: dimethyl benzyl carbinol and its acetate, bromstyrole (traces), methyl octin carbonate, cinnamyl acetate; and, for rounding off the composition, when costing limits permit, hyacinth absolute. There was at one time, incidentally, an absolute of wild hyacinths (bluebells) available, but despite its remarkable odour properties it proved too expensive, owing to the high cost of gathering the flowers even before they were treated.

Hyacinth bases have found quite a number of applications in currently popular perfumes, but we feel that there is still further scope for their use, particularly in perfumes with a green note.

Hyacinth No. 1

Lilac No. 3	10
Jacinthone (Givaudan)	20
Cinnamic alcohol	20
Neroli A	5
Jasmonone No. 4a	10
Jasmin chassis ex benzene	4
Hyacinth absolute	5
Phenylacetic aldehyde 50%	6
Hydratropic adehyde	3
Dimethyl benzyl carbinol	2
Hydroxycitronellal	10
Rose de Mai absolute	5
	100

If it is found that the peculiarly piquant note of the natural flower, which we have often compared with the odour of horsaeadish, is not sufficiently emphasised, an added trace of bromstyrole will impart the desired effect.

IRIS

The scent of the iris flower is quite different from that of the dried iris (orris) root, and it varies according to species. Sometimes one observes a note of orange blossomm associated with the odour of orris root; sometimes almost the odour of hyacinth. The bases that are usually employed in attempts to duplicate this rather elusive floral scent are the various ionones and methyl ionones, terpineol, orris absolute and resinoid, anisic aldehyde, myristic acid, etc.

Iris flower bases have not been used very much in recent years, but in view of the diversity in the odour of the different species, it might be worth investigating them and producing compositions that would not longer completely resemble iris but would add to the number and novelty of the 'solid' blending notes available.

LILAC

There is a good deal of variation in odour among the different species and forms of lilac. Persian lilac, for example (Syringa Persica), resembles hyacinth, while purple liac comes closre to heliotrope and vanilla; while yet another species realls hawthorn. The basic components of a lilac perfume are heliootropin cinnamic alcohol, terpineol, phenylethyl alcohol and hydroxycitronellal. Special notes are given by paracresly acetate, phenylacetic aldehyde, anisic aldehyde and cinnamyl acetate. To emphasise the floral quality use is made of rose absolute rhodinol, jasmin, etc. And, to impart 'thrust', benzyl acetate. The green stalk note is always to be observed in a spray of freshly cut lilac; and this may be contributed to the composition by Vert de Lilas notes; phenylacetic aldehyde dimethyl acetal, etc. The special note of Persian lilac is conveyed by means of a natural or synthetic hyacinth.

Lilac was an essential element in some of the classic semi-floral, floral bouquet and sophisticated perfumes of the past. It is still very important. Lilac relly came into its own after the discovery of hydroxycitronellal, and was a basic constituent of such notable perfumes of the Belle Epoque as Floramye and Quelques Fleurs. First of all, a simple lilac:

Lilac Base 1

Hydroxycitronellal	18
Cinnamic alcohol	1.7
Terpineol	7.4
Benzyl alcohol	17
Linalool	1
Phenylethyl alcohol	18
Styrax resinoid	2.55
Jasmin No. 6	9.1
Phenylacetaldehyde	0.1
Anisic aldehyde	7
Indole 10%	2.55
Heliotropin	15.2
	100.00

Lilac No. 2

Lilol (Givaudan terpinedl)	10
Phenylethy alcohol	18
Hydroxcitronellal	33.5
Cinnamic alcohol (ex Stryax)	9
Menthol	0.7

Phenylacetic aldehyede 50%	0.1
Anisic aldehyde extra	0.5
Peru balsam	1
Jasmin No. 2	8
Helio tropin	11
Ethyl phthalate	8.2
	100.0

Lilac No. 3

Terpineol	20.6
Phenylethyl alcohol	26.4
Cinnamic alcohol	7.4
Cyclosia Base (hydroxycitronellalFirmenich0	7.2
Linalool	3.7
Isoeugenol	0.9
Benzyl acetate	5.55
Jasmin absolute	5.6
Rhodinol	0.9
Anisic aldehyde extra	1.3
Phenylacetic aldehyde 50%	0.25
Bitter almond oil 10%	0.1
Phenylacetaldehyde dimethyl acetal 10%	1
P. Cresyl acetate 10%	0.45
Methyl anthranilate 10%	0.2
alpha-Amyl cinnamic aldehyde	0.25
Jasmonone No. 4	0.9
Bulgarian rose oil	1.25
p. cresol 10%	0.45
Ethyl phthalate	3
Ethyl benzoate	5.65
Hyacinth absolute (Polak's Frutal Works)	1.3
Indole 10%	0.1
Helitropin	5.55
	100.00

Lily-of-the-valley

One may readily distinguish between the odours of Muguet des bois and green house-grown lily-of-the valley. A somewhat rough-and-ready way of compoundig a lily-of-the-valley consists of mizing a lilac with a fresh rose compound. By gradually and systematically altering the proportions of both of these consitutens, it is easy to arrive a note similar to that of lily-of-the-valley. Two features of the delicious muguet des bois, the variety found in the woods, are difficult to reproduce; namely the sharp and very fresh lemony top note and the slightly green note at the end. The basic muguet constituents are:

Hydroxycitronellal, rhodinol, citronellol, terpineol, linalool, indole. These must now be added the relatively recent paratertiary Butyl alphamethyl hydro cinnamic aldehyde (e.g. Givaudan's Lilial) and 4 (4 Hydro xy4-methyl pentyl)--3-cyclohexence-10-carboxaldehyde (Lyral of I.F.F.). Both have become important additions to the perfumer's shelves. Lilial is particularly notable for its extreme persistance and unusual diffusive properties. Also deserving of mention is citronellyl oxyacetaldehyde.

The sharp lemony note de depart can be obtained with fatty aldehydes, certain lactones, lemony esters, etc. Violet leaf absolute, some of the 'greener' oakmosses, phenylacetaldehyde and its acetals, and other odourants to give the necessary verdant background effect. Tarragon (estragon) has been suggested as part of such a green note. Some of the carbinols and their esters are also of interest. To impart the impression of freshness that is one of the Finest characteristics of lily-of-the-valley, use can be made of traces of Ceylon citronella oil-strange as this may seem. Or, better still perhaps, small amounts of the product known as 'citronellyl lactone'.

Muguet No. 1

Citronellol	33.7
Rhodinol P (Rhone-Poulenc)	11.3
Phenylethyl alcohol	24.7
Laurine (hydroxycitronellal, (Givaudan)	14.6
Benzyl benzoate	6.7
Ethyl phthalate	4.5
alpha--Amyl cinnamic aldehyde	2.25
Indole 10%	2.25
	100.00

Cuminic aldehyde gives a characteristic touch typical of the muguet note. Hence its inclusion in the next formula. This hint of cuminal has contributed to the success of a muguet compound made famous by a certain firm of synthetic manufacturers. For a different effect it may be replaced by a good grade of cyclamen aldehyde. Lilial, Lyral, etc. may also be introduced on an experimental basis.

Muguet No. 2

Hydroxycitronellal	34.5
Rhodinol	20.7
Phenylethyl alcohol	13.8
Alcohol C11 (enic)	2
Jasmin d'Espange (Givadudan)	6.9
Linalys acetate	3.5
Heliotropin	6.9
Terpineol	3.5
Cuminic aldehyde	1.35
Jasmonone No. 4a	6.85
	100.00

Linden (Lime Blossom)

The lime (linden, tilleul) blossom has a captivating and powerful odour. A synthetic sometimes sold under the name of lime is nothing more than hydroxycitronellal with something of a 'bouquet'. It is. however, quite possible to reproduce the odour of lime blossom, on a basis of hydroxycitronellal linalool, linalyl acetate, ethyl linallol and its acetate, phenylpropyl alcohol, terpineol and farnesol. Small quantities may then be added of ethyl anisate, anisic aldehyde, cyclamen aldehyda, p.-methyl acetophenone, phenylethyl phenylacetate, geraniol, orange blossom, etc.-and a tilleual absolute is produced by some Grasse firms. Persistence is accetentuated with heliotropin, Peru balsam etc. C. 12 (lauryl) aldehyde gives good results in the top note.

Tillual No. 1

Hydroxycitronellal	15
Linalool ex bois de rose	8
Farnesol	6
Bergamot oil	6
Tilleul absolute (Grasse)	18

Nerol	8
Geranium absolute incolore (Charabot)	3
Rose de mai absolute	4.2
Lavender absolute	4.5
Tonka bean hyperessence (Charabot)	1.5
Petitgrain oil, French	8.5
Orangeflower A	2.5
Jasmin absolute	6.15
Jasmin No. 1	6
Peru balsam resinoid	1.5
Phenylethyl phrnylacetate	1
Aldehyde C12 (lauric)	0.15
	100.00

The expensive character of this 'Golden Age' formula will in practice, of course, call for careful and adequate substituation. The apsiring perfumer can learn much from such problems of adaptation.

Magnolia

The magnolia is much appreciated in the United Stated, where the tree is widely scattered and is often used to provided shady promenades. The thick foliage is intensely perfumed with enormous white, fleshy flowers, splashed with a few mauve or pink patches. What is most striking about the perfume of this flower is the contrast between the heavy, warm base note and the very lemony and fresh top note. The base note may be simulated with ylang and cinnamic alcoho, together with Vanilla, vanillin or ethyl vanillin, with a dash of labdanum or incense. The body consists of hydroxycitronellal, nero and various rosy notes. Finally, the top note is given by lemon, citral and alphaamyl cinnamic aldehyde.

Magnolia provides a good starting point for the development of new and original compositions. Among the magnolia bases ae specialities offered by the leading perfumery supply houses. One notes Magnolys, which gives the very special sharp lemony note of the flower, and Magnolia 2471/D. Both are by Firmenich.

Mignonette (Reseda)

The characteristic note of mignonette may be obtained with, methyl octin or heptin carbonate, methy nony ketone, methy nonyl acetaldehyde, dimethyl hdroquinone, phenylpropyl acetate andstyrallyl acetate. The components of the body and base are geraniol, alpha ionone, hydroxycitronellal, rhodinol, cyclamen aldehyde, heliotropin, coumarin and guaiyl acetate. Also of interest are diphenylethy acetal, phenylethy isothiocyanate, sweet basil oil and boronis absolute.

The followng formula incorporates some alternative suggestions.

Reseda No. 1	
Reseda 215 (Firmenich)	10
Reseda absolue hyperessence (Charabot)	27.1
Cyclamen aldehyde	10.9
Muguet No. 2	27.4
Orangeflower A	0.5
Jonquil absolute (Robertet)	1
Rose No. 2	1
Ylang-ylang oil	3.15
Supercitron 50% (Lautier)	0.8
Superportugal (Lautier)	1
Jasmin No. 2	10.9
Jasmin absolute	2.1
Methyl ionone delta	1.5
Violet leaf absolute (Schmoller & Bompard)	0.15
Coriander oil	1
Musk ketone	1.5
	100.0

The mignonette note, once fashionable, could become to again. It blends well with rose the already popular 'green' notes, and deserves to be considered or the elaboration of new-style perfumes.

Mimosa

The base of mimosa is paramethyl acetophenone, isobutyl salicylate phenyl-acetadehyde and anisly alcohol. These form the characteristic note, together with absolute oil of mimosa. There are three types of absolute oil: absolute from the flowers absolute from the flowers and leaves, and absolute from the leaves. The body of the note is obtained with hydroxycitronellal and cinnamic alcohol, and the base consists of coumarin. Lemon, alpha amylcinnamic aldehyde and C.8 or C.10 fatty aldehydes contribute to the top note.

Narcissus

The white flower of the valley narcissus, grown in the Cevennes, extracted and supplied under the name of Narcisse des Montagnes. For simulating the general odour of Narcisse des the narcissus-taking into account the quite wide differences found among the many varieties-one use the following: benzyl acetate, cinnamic alcohol, hydroxycitronellal, terpineol, methyl anthranilate, ionone, eugenol, aurantiol, ylang-ylang and turberose characteristic paracresylic shading of the narcissus note is then provided by paracresyl acetate and phenylacetate, metacresyl acetate and phenylacetate, octylacetae and pheynlacetic acetic aldehyde.

Base Narceine No. 1

Benzyl acetate	12
Phenylethyl alcohol	20
P. Cresyl phenylacetate	7.5
P. Cresyl acetate	3
P. Cresol	0.5
Neroli B	6
Phenylacetic aldehyde	2.5
Hydroxycitronellal	20
Ylang-ylang oil	19
Narcisse des Mantagnes absolute	2.5
Musk ketone	5
Musk ambrette	2
	100.00

Narcissus No. 2

Isoeuenol	6
Eugenol	6.1
Bois de rose oil, Brazil	2.4
Anisic aldehyde	1.2

Base Narceine No. 1	6
Phenylethyl alcohol	14.5
Terpineol	7.3
Hydroxycitronellal	14.5
Cinnamic alcohol	3.6
Methyl ionone	3.9
Bergamot oil	7.3
Neroli A	7.3
Benzyl acetate	7.3
Jasmin No. 1	7.3
Mastic (lentisque) oil:	
Robertet	0.5
Musk ketone	1.2
Indole 10%	2.4
Heliotropin	1.2
	100.0

The narcissus note has been stylised in some well-known and successful perfumes, and lends itself admirable to this type of work.One thinks of the Narcisse Noir of Caron, the Narcisse Blue of Mury, Que Sais-je of patou, etc.

Nadro

Nadro is a Spanish flower quite similar to the Tuberose (q.v.). It is found in abundance is the flower market of the Rambla de las flomes in Barcelona. It perfume is heavier than that of the tuberrose from the south of France, and above all its background note is much more fruity than that of the tuberose and the French gardenia. Nadro perfume is very fashionable in all the Spanish-speaking countries. Its bases are the same as those found in the tuberrose and the gardenia, with a few lighter constituents than in the first two: benzyl acetate, cinnamic alcohol, linalool, hydroxycitronellal, terpineol, cyclamen aldehyde and, above all, there is more accent on the peach note.

New-Mown Hay

The natural odour of new mown hay, though delightful and exhilarating, is not really a flower perfume, although the small blossoms of such flowers as woodruff and alyssum may contribue to it. In some respects it has points in common with fern of fougere andwith clover of tefle (q.v.), but essentially its odour is that of coumarin and tonka beans. There are several interesting foin coupe a absolutes and on coupe distilled oil available; and, also of Grass origin, flouve absolute, extracted from the flowering tops of a special grass, known as flouvre odorante. Other contituents of new-mown-hay perfumes may include lavender, lavandin, clary sage and rosemary oils; acetamisole, dimethyl acetophenone, ethyl anisate, anisic aldehyde and alcohol, dimethl hydroquinone, halitropin, linallol; and small amounts of sandalwood, patchouli, oilbanum.

Nicotiana

Nicotiana tabacum, known as nicotiana or tobacco flower, is another of those plants whose perfume is most pronounced in the evening. Its odour may be simulated by introducing variations on the jasmin theme, i.e. by adding to a typical jasmin flowers base such lily components as Lilial or Lyral, cyclamen aldehyde, etc., together with small quantitites of p.cresl methyl eitehr or p.cresyl acetate.

Opopanax

This is not a flower perfume but is included here because of its general applicability, like many flower perfumes, in forming part of the background structure of a complex composition. Opopanax resins andresinoids come in a variety of types and are of diversified and sometimes unknown origins. Arctander, in his book 'Perfume and Flavor Materials of Natural Origin', has tried to clarify the situation and confirms that, over the years, opopanax seems to have undergone a subtle change in identity. Many opopanaxes sold under the name are nothing but mixtures, even though some are exceedingly well contrived.

The following formula for an Opopanax Art. (i.e. 'artifical') is for a blend that has give consistently good results in many different applications.

Opopanax Art L

Coumarin	9.3
Vanillin	17.6
Heliotropin	5.7
Musk ambrette	3.4
Musk ketone	2.3
Patchouli oil	1.7
Labdanum brun absolute (Lautier)	4.6
Mandarin oil	2.3

Bergamot oil	2.3
Petitgrain oil, French	1.1
Castoreum tincture	3.4
Olibanol (Robertet)	1.1
Hydroxycitronellal	4.6
Geranium oil African	1.1
Vetiver Bourbon oil	4.6
Sweet orange oil, guinea	4.6
Tolu balsam tinctue	5.7
Diethyl phthalate	17.6
	100.0

Orchid (Orchidee)

Orchid, poppy and clover (trefle) are are examples of perfumes that owe more to the perfumer's imagination than to nature. That is not to say that the orchid, for example, has no odour. Onthe contrary, it has many.The scent of orchids ranges from 'some of the sweetest perfumes and most exquistite fragrance to the driest obnoxious taints. Not a few smell like honey, others of Elder, Helitorope, Wild Grape, Sweet Pea, Vanila, Tuberrose, Honeysuckle, Lily-of-the-Valley, Pineapple, Banana; others are spicy. He goes on the list the odours of over 150 orchids, and it is to be noted that a tuberose of salicyalte note is common to many of them.

The base of orchid in perfumery is a combination of the salicylates, formed by the amyl, isobutyl and benzyl esters the relative proportions varying. Very small amounts of the methyl ester may also be incorporated. Besides these products, there are several other worthy of special mention, i.e. alpha ionone, ylang-ylang bergamot, neryl butyrate, rose components, cyclamen aldehyde, terpineol, paracreyl phenylacetate, aldehydes hydes C.8 to C.12, etc.

The basically salicylate Orchid odour has already lent distincition to such perfumes as Trefle Incarnat and certain mossy and Spanish types, and it will doubtless continue to do so in original compositions of the future.

Pansy

If rosemary is for remembrance, pansy (pensee) is for thought. Its scent, on the other hand, is light and fresh, reminding one more of its other name: heart'-ease. The perfumer chiefly recognises in this lowly member of the violet family, Viola tricolor, a violet odour with a rather special green note.

The foundation of a simulated pansy perfume, as was at one time quite fashionable, was essentially similar to that of the violet. It included alpha and beta ionones, methyl ionones, neryl acetate and, optinally, orris absolute. These are associated with phenylethyl alcohol, rose, jasmin: violet leaf absolute, the alkyne carbonate and other green notes: and a sweet persistence is assured by including a bouquet of 'crystallines' harmonising with the gereral tone.

Peony

Peony (Fr. pivoine, Grem. pfingstrose) is not such a well known fragrant flower, perhaps, at is deserves to be. Its varieties have in the main two distinct types of odour. One of the red peonies is not very pleasant-smelling and calls in fact the harsh green scent of the dahlia. On the other hand the white peony, with a few pink patches, and the completely pink peony, have a deliciously fresh odour. When smelling this perfume one has often had the impression of being in the presence of an excellent citronellol. The basic products for simulating the peoony odour are primarily the rose-like odorants: citronellol, rhodinol, phenylethyl acetate, dimethyl benzyl, carbionol, the butyrate and isobutyrate esters of the rose alcohols, and linallil and ethyl linacol. For the base, there are the dervatives of guaiac wood oil, alpha ionone, styrax, ylang-ylang oil, helitropin and vanillin. The green note may be given by styrallyl acetate associated with paracresyl phenylacetate and cinnamyl acetate. The peony is yet another of those flower types which could contribute rather more than they currently do to novel odour combinations.

Phlox

Phlox, a North American herbaceous plant which has become well acclimatised in Europe, includes many odorous species and varieties. Typical is the commonly grown flower with a rather harsh scent reminding one of violets and helitrope. This can be simulated by using a violet base rich in methyl ionone, fixing it with heliotropin and adding a touch of a hazel nut or noisette compound. Although the phlox deserves further investigation as a poiential flower component in perfumery, the fact must not be overlooked that many people find its perfume disagreeable. Thus Eleanor Sinclair Rohde has described Phlox decussate as a hardy perennial 'with a curious scent much disliked by many people'.

Stockes

The odour of night-scented stock, Matthiola biocornis, is as familiar in Europe as that of the closely related wallflower McDonald, referring to the 'balmy odour given off by its brown-coloured flowers' points out that 'it is not necessary to stoop to inhale the perfume, as it pervades the atomosphere for a distance around, towards the close of the day and through the night.' The stock-gilliflowers also include M. annua, M. adoratissima, etc. The odour to some extent resembles wallflower and carnation, but has a mimosa-violet-heliotrope shading.

Sweet Pea

The sweet pea odour is highly regarded in Anglo-Saxona domestic circles but has never been really successful from the perfumery point of view-either in the U.K. or in France. Within the wide range of odour shadings found in the different varieties of sweet pea, the characteristic odour is a slightly honeyed, hyacinthine orange blossom. Basic odorants for its simulations include: phenylethyl phenylacetate, benzyl salicylate, benzyl isoeugenol, methyl acetophenone, and the various orangeflower notes. To these will be added hydroxycitronellal, cinnamic alcohol, terpineol, linalool and, where costings permit, small quantities of rose de mai absolute-as noted below.

Pois de Senteure No. 1

Coumarin	2.85
Neroli A	2
Rose H	4.3
Sandalwood oil, Esst Indian	5.7
Bergamot oil	5.7
Verbena oil, aret	0.85
Lavender oil	1.4
Ionone alpha	1.4
Jasmin d'Espange (Givaudan)	8.6
Sweet orange oil	8.6
Cinnamic alcohol	14.3
Hydroxycitronellal	11.45
Phenylethyl alcohol	11.45

Phenylethyl alcohol	11.45
Rhodinol	4.3
Phenylacetic acid	3.4
Methyl anthranilate	2.3
Heliotropol (Firmenich)	2.85
Jasmin enfleurage absolute (Lautier)	5.7
Phenylethyl phenylacetate	2.85
	100.00

If this type of compound seems a frifle harsh, a small addition of Rose de Grasse absolute willl round off the edges and enhance the desired honeyed note.

Sweet Pea No. 2

Rose H	13.2
Sandalwood oil, Mysore	2.3
Bergamot oil	10.6
Hydroxycitronellal	13.3
Phenylethyl alcohol	13.2
Benzyl acetate	1.3
Wardia (Firmenich)	5.3
Methyl ionone	4.3
Jasmonone No. 4a	16
Pois de Senteure (Firmenich)	15.6
Vetiver oil	0.8
Benzyl propionate	4
	100.0

Syringa (Philadelphus)

The base of the so-called syringe perfume (the true syringa being lilac) is methyl acetophenone. This syringa or mock-orange, which is in fact Philadelphus coronarious, has an odour that also recalls orange blossom and has, in its finer varieties a fresh lemony top note. As Billot wrote.

'The other components, in addition to methyl acetophenone, are hydroxycitronella, cinnamic alcohol, ylang-ylang, alphaionone, phenylethyl alcohol, products with an orangeflower note terpineol, anisic aldehyde, isoeugenol. The freshness of the depart is imparted by lemon oil, fine quality citral and/or octyle or decyl aldehyde.'

The perfume of the mock-orange, and particularly the lemon-scented varietyl is heady, fresh, very agreable. This is a floral odour that could be effectively used as the flower bouquet, or part of the flower bouquet, of new and attractive perfumes.

We give only a single formula for a syringe composition, but precede it with a special formula for a aldehydic blend that serves not only to give the fresh, sharp to note but has also proved widely useful in compounding other perfume types.

Aldehyde G Blend

Sweet orange oil (Guinea)	42.6
Super-Portugal oil (Guinea, UOP)	8
Aldehyde C.8 (10% in diethyl phthalate)	2
Aldehyde C.9 (10% in diethyl phthalate)	5.5
Aldehyde C.10 (10%in diethyl phthalate)	7.4
Aldehyde C.11 (10%c) (10% in diethyl phthalate)	21.1
Aldehyde C.12 (lauric) (10% in diethyl phthalate)	10.4
Aldehyde C.12 (MNA) (10% in diethyl phthalat)	3
	100.00

Syringa No. 1

Phenylethyl alcohol	15
Folia (bertrand freres)	2
Methyl anthranilate	0.5
Isoeugenol	5
Syringa aldehyde (p.-tolyl acetaldhyde)	4
Anisic aldehyde ex anethole	0.5
Bois de rose oil, Brazil	2.5
Muguet No. 2	2.5
Cassie absolute (Robertet)	1.5
Hydroxycitronellal	15
Jasmonis (Givaudan)	13.5
Jasmonone No. 4a	15
Jasmin absolute	2.5
Amyl salicylate	4
Heliotropin	9
Indole 10%	5
Aldehyde G Blend	2.5
	100.0

Trefly (Clover)

Trefly.clover, loke orchidee (orchid), is one of those important half-floral, half-herbaceous odours founded on the salocylates. One of the famous classic perfumes of the past was the Terfle Incarnat of Piver. Trefle compounds are conventionally based on the salicylates in association with coumarin, lavender, bergamot; with suitable flower notes and aldehydes.

Trefle No. 1

Amyl salicylate	20.0
Isobutyl salicylate	22.0
Benzyl salicylate	8.0
Bergamot oil	12.0
Coumarin	17.0
Isoeugenol	2.5
Vetiver oil	1.5
Ionone alpha	2.5
Ylang-ylang oil	2.5
Oakmoss absolute	0.5
Methyl nonyl acetaldehyde (1%)	0.6
Musk ambrette	2.2
Lavender oil	2.0
Rose oil art. (Bulgarian Type)	1.5
Jasmin absolute art.	2.5
Hydroxycitronellal	2.5
Birch bud oil	0.2
	100.0

Tuberose

The tuberose, though not highly regarded as a flower, has nevertheless found widespread use in perfumery. This applied both to the natural absolute and to 'tuberose artificial'. As a dominate theme it is especially appreciated in eastern countries and in territories under Spanish influence. More generally it finds application as a floral support capable of conferring body and persistence. Its basic components are:

Ylang-ylang oil, phenylpropyl alcohol benzyl salicylate and acetate, benzoin resinoid, peru balsam, tuberose absolute, tuberose pomad absolute and-this is indispensable-methyl saliylate or oil of wintergreen in very small quantities. To give a flower touch one uses C.12 laury aldehyde or other alphatic aldehydes, in association with orange blossom jasmin and a mere suggestion of styrallyl acetate.

Spanish taste has inclined towards their own more pungent and fruity type of tuberose, namely Nardo (q.v.)

As we have implied, tuberose can prove invaluable as a secondary floral adjunct able to impart substance and 'backbone' to a wide range of perfumes. Three formulae follow, the two being for bases which can serve as points of departure for individual experimentation.

Base Tuberose No. 1

Jasmin absolute ex chassi (benzene)	1.6
Tuberose absolute	1.2
Wintergreen oil, natural	4
Methyl salicylate	8
Benzyl acetate	24.5
Benzyl alcohol	22.5
Methyl anthranilate	22.2
gamma Nonyl Lactone	8
peach synthetic (Givaudan)	8
	100.0

Base Tuberose No. 2 (Tuberic Alcohol)

Tuberose absolute (Robertet)	1
Hydroxycitronellal	29.5
Benzyl benzoate	3
Isobutyl salicylate	10
Methyl salicyate	23
Ionone alpha	20
Aldehyde c. 12 (lauric)	10
Alpha -Amyl cinnamic aldehyde	7
Heliotropin	16.5
	100.0

Tuberose No . 3

Tuberic alcohol (or base tuberose no.2)	10.8
Ylang- Ylang oil	10.7
Methyl benzoate	1.7

Geraniol extra	8
Methyl anthranilate	2.6
Methyl; salicylate	2.2
Benzyl acetate	7.6
Nerol	5.4
Rhodinyl isobutyrate	3.2
Cistus absolute	1.1
Alpha- Amyl cinnamic aldehyde	2.2
Isoeugenol	3.3
Heliotropin	5.4
Musk ambrette	1.1
Linalool	21.5
Peru balsam clair (lautier)	10.6
Methyl methylanthranilate	2.6
	100.0

Verbeana

Verbeana has a type of odour which pleases men. It is simple, refreshing and comes midway between what one may term 'hygienic' perfumes, as used in toilet preparations for personal hygiene, and the more frankly perfumed toilet waters of the cologne type.

Verbeana Oil, as distilled from the true verbena, Lippiacitridodora, is now extremely rare, and most of the oils referred to under this in current price lists would seem to owe something to the so-called spanish oil (fromthymus hiemalis) or to oils of lemongrass, litsea cubeba, etc.and of course, citral.

Verveine No .1

Supercitron (Lautier)	3.5
Grapefruit oil	15.55
Cassie synthetic (Givaudan)	7.2
Geraniol extra	9.1
Geranium Bourbon oil	6
Verbean oil, Grasses, rectified	31.1
Citral extra	15.55
Verbemol (Firmenich)	3
Bergamot oil	3
Sandalwood oil, East Indian	1.2
Opopanax-L	4.8
	100.0

Wall Flower

In nineteenth- century perfumery, especially at the beginning, the wall flower (giroflee) enjoyed great favour. The odour of this flower is fresh and agreeable. The base consists of eugenol, isoeugenol and acetyl isoeugenol, associated with benzyl salicylate, amyl salicylate and anishic aldehyde, to which there may be added small quantities of oils of cloves, pimento, bay, or even pepper, and a trace if methyl paracresol. The 'filler' consists of terpioeol, hydroxycitronellol, cinnamic alcohol, phenylethyl alcohol, linalol, geraniol, rhodionl, nerol, dimethyl benzyl carbinyl acetate, to which there may be added an ionone or its derivatives and for the flowery touch, Lilial (Givaudan) and neroli too. The lower notes comprise heliotropin, vanillin, ethyl vanillin, methyl naphthyl ketone, and a little mace or mastic oil or guaiyl acetate.

The wallflower note, orientated towards the basic carnation-salicylateaubepine base, could well contribute to the development of an interesting perfume.

Wistaria

The wistaria, wisterial or glycine, grown for its climbing habit and its attactive drooping racemes of blossom, has a sweet and diffusive odour of rather honeyed type, suggesting orangeflower, lily and mimosa. The odorants chiefly entering into the composition of artificaial wistarias are hydroxycitronellal, benyzyl salicylate; geraniol, phenylethyl alcohol and othe rose alcohols; ylang-ylang, mimosa absolutes, isoeuegenol, terpineol, methyl napthyl ketone, methyl anthranilate, isobutyl phenylacetate, paramethyl acetophenone, p.-methyl totyl ketone, p. cresyl acetate.

Ylang-ylang

The essential oil of ylang-ylang is one of the most widely used of natural materials in perfumery. Formerly, there were types of natural products; ylang from the Bourbon islands of Madagascar, ylang from Manilla and canaga from the Java islands. To-ylang from Manilla has almost entirely vanished. This is a pity, for it had a very special note, more like orange-bloom than ylang reunion and lighter, too with, too with the base more like tuberose. Ylang is so useful that there have been numerous attempts at synthesizing it. Some artificials' are in fact quite close in odour to natural ylang. For Bourbon ylang, the basic products are methyl paracresol and paracresol. The very powerful products are only present in small quantites. Associated with methyl benzyl, benzyl benzoate, eugenol and isoeugenol, thery from characteristic part of this note. The body consists of terpineol, geraniol, linalool and alpha ionone.

This original note has certainly not been fully utilised; it is powerful and heady, especially in the case of Manilla ylang, which is less violent but otherwise similar. Here must be added an orange blossom note (natural or oil of synthetic) methyl anthranilate, and a tinge of methyl salicylate or oil of wintergreen. As a rule, when it is desired to give a 'bouquet' to a composition, it is considerably more advantageous to use natural essential oil-and, moreover, the finest quality that costing will permit.

There are very few fine quality perfume compositions in which ylang-ylang does not or could not enter as a valuable constituent. Here is a formula for an artificial version of Ylang-ylang Bourbon.

Ylang No. 1

Bois de rose oil Brazil	10.5
Linalool ex bois de rose	15.7
Linalyl acetate	8.65
Benzyl acetate	11.35
Vanilla tincture	10.55
Methyl paracresol	6.9
Palmarosa oil	8.6
Nerol (Lorena, Firmenich)	2.6
Benzyl alcohol	4.3
Orris concrete (10% on benzyl benzoate)	5.2
Isoeugenol	4.35
Peru clair (Lautier)	3.5
Coriander oil, Russian	3.5
Methyl benzoate	1.75
Estragon oil (p. Chauvet)	0.85
Methyl anthranilate	0.8
Methyl salicylate	0.8
Canage oil, terpeneless	0.1
	100.00

The general reader should appreciate that, in the case of many if not most of these flowers, there is not actual essential or absolute oil available and, even when there is, it inevitably loses something in the course of distillation of extraction and its odour therefore falls for short of that of the lovong flower.

We have tried to make this chapter on flower perfumes as representative as possible, but realise that it is far from complete, it only on account of the limited space at our disposal and the many regions of the world and their perfumed flora that we have not even touched upon in this survey. But in the future as in the past, it is certain that flower perfumes will be used to give rise to novel fantasies and that, in effecting these changes, they themselves will be altred and modified often by the exaggeration of one or more characteristic notes. It is this fact that underlies the importance of floral compositions.

Sophisticated Perfumes

Sophisticated or fantasy perfumes: in other words, this chapter is devoted to what in France it quite simply called 'la Grande Perfumerie'. A difficult task faces us here, in that we must seek to hold the interest of the reader without exposing ourselves to charges of revealing too much or breaching confidences. This is a particularly delicate situation when currently fashionable perfumes are the subject of discussion.

We shall restrict ourselves to being as objective as possible, but in so doing will offer guides to creation and some formulae, as examples, to facilitate basic research.

Perfumes of Fantasy (as we may call them for want of a better name) are roughly divisible into six categories:

Floral perfumes

Aldehydic perfumes

Chypre types

Oriental types

Green types

Perfumes with a distinguishing dominant note.

These types may and do, of course, overlap. And, independently of the notes that characterise perfumes in each group, one of three, namely light, medium and heavy.

Before quoting examples of these different groups, we give formulae for certain bases, both of a general and more specific nature, that can be utilized in a variety of formulae, just as can many of the floral bases already discusses in paret 3. Here is a representative of the very interesting bergamotvanilla bases:

Bergamot-Vanilla Base

Bergamot oil	100
Vanillin	5
Aldehyde C.12 (MNA) 10%	1
Aldehyde C.8, 10%	0.3

In the formula that follows the cedrat oil, once a natural product, may be replaced by the now conventional artificial blend of lemon, bergamot and orange oils.

Aldehydic Base A. 1

Aldehyde C.8	0.50
Aldehyde C.9	1.25
Aldehyde C.10	2.50
Aldehyde C.11 (undecylenic)	1.25
Aldehyde C.12 (lauric)	2.50
Aldehyde C.12 (MNA)	1.50
Bergamot oil	12.50
Bergamot oil, sesquiterpeneless	6.20
Superorange (Lautier) 50%	10.00
Supercitron (Lautier) 50%	1.90
Lemon oil	1.25
Cedrat oil	3.75
Neroli A	3.10
Folia (Bertrand freres)	0.60
Ylang-ylang oil	37.50
Opopanax L.G. (Givaudan)	1.25
Cosus absolute	0.60
Musk tincture No. 1	2.50
Rose No. 2	6.20
Sandalwood oil	3.15
	100.00

Aldehydic Base A. 2

Aldehyde C.12 (lauric)	1.30
Aldehde C.11 (undercylenic)	0.78
Aldehyde C.10	0.39
Vanillin	1.95

Coumarin	9.75
Gydroxycitronellal (Laurine (Givaudan)	9.75
Phenylethyl alcohol	14.30
Rose oil, Bulgarian	2.60
Geraniol 100% extra (Firmenich)	6.50
beta-iso Methyl ionone (Raldeine D)	6.50
Benzyl acetate	4.55
Jasmin absolute	3.90
iso Eugenol	6.50
Anisic aldehyde	7.80
Ylang-ylang oil	6.50
Linalool ex bois de rose Brazil	13.00
Sandalwood oil	11.70
Dimethyl phthalate	22.23
	130.00

Curacao Base

The 'Orange curacao' note is very characteristic and the actual Curacao orange oil virtually unobtainable. For that reason the following formula will often prove useful.

Bitter orange oil (Guinea)	37.50
Bitter orange oil, deterpenated	7.45
Anethole	4.65
Citral	3.70
Coriandrol (from Russian corander oil)	2.70
Aldehyde c.8	2.00
Aldehyde C.9 10%	5.00
Aldehyde C.10	7.00
Aldehyde C.11 (undecylenic)	18.30
Aldehyde C.12 (MNA)	3.00
Aldehyde C.12 (lauric)	8.70
	100.00

Leather or 'cuir' bases have continued to be popular and are widely utilised in perfumery at the time of writing. They are indispensable in certain fashionable perfumes and are particularly of interest in perfumes for men.

Cuir Base C. 1

Bergamot oil	1.5
Framboisis (de Laire)	7.5
Coromia (Givaudan)	40.0
Corinal (Firmenich)	14.0
beta-Methyl ionone	4.5
Jasmin No. 2	2.4
Mandarin oil	1.5
Cedrol	12.0
Lilac No. 2	9.0
Musk ketone	1.8
Musk ambrette	1.8
Neroli B	0.9
Coriandrol	0.3
Cedrat oil	0.8
Vanillin	1.5
Dimethyl phthalate	0.5
	100.0

Cuir Base 2

Alliantone (Givaudan)	14.0
Hyacinth absolute (Polak's Frutal Works)	9.0
Aldehyde C.11 (undecylenic) 10%	10.0
Aldehyde C.10, 10%	4.0
Hydroxycitronellal	4.0
Angelica root oil	2.0
Musk ketone	3.0
Ethyl vanillin	6.5
Costus absolute, 10%	2.5
Birch tar oil, rectified	10.0
beta-Methyl ionone	15.0
Ionone extra	10.0
Terpineol	10.0
	100.0

The woody note is often employed in association with other notes, not only to confer its own characteristics but to soften and round off the finished composition.

Woody Base B.1

Linalyl acetate	27.00
Bergamot oil	12.35
Rose de Grasse absolute	12.20
Jasmin absolute	6.90
Bois de rose oil, Brazil	6.00
Lilac No. 2	5.70
Muguet No. 1	5.25
Vanillin	4.95
Coumarin	4.95
Sandalwood oil	3.90
beta Methyl ionone	2.70
Neroli oil	1.95
Bitter orange oil, Guinea	1.95
Labdanum absolute	1.20
Patchouli oil	1.05
Vetiver oil, Bourbon	1.05
Hyperessence orange (Charabot)	0.90
	100.00

The moss note plays a very important part in perfumery. It sustains the head notes of 'green' compositions, which are currently fashionable; but long before this is found other applications. That great perfumer Roudnitska has contributed significantly to the popularity of the moss note, and perfumers everywhere know the famous mossy base, made by one of the leading synthetic houses and bearing the name of a German province.

The day when oakmoss was first associated with the synthetic odour of isobutylquioline was indeed a landmrk in the history of perfumery. It opened a new and broad avenue of perfume creation, and especially so when homologous odourants became available to vary the original accord and multiply the possibility of further combinations.

In their basic notes these mossy compositions afford admirable support for special fruity effects, on condition that they are accompanied by a more 'human' note, as it were, such as musk, amber, civet etc.

Moss base M. 1

Sandalwood oil	10.20
Bergamot oil	10.25

Bulgarian rose oil	2.40
beta-Methyl ionone	9.10
Coriandrol	0.25
Jasmin No. 4	2.40
Patchouli oil	6.70
Thyme oil, red	0.35
Vetiver oil, Bourbon	5.30
Ciste absolute	5.50
Oakmoss absolute	5.30
Castoreum	11.30
Neroli A	0.95
Musk ambrette	0.75
Caraway oil (Flebo)	17.65
Superorange (Lautier)	11.60
	100.00

In the following formula readers should note that vetiver acetate does not mean vetiveryl acetate. The former-with its own distinctive odour-results from the acetylation of the oil itself, with naturally involves not only the acetylation of the oil's vetiverol but also that of the other alcohols present in the oil. Vetivery acetate, on the other hand, is prepared by the simple acetylation of vetiverol.

Base 1. S

Opopanax L. G. (Givaudan)	30.0
beta-is Methyl ionone	13.5
Hydroxycitronellal	7.5
Ylang-ylang oil	2.5
Ionone alpha	5.0
Rose Bulgarian oil (10%)	10.0
Jasmin absolute	5.0
Vetiver oil, Java	1.0
Musk ambrette	2.6
Coumarin	1.0
Vanillin	2.0
Base Claveline No. 1	2.5
Muguet No. 2	10.0

Vetiver acetate	5.0
iso Butylquinoline	2.5
	100.0

Moss Base M. 2

Sandalwood oil	16.60
Rose de Mai absolute	3.80
beta-Methyl ionene	4.50
Neroli oil	1.50
Jasmin absolute	3.80
Thyme oil	0.60
Patchouli oil	1.55
Vetiver oil, Java	7.60
Ciste absolute	4.15
Tree moss absolute	9.10
Castoreum tincture	2.65
Opopanax L	2.65
Musk ambrette	1.15
Tincture of musk	1.50
bergamott oil	32.70
iso Butylquinoline (50%)	4.60
Supercitron (Lautier) 50%	0.75
Superorange (Lautier)	0.40
Coriandrol	0.40
	100.00

This subject has also been discussed in part 2 under Green, Fruity and other special notes. In addition to the newer 'green' odorants marketed as pure chemicals, others have been introduced as proprietary bases. In most Instances these bases have been well contrived, So as to permit their introduction into standard formulae without causing any undue imbalance of interference. They nevertheless give to effects that are quite disitinctive and different from those that precedes their introduction. The auxiliary notes so introduced may of course be pleasing or displeasing, but the possibility of producing novel and intersting effects cannot be overlooked.

Moss notes may be more or less 'fruity' in type, according to taste. Moss Base M. 2 can very easily be reorientated in this fashion.

A certain number of odorants are capable or suggesing the sea and the open air, faintly suggesting the odour of ozone. Givaudn's Alliantone, Laserson's Aldehyde Mer and Robertet's Absolu Marin are among the products of this type that strike a note of originality and may well introduce effects that appeal to outdoors enthusiasts, the masculine market, and perhaps a still wider market. This type of perfume could well be the subject of to morrow's success story.

We now turn to the various general types of perfume indicated in our earlier classification.

Floral Bouquest Perfumes

Perfume QH Np.1	
Lilac No. 2	50.00
Hyacinth absolute (Polak's Frutal works)	0.10
Aldehyde C.12 (MNA) 10%	0.25
Aldehyde C.12 (Lauric) 10%	0.10
Citronellyl lactone (I.F.F.) 10%	0.05
Amyl salicylate	5.00
Sandalwool oil	1.55
beta-Methyl ionone	5.05
benzyl acetate	3.90
Rose No. 3	4.00
Jasmin absolute	2.00
Cedrat oil	7.00
Bergamot oil	5.00
Ylang-ylang oil	10.00
Musk ambrette	1.00
Musk ketone	1.00
Vanillin	2.00
Ambrophore (Firmenich)	2.00
	100.00

The next flower perfume (AO) is characteristic of kind of bouquet which had a great sucess at the end of the nineteenth century. As an essential part of its structure it contained a base termed Bouvardia, which had then and still retains a wide acceptance among perfumers. For that reason we first give a formula for a base of this general type.

Bouvardia BM

Ylang-ylang oil	20.00
Geraniol extra	5.00
Jasmin absolute	3.75
Base Tuberose No. 1	2.50
Neroli B	12.50
beta-Methyl ionone	2500
Bois de rose oil, Brazil	25.00
Hyperssence orangeflower (UOP)	6.25
	100.00

Perfume AO

Mimosa flower absolute	1.7
Rose de mai absolute	3.4
Hyperessence orangeflower	5.0
Naricisse des Montagnes absolute (Camilli)	2.0
Base Tuberose No. 2	4.0
Jasmin absolute	3.4
Jasmonone No. 4a	1.0
Ylang-ylang oil, Manilla	3.0
Heliotropin	2.0
Acacia 200 (Firmenich)	8.5
Bouvardis BM	4.0
Bouvardia 100% (de Laire)	3.0
Bergamot oil	10.0
beta-Methyl ionone	8.0
Anisic aldehyde	6.0
Methyl anthranilate	1.0
Linalys acetate	2.0
Ionone alpha	2.0
Ambrophore (Firmenich) 3%	20.0
Civet tincture	10.0
	100.0

The following perfume is distinguished by its association of a lilac type of composition with the atmosphere of the sea.

Perfume TL

Musk ketone	1.2
Rose No. 1	2.0
Hyacinth No. 1	5.6
Lilas Isobutaflor (Robertet)	7.7
Jasmin absolute	10.0
Lilac No. 3	72.0
Aldehyde Mer (Laserson & Sabetay)	0.5
Hyacinth absolute (Polak's Frutal)	1.0
	100.0

Perfum F

Ylang-ylang oil	12.70
Jasmin absolute	3.40
Narcisse des Montagnes absolute (Camilli)	2.10
Lilac No. 3	21.50
Paracetone (Givaudan)	22.70
Gardenia 9058 (Givaudan)	10.25
Heliotropol (Firmenich)	4.20
Jasmin No. 4	4.20
Grapefruit oil	5.10
Bergamot oil, sesquieterpeneless	3.40
Neroli A	3.40
Base Cuir C. 1	2.10
Coumaria absolute oil	1.00
Coumarin	1.70
Rose No. 1	1.00
Pollenol (Firmenich)	0.50
Hyperessence reseda (Charabot)	0.15
Aldehyde C.12 (MNA) 50%	0.05
Phenylacetaldehyde dimethylacetal 50%	0.05
Cyclopentadecanolide	0.35
	100.00

Perfume HB

Jasmin No. 2	7.50
Bergamot oil	10.00

Lavender oil	7.45
Opaslaunax (Ets. Hasslauer)	7.50
Methyl anthranilate	6.70
Orange oil	4.10
Lilac No. 1	3.60
Rose No. 1	3.00
Methyl ionone	2.20
Jasmin absolute	2.20
Muguet No. 1	2.00
Neroli A	1.40
Claveline Base No. 1	1.30
iso Eugenol	1.30
Sandalwool oil	1.30
Heliotropin	1.30
Ambreine S (Firmenich)	0.80
Vanillin	0.80
Coumarin	0.75
Orangeflower water absolute	0.80
Ylang-yland oil	0.65
Anisic aldehyde	0.45
Cedarwood oil, Virginia	0.40
Merisia (Descollonges)	0.40
Orris absolute P.V.	0.20
Benzyl acetate	0.20
Zdravetz oil, 10%	0.90
Cinnamon oil, Ceylon 10%	0.40
Framboisis (de Laire) 10%	0.20
Peru balsam Tincture	13.00
Civet tincture	13.00
Musk No. 1 tincture	4.20
	100.00

Perfume AR

Jasmin No. 4	1.10
Jasmin No. 2	3.95
Jasmin absolute	2.65
Rose de Grasse absolute	1.60

Rose No. 1	2.10
Ylang-ylang oil	1.60
Arhenol (Firmenich)	7.10
Hydroxycitronelhal	6.10
Daturol (Firmenich)	0.55
Lilac No. 1	5.10
Methyl ionone	3.60
Irophore (Firmench)	0.30
Bioflor (Synarome)	6.65
Linalool	2.60
Bois de rose oil, Brazil	1.15
Nerol	0.55
Teprene (Synarome)	6.15
Muguet No. 1	10.00
Bergamot oil	13.00
Aldehydic Base Al	3.20
Aldehyde C.11 (undercylenic) 10%	0.40
Oakmoss absolute decoloree (Robertet)	1.10
Cyclopentadecanolide 1%	0.80
Vanillin	0.55
Musk ketone	1.20
Musk ambrete	1.10
Heliotropin	0.95
Civet tincture	3.70
Must No. 1 tincture	3.20
Vanilla tincture	5.25
Castoreum tincture	1.10
Cuir Base C. 1	0.80
Castoreum Anhydral (Givaudan) 1%	0.80
	00.00

Aldehydic Perfumes

Perfume VN

Bergamot oil	5.30
Bitter Orange oil	4.25

Aldehydic Base A2	3.00
Ambreine S (Firmenich)	3.25
Methyl ionone	4.25
Cinnamic aldehyde	3.40
Jasmin de provence (Descollonges)	3.00
Petitgrain oil, French	2.20
Jasmin absolute	2.20
Sophora (Givaudan)	2.80
Lavender	1.40
Neroli	1.15
Jonquil absolute (Charabot)	0.50
Hydroxycitronellal	2.70
Sandalwood oil	0.60
Benzoin Gomodor (UGP)	0.60
Opepanax vrai resine (Haslauer)	3.00
Elemi resinoid	2.00
Rose No. 1	2.20
Civet tincture	30.60
Musk tincture	12.45
Peru balsam tincture	5.15
Castoreum tincture	4.00
	100.00

Perfume C

Rose No. 2	0.40
Lilac No. 3	4.20
Jasmin No. 2	6.70
Neroli B	0.15
Hydroxycitironellal	6.30
Terpineol	3.20
Cinnamic alcohol ex styrax	0.50
Methyl ionone	3.20
Amarante (Givaudan)	5.00
Oakmoss absolute	1.25
Opopanax L	3.75
Base 1. S.	2.60
Liquidambar 11	0.10

Mousse de Saxe (de Laire)	5.00
Thyme oil	0.30
Vetiver oil, Java	1.90
Pachouli oil	3.00
Sandalwood oil	3.00
Coriander oil, Russian	4.00
Cedrat oil	1.00
Bitter Orange oil	2.00
Lavender oil	3.00
Bergamot oil	10.00
Linalyl acetate	5.00
Amberime S. (Firmenich)	4.50
Dimethyl phthalate	0.60
Ethyl vanillin	0.88
Musk ketone	0.50
Musk ambrette	1.00
Cyclopentadecanolide	3.00
Coumarin	3.00
Aldehyde C.11 (undercylenic)	0.42
Aldehyde C.12 (lauric)	0.36
Aldehyde C.12 (MNA)	0.27
Tincture of civet	1.50
Tincture of castoreum	8.50
	100.00

Fairly frequent reference is made in these formulae to the natural resin, Liquidambar. This balsamic product of very dark bituminous aspect is not used as such but is appropriately treated to yield three different fractions. The first of these has the strongly gassy styrene odour; the second has a labdanum odour and an 'animal' note; while the third has the animal note in a even more marked degree. In fine perfumery only the second and third fractions are normally used; and these are referred to in the various formulae as Liquidamber II and Liquidember III.

Treatment of raw materials in this way may be carried out in the perfumery laboratories if they happen to include a suitable chemical laboratory adequately staffed. Alternatively arrangements can often be made with an outside laboratory to carry out this and other collaborative work.

Perfume SP

Opopanax L	2.20
Opopanax 18 (de Laire)	0.90
Cyclamen aldehyde	0.10
Amyl salicylate	0.25
Costus resinoid (Camilli)	0.15
Bergamot oil	3.20
Patchouli oil	2.40
Grisambrol (Firmenich)	0.80
Labdanum oil (Schmoller)	0.25
Moss Base M2	0.40
Oakmoss absolute superessence (Yugoslav)	0.90
Liquidamber II	0.05
Mousse 1026 (Roure Dupont)	2.15
Musc BRB (Rhone-p;oulenc)	0.10
Cyclopentadecanolide	0.15
Ethyl vanillin	0.10
Thibetine (Givaudan)	0.60
Animalis (Snarome)_	0.30
Civette RP No. 2 (Rhone-poulenc)	0.10
Elecampane oil	4.50
Sandalwood oil	0.20
Methyl ionone	3.20
Jasmonone No. 4	5.70
Gardenia 9058 (Givaudan)	19.70
Gardenia No. 1	4.50
Cardamom oil, Naardenised (Naarden)	0.25
Hydroxycitronellal	2.40
Corona (Roure Dupont)	1.70
Hyacinth absolute (Polak's Frutal)	1.60
Phenylacetaldehyde	0.05
Camomile absolute (Schmoller)	0.15
Lavender oil, Barreme (42% esters)	1.30
Linalool ex bois de rose	4.50
Ylang ylang oil	0.25
Styrallyl acetate	2.10

Aldehyde C.8	0.10
Aldehyde C.9	0.10
Aldehyde C.10	0.60
Aldehyde C.11 (undecylenic)	0.60
Aldehyde C.12 (leuric) 50%	0.70
Opopanax resin tincture	6.30
Peru balsam tincture	20.00
Vanilla tincture	1.10
Castoreum tincture	2.70
	100.00

Chypre Types

Chypre perfumes have always found great favour among women and, indeed, among me. Witness the famour Chaypre of Coty, about which and its constituents so much has been written.

Characteristic of the Chypre odour, in addition to its conventional notes of bergamot, oakmoss, civit, linalyl acetate, amyl salicylate, rose, neroli, vetiver, sandalwood, labdanum and the little rustic or herbal notes of red thyme, tarragon and basil, etc. is a note of safrole or isosafrole. Others will see in this very special note, which assures the perfume's success, a celebrated composition of the German firm Heine, known under the name of product EM and probably base on oakmoss labdanum, liqoidamber, linalyl acetate-and various floral elements.

Many Chypre variants have been introduced, each with its slightly different note or emphasis which distinguishes it from the other members of its class.

When a perfumery house lacks imagination enough to devise a really new perfume, it tends to falb on a 'special: this being a more or less safe bet, in that it is most unlikely to prove an object failure. This 'policy of the least effort' effort' provoked Maurice Chevron to remark; 'It is simply beef steak.'

During the past few years aldehydic chypres have made headway. The following examples are given as typical of this class.

Perfume C. 2

Rose No. 1	1.80
Ysminia (Firmenich)	15.00
Jasmin absolute	15.00
Oakmoss absolute superessence,	

Yugoslay (Sehmoller)	0.60
Bergamot oil	4.20
Oakmoss absolute (Camilli)	4.35
Jasmin No. 1	4.00
Geranium sur rose oil	1.80
Methyl ionone	11.30
Vetiver oil	3.60
Sandalwood oil	1.30
Linalool ex bois de rose	1.80
Dianthine (Firmenich)	7.60
Eugenol	0.75
Hydroxycitronellal	0.75
Gardenia 9058 (Givaudan)	4.00
Costus absolute 10%	2.10
Mace oil	0.15
Florizia (Firmenich)	3.15
Tincture of Musk, 3%	7.60
Tincture of Civet 3%	1.00
Musk ambrette	0.70
Musk ketone	1.40
Coumarin	0.80
Vanillin	0.15
Aldehtde C.10, 1%	0.80
Aldehyde C.11 (Mndecyolenic) 1%	1.20
Aldehyde C.12 (MNA) 10%	3.60
	100.00

This is typical of Aldehydic Chypre. The following Chypre Base is also, in its way, very characteristic.

Base Chypre H

Coumarin	8.70
Vanillin	4.60
Ethyl vanillin	2.90
Heliotropin	1.80
Methyl ionne	1.20
Musk ketone	0.75
Rose H	0.60
Orange oil, better, Guinea	4.50

Geraniol extra	2.90
Bois de Rhodes oil (Chiris-UOP)	1.00
Noisette (de Laire)	0.20
Sandalwood oil	2.80
Benzoin Supergomodor (Chiris-UOP)	0.45
Liquidambar II	2.90
Labdanum Clair (Lautier)	5.80
Linalool ex bois de rose Cayenne	0.75
Linalyl acetate ex bois de rose	2.90
Terpinyl acetate	8.80
Benzyl acetate	2.90
Vetiver acetate	0.09
Estragon (tarragon oil 5%)	0.54
iso Butylquinoline 5%	0.75
Ysminia (Firmenich)	1.20
Bergamot oil, sesquiterpeneless	34.97
Bergamot oil	6.00
	100.00

Perfume MD

Opopanax L	2.60
Hydroxycitronellal	2.60
Cyclamen aldehyde	0.40
isobuty salicylate	1.70
Costus oil	0.90-
Bergamot oil	4.22
Cyclosia Base (Firmenich)	2.00
Patchouli oil	18.10
Vetiverol	4.82
Jasmin No. 1	4.23
Ylang-ylang oil	5.07
Muguet No. 1	4.22
Paracetone (Givaudan)	4.22
Lavender oil	1.70
Hyacinth absolute (polak's Frutal Work)	0.45
Gardamine (Synarome)	4.22
Gardenia No. 1	6.07

Galbanum oil (Robertet)	1.70
Oakmoss absolute superessence (Schmoller)	2.60
Base tuberose No. 1	0.85
Rose No. 2	0.45
Cardamom oil	1.70
Ambre 83 (de Laire) 10%	0.85
Grisambrol (Firmenich)	2.25
Ethyl vanillin	0.45
Musk ketone	4.22
Musk BRB (Rhone-poulenc)	0.85
Coumarin	3.37
Cyclopentadecanpliiode	0.90
Civetinae (Firmenich) 100%	0.90
Musk ambrette	4.22
Ambrophore (Firmenich)	2.87
Animallss (Synarome)	2.15
Aldehyde C.11 (undecylenic)	1.70
Aldehye C.12 (lauric)	0.45
	100.00

The number of chypre variations is very great and it would be impossible for us to offer examples of a comprehensive range of them in the necessarily restricted space available to us. The following however, reveals the incorporation of a distinctively 'animal' note in a chypre base.

Chypre 1. D.

Oakmoss asbolute hyperessence (Charabot)	0.30
Jasmin absolute	0.90
Muse VH (Ets.Hasslauer) 10%	20.15
Muse baume epure (payan & Bertrand) 10%	10.00
Ambergris tincture	18.80
Civet tincture	29.00
Musk ketone	0.30
alpha-Methyl ionone	0.90
Sandalwoold oil	0.40

Vetiver oil	0.90
Bergamot oil	4.75
Rose No. 3	3.75
Bouvardia CNC (Firmenich)	4.75
Carrot Clair (Lautier 10%)	2.05
Celery Clair (Lautier) 10%	1.25
Tobacco W (I.F.F.)	0.55
Aldehyde C.11 (undercylenic) 10%	0.25
Cyclopentadecanolide 1%	0.15
Orange oil superdeterpence (Charabot)	0.35
Celery seed oil	0.35
Angelica root oil	0.15
	100.00

The following formula is for a modified chypre with a peach type of top note.

Perfume V.W.

Ysmina (Firmenich)	3.00
Wardia (Firmenich)	2.00
Benzyl acetate	9.00
Orange oil sweet	3.00
Jasmin absolute	1.25
Vetiveryl acetate	4.50
Cedryl acetate (Givaudan)	4.00
Sandalwood oil (Mysore)	2.50
Lavender oil, Barreme 42% esters	6.00
isoEugenol	1.75
Amyl salicylate	1.50
Bergamot oil	12.00
Lemon oil, Guinea	3.50
Methyl ionone	5.00
Ylang-ylang oil	3.50
Oakmosss decoloree (Robertet)	3.50
Patchouli oil	2.50
Petitgrain oil, paraguay	4.00

Indole	0.15
Citral	1.50
Citral	0.50
Aurantiol	4.00
Dimethyl benzyl carbinol	3.00
Hydroxycitronellal	3.00
I-citronellol	2.00
Geranium extra	2.50
Fennel oil	0.75
Black pepper oil	0.75
Coumarin	2.60
Musk ketone	1.50
Civettone	0.20
Ambrettozone (Haarmann & Reimer)	0.40
Ambrarome Absolue (Synarome)	0.25
Clove bud oil	0.30
Aldehyde (pseudo) C.18, 10%	0.40
Aldehyde (pseudo) C. 16, 10%	0.20
Aldehyde C. 14 ('peach'), 10%	5.00
	100.00

The principle underlying the creation of so-called perfumes is to utilise balsams and resins of all kinds as the base, e.g. peru balsam, benzolin, opopanax, olibanum, labdanum, etc., accompanied by musk and civet, etc. natural and artificial. The conventional Crystalline 'fixatives' are also used according to taste. The desired objective is to obtain a perfume with warm and even seductive tonalities. The Typically oriental base is 'floralized' by means of heady flower odours such as jasmin, tuberose, magnolia, gardenia, honey-suckle, syringa, etc.

Due note must be taken of the fact that all the basic raw materials are heavy in character and slow to be released into the atmosphere. It is therefore necessary to use, with them, a sufficiency of citrus type oils, etc. acetates and other synthetics of a light nature, in order to entrain and disperse them.

By way of example we give a base that may serve as a starting point for these types of perfume.

Base S.H.

Tonka beans hyperessence (Charabot)	1.75
Peru balsam rectified (hasslauer)	3.30
Castoreum anhydrol (Givaudan)	2.55
Ethyl vanillin	2.50
Bergamot oil	51.25
Orange oil, bitter (Guinea)	8.70
Orange oil, sweet	8.70
Lavender oil, Barreme	4.40
Ondatrol (Descollonges)	0.75
Linalyl acetate ex shiu oil	16.40
	100.00

Here is another oriental perfume:

Perfume J

Coriandrol (Robertet)	10.85
Vetyrisine (Firmenich)	7.30
Opaslaunax (Hasslauer)	7.30
Humuscol (Descollonges)	5.82
Vanillin	3.90
Heliotropol (Firmenich)	0.35
Coumarin	3.65
Sandalwool oil	3.65
Lavender oil, Barreme, 42% esters	3.65
Bergamot oil	3.65
Coriander oil, U.S.S.R.	2.91
Gardenia 9058 (Givaudan)	3.65
Neroli	2.54
Supercuracao (Lautier)	2.59
Clary sage (Chiris-UOP)	1.48
Jasmin absolute	1.48
Pasmin oil	0.74
Musk ambrette	0.74
Ylang-ylang oil	0.37
Rose No. 1	0.37
Wintergreen oil	0.14
Peru balsam rect. (Hasslauer)	2.50
Cyclopentadecanolide	0.92
Anhydrol Castoreum (Givaudan)	0.37
Civettone 100%	0.37
Musk tincture No. 1	28.71
	100.00

Green Perfumes

For some years there has been a growing demand for perfumes with a more of less pronounced note of greenery or verdure. It could of course be said that the original perfumes with a type of green note were the ferns or fougeres, led by the famous Fougere Royale of Houbigant. Other fougeres were quick to follow, and all helped to popularize the fern note, which is really one of forest trees and undergrowth rather than a truly green leaf note. After this came a profusion of 'green' perfumes, and the fashion still endures.

Here is a hyacinth-green base which can be of considerable service in the creation of green perfumes.

Hyacinth Green Base No. 10

Hydroxycitronellal (Cyclosia, Firmenich)	3.60
Phenylethyl acetate	1.80
Phenylethyl alcohol	43.00
isoEugenol	3.50
Cinnamic alcohol	16.60
Phenylacetaldehyde 50%	0.85
Phenylacetaldehyde dimethyl acetal	0.50
Folial (Firmenich)	0.05
Hyacinth absolute (Polak's Frutal)	1.25
Benzyl acetate	1.80
Phenylethyl formate	0.50
Terpioneol	3.10
Rhodinol	1.20
alpha-Amylcinnamic aldehyde	0.30
Paracetone (Givaudan)	0.20
Rose No. 2	0.06
Jasmin absolute	0.20
Hosaldeine (de Laire)	0.79
Framboise 2222 (Firmenich) 10%	0.24
Dimethyl phthalate	20.40
	100.00

The green note is rather more restrained in the formula that follows:

Perfume P. No. 2

Jasmin No. 1	12.65
Jasmin absolute	5.60
Lilac No. 3	22.90
Vetiver oil, Java	2.45
Orangeflower No. 4	4.95
Rose No. 1	4.95
Narcisse des Montagnes absolute (Camilli)	4.95
Methyl cinamate	2.40
Phenylacetaldehyde	2.45
Narcissus No. 2	25.65
Phenylacetaldehyde dimethyl acetal	0.26
Vett de Lilas (De Laire)	0.94
Coumarin	3.70
Musk ketone	1.20
Oakmoss absolute, Yugoslay, Superessence (Schmoller)	3.75
Liquidambar 11	1.20
	100.00

Other suggestions on the subject of green note are to be found in part-2.

Dominant note types

These are perfumes which have a well-defined characteristic not produced by a synthetic odorant or a group of two or three ordorants, natural or synthetic.

It is enough to obtain in perfumery what, in painting, one terms a grisaille: in other words a soulless overall tint, which shades off into a heavy and nondescript mist. To avoid this one experiments with a restricted number of odorants in order to arrive at a note that novel and, as we have said well-defined.

Here is a formula in which the dominant note is formed by an accord of four principal odorants: ambergris, Arhenol, boronia and cassics:

Perfume D

Boronia absolute oil (Plaimar)	375
Cassis bud absolute incolore	3.00
Oakmoss absolute incolore	2.50
Jasmin absolute Butaflor	
(Roberter)	1.25
Vetiver oil, naardenised (Naarden)	7.38
Carrot oil, naardenised	0.07
Paracetone (Givaudan)	9.80
Benzoin Supergomodor	
(Chiris-UGP)	2.00
Rose No. 1	1.87
Cinnamon oil, naardenised	3.50
(Naarden)	1.25
Clay sage oil, naardenised	3.50
Clay sage oil, natural	3.50
Sandalwood oil	4.00
Hydroxycitronellal	4.50
Arhenol (Firmenich)	4.50
Pollenol (Firmenich)	3.00
Ambrarome (Firmenich0	7.38
Onetroll (Descollonges)	3.50
Aldehyde C.10, 10%	0.03
Alcohol C-11 (undecylenic)	0.62
Linalool ex bois de rose Brazil	3.75
Bergamot oil, sesquiterpeneless	15.50
Mandarin oil	0.75
Moskene (Givaudan)	0.25
Ethyl vanillin	2.50
Benzyl acetate	2.25
Opopanax tincture	4.00
Castoreum tincture	3.60
	100.00

The Ambergris Note

When it comes to using this composition for preparing a perfume of chosen concentration, the quantity of tincture of ambergris that should be added is calculated in the proportion of 100 parts of the concentrate to 73.5 parts of ambergris tincture-with the balance made up of perfumery alchol. As an example suppose that what is wanted is a perfume containing 15 per cent of concentrate. Then to 15 parts of the concentrate we add 11 parts of tincture of ambergris, and complete the formula by adding a sufficiency of alcohol at 95 to arrive at a total volume of 100 parts.

Tincture of ambergris at 3 per cent concentration may be replaced by much less expensive synthetics: vide the section of Animal Notes in the chapter on synthetic odorants. In this particular case excellent results, possibly even superior to those yielded by the natural product, may be obtained with a 3 percent tincture of Ambergris Synthetique (Givaudan).

Another example of a formula in this category may be given.

Perfume BM

Arhenol (Firmenich)	5.40
Sophora (Givaudan)	20.00
Gattleya (Givaudan)	3.60
Jonquile alpha (de Laire)	6.00
Hydroxycitronellal	23.00
Orangeflower A	0.30
Folia (Bertrand greres)	2.00
Methyl ionone	1.00
Paracetone (Givaudan)	3.00
Cinnamic alcohol ex styrax	9.78
Benzy acetate	2.00
Phenylethy alcohol	0.80
Rose No. 1	3.20
isoEugenol	0.80
Citral	0.40
Orange oil, bitter	4.00
Orange oil, sweet	1.60
Cedrat oil	2.00
Aldehyde C.12 (MNA)	0.03
Aldehyde C.11 (undecylenic)	0.02
Patchouli oil	0.27
Goumarin	3.00

Ethyl vanillin	0.80
Jasmonone No. 4A	3.00
	100.00

The formula for the finished perfume is made up as follows:

Perfume concentrate as above	
(Perfume BM)	15 kilos
Tincture of musk NO. 2	4 litres
Alcohol at 95	81 litres

After chilling and filtration oe obtains 100 litres of perfume.

Many simple, small-scale chemical processes may be profitably used by the perfumed of his associates. One thinks of the fractional distillation of Virginian cedarwood oil, for example, or the interesting end-product of distilling bergamot oil over oakmoss, just as the larger supply houses have distilled geranium over rose flowers and petitgrain over orange flowers. The separation of a determined portion or protions of a known essential oil can also yield an attractive result. Nothing should be overlooked in fact, that may contribute a novel and perhaps an inimitable note to a new perfume.

Manufacturing Processes

No perfume can be better than the concentrate from which it is prepared. Hence the necessity not merely of ensuring the result in conception and formulation but also of taking every possible care in the selection, purchase and storage of raw materials. A constant standard of quality is essential.

Citrus oils are among those materials which deteriorate relatively rapidly. Stocks should therefore be used by accordingly and any falling off in quality duly noted and acted upon. Storage basements, etc., should be dry, shaded and well ventilated. They should afford adequate protection against normal fire risks. Storage should preferably be in glass, although internally lined aluminium, cans provide one of the permissible alternatives. Some oxidation prone essential oils are often treated on the production site with traces (e.g. part in 20,000) of antioxidants, but the practice of adding such materials should be kept to a minimum and not knowingly encouraged in fine perfumery. A first-grade fresh oil is always superior to a comparable treated oil.

A few ordorants, e.g. myristic aldehyde, should note be stored in the cold. This particularly aldehyde tends to polymerise if kept below room temperature.

When weighting-out, the formula may conveniently be typed on a Celophane-wrapped card and clipped into a holder having a movable wide flat strip, designed to indicate clearly the actual line that is to be weighed.

Much thought should be given to the containers and other utensils, in respect of the metals from which they are fabricated (e.g. good quality tinplate) and their design (e.g. with spouts for drip-free pouring and bases suitable for use on a steam bath or hot plate).

Accurate weighing is essential, and especially so in the case of very small quantities, which may have to be weighed separately on a more sensitive balance or used as a 10, 4 or 1 per cent solution in ethyl alcohol, benzyl benzoate, diethyl phthalate or other appropriate diluent. A very serviceable type of balance is one that incorporates deluent.

A very serviceable type of balance is one that incorporates a zero resetting device and a calculator which shows automatically, at the end of the weighing, the same total as that shown in the typed formula.

Most mixtures are prepared in the cold, but some require gentle heating to promote through solution. Senstitive materials such as flower absolutes and fatty aldehydes should be added only after such dissolving-with-heat has been effected and the blend allowed to cool.

Modern mixing equipment offer many improvements on the old-fashioned hand method once used in the perfumery industry. The steps that follows comprise the maturation of the concentrate on storage and (in the case of spirituous perfumes) its subsequent reduction or dilution with alcohol; its chilling, filtration and filling into bottles.

Probably the best way of preparing a finished perfume consisting of the compounded odourants known as the perfume concentrate, together with alcohol and water, is to pre-mix the concentrate with an equal quantity by volume of the distilled water, allow to cool completely, and then add the concentrate-plus-alcohol with renewed stirring. This method tends to prevent colloidal precipitation of part of the concentrate, which one gets by adding the concentrate to the main bulk of the conentrate, which one gets by adding the conentrate to the main bulk of alcohol initially, or the difficulty in solubilisation that may arise when the concentrate is added last of all.

After the lapse of some 24 hourse the alcoholic batch is chilled (0.4 to 0.6°C) and filtered. Where filter aids are used, as in the case of weakly alcoholic solutions, asbestos wool and distomaceous earth are preferred to the mildly alkaline magnesium carbonate.

Alcoholic Strengths

As we mention in the chapter on eaux de Cologne, the perfume content of Colognes, eaux de toilette, eaux de parfum and other fancifully named 'dilute perfumes' may range from 3 to 8 per cent, although in some few cases this figure has been found to exceed even 10 per cent. There seems little point in marketing as a toilet water what is, in fact, a perfume-unless its wter solubility hs been artificially enhanced for the purpose.

Perfumes themselves range from the perhaps old-fashioned 'low' of 10 per cent to 15, 20, 25 and even, quite irrationally, 35 per cent. The aqlcoholic strength may lie between 85° and 95°.

Inexperienced perfumers, and some captains of industry in the perfumery world who are not perfumers, seem occasionally to believe that higher perfume concentration means enhanced strength and tenacity. This is not so. Sometimes the tenacity may be slightly increased but, beyong a certain optimum level, the strength is not increased. Indeed, too high a concentration lowers the tonality of a perfume and flattens it out, curtailing its ability to expand. With a very high concentration dull, non-diffusive perfumes result, and one of the most valued properties of a good grade of ethyl alcohol is wasted.

Control

Adequate checking and control methods are of course essential at all stages of perfume production: from the intake and assay of raw materials, through storage and processing to filling and packaging. The variability of certain materials because of batch or climatic deviations, etc., is an additional obstacle in the way of producing a uniform series over a period of time. The perfumer should be closely concerned with the provision and use of standard samples for odour checking and comparison. These standards must be kept in optimum conditions, i.e. where possible in sealed ampoules or under nitrogen. Watch should also be kept on the exact matching of colour shades.

Ethyl Alcohol : Coversion from Gay-Lussac to equivalent degrees Proof, U.S. and U.K., and compared with percentage Alcohol by Volume.

Gay-Lussa (15°C)	%Alcohol by volume (60°F)	Equivalent specific gravity in air (60° F/60°F)	Degrees overproof (U.K.)	U.S. Proof at 60°F (approx.)
85	84.71	0.8503	48.49	170
86	85.71	0.8472	50.25	172
87	86.72	0.8442	52.01	174
88	87.72	0.8411	53.78	176
89	88.73	0.8378	55.55	178
90	89.74	0.8346	57.31	180
91	90.75	0.8312	59.08	182
92	91.75	0.8278	60.85	184
93	92.76	0.8243	62.62	186
94	93.76	0.8206	64.38	188
95	94.76	0.8168	66.15	190
96	95.76	0.8129	67.91	192
97	96.76	0.8087	69.67	193
98	97.77	0.8043	71.44	195
99	98.79	0.7996	73.20	197
100	99.78	0.7947	74.97	199
100.2	100.00	0.7936	75.35	200

Notes: (1) Equivalent specific gravities in air at the now standard temperature of 20° C are given in the specific Gravity of Spirits tables published by H.M. Stationery Office, London, 1954. (2) Degrees overproof may also be stated as 'percentage of proof sport',in which case 48.49, for example becomes 148.49. (3) It will be seen that the gay-Lussac figures are in closes approximation to those given for percentage alcohol by volume. They are in fact derived from the volume of alcohol measured at 15° C contained in 100° CC of the alcohol-water mixture also at 15°C.

It is frequently necessary to dilute 95 per cent alcohol to 90, 85, 80, 70 per cent of even lower strengths. To determine the quantity of required to reduce the proof of alcoholic solutions by a definite amount, one divides the percentage by volumeof alcohol in the given proof by the percentage by volume of alcohol of the desired proof. The quotient is multiplied by the percentage by volume of water in the desired proof, and from this one substracts the percentage by volume of water in the given proof. The remainder is the number of volumes of water that must be added to 100 volumes of the given proof to produce a solution of the desired proof. The resultant volume of the diluted alcohol will be the quotient first obtained multiplied by the original volume.

Thus if 13.38 vols. of distilled water are added to 95 per cent alcohol the resultant solution will be 85 percent alcohol.

90 per cent alcohol may be prepared by diluting 947 ml of 95 per cent alcohol with waer to 1000 ml.

80 per cent alcohol results from diluting 82 ml of 95 per cent alcohol to 1000 ml.

70 per cent alcohol is obtained by diluting 737 ml of 95 per cent alcohol; 60 per cent by diluting 632 ml, 50 per cent by diluting 526 ml, and 45 percent by diluting 474 ml to 1000 ml with purified water (7.)

Contraction of volume and rise of temperature occur when ethyl alcohol and water are mixed. The final adjustment of volume, when preparing these dilutions, is therefore made at the same temperature as that at which the 95 percent alcohol is measured, i.e. about 20C.

3

Perfumes for Many Purposes

The uses of perfumes

'We live in a world of odour, just as we live in a world of light and sound'. In the big cities we are never far removed from the manifold activities of the perfumery industry. To compile list of perfumery application is virtually impossible, because new applications are being discovered almost daily. The following list, though far from complete, will at least serve to indicate something of the range of perfumery uses in a modern industrialised society.

(a) Household Products

Soaps and synthetic detergents
Miscellaneous cleansers
Disinfectants
Polishes
Paints
Adhesives
Air (space) deodorants etc.

(b) Personal Products

Cosmetics; make-up preparations
Toilet and beauty preparations
Perfumes, toilet waters
Pharmaceutical prepartions etc.

(c) Industrial products

Dry cleaning
Leather and rubber articles
Artificial leather
Linoleum
Plastics
Printing inks, perfumed board and paper
Textiles etc.

(d) Agricultural Products

Insecticides
Insect and animal repellants
Animal baits and attractants
Veterinary products
Cattle feeds
Farmyard 'masking' odorants etc.

(e) Flavours

Beverages
Foods
Medicines etc.

While the unspoken aim of every ambitious perfumer must surely be to create a true perfume-by which one means an alcoholic extract-that will attain a satisfactory measure of international celebrity, it must be admitted that few perfumers ever realise this aspiration. Yet many become well known to their contemporaries as the creators of this or that soap perfume. Still others devote most of their creative activities to the preparation of attarctive, stable and otherwise satisfactory perfume compositions for use in the various toiletries, industrial products etc. listed abvoe. The problems which they encounter in this work are many, and some of them are considered individually in the remaining pages of this chapter.

Perfumes for Soaps

Perfumes of outstanding performance in soap are the exception rather than the rule, adding as a corollary that many perfumes which give excellent results in a variety of other preparations will be failures in soap.It will probably be conceded by most perfumers and soap makers that their most successful perfumes have been the result of considerable trial and error. Years of experience will have shown which individual ingredients give strong and lasting effects in soap, but in certain combinations or blends even these otherwise successful items will fail to produce the anticipated effects.

Four attitudes to soap perfuming should be taken into account in order to ensure the production with the minimum waste of time and effort of a successful soap perfume. They are (1) psychological and aesthatic; (2) economic; (3) technical and (4) chemical. The fourth term is loosely used in this context to cover physical-chemical and biochemical as well as straight forward chemical reactions.

The governing factors are, or should be, those of a psychological, aesthetic and artistic character. While it is most desirable that the soap perfumer should have a sound scientific knowledge of the probable behaviour of aldehydes, ketones, esters and so on, when they are incorporated in a soap base, it is even more essential that he shall be an artist in perfumery, able to understand, anticipate and satisfy changing fashions in the public taste for perfumes. In addition to this, he ought to be capable of selecting and using his raw materials to the best economic advantage. The techniques that he employes in his work are likewise extremely important, for they should be adopted and modified in such as way as to save him the maximum amount of time and trouble, both during the creation and compounding of the perfumes and its subsquent shelf-testing in soap.

The soap perfumer is never allowed to forget that the perfume soap system presents certain unique and sometimes unpredictable behavioural phenomena. For that reason he is obliged to test his perfume in a standard soap base, and not merely on smelling-strips, at all stages of its development. He tests his raw materials in this way, often at the level of 1 percent in soap and may similarly test partial blends in soap before finally completing his perfume and testing that. The small perfumed soap tablets may be examined immediately, stored wrapped of unwrapped and then re-examined, or subjected to acceleration tests with U.V. light etc.In this way it is possible to assess odour and colour effects and record them over a prolonged period, filling the information so obtained for future reference.

The keeping properties of perfume in soap are governed by various physico-chemical phenomena, specifically mentions the absorption of perfume by soap. evaporation of perfume; the autoxidation of both soap and perfume; and th reactivity of soap due to the equilibriym:

RCOONa + HO = RCOOH + RaOH.

In regard to the first two factors, work shows that some perfumes will tend to remain in the aques phase: some will probably be absorbed on the outer surface of the soap micelle; some may be absorbed between the methyl tails; and some apparently become oriented in the micelle, forming a more of less stable complex.

With the esters there is no association, hence no soluilisation, and as a direct consequence the esters gie in soaps a more intense odour than do the alocohols. Decyl alcohol gives a feeble odour; decyl acetate a strong odour; geraniol a feeble odour; tetra hydrogeraniol which is a saturated compound and thus more soluble, gives a very weak odour;

while geranyl acetate gives a very strong odour. So if we mix geraniol and geranyl acetate in a soap, it is the aetate which will cominate, whereas in and alcoholic solution the reverse will hold good. These results are valid for so-called anhydrous soaps which actually contain a certain proportion of water (5-10 percent).

Esters vary considerably, one from another, in their stability and odour yield in soap; but as a group they are valuable contituents of soap perfumes. Among the carbinol esters styrallyl (methyl phenyl carbinyl) acetate is outstanding.

Alcohols: As we have seen, alcohols tend to give uniformly lower odour values in soap than do the corresponding esters, but for the same reason they usually remain well 'fixed' in the soap and their odours though mild are persistent. Fatty alcohols have weak odours, but unsaturation in the chain improves the odour performance. Of terpene alcohols the most important are lineolol and terpineol. Anisic alcohol is useful in lilac and muguet.

Ketones: In this group performance varies considerably. Among those substances with a good odour yield in soap are the ionones, benzophenone, p.methoxy and p.methoxyle acetophenones and ethyl amyl ketone.

Aldehydes and Acetals: Many aldehydes-aromatic, terpene and aliphatic are widely used in soap perfumery, despite their reactivity and relative instability as a class. Cyclamen, amyl cinnamic lauric aldehydes are among these which can give very satisfactory results. In some cases the aliphatic aldehyes are pre-mixed with the corresponding alcohols, with the intention of imporving their stability by faclitating the formation of hemi-acetals.

Dimethyl and diethyl acetals cannot be used as simple substitutes for the corresponding aldehydes. Their odours are different and their performance not always encouraging.

Other constituents: Of the ethers, several are distinguished by their satisfactory odour effects in soap. Examples are amyl benzyl ether, p. cresol methyl ether and diphenyl oxide Terpenes can give quite interesting results. As one would expect, the odour yield of phenols ranges from moderate to poor. Eugenyl acetate gives a stronger odour than eugenol or isoeugenol, but it discolours and is not entirely stable. The effect of methylation, as in eugenol methyl ether, is to enhance the strength of odour. Of the lactones one may note such useful items as gamma-nonyl lactone, gamma-under-alactone and coumarin.

'The soap perfume of to-day,' 'would look askance at some of the perfume formulations used years ago. A typical formula contained large percentages of such natural products as neroli, cassia, cloves, geraniym, lavender, patchouli, rosemary, sandalwood and vetiver, with only small proportions of coumarin and a few other synthetic aromatic chemicals and isolates.' This was indeed the picture up to the beginning of World War II. A French soap perfume formula used in the late 1920's included, for example, six different essential oils, four resins and resionoids, one concrete oil and three straight synthetics (amyl salicylate and two nitro-musks). To-day the cost of such a perfume would be prohibitive and, in the case of a widely distributed soap, a sufficiency of some of the natural materials might not always be available. Advances in synthetic chemistry have provided the soap perfumer with an ever-increasing range of synthetic odorants, from which he can select products of good odour and colour stability, capable of creating new perfume effects. At the same time the production of synthetic odorants aids materially in standardising quality and stabilising costs. Even so, the utility of the natural products should not be underestimated. Although one is now frequently obliged to reverse the practice so reasonably recommended by Spencer in the Twenties ('concentrate on natural products and add to their effect by the use of isolates and synthetics'). It is still true to say, as he did then, that Peru balsam, styrax, olibanum and other resinoidscan from the backnone of many soap perfumes which, indeed, could scarcely exist without them.

Soap perfumery fashions: It is essential for the creative soap perfumer to keep in touch with changing fashions, not only in his own country but throughout the world.

White toilet soaps with restrained 'clean'-smelling odour were made fashionable in the 1935-1945 period. Since then soaps have become more colourful and their perfumes more pronounced, distinctive and even exotic. Colour in soap is not merely decorative: it also successfully conceals any slight discoloration caused by the use of certain odorants, which for this reason would not be acceptable in pure white soaps. Perfumes are also used, in some brands atleast, in higher concentration or at higher intensity-this serving to perfume the skin after the bath or showewr. Greater care is also taken to avoid the use of perfumery materials known to irritate sensitive skins.

It is recommended that soap perfumes should frequently consist of the smallest possible number of ingredients and that above all, each odorant should be selected for its strength of odour and stability in soap base. What is not wanted is a formula containing 'passengers' which do not contribute effectively to the final result and which reduce the perfumes overall intensity.

Perfuming Synthetic Detergents

The perfumes used in blended synthetic detergents have a dual role: they mask the inherent odours of the raw materials and impart a type of fragrance which meets the special requirements of the finished product. There are, in general, five different types of off-odour associated with detergent materials, and these must be masked when they become perceptible:

(a) Odourous substances such as petroleum derivatives occuring with alkyl-aryl sulphonates; also slight petroleum odours present in nonionics.

(b) Fatty odours originating from aliphatic alcohols found in alkyl sulphates.

(c) Sulpher odours sometimes originating from such detergents as nonyl phenol sulphonate made from propylene trimers and terramers, which may contain sulphur derivatives.

(d) Odours formed as the result of slight oxidation of certain alkyl-aryl detergents. To avoid this condition, various antioxidants have been recommended.

(e) Odours resulting from pyrolytic action when detergerts are overheated during the drying processes.

The formulator is rarely content to mask such off odours. He will aim at a combined job of odour-masking and definite perfuming. Here he is faced with the type and end-use of the detergent. So-called light duty detergents for washing dishes should have clean, fresh odours that do not conflict with food odours and do not persist after the detergent has been used. Nobody wants a perfume to adhere to china and glassware after there utensils have been washed. Hence the current popularity of lemon odours for this purpose. For the type of light duty textile detergent, as used for washing delicate fabrics and feminine garments, a more sophisticated perfume may be demanded-and even one that leaves behind it a faint but pleasant residual odour. Yet another problem is posed by the heavy duty laundry detergents and other products of high pH, for whose perfuming it is necessary to conentrate on the more alkale-resistant odorants. Then there are detergent disinfectants to be considered, in which convention may restrict the choice topine, lavender, resemary etc.

Experiments to determine the stability over a period of one year, in an alkalineperborte-containing detergent of a number of conventional perfumery chemicals, have been done. For this purpose 100 mg of each odorant was intimately mixed with 100 g of a commercial detergent containing 5 per cent of sodium perborate and having a pH in 1 per cent solution at 20°C of 0.5. After the lapse of a year each sample was examined for odour, and in 1 percent aqueous solution was compared with a freshly prepared sample of the same strength. The sample under test was again re-examined after boiling for 30 minutes and for one hour. The following odorants showed good stability under all these conditions.

Cineole, linalool, menthol, linalyl acetatem phenylethyl acetate, methyl salicylate, acetophenone, methyl ionone, musk ketone, p.methoxy and p.methyl acetophenones, acethole, diphenyl oxide, cyclamen aldehyde. (Anethole undergoes limited oxidation but is otherwise satisfactory. Vanillin is transformed to its sodium salt, loses odour intensity, and acquires a rubber like note).

The methyl and ethyl ethers of beta-napthol could be added to this list, as well as most of the odorants once used in perfuming the so-called cold prcoess soaps.

Examples of a lingering perfume for adding to wash-day fabric cleaners anda more evanescent perfume for use in a dishwashing detergent have been suggested. The former contains from 3 to 10 per cent of such long-lasting odorants as styrax, amyl cinnamic aldehyde and cedryl cetate, together with 10 per cent of heliotropin; while the second formula is based largely on relavity transient esters and unobtrusive alcohols. Asked to devise a household laundry detergent perfume which would leave behind a suggestion of 'clean linen', one of the present authors took 15 per cent each of benzophenone and lauric alcohol, together with smaller quantities of cyclamen aldehyde, musk ketone, heliotropin, coumarin nd oil of patchouli etc., rounding off the complex with pheynylethyl acetate and other rose-type esters and alcohols. Many alternatives will occur to the practising perfumer.

Among the household cleaning aids which are nowadays sent to market with the added incentive of a pleasant perfume are scouring powders, carpet and other specialised cleansers, starches and bleaches. Lavatory bowl cleaners are also perfumed, whether they are based on alkalis or on sodium acid sulphate. Liquid cleaners based on ammonia and window cleaners sometimes incorporating both ammonia and isopropanol, may likewise be perfumed--and, indeed, compounded perfume compositions of good stability and all-round performance are specially produced and marketed for all these purposed.

Perfumed Disinfectants: 'Why should disinfectants smell like disinfectants' asked Dr. F.W. Brown in an article published in 1930. Since that time most disinfectants intended for domestic use have lost their former malodorous character. Some have still a recognisably disinfectant odour of chlorocresylic type, despite the fact that they usually contain perfumery materials; whereas others have undergone a complete transformation and are marketed as floral bouquet disinfectants.

Perfumes can in fact exert a dual function in disinfectants and antispeptics; and in similar fashion can act as preservative agents in a wide variety of products, ranging from emblaming fluids to cosmetics. Odorants as a class possess antifungal and antibacterial properties. The various group of perfumery chemicals, of which they tested a sample range of 230 items, exhibit the following order of decreasing antibacterial activity: aldehydes, alcohols, acids, lactones, ethers, ketones, esters and acetals. Of the few phenols tested eugenolwas the most active. It is curious, perhaps, to find acetals at one extreme of the list andthe parent aldehydes at the other. Benzaldehyde and undecylenic aldehyde inhibited growth of B. subtilis, E. coli, S. aureus 10390 and S. aureus Ox-H at concentrations ranging from 1 in 500 to 1 in 2000. Methyl acetophenone also showed a broad spectrum of effectiveness at 1 in 500. Octyl and decyl alcohols, cinnamic aldehyde, heptyl formate, cedrol, methyl heptin carbonate and eugenol were highly effective against some but not all of the bacteria cultured in these tests.

Scuebtusts had previously tested 136 essential oils against five different fungi. F. oxysporum f, lycopersici, C. albicans, R. nigricans,P. betae and S. cerevoseae. Only the vapours from the oils were allowed to come in contact with the broth cultures, oils itself being kept for five days at a distance of 5mm from the surface fo each petridish. The vapours of the following essential oils showed the greatest activity against the test organisms, this short list again being given in decreasing order of effectiveness; cumin, garlic, eucalyptus, tarragon, sweet birch, spearmint, caraway. The four clove oils examined were derived from bud, leaf and sterm. They showed remarkably low activity, considerably lower-for example than coriander. Black pepper and pinus pumilio oil vapours showed virtually no inhibitory action on any of the fungi. Vapour pressures and other physical, as well as chemical factors must obviously come into play here. Scientists who carried out an earlier series of tests on fungi of 200 essential oils were of the opinion that the vapours of essential oils are often more active against bacteria and fungi than the oils in liquid form and found Spanich hop oil unusually effective against staphylococci and strentococi. Of the 106 essential oils tested by Researchers the most generally effective as antibacterial agents were lemongrass, Ceylon cinnamon, cassia and coriander. The findings are unusual in that they relate in part to some of the more expensive flower oils and do not seem, in other respects, to support the conclusions of the investigators whose work has already been cited. Their descending order of antifungal effectiveness reads as follows: sandalwood vetiver, rose, neroli, citronella, geranium, bay, patchouli, jasmin, anise, ylang-ylang and lemon.

Considerations of cost restrict the more widerspread use of essential oils and perfumery chemicals as preservatives, antiseptics and disinfectants. Wedoerburn points out, more-over, that the essential oils are by their nature volative and their effectiveness tends to diminish with time. Even so, they are frequently used to support the main antibacterial, antifungal action, thus helping to make the product in which they are used both more attractive in odour and less liable to micro-organic attack.

Cholrophenolic disinfectants have commonly been improved in odour by the incorporation of such odourants as terpineol, benzyl acetate, diphenyl methane, diphebyl ether, terpinolene, safrole, bornyl acetate; together with such essential oils as citronella lemongrass, steam-distilled pine, camphor and cinnamor leaf. In the following type of basic perfume compound, the terpineol acts not merely as odorant but also as a solvent or coupling agent and as an auxiliary antibacterial agent:

Terpineol	50 parts
Lemongrass oil	10
Pine oil, steam-distilled	10
Benzyl acetate	8
Terpenolne	7
Citronella oil	10
Bornyl acetate	5

At one time the Australian ti-tree oil, distilled from the leaves and terminal branchests of Melaleusa alternifolia, became popular as a constituent of disinfectants. This oil has a pungently spice-like odour, somewhat reminiscent of nutmeg, and a high antispetic value.

Disinfectants based on quenternary ammonium compounds, e.g. cetrimide, are particularly well adapted for perfuming. One British brand is marketed as a floral bouquet disinfectant an as lavender, carnation, gardenia etc. In developing perfumes of this type it is necessary to study the solubilision sation of perfumery materials, the relative 'emergence' of odours from mainly aquenous solutions, and the mechanism of complex formation in mixed cationic/nonionic products.

The hypochlorite disinfectamts and bleaches, inculding the french eau dejaval, and considerably restricated in us by their disagreeable odour, Effective covering of the odour is said to have been achieved with the aid of two alternative mixtures consisting of 1 gram of either musk xylol or nerolin 11(B- naphthol methyl ether, or yara yara) dissolved in 10 mls of carbon tetraachloride, 15,mls of sulphonated castor oil and 1.5 grams cethyl alcohol, made up to a total of 100 mls with water. The dilution required is 1 mls either mixture to every 100 mls of percent hypochlorite solution. Both blends were reported to ensure adequate odour masking, coupled with resistance to the chemical action of the hypochlorite, nontoxicity in the required concentration, and non-interference with bactericidal action.

In our previously quoterticlw we suggested some simple basic perfume formules suitable for addition in small proportions to a nonreacting disinfectant base. One of these reads as follows:

Citronella oil	25 parts
Thyme oil, red	25
Sassafrass oil artificial	25
Terpineol	25

Most perfumers would probably want to bring such a formula up to date, by part replacement of some of the constituents and the introduction of other, newer synthetics: or at least by adjusting the started proportions in order to get the optimum odour- effect.

Perfuming the air

Room sprays of the aerosol air freshener type representthe latest development in a whole series of products that inculde the old- style cinema sprays, perfumed sickroom sprays, specialised air disinfectants and deodorisers, and wick- type air freshners. Also in the same general category may be included incense cones, pastilles or papers: the joss sticks known as agarbatties: and even fumigant candles and lavatory deodorant blocks.

Perfumes for aersoal air freshners and similer purposes may have a light, refreshing floral odour, or they may be 'green' minty, herbal, spicy or woody. They offer considerable scope, in fact, for the enterprising and ingenious perfumer because they should be fairly persistent (as covering or masking agents for kitchen smells) and yet light and unobtusive. Citrus and lime blossom notes can be be attractive. Pine, pine needle, cedarwood and cedar leaf oils have the requisite pungency, and blend well with other useful odorants such as terpineol, terpinyl actetate, borneol, bornyl acetate, thyme, rosemary, spike and lavender.

The leading aerosol air freshner in the Indian market was at one time a blend of orange, cologne, verbene, lavender and clove. Others that achieved varying degrees of popularity were lemon and pine, lavender and pine, lemon and varying eucalyptus, lavender, honeysuckle, jasmin, floral and pine,oriental, jasmin-lilac, rose and spicy-floral. The leading wick type room deodorants were said to have lemon-pine and camphor-pine odours.

Three types of odorant come into consideration:those that temporarily inactivate or anaestheise the olfactory nevers and thus lessen sensitivity to malodours: and those that act by pairing with specific malodorants to lessen the combined odour-intensity. Most of the odorants used in practice come into the first category. A few, such as formaldehyde, acetaldehde, etc. are to be found in the second category. Those in the third group, being limited by the specify city of their action, are similarly limited in number. 'Some of the more interesting pairs of odours compensating each other are: skatole and coumarin, ethyl mercaptan and eucalyptol.' Musk could ' neutralise' the odour of bitter almonds, cedarwood the odour of rubber, Tolu baksam that of beeswax.

Room deodorants containing formalin (solution of formalldehyde) need also a covering agent capable of disguising formaldehyde odour. Perfumery supply houses, aware of this need, have perfected blends stable in the presence of the aldehyde and possesing such odours as fruity, heliotrope, sweet vanillin, jasmin, lavender, lilac, pine. These are normally used at the rate of 1/2 oz to the gallon of formalin. Similar blends are specially compounded as 'cover' for the odours of isoprohyl alchol, acetone and para dichlorobenzene as used in various household cleaners, polishes, lavatory deodrants etc.

Incense and fumincs

Incense and fumigants represents the oldest method of perfumer realease: the buring of fragrant woods, spices, resins and balsams, a parctice which in itself gave rise to the word perfume (per, fumum= through,, smoke). The burning of these fragrant material has persisted through the ages and is extremely widespread geographically. Among the odorants commonly used in incense cones, joss sticks, agarbatties, Armenian papers and fumigants of all types-often in association with charcoal, saltpetre and ammucilaginous binding agent are:

Olibanum (incense] frankincense), nenzoin, myrrh, labaanum, styrax, mastic elemi, tolu, Peru and other oleoresins and balsams: sandal, agar, deodar, cedar, cascarilla and other woods; clovesand cinnamon bark; vetiver, patchouli, sandle, cedear and various other essential lils; and, finally, a number of crystalline synthetics of sweet, persistant odour, including vanillin, coumarin, heliotropin, rose crystals and the nitro-musks.

Perfumed Candles

The most popular type of scented fumigant in India is currently the so-called fragrance candle. Candles which give off a pleasant aroma, whether they are lit or unlit are helping to lift the sales of the 'gift candle' even above its present annual level of over Rs. 150 million. Seven firms appear to account for most of the market. The perfume, which must be soluble in the waxstearic acid candle base, may be present in proportions ranging from 2 to 5 per cent or even, exceptionally, 7 or 8 percent. Of these the most successful seem to be these with floral-fruity, spicy, strawberry, coconut and vanilla notes, but special praise is accorded to Avon's Charisma and Moonwind, which are attractively perfumed when unlit and 'strong and true' when bunring.

Paints and Polishes

The paint industry has introduced a host of new and useful products during the second half of the twentieth century, but the problem of paint's inherently malodorous character still remains. The worst offenders are solvents and thinners, oils and resins, as well as certain of the more specialised constituents such as anti-skinning agents. Vanillin andcoumarin are much used in much used paint and lacquer 'deodrants' (ie. as masking agents and reodorants). Sweet woody bouquets, violet vanilla, oriental and sweet citronella compositions, have found favour in this respect. An Indian patnet suggests the following formula for a Paint Deodoriser: amyl butyrate 6 parts, benzyl acetate 21.6, phebylethyl alcohol 31.2, citral 5.6, geraniol 20, phenylacetic acid 7.8, coucarin 7.8, while this is of some interest as a specific reference, few industrial perfumers would feel unable, we think, to improve upon it, and to do so without infringing upon the patentee's claims in any way.

Much thought has to go into the divising of paint odorants. Too much perfumer, or perfume imperfectly compatible with the formula, may spoil the consistency, levelling, drying or even the adhesion or durability of the paint. The perfume should therefore have a good odour yield, even on dilution. Its various components should be able to mask the more volatile malodours of the solvents and the more persistent lower notes of synthetic resubs, oils etc. A typical perfumery supply house markets not only a series of solvent masking odorants and a matching series of resin-oil masking agents, but also special deodorant-perfumes for perosol paints and lacquers and 'masks' for sealers, primers and paint removers. A cosmetic house once supplied a perfume lacquer for painting inside chests of drawers and on the under-surface of chairs, small tables etc., in order to create an eclusive, long-lasting odour effect in the boudoir.

Polishes no longer reek of kerosene, paraffin or even oil of mirbane. Their basic ingredients are in general less malodorous than they were in the past. Pince, cedar, lavender and citrolella types of perfume are among those used for the improvement of furniture polish odours. Among the odorants commonly used are safrole, bornyl acetate, terpinolene, terpineol, steam--distilled pine, oil, spike and lavandin oils, coumarin, musk xylol. Shoe polishes still tend to smell of bitter almonds but cuir de Russie, lavender, pine, woody and lilac compounds are all on offer to the more enterprising leather polish manufactures.

Other Household Products

Other household products that call for specialised perfuming are adhesives of various types (e.g. with minty lilac or carnation clove compounds), laundry starch, paradichlorbezene blocks, lavotry bowl cleaners, plastive sheeting, paper tissues and dry cleaning fluids. With the adevent of micro-encapsulated perfumes the range of 'reodorisation' has been further extended to cover reactive products in which some normal, unprotected odorants would be unstable.

Perfuming Cosmetics

Perfumes devised for use in cosmetics and toilet preparations have to be dermatologically acceptable as well as aesthetically appealing and chemically and physically compatible. In one of our several studies on the perfuming of cosmetics and particularly of cosmetic emulsions, i.e. creams of both solid and liquid types, Pandaetal has introduced the subject in the following terms.

'So far as handkerchief perfumes are concerned, the technologist has relatively few problems, except, of course, to produce a food and economical perfume. In the field of cosmetics the difficulties are more numerous and often very complex. Creams containing alkali, even when neutralised by fatty acids, present problems of stability and discoloration. Many perfumery ingredients darken on exposure to light, or form coloured compounds with other substances. In the presence of soaps this discoloration may be accentated. In lotions the colour question may still exist, but the problem of emulsion stability is more vital. Emulsions are adversely affected or modified by certain perfumery ingredients. This effect holds good for firm creams but is less apparent, and a considerable time may elapse before signs of changes in consistency are observed.'

Much has been written on the subject of perfumes that can give rise to primary irritation (these being very few in number and best avoided in cosmetic practice) and those that may provoke reactions of an allergic nature on certain hypersenstive skins. Perfumes and perfumed cosmetics are nowadays increasingly subjected to stringent dermatological 'prophetic *ptch*', 'repeated insult' and other specially devised tests before they are distributed for sale to the general public. 'Allergic reactions due to cosmetics and especially to perfume oils are extremely rare, and notably so if one relates them to the amounts used daily.'

Adapting the perfume to the vehicle

All perfumers know, that odorants and combination so odorants and exhibit variable odour characteristics according to the medium in which they are used. 'A given composition, when incorporated in a hair oil, reveals a quite different odour from that which its has when used in a powder or as a simple alcoholic solution. A similar type of odour shift occurs when the perfumed product is put to use, i.e. when the cream or lotion is applied to the hair.' The wish on the part of a manufacturer to produce a range of cosmetic products with an identical odour confronts the perfumer with problem, namely that each of the products will have a separate effect on the perfume. In order to achieve the same odour to achive the same odour effect (e.g. with a water base, a water-alcohol solution, an oil-in-waer emulsion,an anionic shampoo, a water-in-oil emulsion and a clear ol bas) it is necessary to balance the perfume composition for each and every preparation.'

In some cases the variation in odour, using a simple standard formula in several different vehicles, may not be excessive, but in most cases some special modifications will have to be made in the standard perfume formula in order to ensure a constant level, throughout the series, of characteristic odour effect and intensity. The odour yield or relative intensity of anisic alcohol or phenylethyl alcohol in a watery base is much lower that of the more water-insoluble amyl salicylate or geranyl acetate. Jellinek has suggested a classification of odorants on these lines and has shown, in two specially devised formulae, how two parts of coumarin in a mineral oil base will have to be replaced by six parts in a water base, if the same apparent odour effect and intensity are to be obtained. The respective figures for phenylethl alcohol area 10 and 30, but in the case of amyl salicylate the effect is reversed and they become 10 and 1.5, while for geranyl acetate they are 10 and 0.6 and for alphaionone 2 and 0.3.

Perfuming Creams

Work on the surface activity of odorants has helped materially to show how and why such substances can, according to their exact chemical type and structure, interfere more or less-and sometimes deleteriously-with the structure of cosmetic emulsions. Thus terpineol is an extremely active substance and can make or break an emulsion. It has an adverse effect upon certain work-in-oil emulsions and in many cases will break a cream in which wool wax is the emulsifying agent.' Moreover, 'benzyl alcohol tends to splubilise or peptise emulsifiers and greatly change the nature of an emulsified product'. With a fore knowledge of such reactivities and of the behaviour of conventional cosmetic emulsifying systems anionic, cationic, nonionic etc. it is possible to avoid most of the pitfalls and formulate cream perfumes which will not unduly affect either viscosity or stability.

Apart from dermatological and physico-chemical consideration, the perfumer has also to take into account the type of perfume to be used in a cream and the level at which it should be incorporated. Simple floral perfumes are not so widely used as formerly, although rose-bsed bouquets, being satisfactory from so many points of view, are still justly popular. The proportion of any perfume used in a cream is best arrived at by joint decision of the perfumer and the cosmetic chemist, but in general it will lie betwen 0.15 and 0.6 per cent of the total formula.

Perfuming Powders

The perfuming of cosmetic powders is one of the most difficult tasks confronting the perfumer. Powders are usually mixtures of materials, each with different structures and absorption characteristics. The separate constituents may and often do differ from source to source or even from delivery to delivery. Talc is a notable case in point. Changing the grade of talc can readily modify the perfume odour and increase or decreases its intensity. Such phenomena call for the closest co-operation between perfumer, cosmetic chemist and the quality control laboratory.

When a perfume is intimately distributed throughout a powder of fine particle size, the exposed surface may be very great and the likelihood of evaporation and oxidation correspondingly increased; particularly when a pack has been opened and the contents exposed. This calls not only for careful selection of perfumery materials and expert compounding but also for equal care in the choice of re-sealable containers such as talcum canisters. If plastic packs are used in place of metal adequate tests have to be carried out to ensure that the plastic is one which does not allow too marked a loss to take place through it. The rate of vapour loss of individual odorants through the plastic walls of a container varies, with the result that a blended perfume subjected to loss of this kind soon becomes unbalanced and of altered character.

Talcs, kaolins and diatomaceous earths have their own, often earthy odours and an inadequate powder perfume will sometimes allow this inherent offodour to 'show through'. Much pre-testing of odourants in these bases is often desirable before compounding and testing perfumes for use in face, talcum, body and baby powder to Typical proportions of perfume range from 0.2 per cent for baby powders to 1.5 or even 3 per cent for face powders.

Perfuming Lipstick and Nail Laquer

Lipstick perfumes must to some extent be flavours, but the general aim is to make them have a pleasant taste without actually suggesting flavour-appeal. There are many odorants with a bitter or othersise objectionable flavour, and these are to be avoided.

The banana or pear odour of nail lacquers based on nitrocellulose and volatile solvents is not invariably liked, but the masking of this odour is difficult in view of both the volatility and strong odour of the vehicle. It is relatively easy to devise a perfume which will persist on the nails after the lacquer film has dried, but what the nail varnish manufacturer would prefer to have, is a nail lacquer which has a pleasant odour in the bottle and while drying leaves behind a film which isodorless.

Hair Preparation Perfumes

The thioglycollates present in hair waving and depilatory formulae have the disadvantages, from the perfumery point of view, of possessing strong and unpleasant odours of their own, of liberating sulphutous odours upon reaction with the hair or skin, of being reactive with some perfumery chemicals; and of involving alkaline condition which of themselves are unfavourable to certain odourants. Some helpful suggestions are to be found in the perfumery literature, relating to the behaviour of some 200 odorants in ammonium thioglycollate solution, and to the suggested perfuming of depilatories with combinations of camphoraceous woody and herbal notes, rosemary, patchouli, spicy, ambered and musky botes etc.

Shampoos must have a pleasant odour in the bottle and also leave behind an attractive aura, more or less persistent on the dried hair. Some perfumes have a marked and, of course, undesirable softening effect upon hair lacquer films. Perfumes for use in hair sprays should not contain excessive amounts of osorans (e.g. terpenol) having a solvent action on the resin content; they should not, moreover, contain more than a limited proportion of highboilong' constituents, as these can unduly prolong the drying time.

Bath salts and bath oils are often highly perfumed. The former may have to be alkali-resistant.

Perfumed Aerosols

The traditional handkerchief perfume consistuents of a number of odorous constituents dissolved in alcohol. its aerosol or pressure-packed equivalent exists as an alcohol-odorants solution in association with a liquefied propellant, usually of the halogenated hydrocarbon type. Consideration of the stability of perfume packaged in such a pressurized container should take into account the influence of the propellants (Freon II being the least satisfactory of this series for the purpose), the influecne of other constitutents of the aerosol formula the effect of the valve matertial and the effect of the metal container. In a chromatographic study of the action of propellants on the perfume constituents of aerosols, Aime and peyron found that only certain aldehydes (hydroxycitronellal, decanal and undercanal) under went chemical modification, viz. acetalization, under the conditions of testig, and then onlu in Freon II conventionally stabilised with nitromethane. Hydrocarbons, a alcohols, carbinols, esters, ethers, ketones, lactones and nitro-compounds were apparently unaffected. Even the modified aldehydes remained unchanged when the nitromethane stabiliser in the Freon II was replaced by 1 in 10,000 of morpholone, o-tolyl biguamide or diphenylamine.

In one of the most comprehensive studies of aerosol perfumes, it is suggested that propionates and lemon oil should in general be avoided, and ionones and orange oil chosen with care.

Perfumes in non-alcoholic vehicles include the perfumed candles already discussed; also other solid perfumes such as perfumed pomades, solid Colognes, and the briquetted used as moth repellants and to impart an elusive odour to linen cupboards. The perfumed made was the forerunner of the solid cream sachet and this, in turn, gave rise to the liquid cream sachet. Liquid sachets may contain up to 10 or 12 per cent of perfume oil, and this naturally gives rise to problems of stability. The perfumer will avoid readily hydrolysable odorants and other materials likely to favour emulsion breakdown and discoloration, and in this may be assisted by keeping the emulsion on the acid side, at a pH betwen 5 and 6. The old-style European Sachets were of course small cushion-shaped bags ofgragrant pourri. So called solid Colognes usually have a high content of menthol.

In Pharmacy and Medicine

We have already asked why disinfectants should smell like disinfectants. And 'should liniments smell like liniments?' making a plea for non-malodorous sembrocation, liniments chest rubs and sports lotions, he suggests not only the use of less pungent active ingredients but also the incorporation of such odorants as clove, thyme, rosemary, lavender, camphor, sassafrass, cedar and cedar leaf, aniseee, eucalyptus, mint and other essential oils, as well as isolated and synthetics.Capsicum oleoresin and tincture are among the odorants materials which also function as rubefacients and counter-irritants.

Nasal douche tablets, sprays and inhalants commonly contain odorants. T-M-E- nasal sprays in India are based on thymol, menthol and eucalyptol.

Perfumes have in fact been used. for centuries in medical and pharmaceutical (not to say alchemical) practice Certain odorants are of special utility, quite apart fro their odoraiferous character, as antiseptics bacteroustats, fungistants, carminatives, anodynes, mild local anaesthetics and cooling agents, fumigants, inhants, counter-irritants etc. Some essential oils promote expectorationby direct stimulation of the respiratory tract. The most effective oil for this purpose was anise, the runners up being oils of turpentine, pineeecucalytus and lemon.

The impact of perfumes and odours upon medicine dates back to the times when the burning of malodorous substances around a sick person was thought to be a means of driving out demons, and when odorants were used as disinfectants, carminatives, primitive transquillisers and of course, emblaming agents. Odour can be helpful, too, in diagnosis. Some diseases have distinctive odours. Attention has been given to the psychological and physiological excepts of odours and odorants, but even so the subject is still largely unexplored and could well repay serious investigation.

Industrial Perfumes

Perfumed gloves go back through the ages. Perfumed textiles are as old, in origin, as the wax and resin treated cere clothes used in embalming. In the 1930's Harris Tweed perfumes were devised for imparting to less expensive tweeds the characteristic mossy, peaty, healthery odour of the genuine Harris material. In 1938 perfume were devised for covering the off-odours imparted by dyes and other additives to crush-resistant velvet. At about the same period, in a blind test involving 1000 women it was shown that, from four pairs of stockings taken from the same batch, the one pair that had been faintly perfumed was considered by 96 per cent of the women as the best in quality, although nobody actually commented upon the odour. Women were concurrently being offered perfumed ribbons and plastic floral ornaments.

Perfumes for Textiles

Perfumes for textiles should be substantive to the material to be treated and yet sufficiently volatile to be readily perceived. That some odorants are remarkably persistent in these conditions may be appreciated when smelling a face cloth that has been used for soap-and-water washing for a deliberately prolonged period of several weeks. Notably persistent for example, are many of the synthetic musks, patchouli, gamma-undecalactone and methyl nonyl acetaldehyded. Some compounds may have to withstand unsually high processing temperatures. Others may be expected to resist several washes.

Covering the solvent odour is the main function of reodorants devised for addition to dry cleaning fluids, although such masking agents may also be required to leave behind a faint residual perfume on the treated fabric or garmebt. In all cases adverse reactions between odorants and fabrics, dyes, finishing and profing agents etc. must be avoided.

Perfumed Ink and Paper

The perfuming of printing in has been given a good deal of attention and special perfumes have been devised to blend well with all kinds of printing inks without determent to the various printing processes. The proinks of perfume tends to range between 0.3 and 0.5 percent of the quantity of ink used, in the case of absorbent newsprint, to 1 per cent for normal effect is required.

Paper in many forms may be subjected to the perfumers techniques: not only paper perfumed by means of printing ink but spray-perfumed cards, programmes, stationery; as well as waxed wrapping papers, towels, tissues, toilet paper etc. According to one supply house oneof the most important uses of masking odours in the paper industry is in gummed papers.

Widely used in nearly all industries, gummed tapes have normally, an almost universally unpleasant odour and taste. A number of companies have endeavoured to eliminate either or both of these undesirable factors, and with the help of the perfume and flavour chemist very satisfactory results have been achieved. Masking odours of a peppermint or spearmint, sassafras, vanilla or spice type are commonly used and can be prepared in either oil or water-soluble form, depending upon the manufacturing process. In such instances it is usually an animal base glue that is the factory culprit, and this achesive is normally applied ho at around 130° to 140° F, although some so as high as 350° for a brief, finishing process. This requires an odour and/or flavour that will withstand such temperatures.

The masking compounds must possess unsusual stability, as the product is sometimes stored for as long as two years before actual use.

Clove 1 oil, safrol and methyl salicylate ae sometimes used but most satisfactory are spedifically developed compounds that give the proper coverage and stability together with the distinctiveness of a tailor-made product. Cost is an important factor and must be kept to a minimum. Compounds developed can usually be applied ina proportion of 0.1 per cent. Taped used in the food industry, particularly, are often masked, owing to the food industry, particularly, are often masked, owing to the unpleasant odour associated with the animal glue involved and for this application usually a nutralised effect, rather than a perfumed one, is desired.

Masking Malodours

The perfuming of wallpaper as a means of masking or offsetting any inherent malodour of the paper of adhesive is probably is a more attractive ideal than that of seeking to impart a noticeable and persistent odour by this means.

Synthetic rubber emulsions, widely used in industry, are distinguished by their offensively ammoniacal odour. This is frequently masked by specially prepared compounds. Natural rubber products such as rubber glue rubberised textiles, carpet and upholstery backings and shoe components, are also improved by the skills of the industrial perfumer. The same applies to plastics and other man-made materials and fabrics.

Perfume in Agriculture

Agricultural and hotricultural products, including fertilizers and insecticide sprays as well as cattle feeds and veterinary products, have been improved upon by the perfumer's art. as far back as the 'Fifties certian Indian perfumery laboratories were being asked to solve the problem of making sulphuric acid-treated phosphate rock less repulsive in odour. The residual odour of the finished superphosphates was successfully covered, one firm acclaiming to have produced as masking compound of so concentrated and economic a character that it was satisfactory when used at the level of 0.02 percent. This achievement gave impetus to the odour masking and 'reodorising' of all other types of commercial fertiliser, including those based on urea, fish solubles, activated sludge, dried bone meal, animal manure, tankage and meat offal.

The level of perfuming usually runs from 01. to 0.3 per cent. Odour intensity, masking ability and low price level are essential requirements.

Most odour-masked fertilisers are more likely to be found in horticultural consumer type packs, put up specially for home gardening, rather than in the average farmyard. Big farms have associated problems, however. One of the authors was consulted some years ago by a firm controling large-scale piggeries in the Western contry of England. Public complaint had been made of the wind carried odours from one of these piggeries. After laboratory tests with pig dung, urine, straw water and variety of odorantsm and the preliminary utilisation of a fan and wind tunnel, some suitable formulae were contrived. Thereafter, and for several years until the piggery was redesigned and later removed from the site, the through areas were sprayed with an emulsified solution containing such odorants as dimethyl hydroquinone, benzyle and bornyl acetates, methyl salicylete, citronella terpenes, terpinolene, diphynyl oxide etc., and what was then an inexpensive grade of Peru balaam.

Liquied fertilisers in bottles and powder fertiliser in bags or cartons may simply include a proportion of odour-masking compound or else may give a suggestion of a new mowm hay apple lot, fougere or moss odours. Some firms are said to have used rose, citrus, pine and vanilla compositions.

Perfumed Insecticides

The perfuming of insecticides is not likely to affect their insecticidal activitym, but this factor must nevertheless be considered. In most cases it is necessary to make the disagreeable odours of the active agents and/or solvents Pheromone research had led to the experimental production of both insect attractants and insect repellnts, based of course on species-specific odourous substances or compounds. Moreover, some essential oils have been proved to act synergistically, when added to fly sprays, by increasing the normal effectiveness of the effectiveness of pyrethrins in fly sprays tbe following were most suitable; Backhousia myrtifolia, Zieria smithii, Melaleuca bracteata and Huon pine (Dacrydium franklinii). Oil of backhousia is said to have proved more effecient than sesame oil, a widely accepted activator. Any capable perfumery supply house could, if requested, incorporate such oils in a pleasantly attractive perfume compound.

Many other uses

At least half a century ago perfumes were spraryed into cinemas in order to add another dimension, as it were, to the screened performance. Since that time special devices have been used to produce 'scented movies'. These include mechanical sprays for injecting perfumes in to the ventilating sustem, aerocols and electronic precipitators. Two proprietary processes are styled respectively 'Smell-O-Vision' and 'romarama'.

The perfuming of the Bombay Metroiin the 1950's a appeared to open up tremendous prospects of or the introduction of similar deodourant-reodorants and recently into other underground railways, but little enough in the event seems to have come of the idea.

Readers familiar with the buying of chemistry set for school boys may yet be unaware that, inthe late 1030's a perfume chemistry set was on sale in the U.S.A. The dit included 14 basic perfume chemicals, measuring and mixing aids, smelling slips and spare bottlesets., aopether with a book of instructions designed to team the student 'how to make perfume of various types'. At the other end to the time scale we find an expert on emblaming fluids refering to the use, on pre-treated cadavers, of oil of cedar, myrrh cinnamon and other aromatic substances.

The introduction of spray-dried and micro-encapsulated perfumes and flavours has further extended the scope of perfume application.

The smell Society, formed in London in 1935, had as its avowed objective 'preventing pollutionof the air and safeguarding the sense of smell. By the encouragement of good smells life will become a fuller and lovelier thing'. To which may perhaps be added the after thoughts 'Perfumes that persist on the skin: perfumes, even the most persistent, are volatile by definition and sufficiently evanescent in the conditions of use. Unfortunately in India we have not yet able to start such society.

Flavours as Perfumes

Finally one comes to the important use of odorants, both natural and synthetic, in the perparation of flavourings. The flavour of a good or beverage is a perfume plus as taste. That is why in a book on perfumery one must glance however briefly, at the subject of flavours. Taste is perceived by receptor spots or 'buds' on he tongue and elsewhere in the mouth, whereas the odour part isperceived by the nose and, 'Most of the discrimination attributed to the palate is really performed by the olfactory membrances'. The statistical occurrence of the true gourmet among perfumers and flavourists, food and wine tasters and chefs de cuisine, is likely to be at a higher level than one would find in the traditional ranks of bibulous clubmen and boardroom epicures.

Properly speaking the term 'flavouring' should be used to describe a substance employed to give a flavour. In 1970 the Council of Europe's working party on flavour proposed the following definitions 'a flavouring is a substance...which has predominately odour-production properties and which possibly affects the taste'. It is not mere coincidence that the world's most active and knowledgeable producers of synthetic odorants for perfumery also occupy approximately the same pre-eminent position in the field of artificial flavorings.

Biological and toxicological factors necessarily restrict the number of odorants that can be regarded as permissible for use in flavourings. Reference may be made in this respect to the GRAS (Generally Recognisd as Safe) list issued by the Flavouring Extracts Manufacturers' Association of America, and also to current information on international legislation as it affects flavourings.

The I.O.F.I. (International Organisation of the Flavour Industry), has initiated work on the evaluation of flavouring materials form the public health point of view.

The formulation classification and analysis of flavours have been interestingly discussed during the past decade. Among the flavourings thus dealt with in detail are fruit, beverage, liquerur, cordial and confectionery flavours; herbs, spices, sauce and curry flavours; tobacco, toothpaste and pharmaceutical flavours; and, of course, flavours for all types of 'convenience foods' and protein replacements.

4

Infrared Spectra of Some Naturally Occuring Sequiterpene Hydrocarbons

Sesquiterpene hydrocarbons occur in most of the essential oils. They are generally found as complex mixtures of closely related isomers. Identification of partcular sesquiterpene hydrocarbon and its quantity help us to formulate speciality cosmetics and fragrance compounds. The purity of the each compounds isolated was checked by gas chromatography. Fig. 1-36.

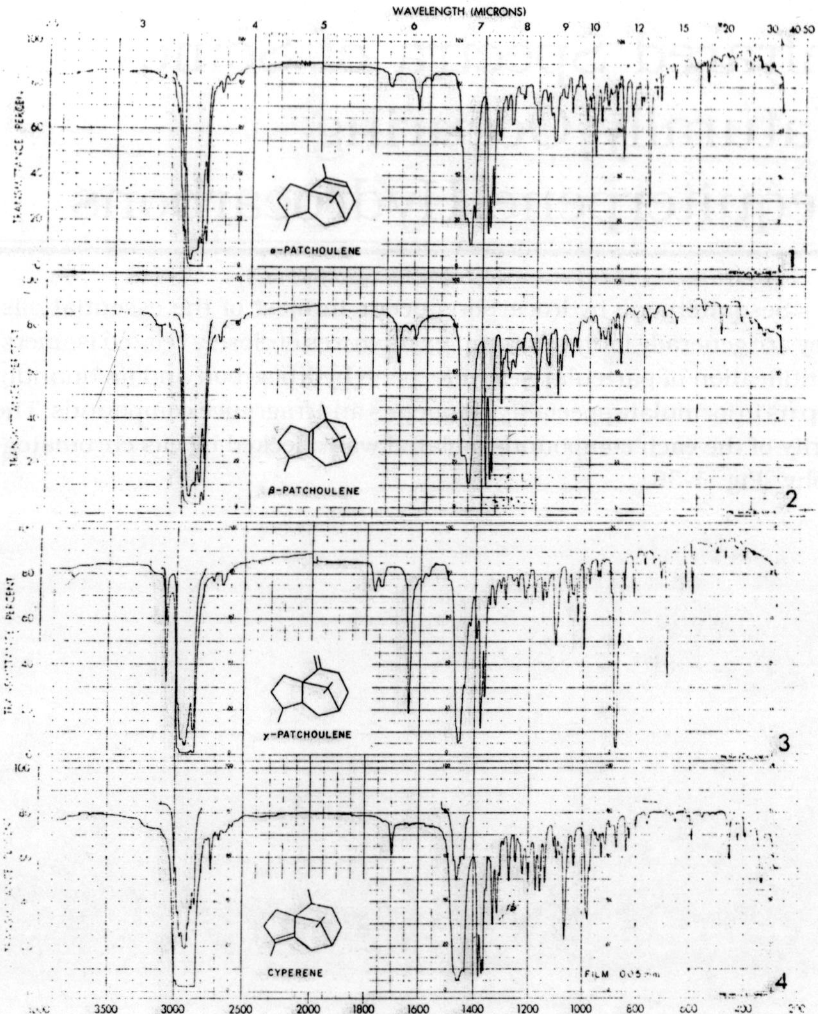
WAVELENGTH (MICRONS)
TRANSMITTANCE PERCENT
α-PATCHOULENE
1
β-PATCHOULENE
2
γ-PATCHOULENE
3
CYPERENE
FILM 0.05 mm
4
FREQUENCY (CM⁻¹)

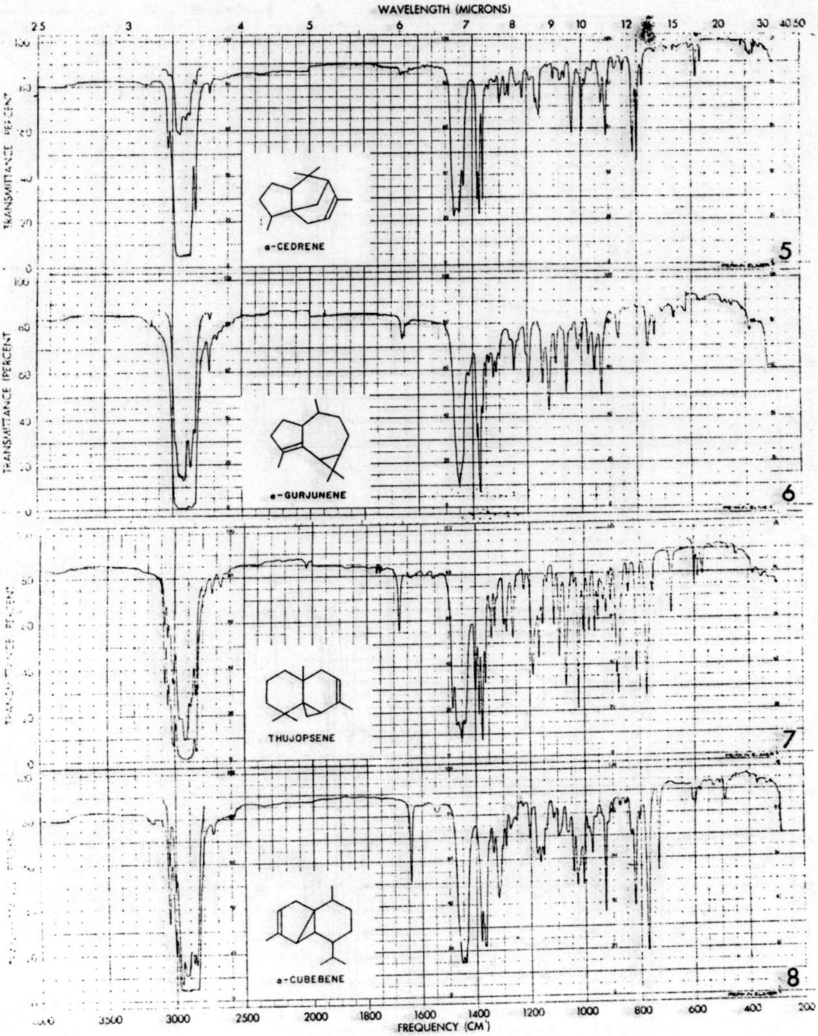
WAVELENGTH (MICRONS)
TRANSMITTANCE (PERCENT)
α-CEDRENE
5
α-GURJUNENE
6
THUJOPSENE
7
α-CUBEBENE
8
FREQUENCY (CM⁻¹)

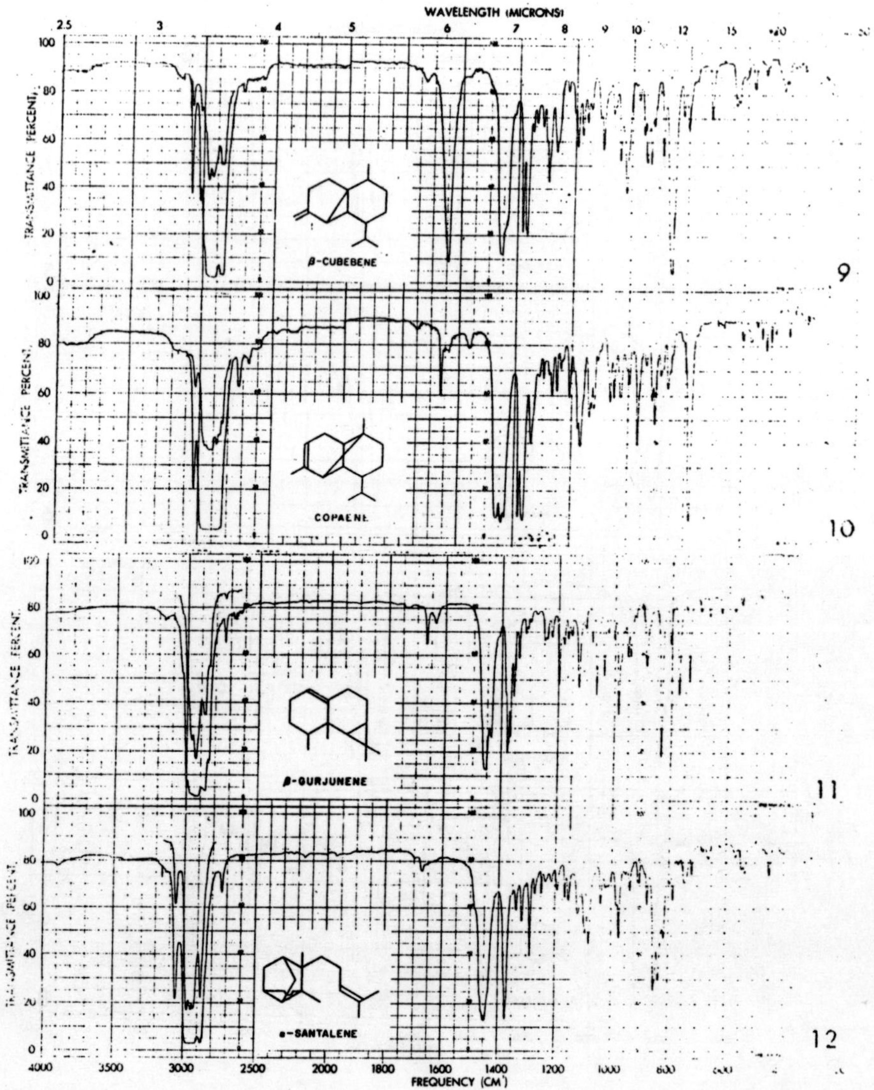
WAVELENGTH (MICRONS)
TRANSMITTANCE PERCENT
β-CUBEBENE
COPAENE
β-GURJUNENE
α-SANTALENE
FREQUENCY (CM⁻¹)

9

10

11

12

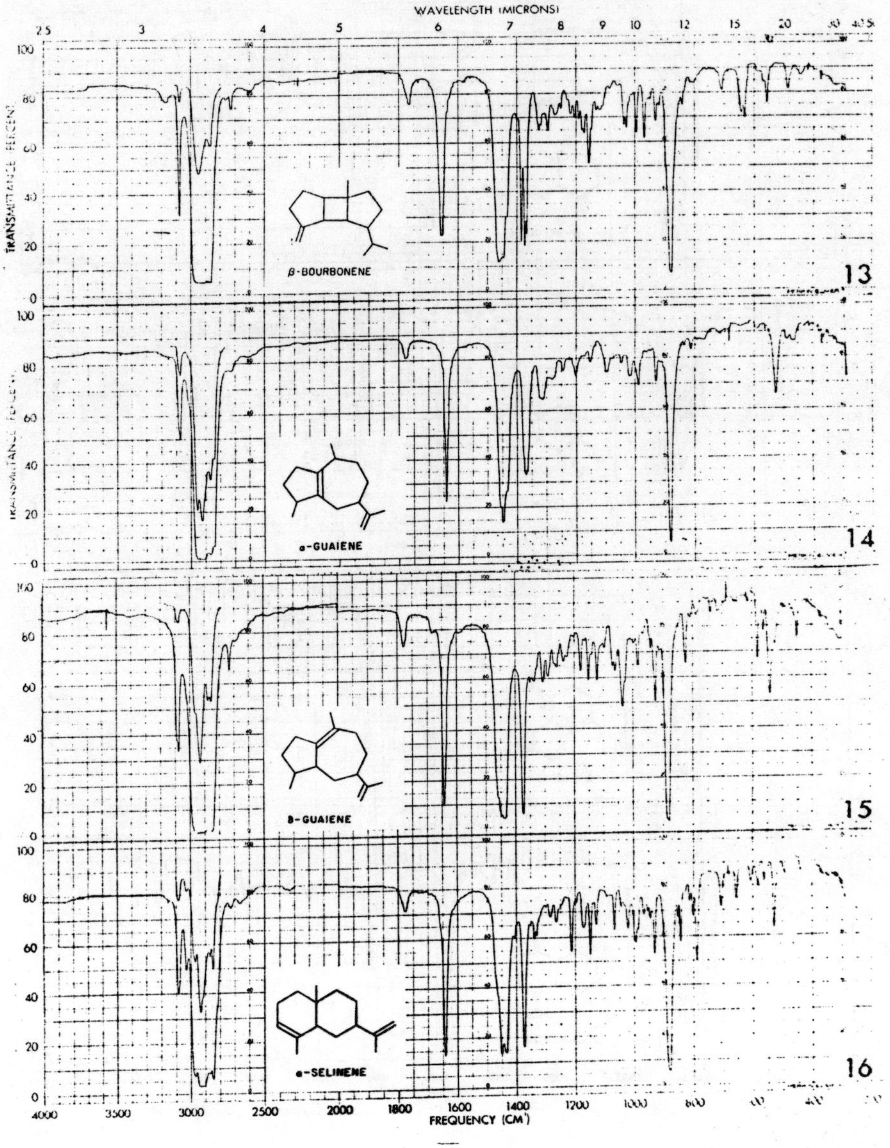
WAVELENGTH (MICRONS)
TRANSMITTANCE PERCENT
β-BOURBONENE
13
α-GUAIENE
14
β-GUAIENE
15
α-SELINENE
16
FREQUENCY (CM⁻¹)

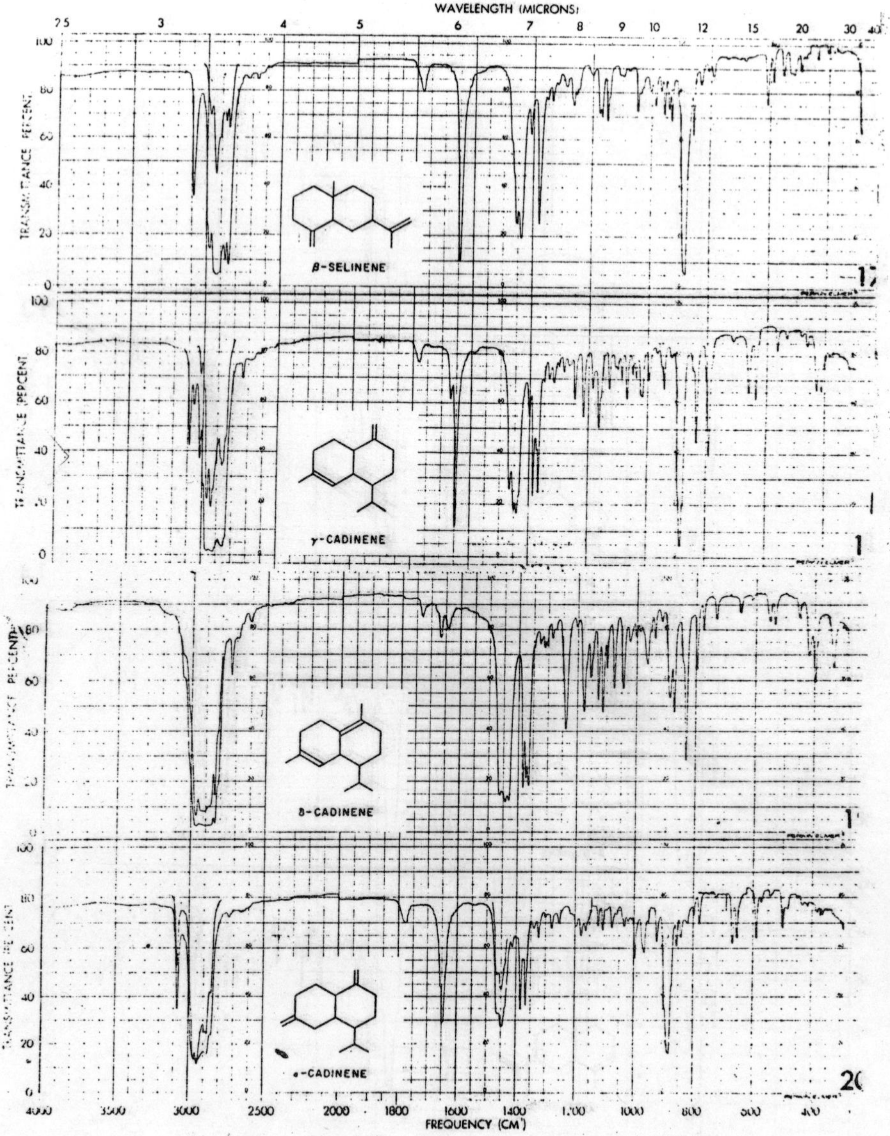
WAVELENGTH (MICRONS)
TRANSMITTANCE PERCENT
β-SELINENE
γ-CADINENE
δ-CADINENE
ε-CADINENE
FREQUENCY (CM⁻¹)

Infrared Spectra of Some Naturally Occuring Sequiterpene Hydrocarbons

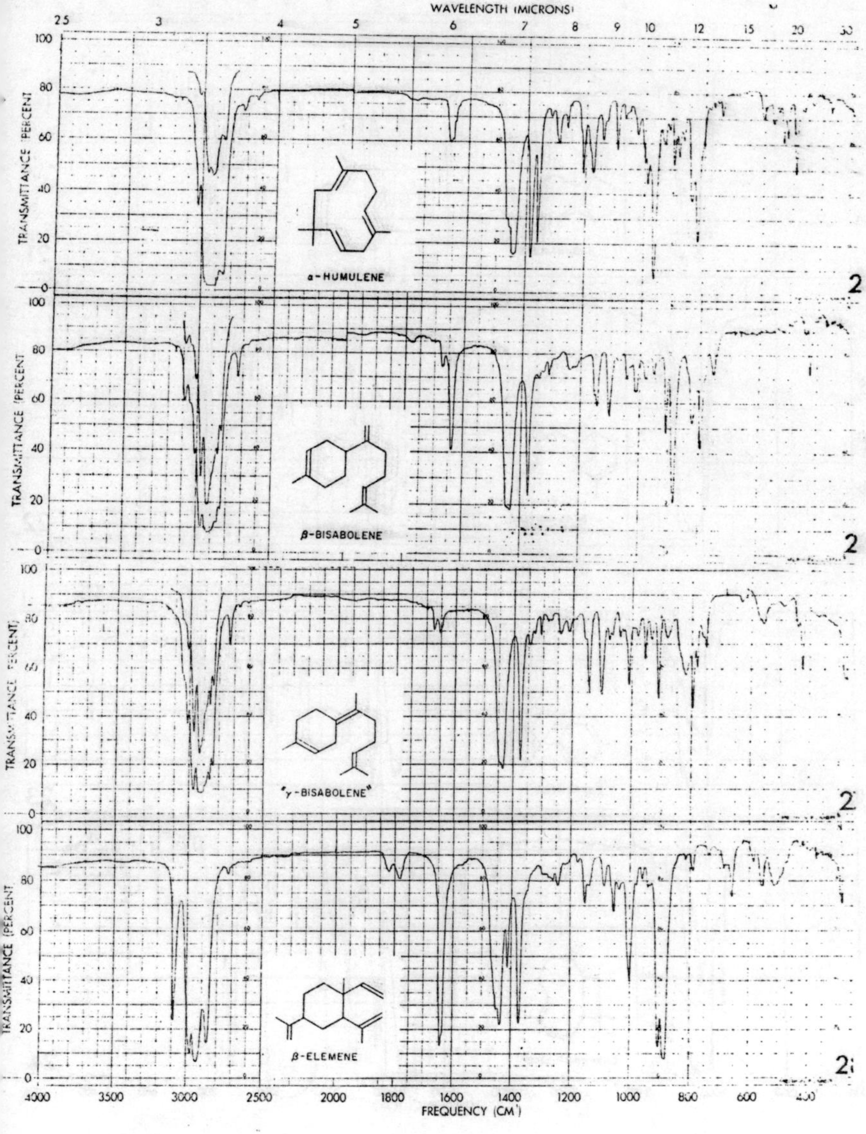

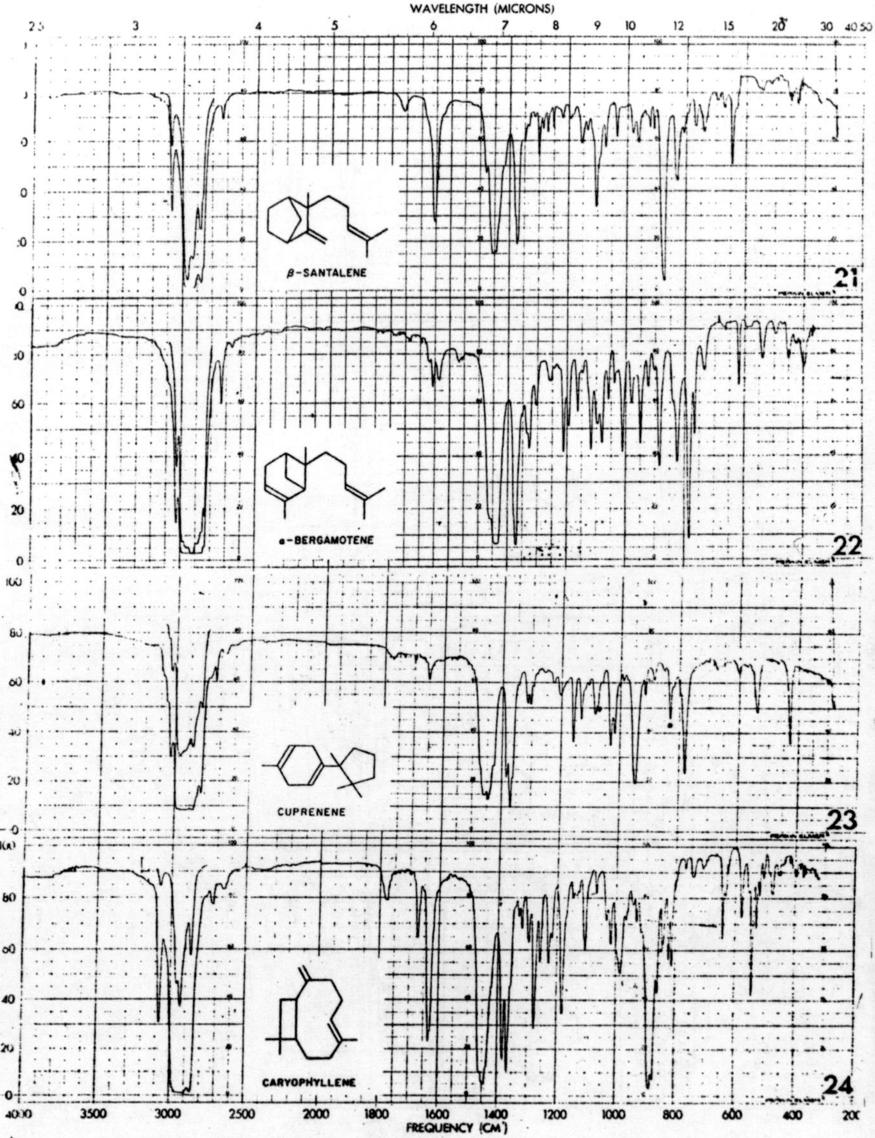
WAVELENGTH (MICRONS)
β-SANTALENE
21
α-BERGAMOTENE
22
CUPRENENE
23
CARYOPHYLLENE
24
TRANSMITTANCE
FREQUENCY (CM⁻¹)

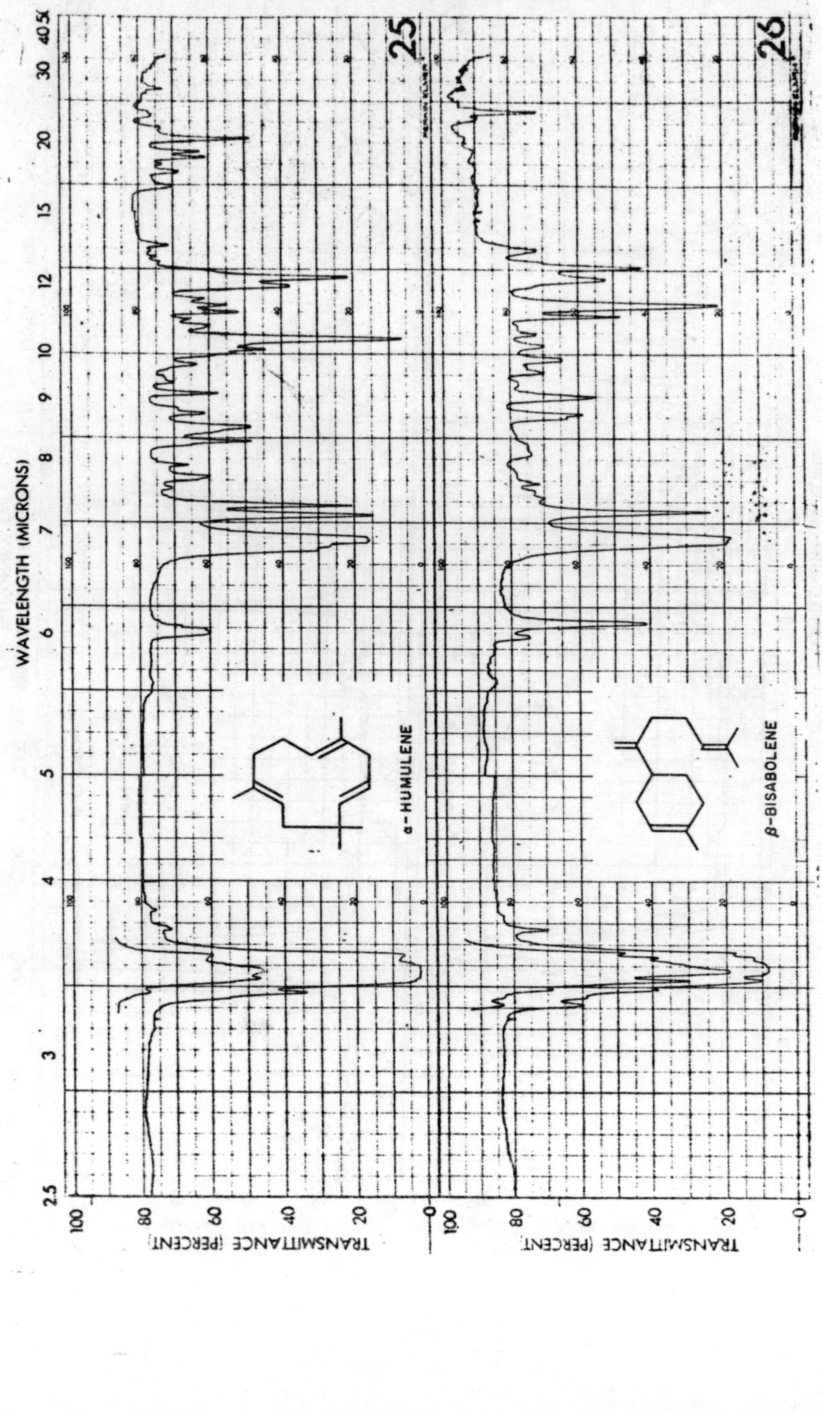
WAVELENGTH (MICRONS)
TRANSMITTANCE (PERCENT)
25
α-HUMULENE
26
β-BISABOLENE

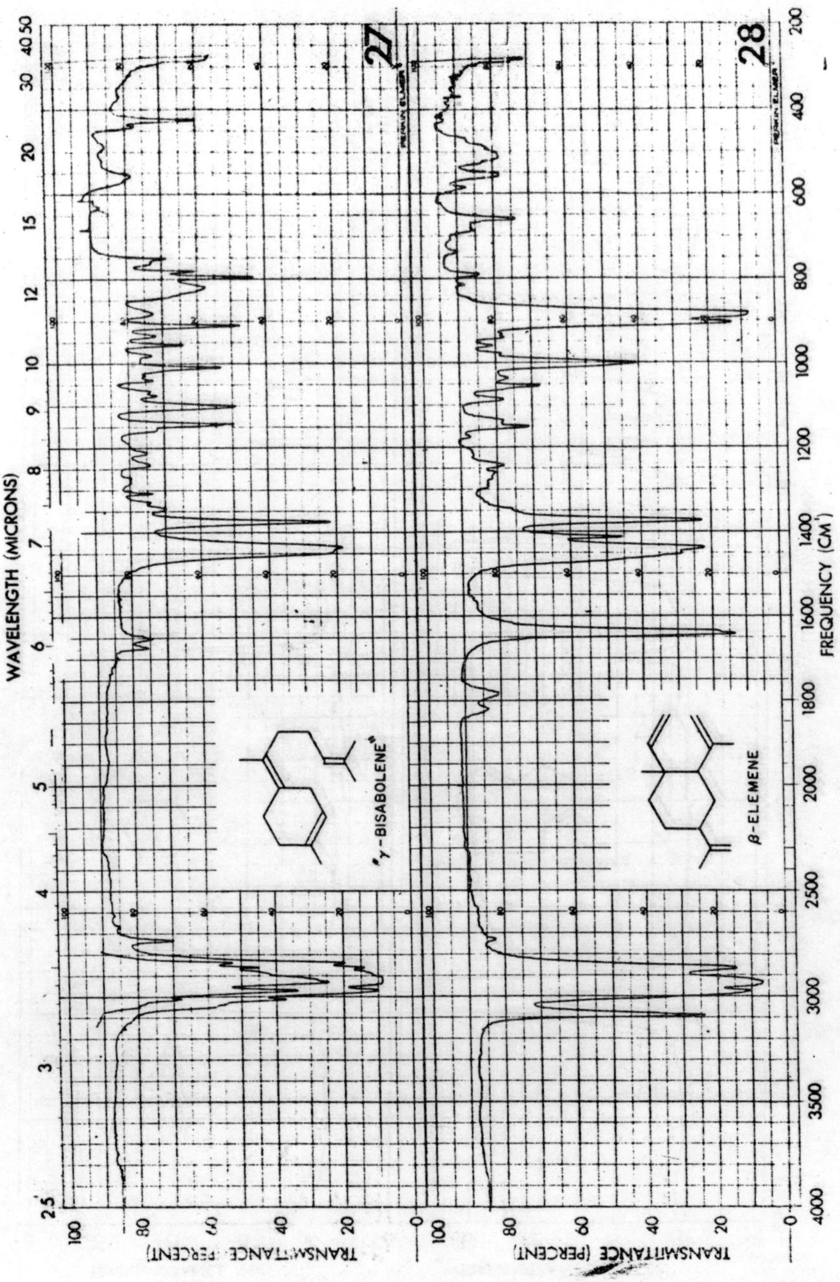
WAVELENGTH (MICRONS)
FREQUENCY (CM⁻¹)
TRANSMITTANCE (PERCENT)
27
28
"γ-BISABOLENE"
β-ELEMENE

5

Infrared Spectra of Fragrance Compounds

The routine analysis of a fragrance oil by a combination of gas liquid chromatography (GLC) and infrared spectroscopy (IR) requires a number of standard IR spectra to enable the analyst to identify the fragrance compounds isolated. For this purpose, we have compiled a library of standard IR spectra of fragrance compounds. Fig. 1-99. In the past, difficulty was frequently encountered when we tried to identify an isolated fragrance compound by direct comparison with the IR spectra of commercial products. Upon examination of some of these commercial fragrance compound we found that they were frequently mixtures of 2 or more components. The IR spectra obtained from these commercial samples are often, therefore, not suitable for identification purposes. For this reason, the decision was made to compile a library of IR spectra of GLC purified fragrance compounds.

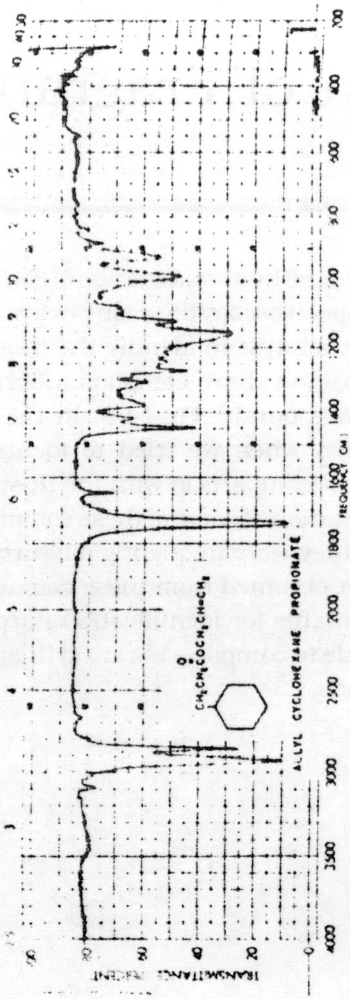
ALLYL CYCLOHEXANE PROPIONATE
FREQUENCY (CM-1)
TRANSMITTANCE (PERCENT)

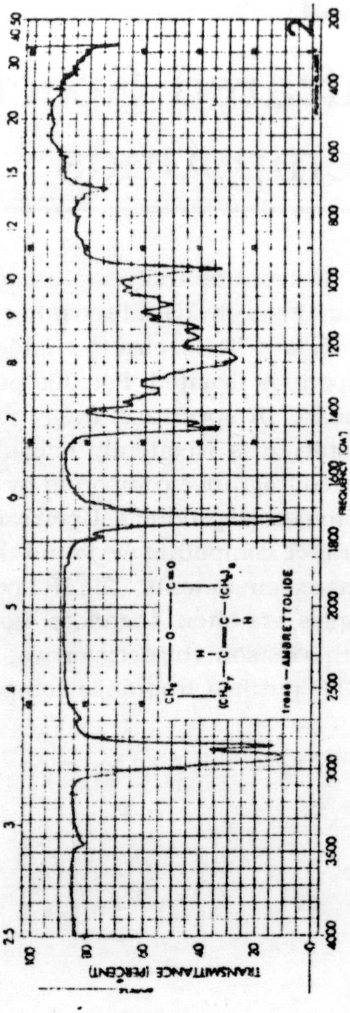
trans—AMBRETTOLIDE
WAVELENGTH (MICRONS)
FREQUENCY (CM-1)
TRANSMITTANCE (PERCENT)

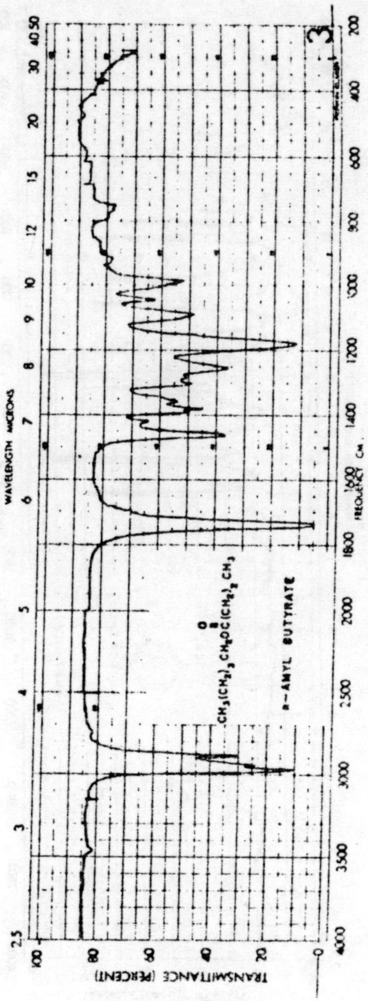
WAVELENGTH MICRONS
TRANSMITTANCE (PERCENT)
FREQUENCY CM.
n-AMYL BUTYRATE
3

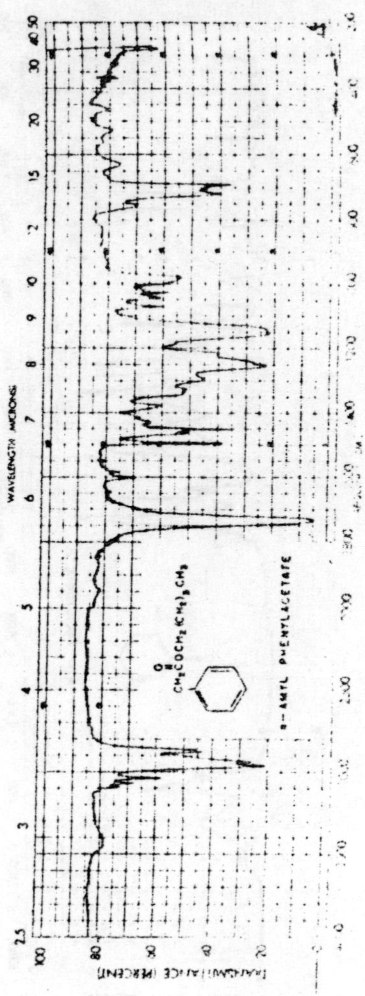
WAVELENGTH MICRONS
n-AMYL PHENYLACETATE
4

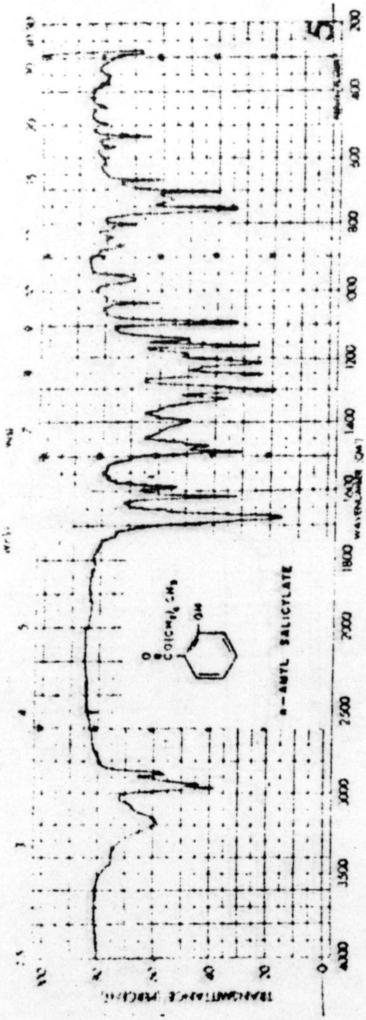
n-AMYL SALICYLATE

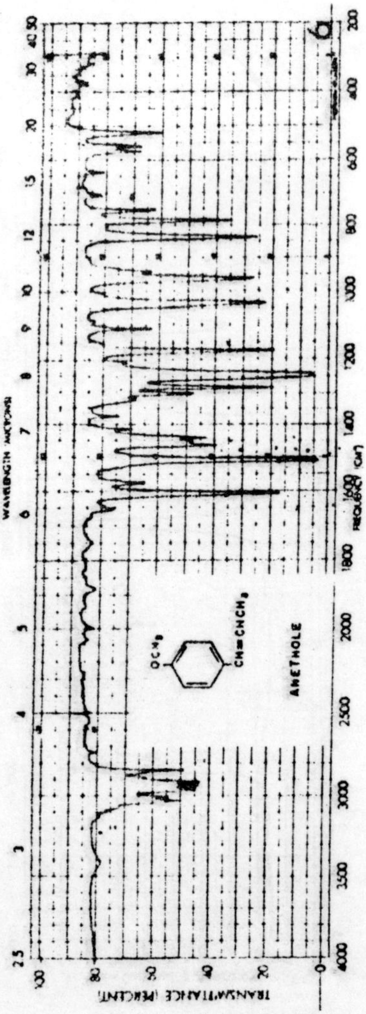
ANETHOLE

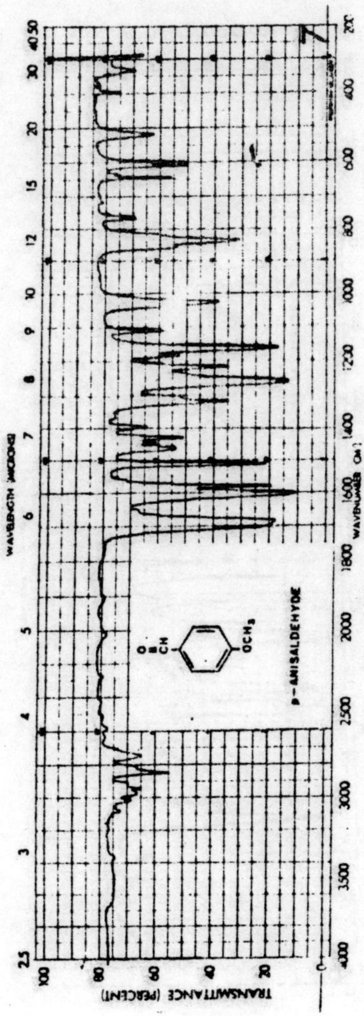
WAVELENGTH (MICRONS)
WAVENUMBER CM-1
TRANSMITTANCE (PERCENT)
p-ANISALDEHYDE
7

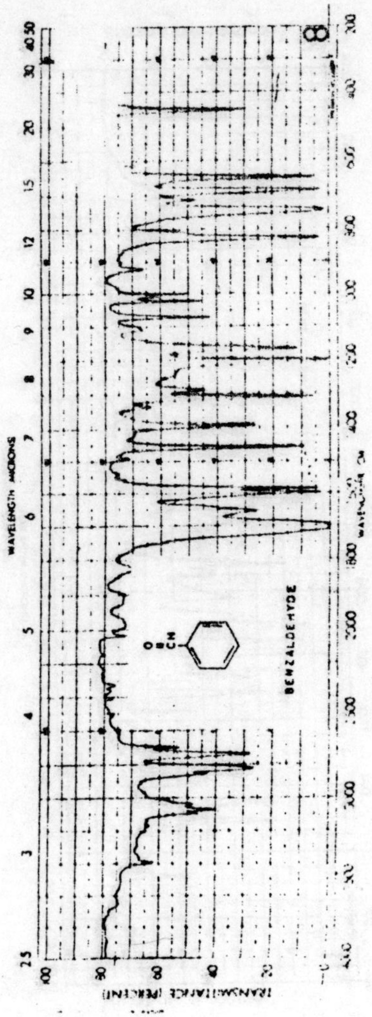
WAVELENGTH (MICRONS)
TRANSMITTANCE (PERCENT)
BENZALDEHYDE
8

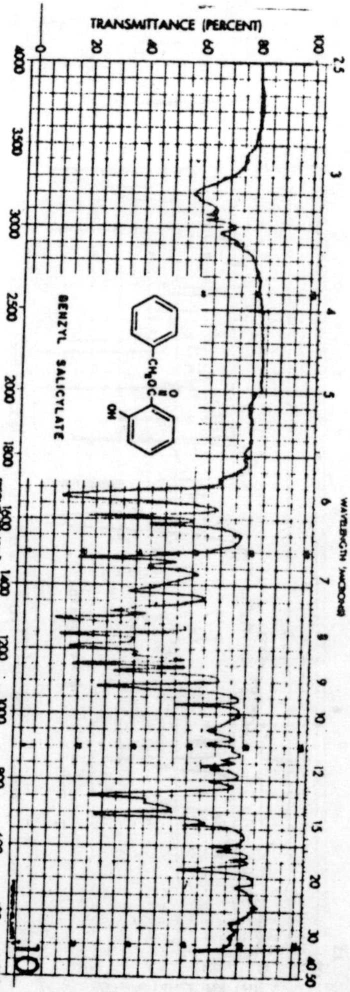
TRANSMITTANCE (PERCENT)
BENZYL SALICYLATE
WAVELENGTH (MICRONS)
FREQUENCY (CM-1)
10

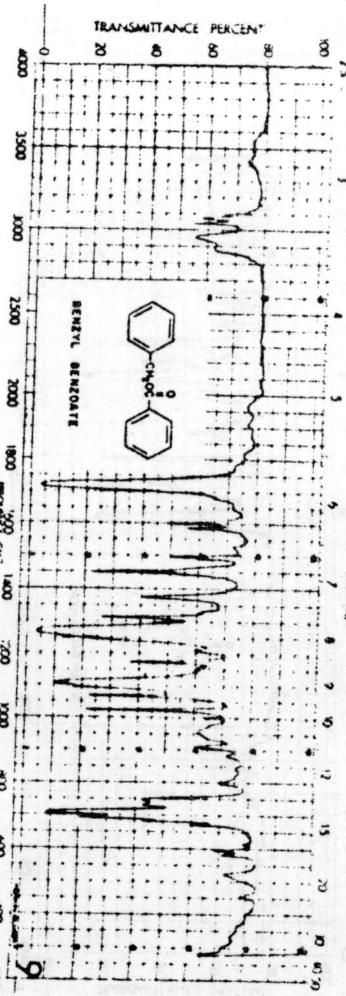
TRANSMITTANCE PERCENT
BENZYL BENZOATE
FREQUENCY (CM-1)
9

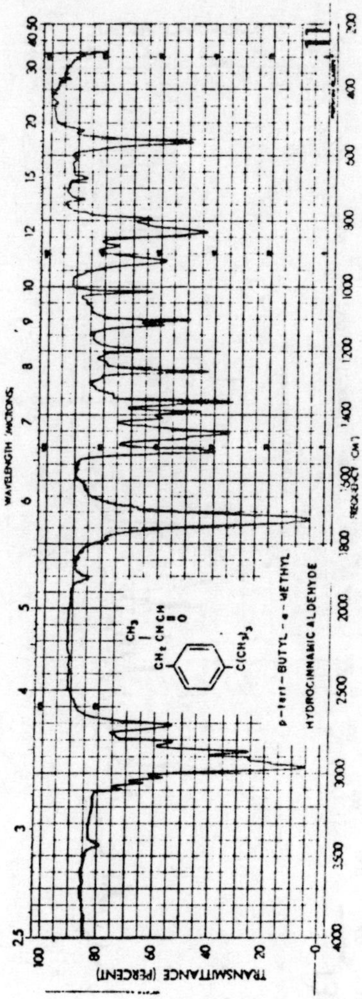
WAVELENGTH (MICRONS)
TRANSMITTANCE (PERCENT)
FREQUENCY (CM⁻¹)
p-tert-BUTYL-α-METHYL HYDROCINNAMIC ALDEHYDE
11

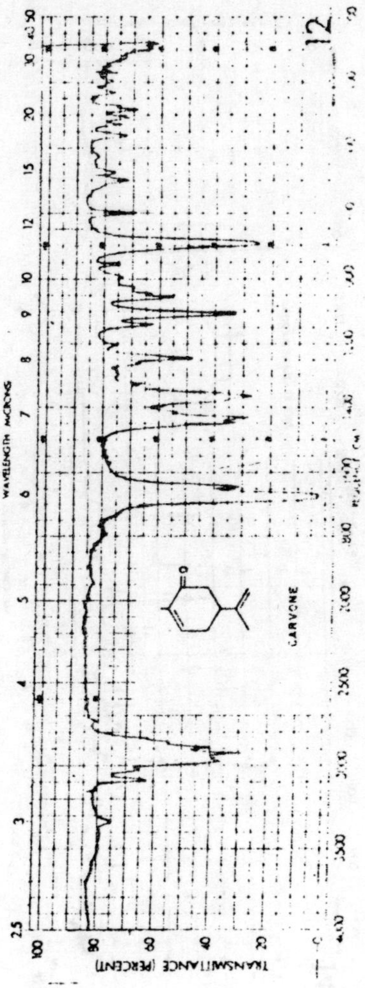
WAVELENGTH (MICRONS)
TRANSMITTANCE (PERCENT)
CARVONE
12

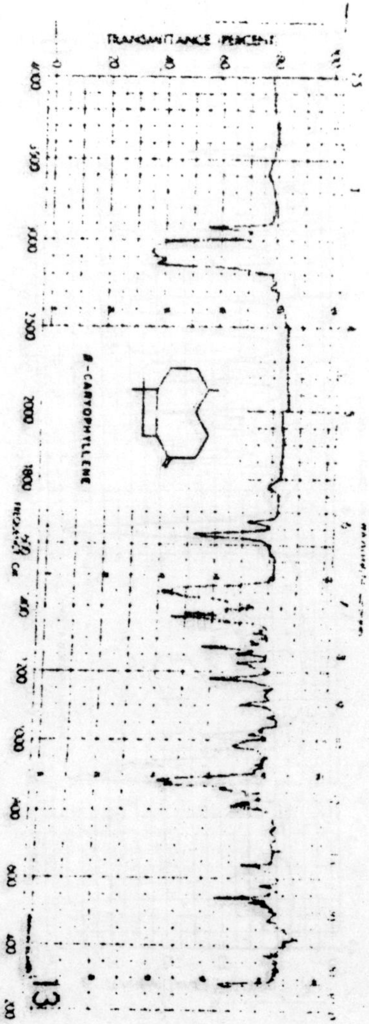
TRANSMITTANCE (PERCENT)
β-CARYOPHYLLENE
13

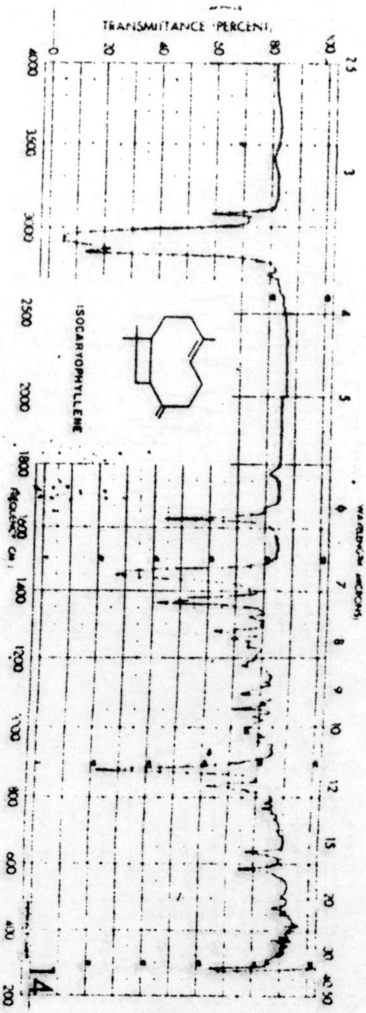
TRANSMITTANCE (PERCENT)
WAVELENGTH (MICRONS)
ISOCARYOPHYLLENE
FREQUENCY (CM⁻¹)
14

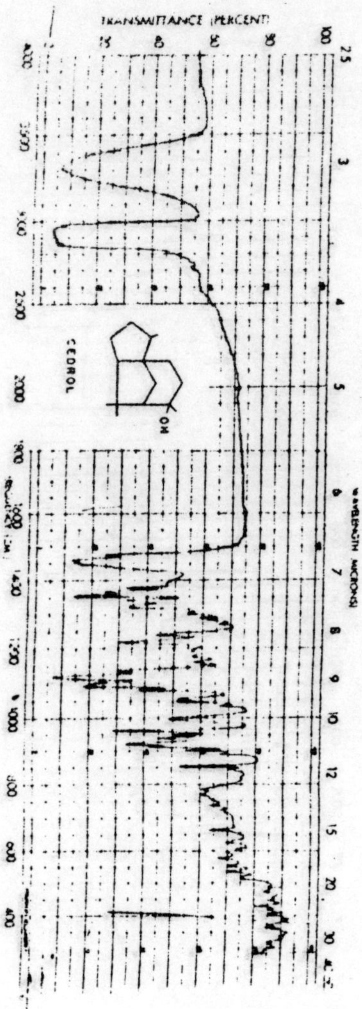
TRANSMITTANCE (PERCENT)
WAVELENGTH (MICRONS)
CEDROL
OH

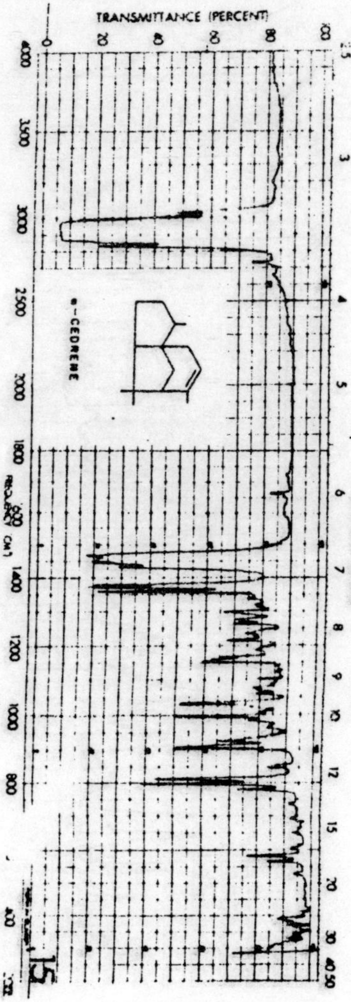
TRANSMITTANCE (PERCENT)
WAVELENGTH (MICRONS)
FREQUENCY (CM⁻¹)
α-CEDRENE

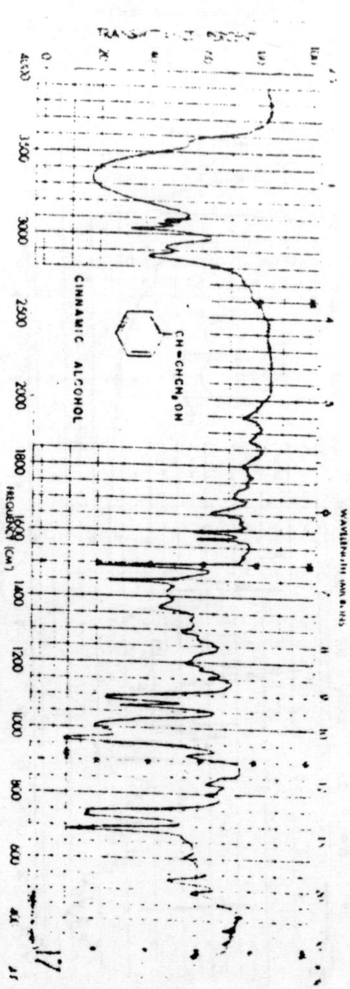
TRANSMITTANCE PERCENT
WAVELENGTH (MICRONS)
FREQUENCY (CM⁻¹)
CH=CHCH₂OH
CINNAMIC ALCOHOL
17

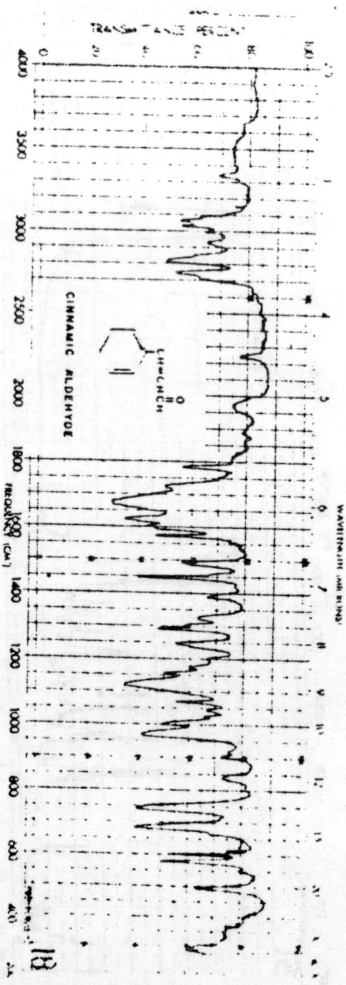
TRANSMITTANCE PERCENT
WAVELENGTH (MICRONS)
FREQUENCY (CM⁻¹)
CH=CHCH
CINNAMIC ALDEHYDE
18

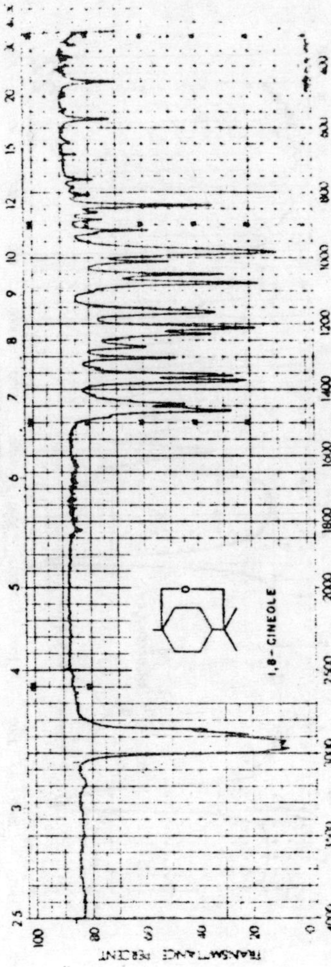
WAVELENGTH (MICRONS)
FREQUENCY (CM⁻¹)
TRANSMITTANCE (PERCENT)
1,8-CINEOLE

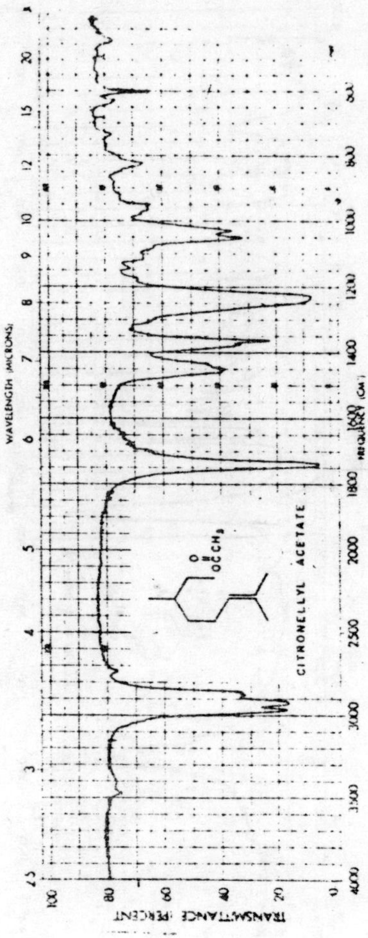
WAVELENGTH (MICRONS)
FREQUENCY (CM⁻¹)
TRANSMITTANCE (PERCENT)
CITRONELLYL ACETATE

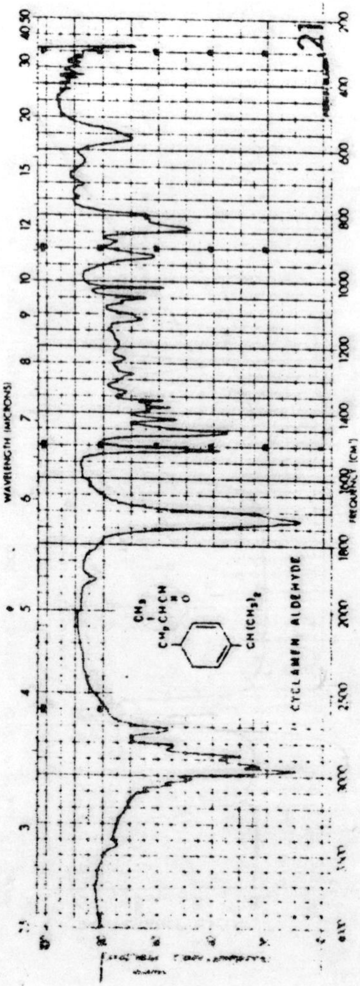

21
CYCLAMEN ALDEHYDE
WAVELENGTH (MICRONS)
FREQUENCY (CM⁻¹)

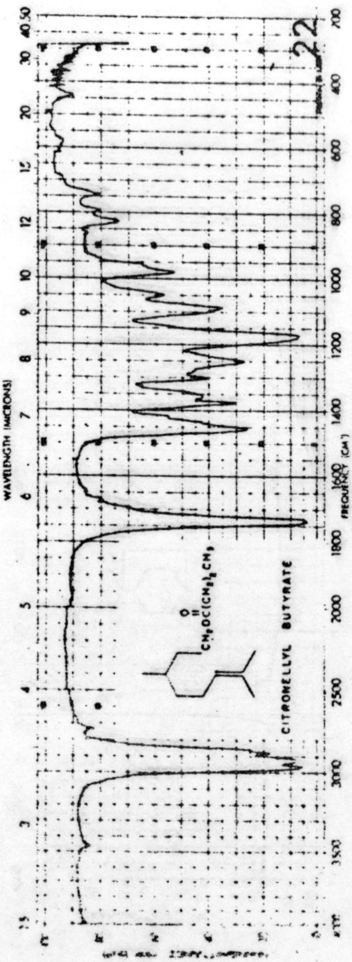

22
CITRONELLYL BUTYRATE
WAVELENGTH (MICRONS)
FREQUENCY (CM⁻¹)

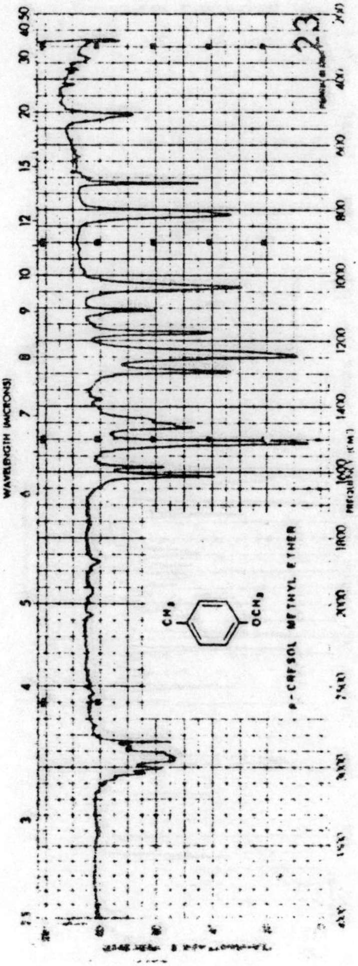
23
P-CRESOL METHYL ETHER
WAVELENGTH (MICRONS)

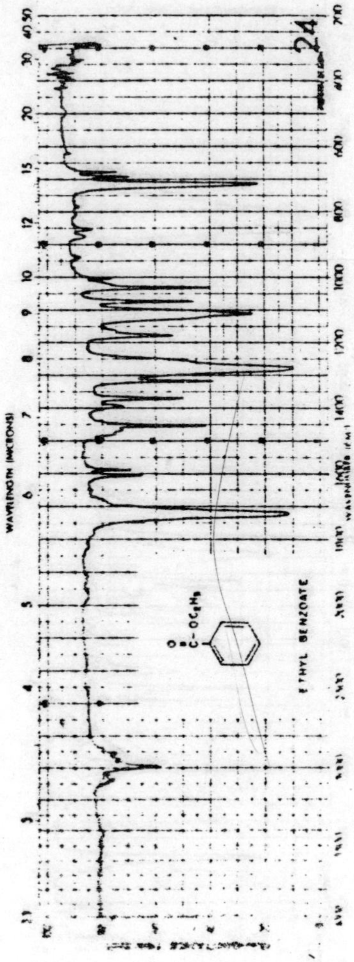
24
ETHYL BENZOATE
WAVELENGTH (MICRONS)

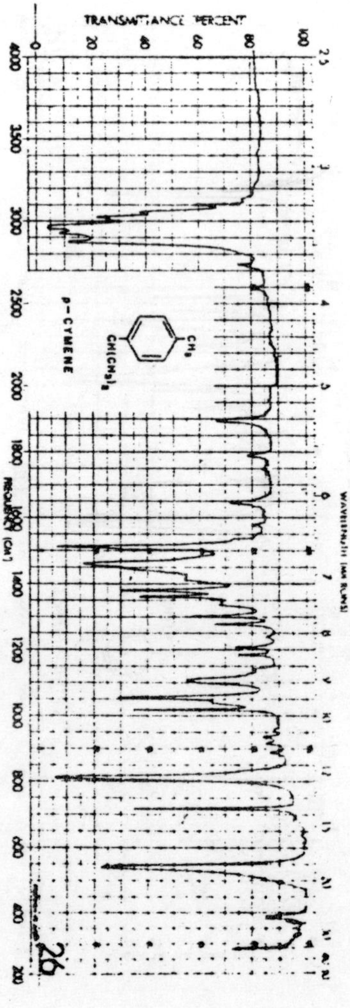
TRANSMITTANCE PERCENT
WAVELENGTH (MICRONS)
FREQUENCY (CM⁻¹)
p-CYMENE
26

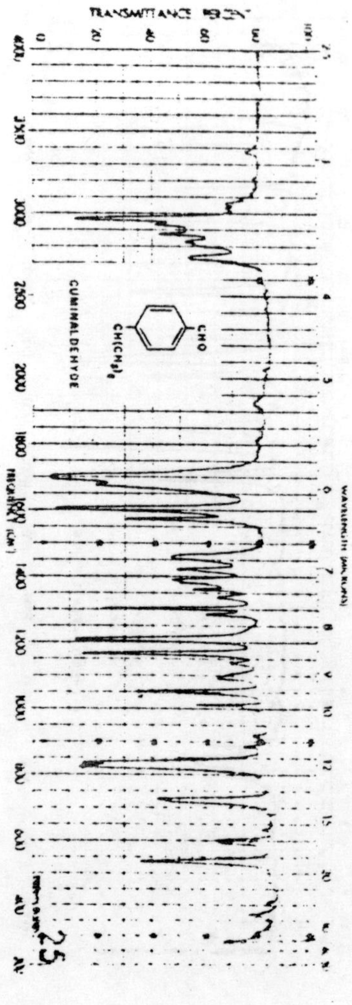
TRANSMITTANCE PERCENT
WAVELENGTH (MICRONS)
FREQUENCY (CM⁻¹)
CUMINALDEHYDE
25

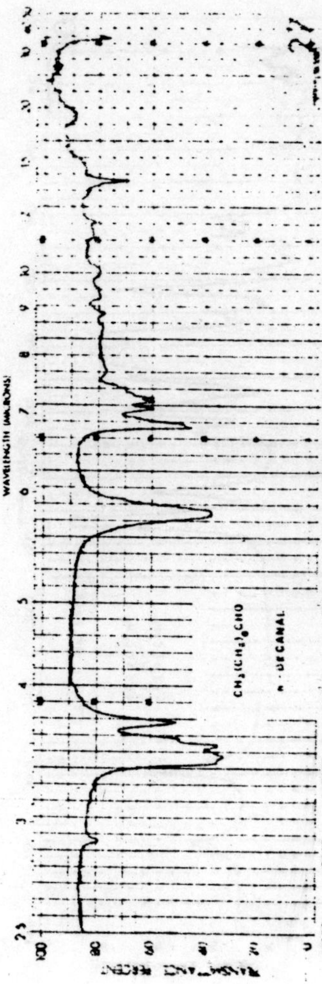
WAVELENGTH (MICRONS)
CH3(CH2)8CHO
n-DECANAL
FREQUENCY (CM-1)
TRANSMITTANCE (PERCENT)

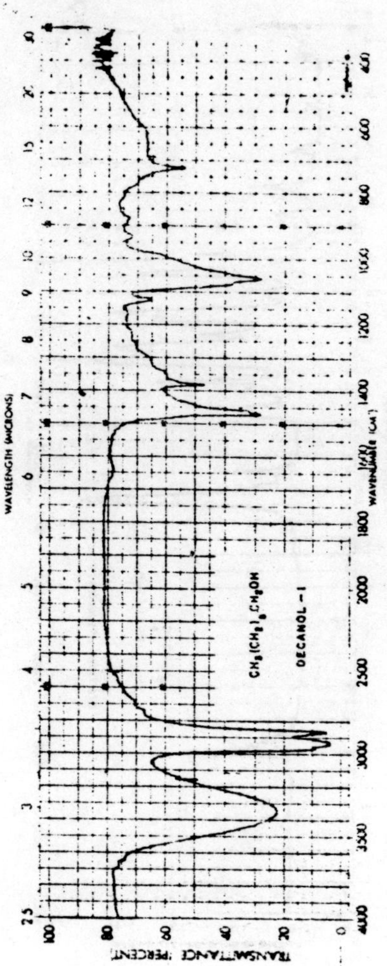
WAVELENGTH (MICRONS)
CH3(CH2)8CH2OH
DECANOL-1
WAVENUMBER (CM-1)
TRANSMITTANCE (PERCENT)

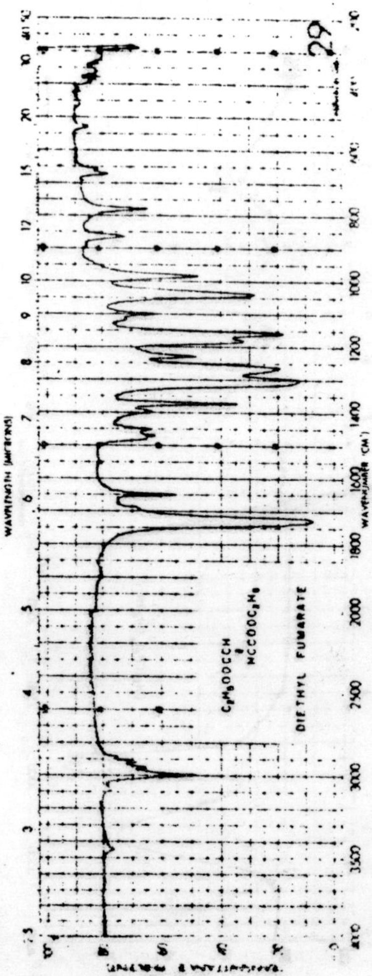
WAVELENGTH (MICRONS)
WAVENUMBER (CM⁻¹)
C₂H₅OOCCH
‖
HCCOOC₂H₅
DIETHYL FUMARATE
29

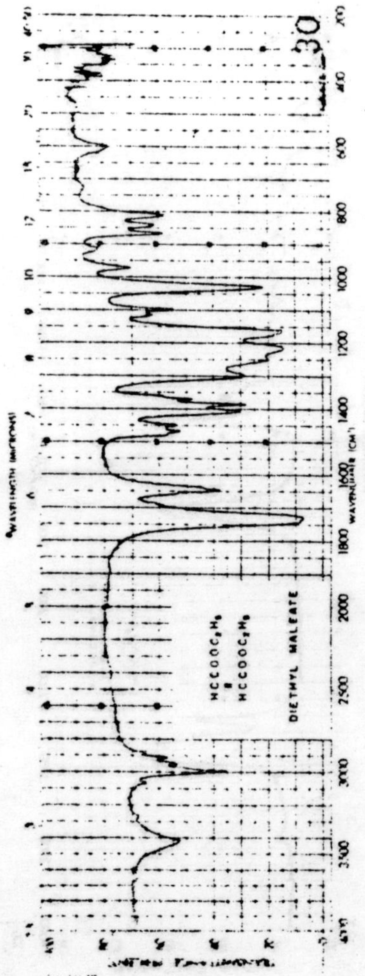
WAVELENGTH (MICRONS)
WAVENUMBER (CM⁻¹)
HCCOOC₂H₅
‖
HCCOOC₂H₅
DIETHYL MALEATE
30

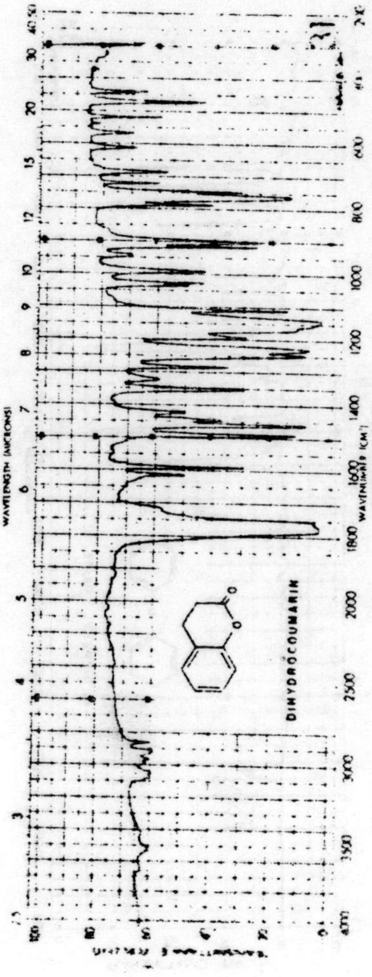
WAVELENGTH (MICRONS)
DIHYDROCOUMARIN

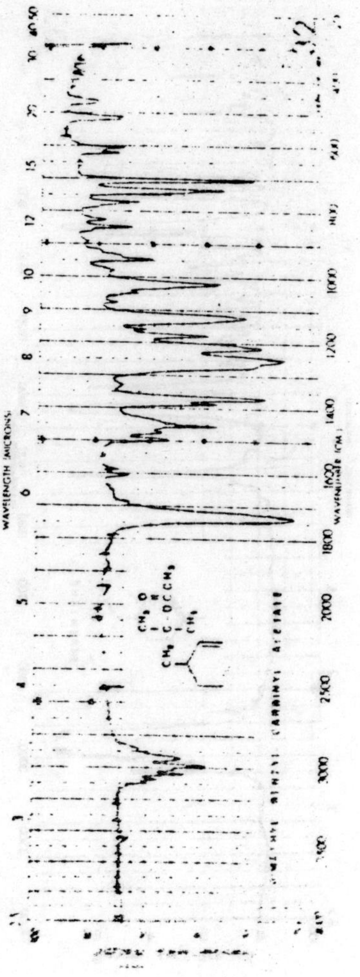
WAVELENGTH (MICRONS)

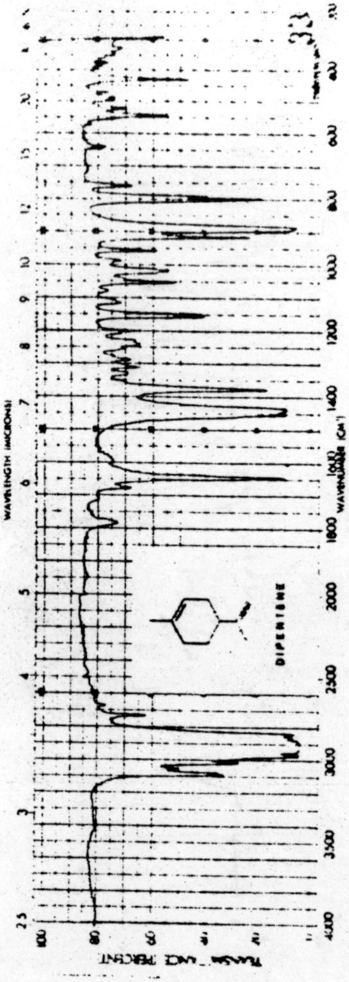
WAVELENGTH (MICRONS)
WAVENUMBER (CM⁻¹)
DIPENTENE
33

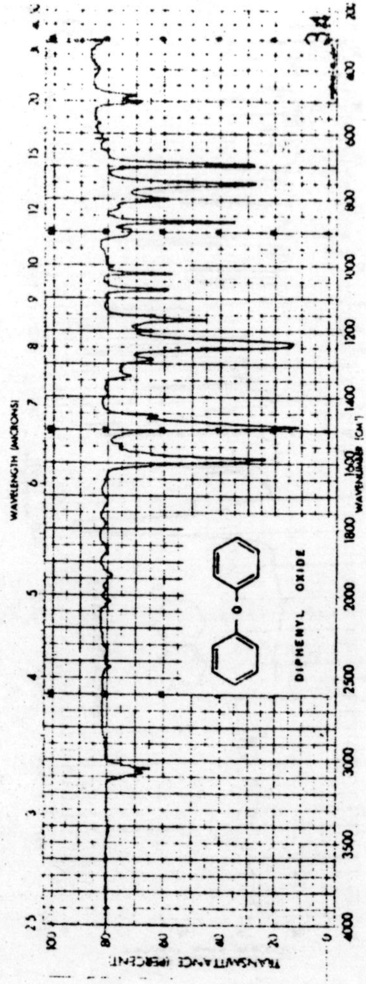
WAVELENGTH (MICRONS)
WAVENUMBER (CM⁻¹)
TRANSMITTANCE (PERCENT)
DIPHENYL OXIDE
34

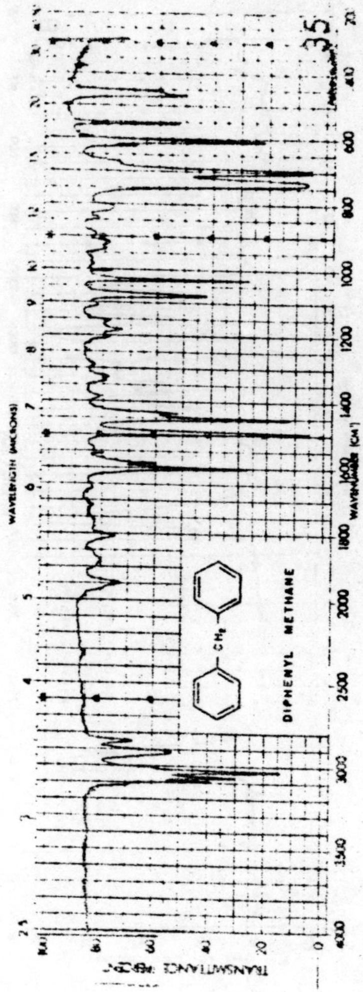
WAVELENGTH (MICRONS)
WAVENUMBER (CM⁻¹)
TRANSMITTANCE (PERCENT)
DIPHENYL METHANE
35

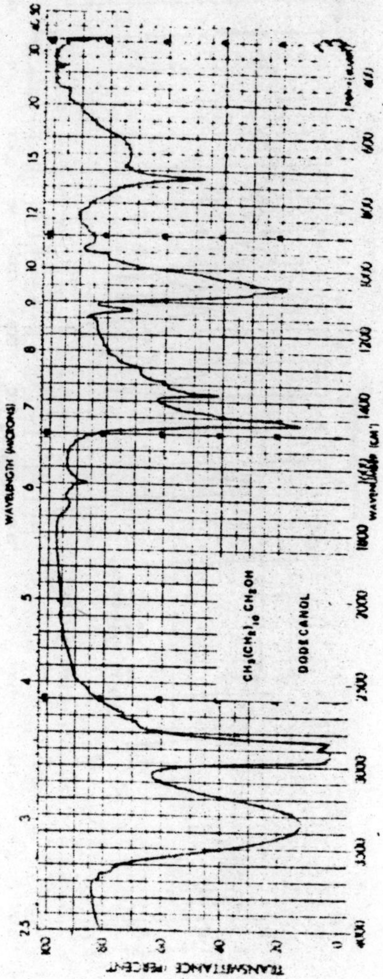
WAVELENGTH (MICRONS)
WAVENUMBER (CM⁻¹)
TRANSMITTANCE (PERCENT)
CH3(CH2)10 CH2OH
DODECANOL

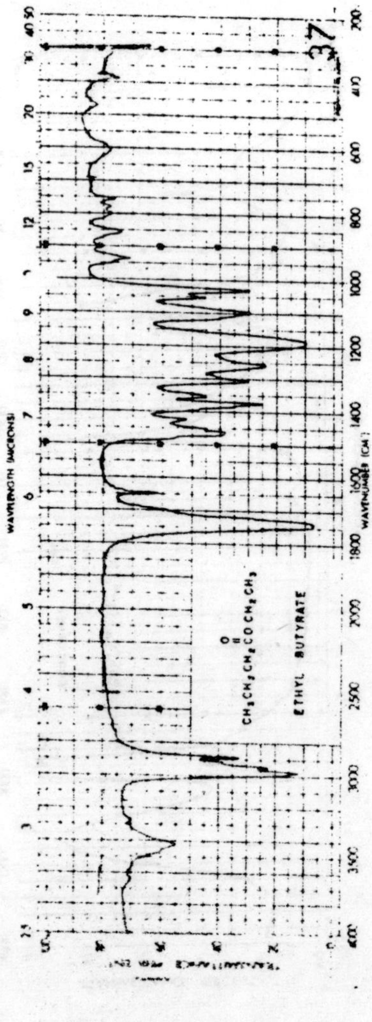
37
WAVELENGTH (MICRONS)
WAVENUMBER (CM⁻¹)
ETHYL BUTYRATE

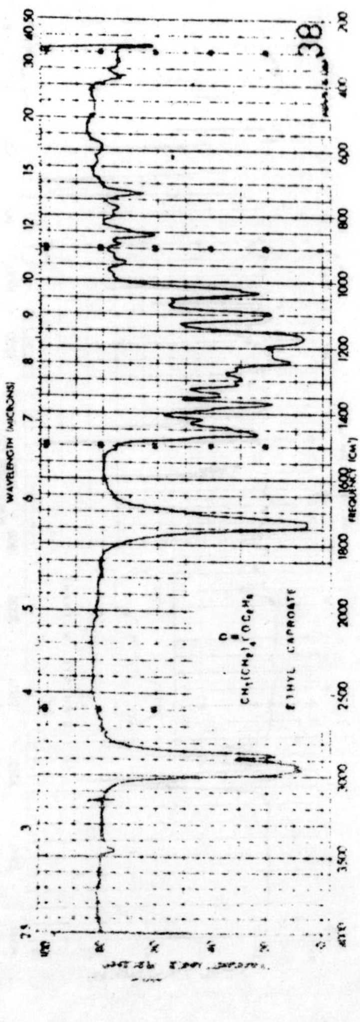
38
WAVELENGTH (MICRONS)
FREQUENCY (CM⁻¹)
ETHYL CAPROATE

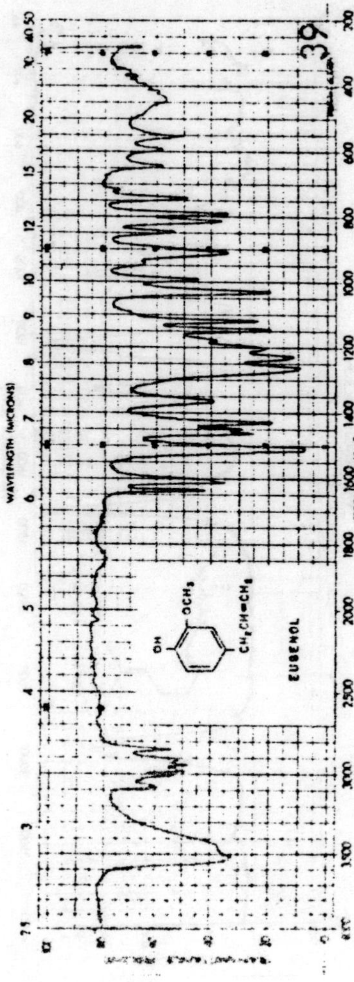
39
EUGENOL

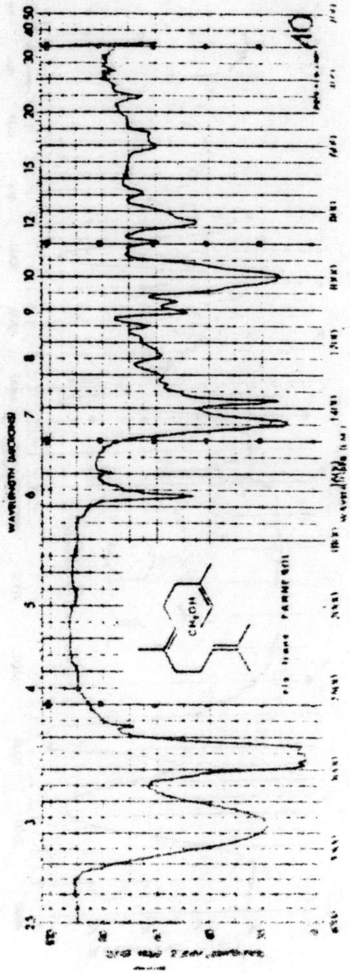

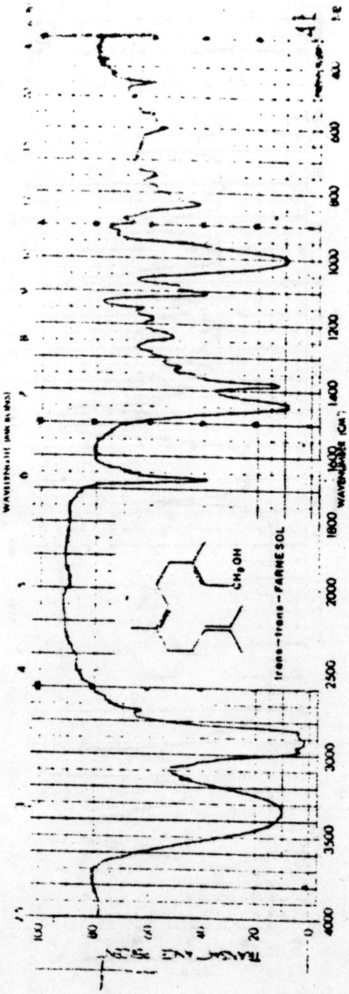
trans–trans–FARNESOL
CH_2OH
TRANSMITTANCE (PERCENT)
WAVENUMBER (CM^{-1})
4000
3500
3000
2500
2000
1800
1600
1400
1200
1000
800
600
400

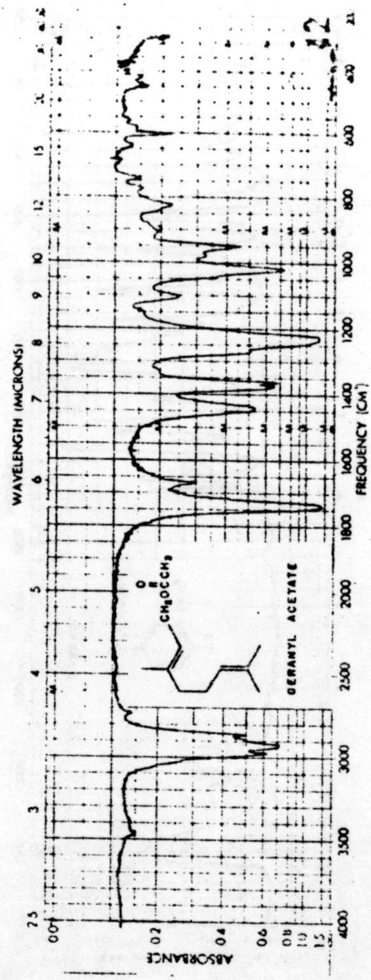
GERANYL ACETATE
WAVELENGTH (MICRONS)
FREQUENCY (CM^{-1})
ABSORBANCE
4000
3500
3000
2500
2000
1800
1600
1400
1200
1000
800
600

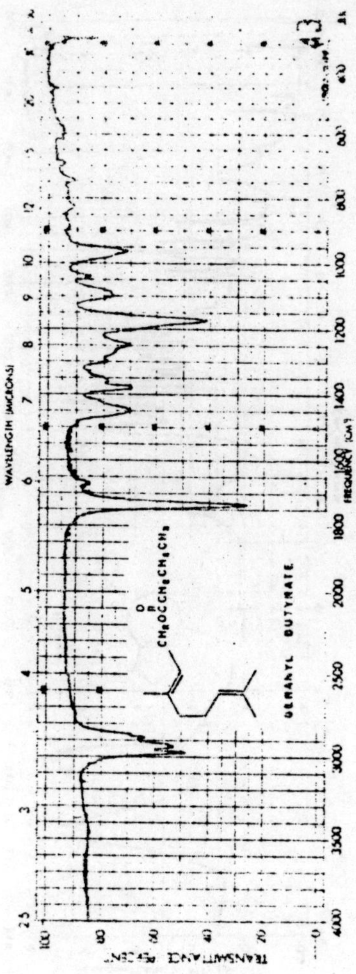
WAVELENGTH (MICRONS)
FREQUENCY (CM⁻¹)
TRANSMITTANCE (PERCENT)
GERANYL BUTYRATE
43

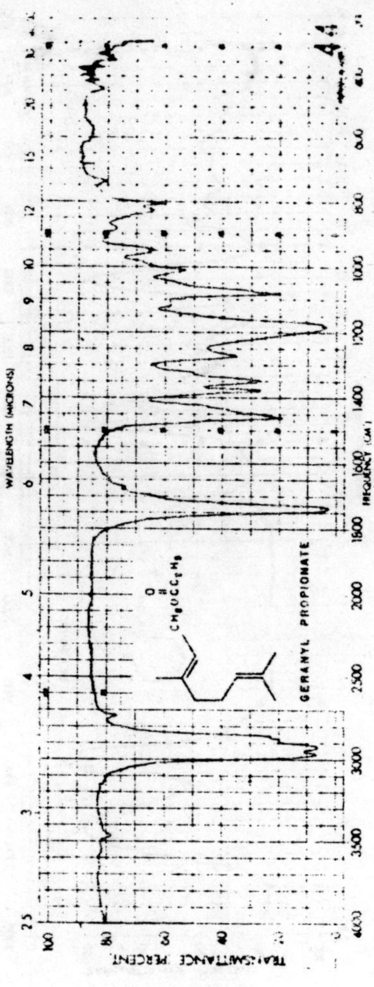
WAVELENGTH (MICRONS)
FREQUENCY (CM⁻¹)
TRANSMITTANCE (PERCENT)
GERANYL PROPIONATE
44

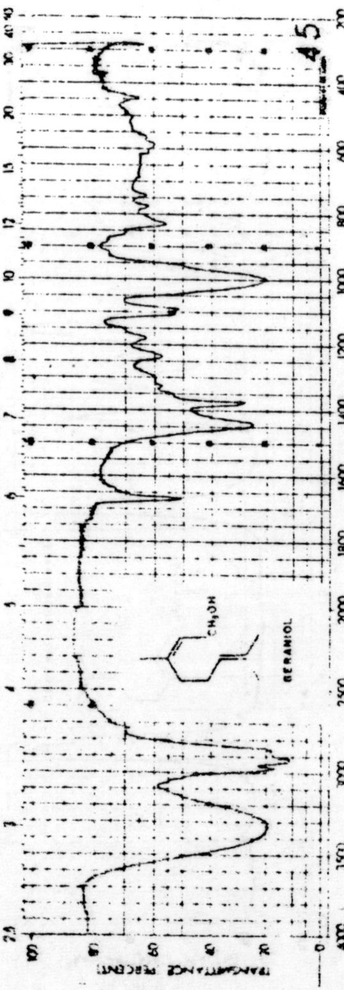
45
WAVELENGTH (MICRONS)
FREQUENCY (CM⁻¹)
TRANSMITTANCE (PERCENT)
GERANIOL
CH₂OH

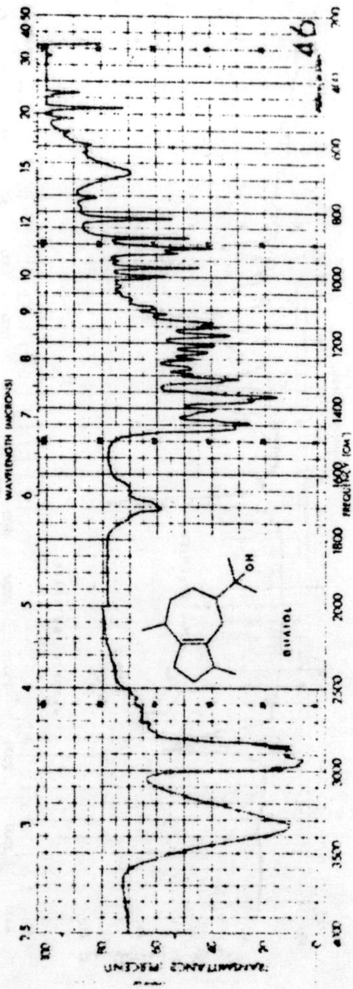
46
WAVELENGTH (MICRONS)
FREQUENCY (CM⁻¹)
TRANSMITTANCE (PERCENT)
GUAIOL
OH

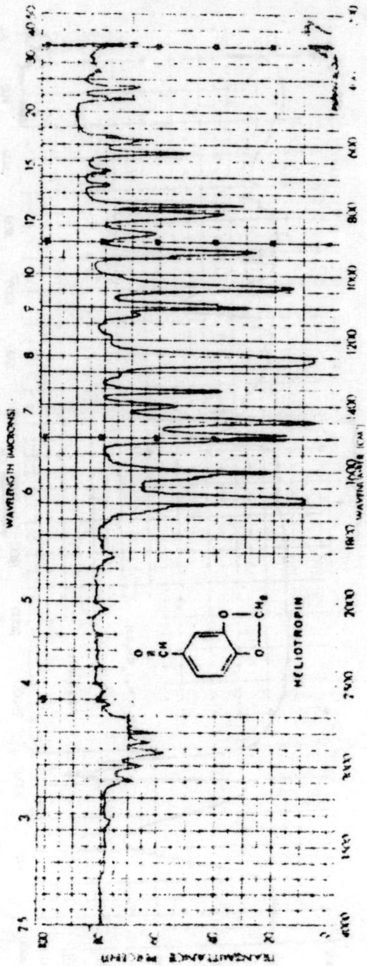
HELIOTROPIN
WAVELENGTH (MICRONS)
47

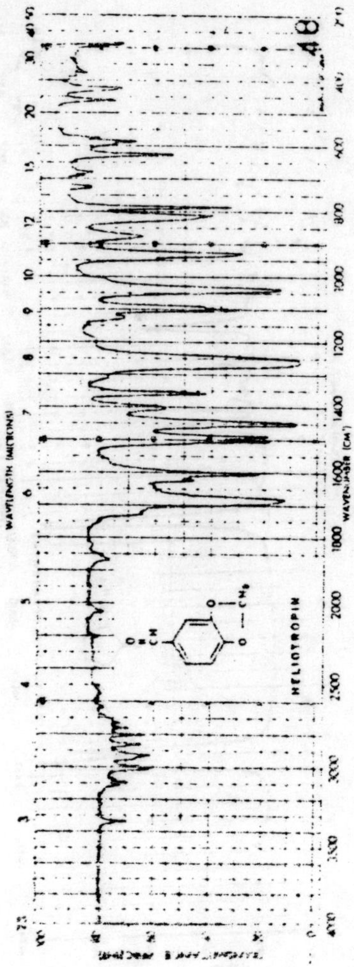
HELIOTROPIN
WAVELENGTH (MICRONS)
48

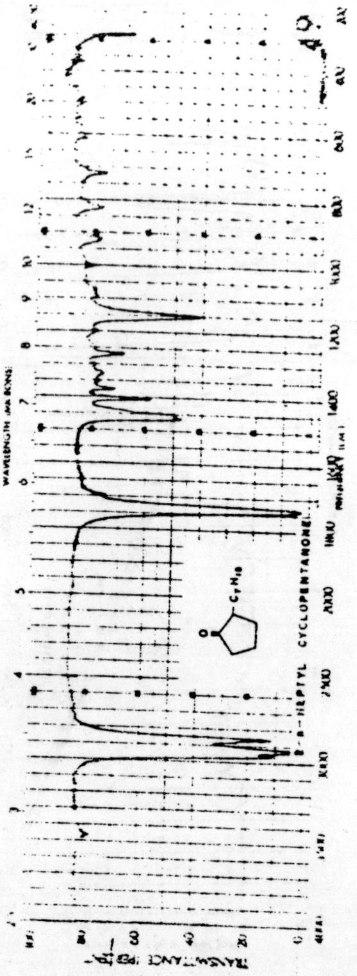
WAVELENGTH (MICRONS)
TRANSMITTANCE (PERCENT)
2-n-HEPTYL CYCLOPENTANONE
49

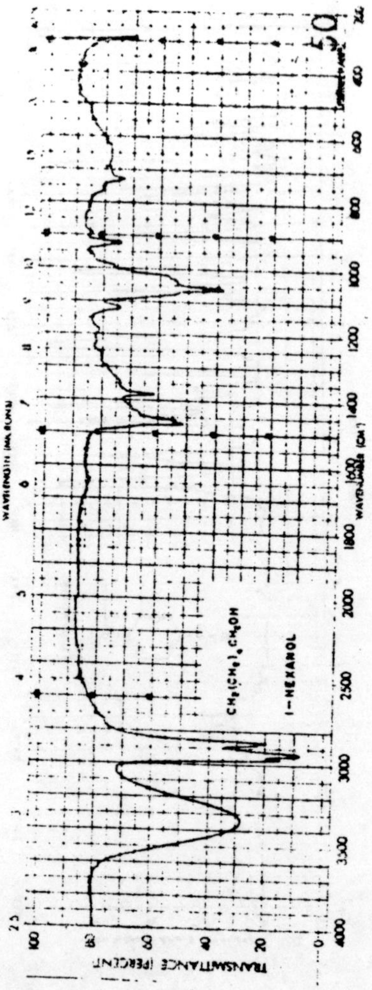
WAVELENGTH (MICRONS)
WAVENUMBER (CM-1)
TRANSMITTANCE (PERCENT)
CH3(CH2)4CH2OH
1-HEXANOL
50

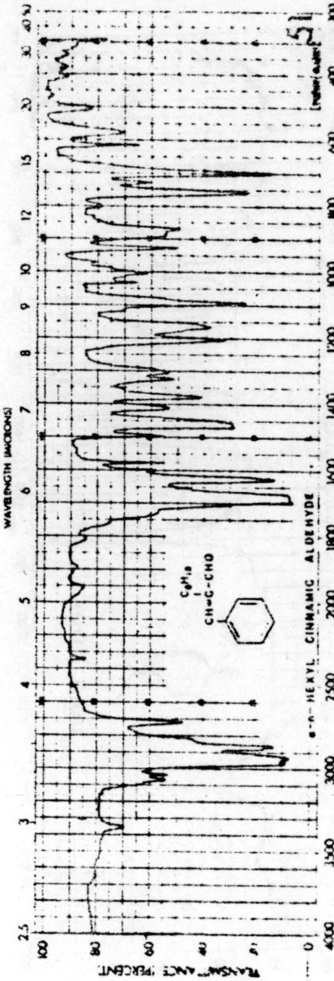

WAVELENGTH (MICRONS)
TRANSMITTANCE (PERCENT)
WAVENUMBER (CM⁻¹)
α-n-HEXYL CINNAMIC ALDEHYDE
51

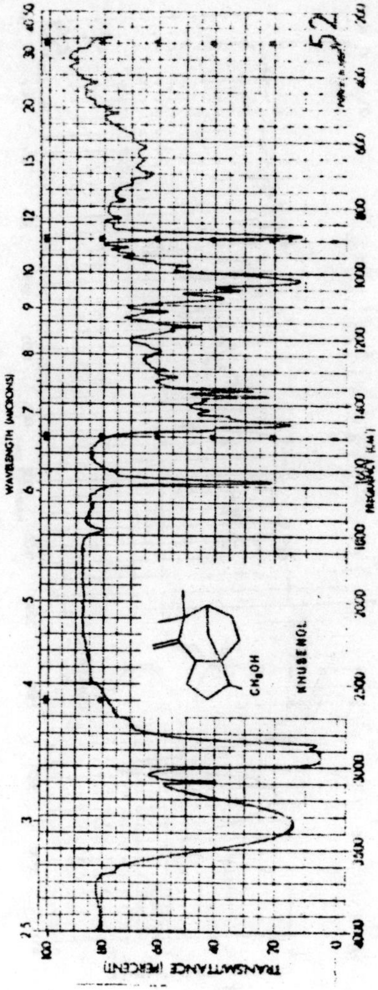

WAVELENGTH (MICRONS)
TRANSMITTANCE (PERCENT)
FREQUENCY (CM⁻¹)
CH₂OH
KHUSENOL
52

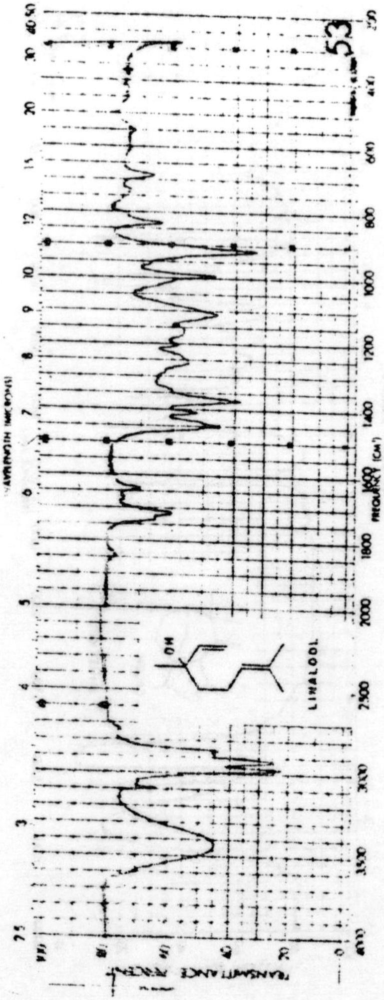

53
LINALOOL

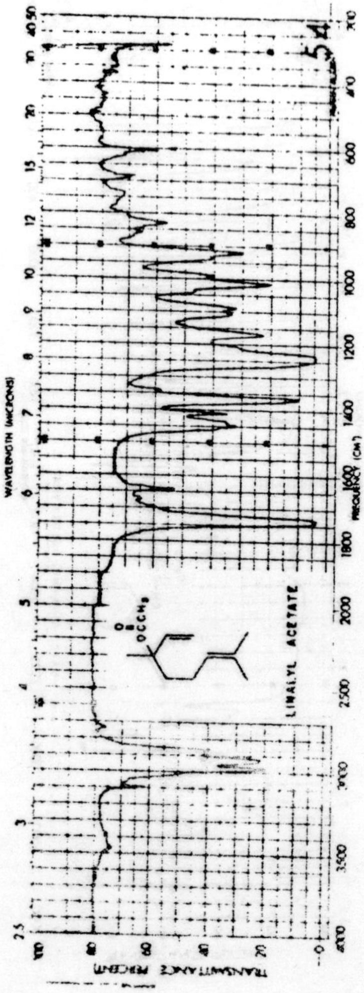

54
LINALYL ACETATE

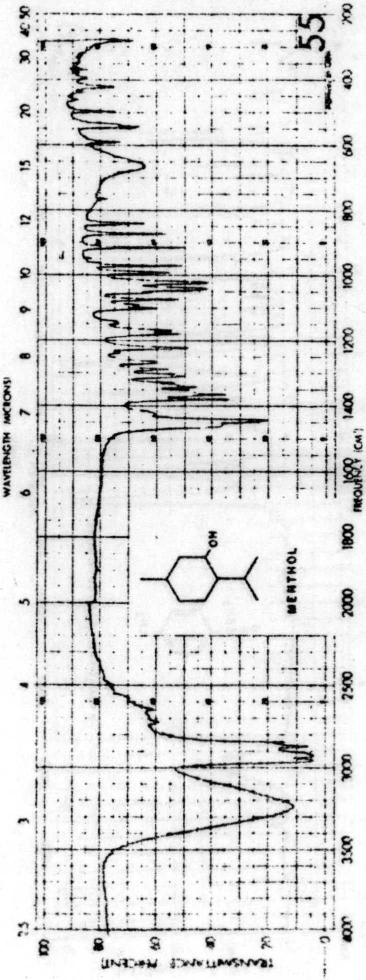
55
MENTHOL
WAVELENGTH (MICRONS)
FREQUENCY (CM⁻¹)
TRANSMITTANCE (PERCENT)

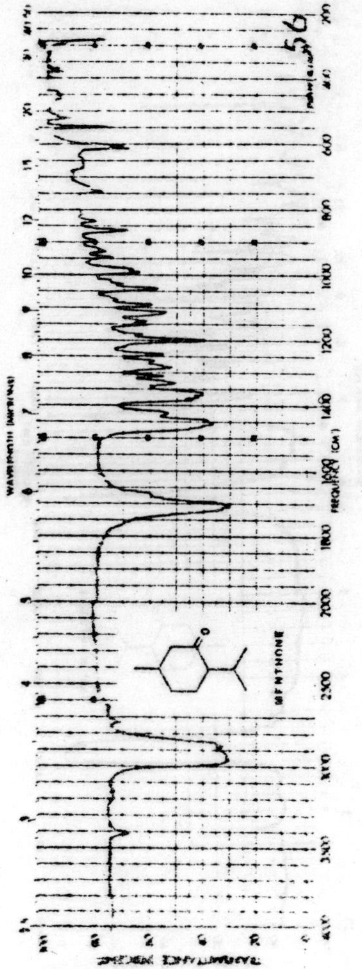
56
MENTHONE

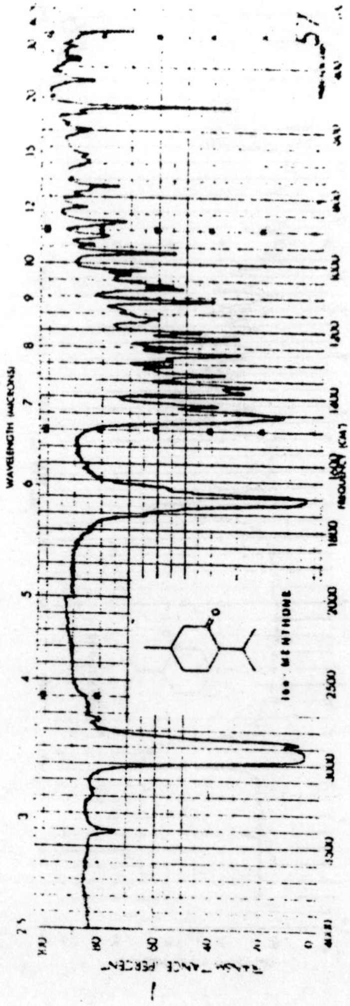
WAVELENGTH (MICRONS)
FREQUENCY (CM-1)
TRANSMITTANCE (PERCENT)
iso-MENTHONE
57

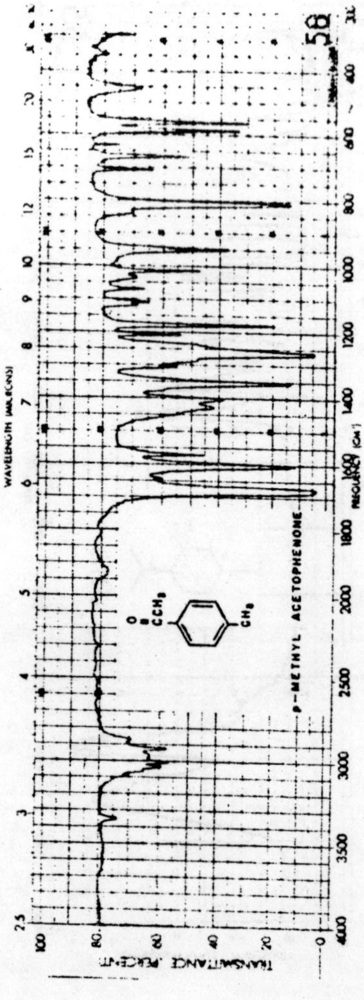
WAVELENGTH (MICRONS)
FREQUENCY (CM-1)
TRANSMITTANCE (PERCENT)
p-METHYL ACETOPHENONE
58

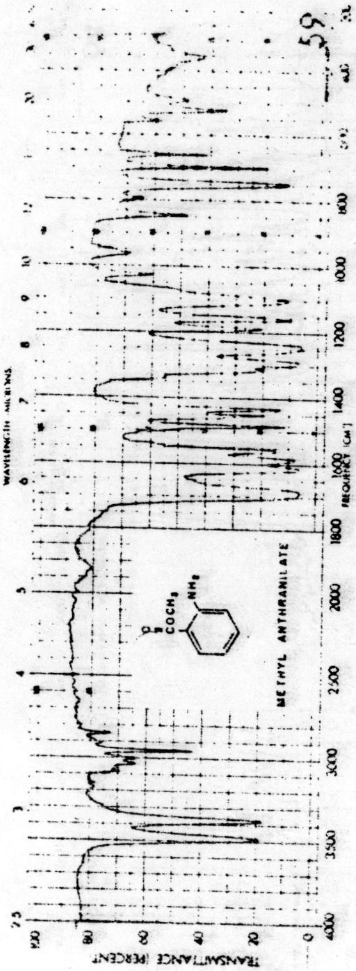
METHYL ANTHRANILATE
COCH3
NH2
WAVELENGTH (MICRONS)
FREQUENCY (CM⁻¹)
TRANSMITTANCE (PERCENT)
59

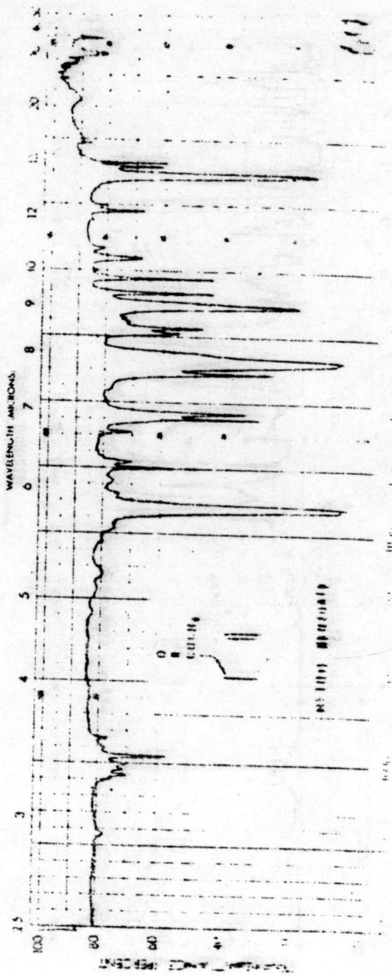
WAVELENGTH (MICRONS)

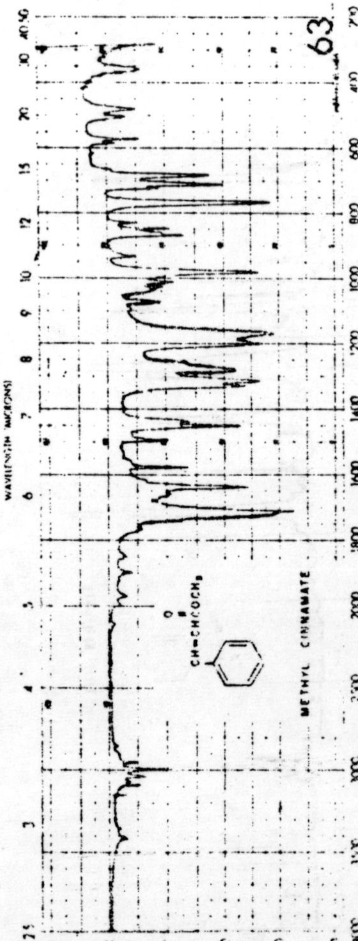
METHYL CINNAMATE
63

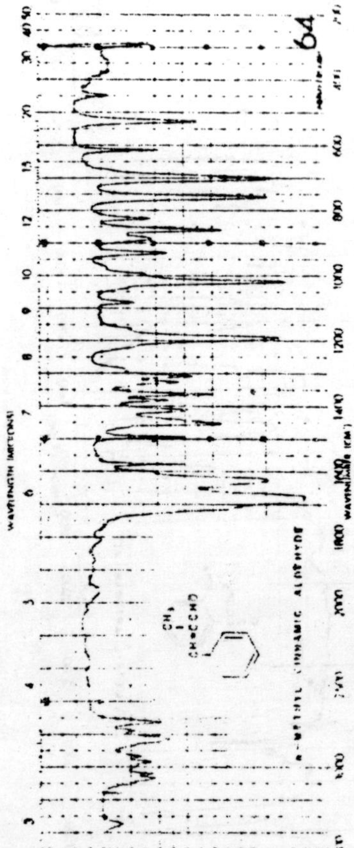
METHYL CINNAMIC ALDEHYDE
64

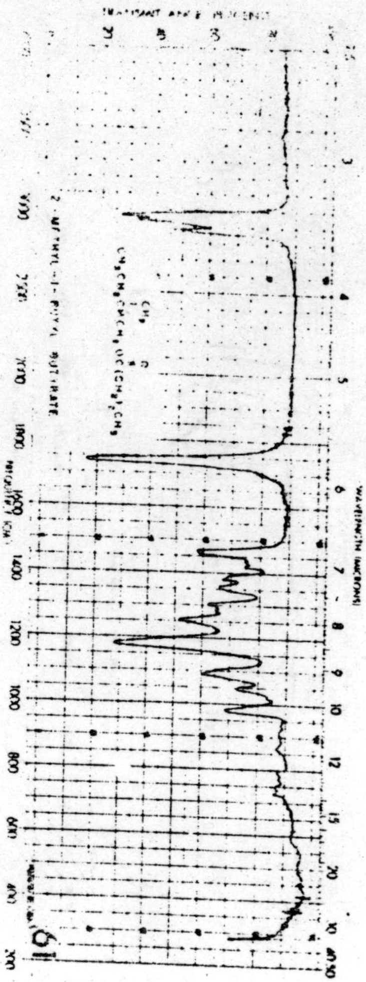
2-METHYL-1-BUTYL BUTYRATE
WAVELENGTH (MICRONS)
TRANSMITTANCE (PERCENT)

61

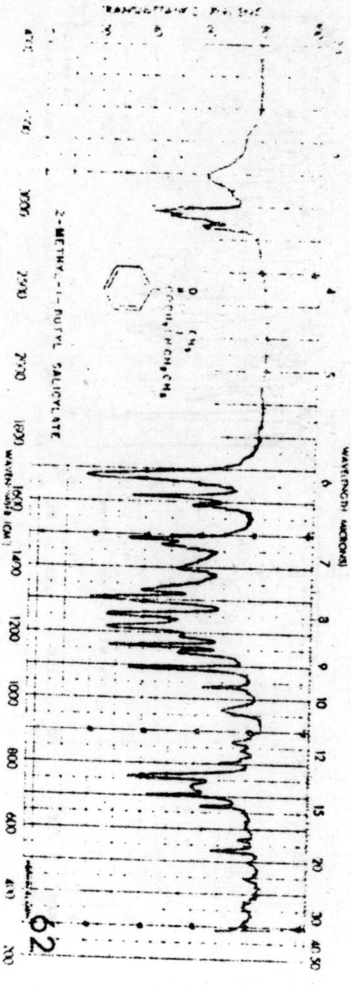
2-METHYL-1-BUTYL SALICYLATE
WAVELENGTH (MICRONS)
WAVENUMBER (CM⁻¹)

62

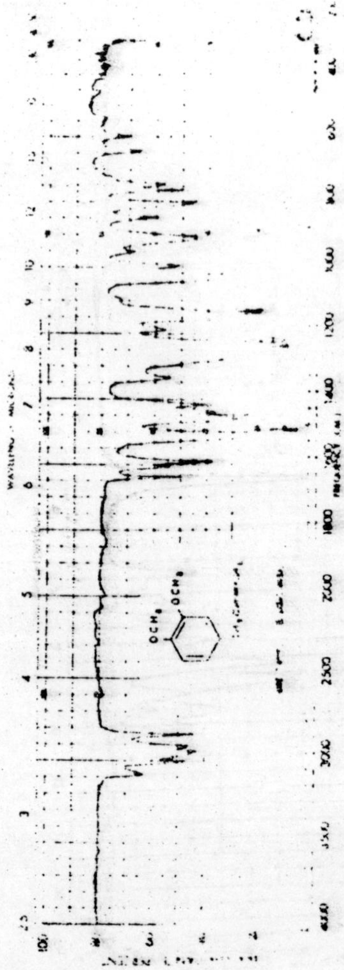

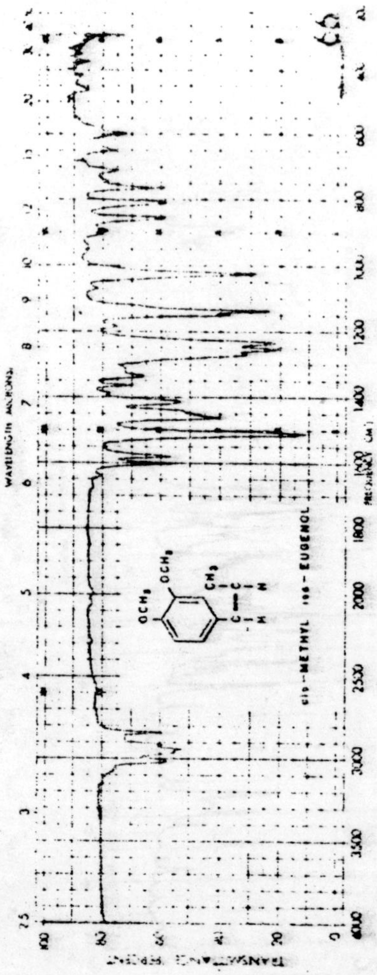
WAVELENGTH MICRONS
FREQUENCY (CM⁻¹)
TRANSMITTANCE (PERCENT)
cis-METHYL iso-EUGENOL

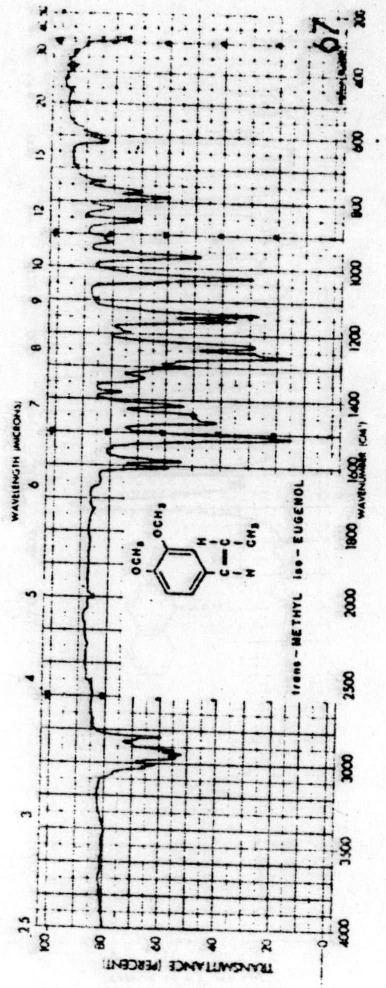
WAVELENGTH (MICRONS)
WAVENUMBER (CM⁻¹)
TRANSMITTANCE (PERCENT)
trans-METHYL iso-EUGENOL

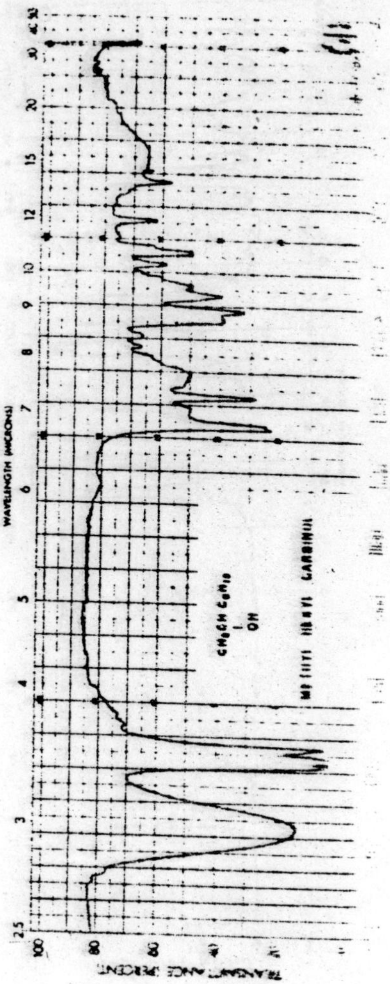
WAVELENGTH (MICRONS)
TRANSMITTANCE (PERCENT)

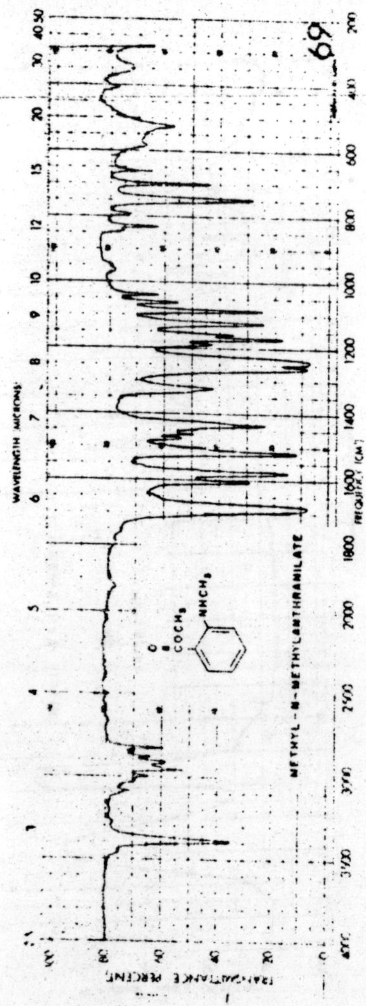
WAVELENGTH (MICRONS)
TRANSMITTANCE PERCENT
FREQUENCY (CM⁻¹)
METHYL-N-METHYLANTHRANILATE
69

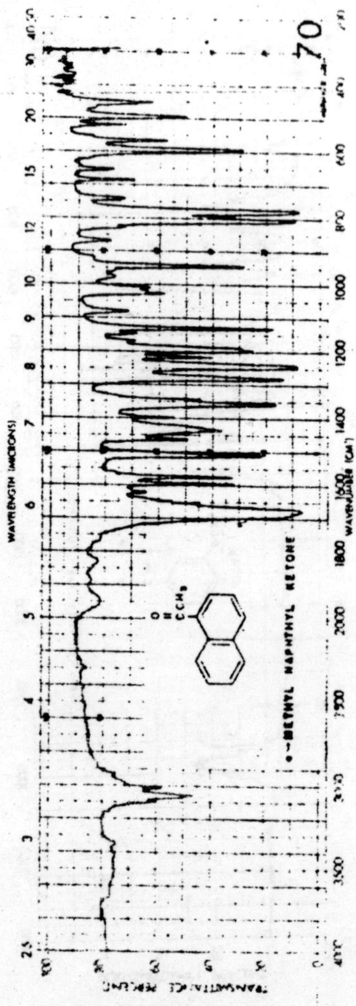
WAVELENGTH (MICRONS)
TRANSMITTANCE PERCENT
WAVENUMBER (CM⁻¹)
α-METHYL NAPHTHYL KETONE
70

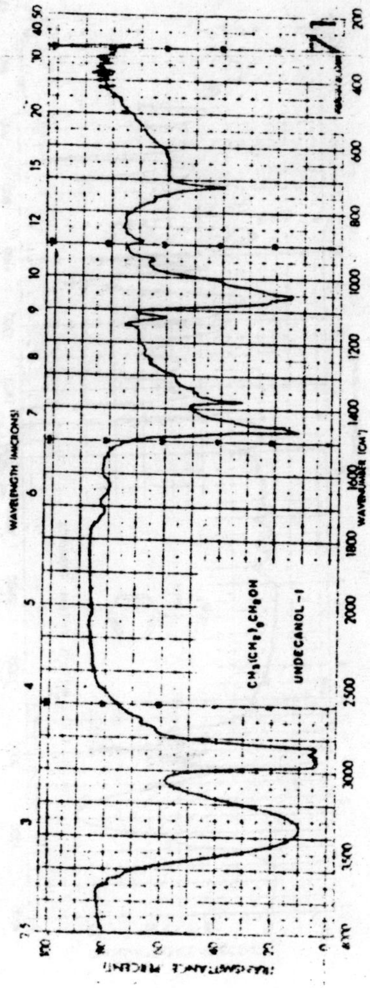
WAVELENGTH (MICRONS)
WAVENUMBER (CM⁻¹)
TRANSMITTANCE (PERCENT)
UNDECANOL-1
71

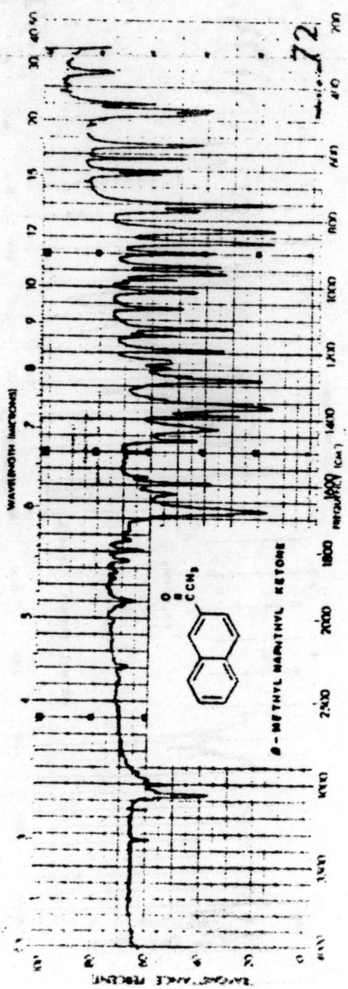
WAVELENGTH (MICRONS)
TRANSMITTANCE (PERCENT)
β-METHYL NAPHTHYL KETONE
72

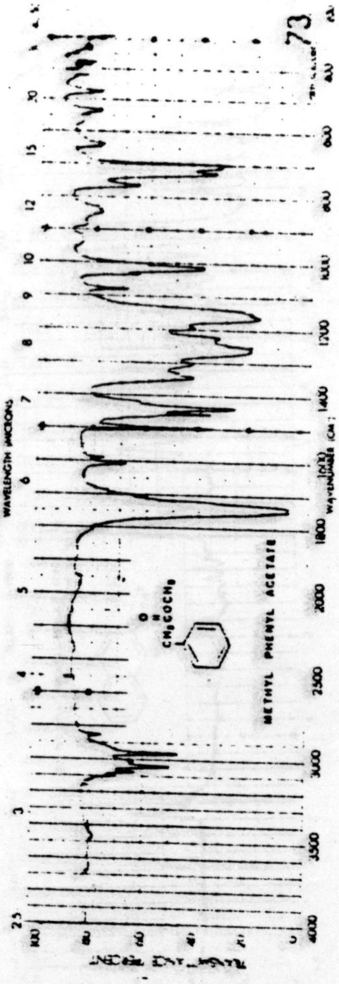
WAVELENGTH (MICRONS)
TRANSMITTANCE (PERCENT)
WAVENUMBER (CM⁻¹)
METHYL PHENYL ACETATE
73

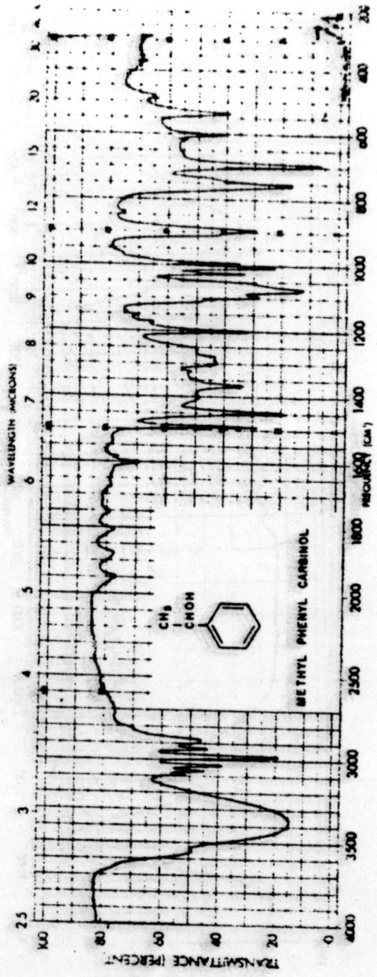
WAVELENGTH (MICRONS)
TRANSMITTANCE (PERCENT)
FREQUENCY (CM⁻¹)
METHYL PHENYL CARBINOL
74

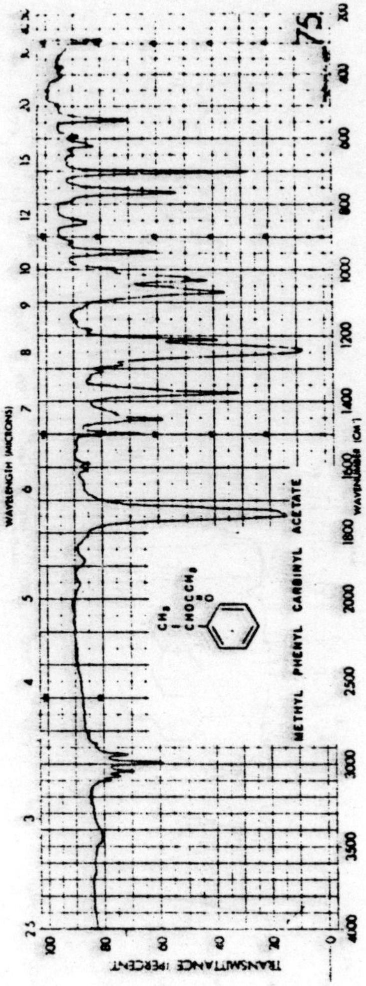
WAVELENGTH (MICRONS)
WAVENUMBER (CM⁻¹)
TRANSMITTANCE (PERCENT)
METHYL PHENYL CARBINYL ACETATE
75

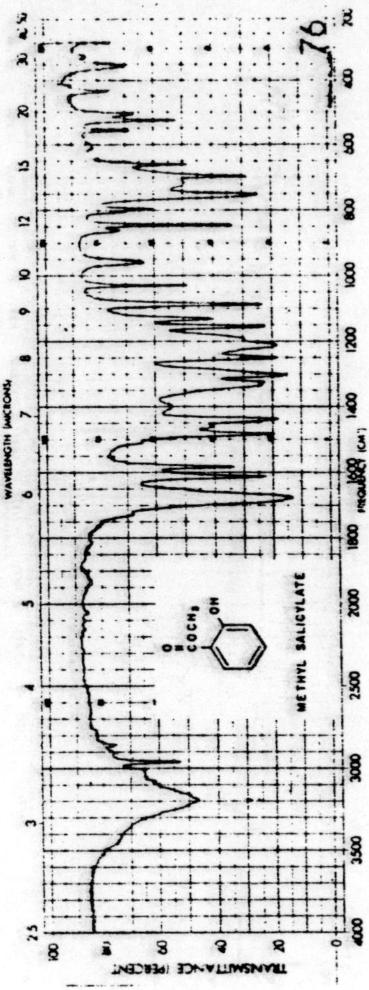
WAVELENGTH (MICRONS)
FREQUENCY (CM⁻¹)
TRANSMITTANCE (PERCENT)
METHYL SALICYLATE
76

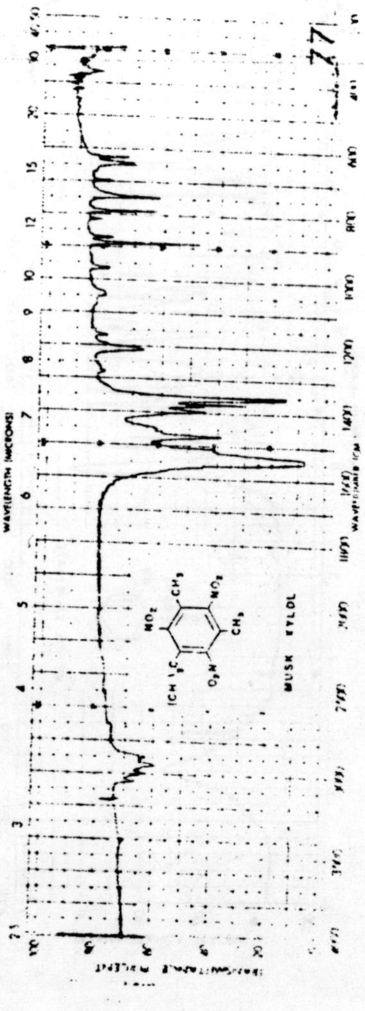
WAVELENGTH (MICRONS)
WAVENUMBER (CM⁻¹)
MUSK XYLOL
77

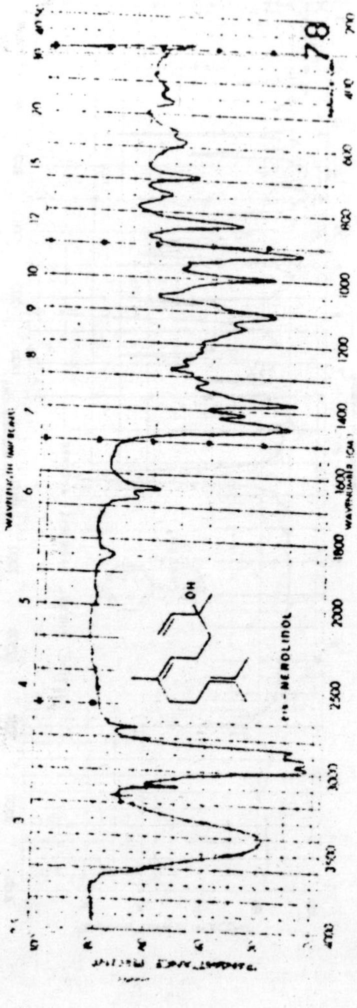
WAVENUMBER (CM⁻¹)
cis-NEROLIDOL
78

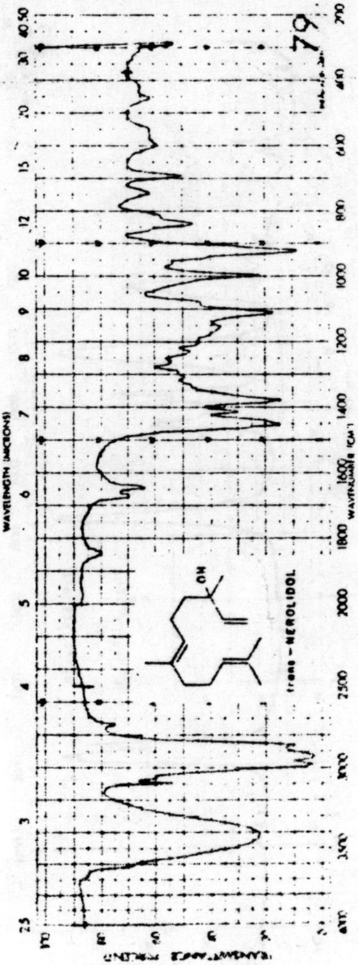
WAVELENGTH (MICRONS)
WAVENUMBER (CM-1)
OH
trans-NEROLIDOL
79

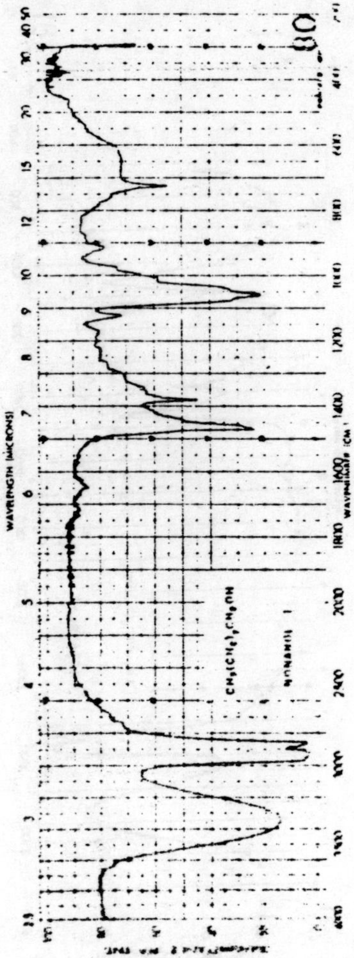
WAVELENGTH (MICRONS)
$CH_3(CH_2)_7CH_2OH$
NONANOL-1
80

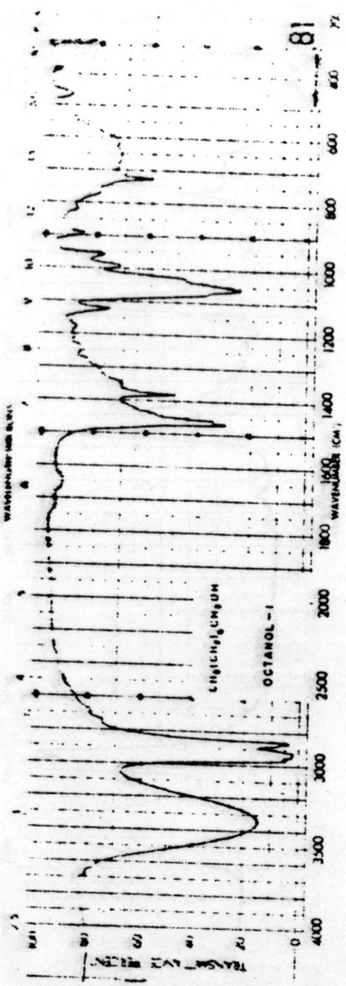
81
OCTANOL-1
WAVENUMBER (CM⁻¹)

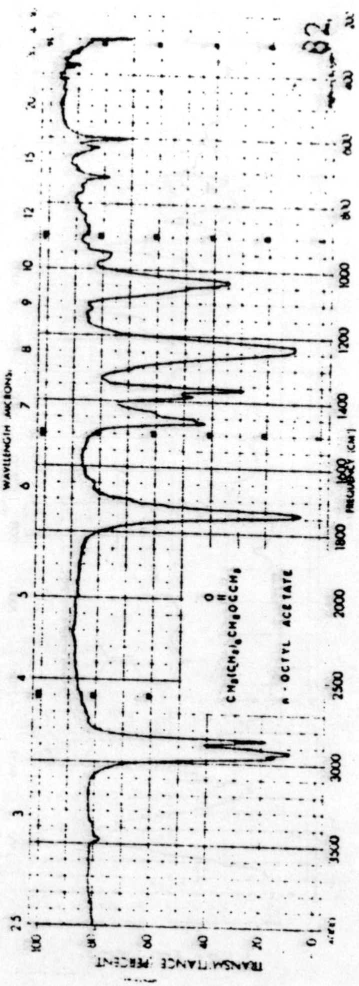
82
n-OCTYL ACETATE
WAVELENGTH (MICRONS)
TRANSMITTANCE (PERCENT)
FREQUENCY (CM⁻¹)

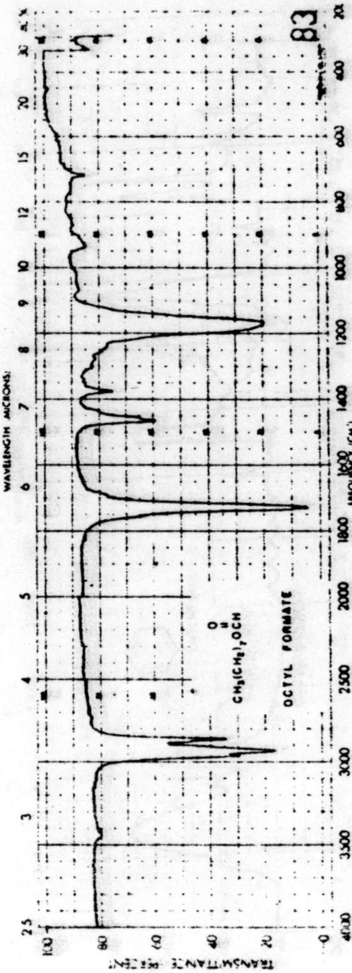
83
OCTYL FORMATE
WAVELENGTH MICRONS
FREQUENCY (CM⁻¹)
TRANSMITTANCE (PERCENT)

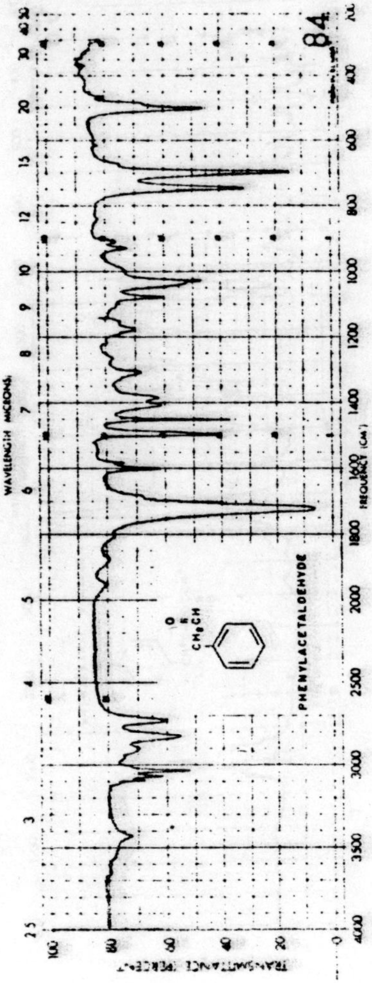
84
PHENYLACETALDEHYDE
WAVELENGTH MICRONS
FREQUENCY (CM⁻¹)
TRANSMITTANCE (PERCENT)

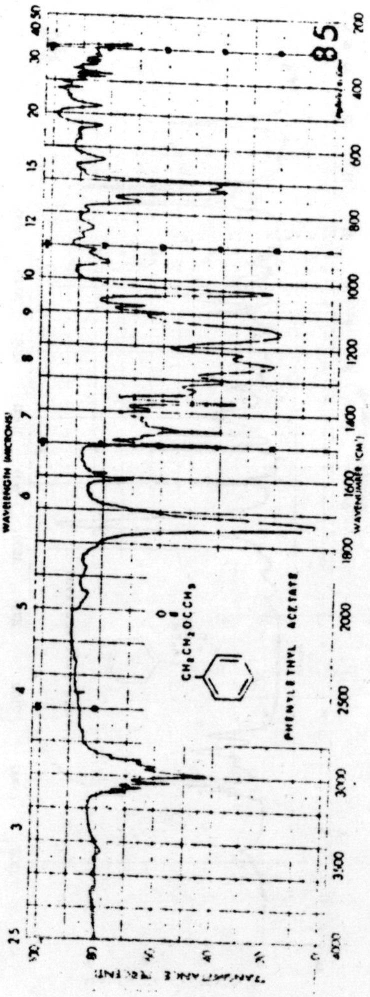
85
WAVELENGTH (MICRONS)
WAVENUMBER (CM⁻¹)
TRANSMITTANCE (PERCENT)
PHENYLETHYL ACETATE

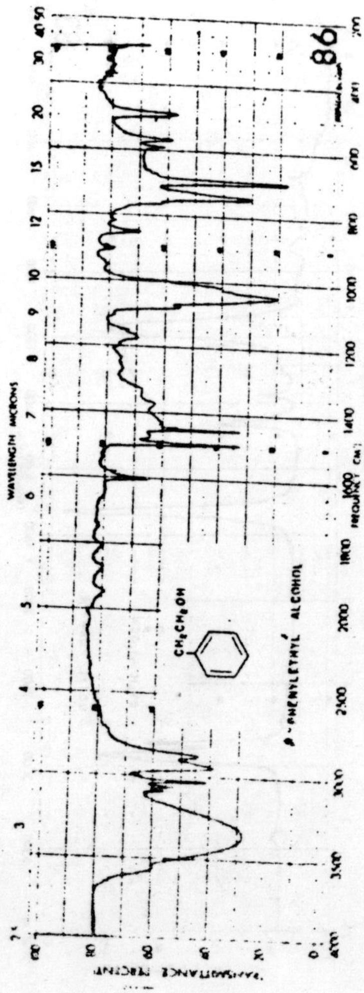
86
WAVELENGTH (MICRONS)
FREQUENCY (CM⁻¹)
TRANSMITTANCE (PERCENT)
β-PHENYLETHYL ALCOHOL

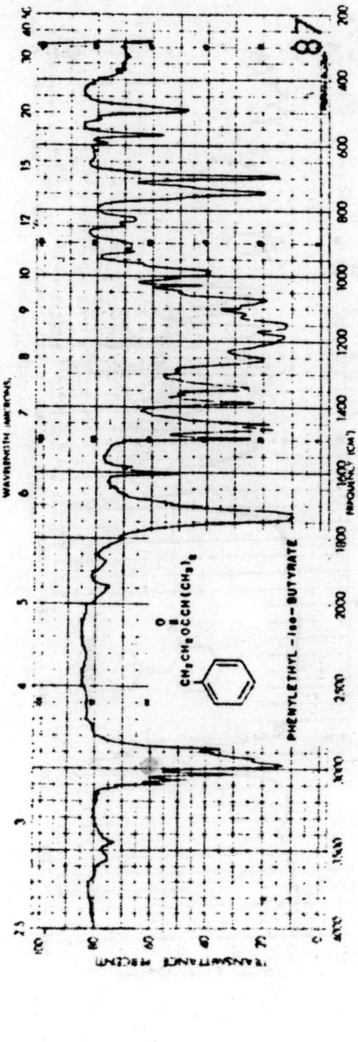
87
PHENYLETHYL-ISO-BUTYRATE
WAVELENGTH (MICRONS)
TRANSMITTANCE PERCENT

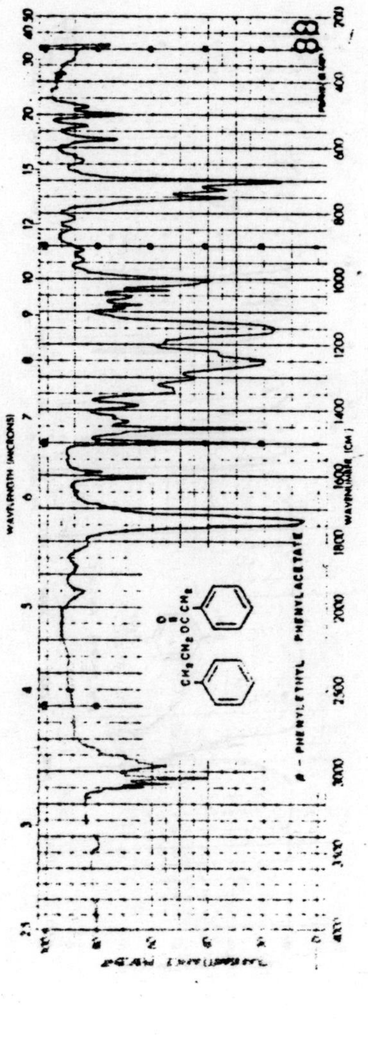
88
β-PHENYLETHYL PHENYLACETATE
WAVELENGTH (MICRONS)

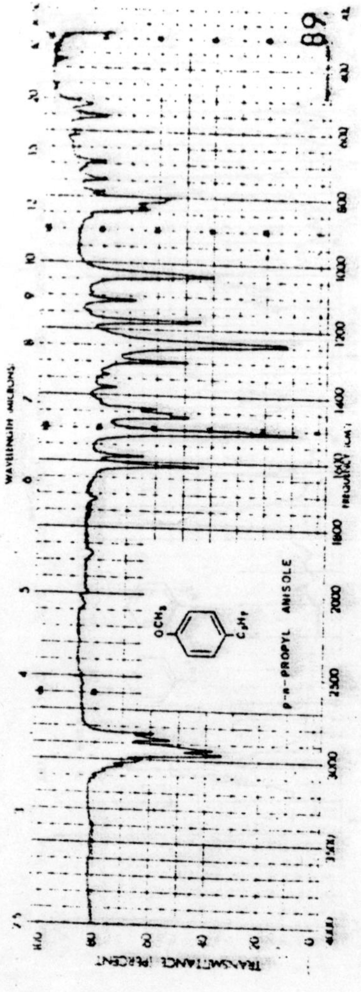
89
WAVELENGTH (MICRONS)
FREQUENCY (CM⁻¹)
TRANSMITTANCE (PERCENT)
P-n-PROPYL ANISOLE

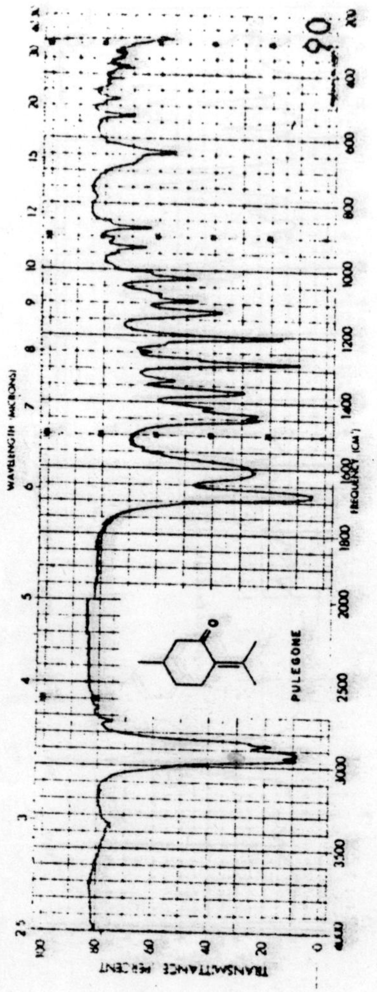
90
WAVELENGTH (MICRONS)
FREQUENCY (CM⁻¹)
TRANSMITTANCE (PERCENT)
PULEGONE

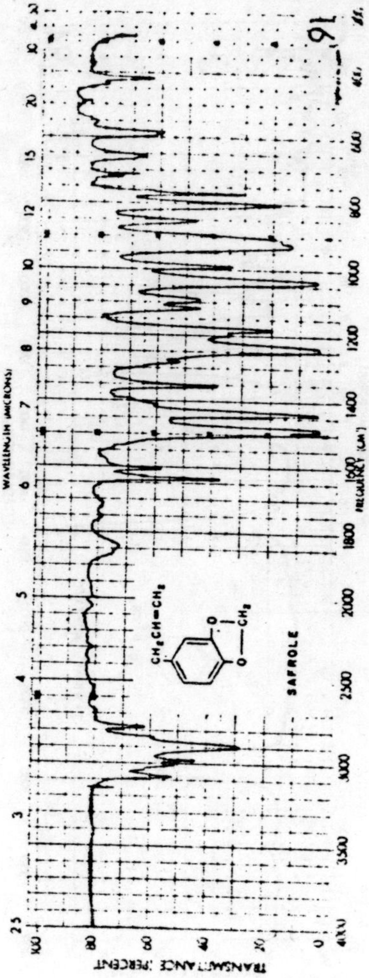
91
WAVELENGTH (MICRONS)
FREQUENCY (CM⁻¹)
TRANSMITTANCE (PERCENT)
SAFROLE

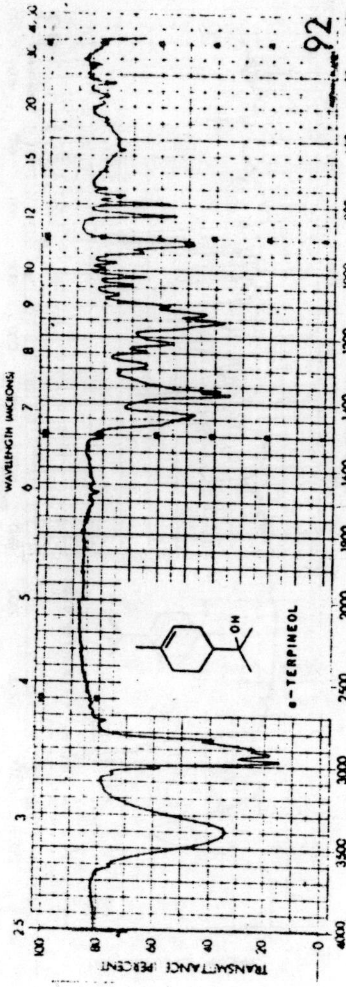
92
WAVELENGTH (MICRONS)
FREQUENCY (CM⁻¹)
TRANSMITTANCE (PERCENT)
α-TERPINEOL

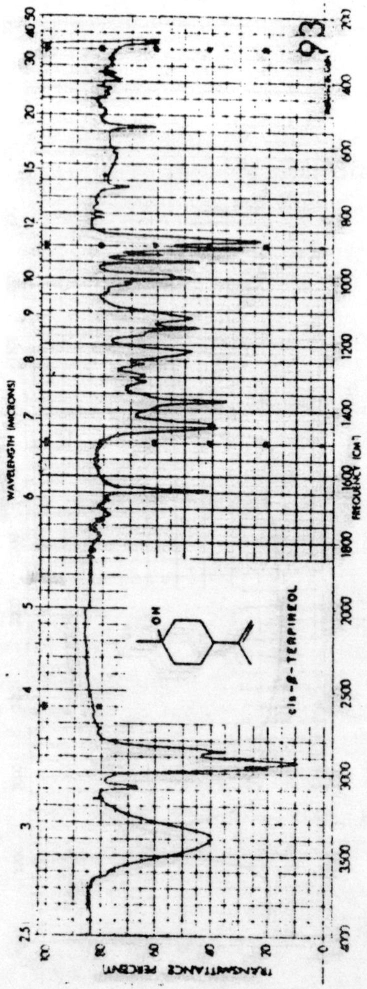
93
WAVELENGTH (MICRONS)
FREQUENCY (CM⁻¹)
TRANSMITTANCE (PERCENT)
OH
cis-β-TERPINEOL

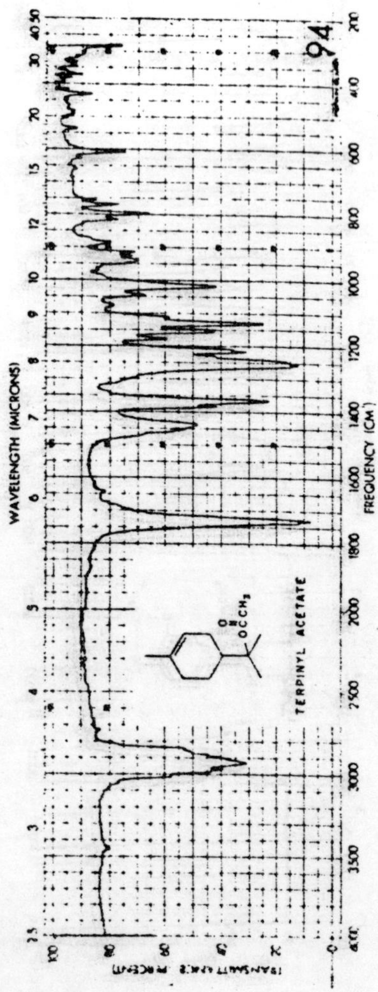
94
WAVELENGTH (MICRONS)
FREQUENCY (CM⁻¹)
TRANSMITTANCE (PERCENT)
O
OCCH₃
TERPINYL ACETATE

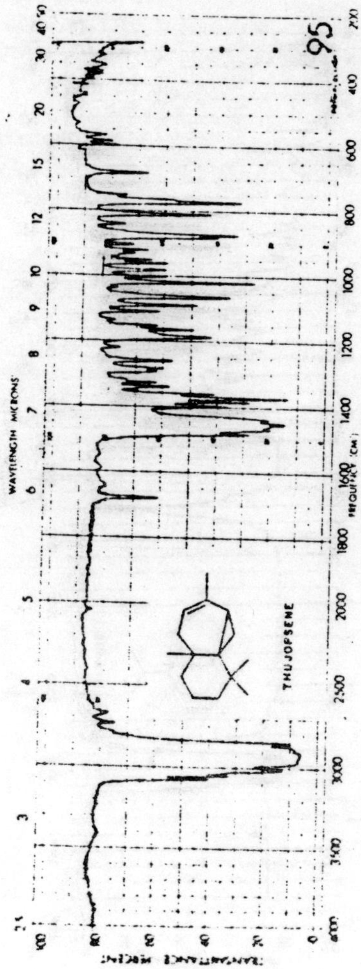
95
THUJOPSENE

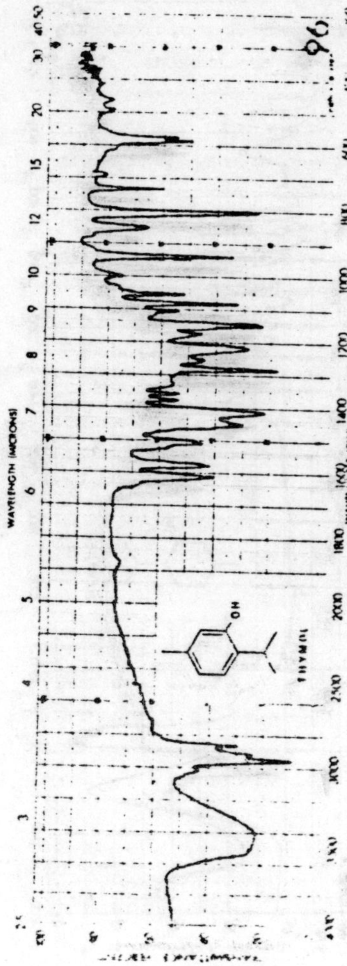
96
THYMOL
OH

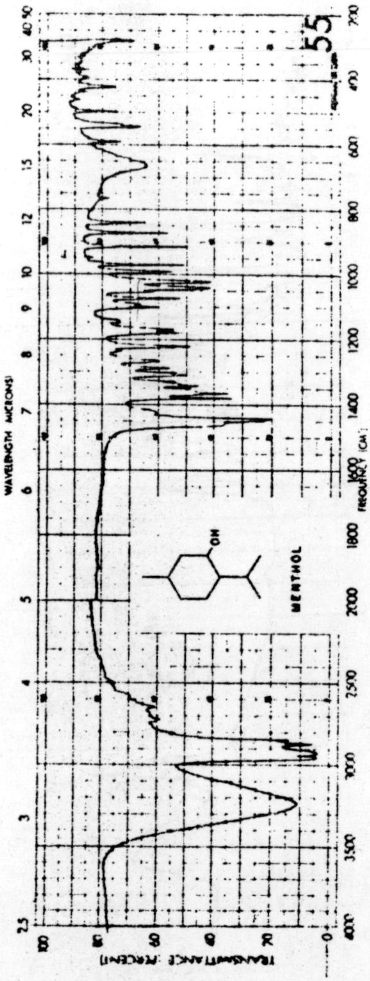
55
MENTHOL
OH

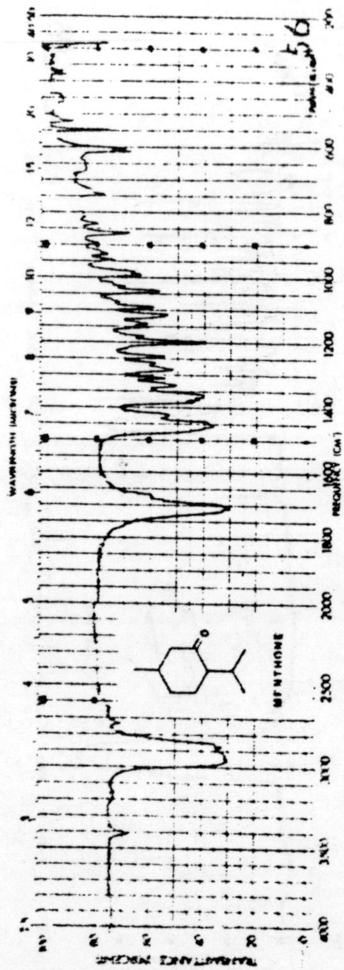
56
MENTHONE
O

6

Analysis of Cosmetics

Lipsticks

A lipstick is a mixture of fatty base materials typically composed of various oils, waxes, glycerol, and oleyl alcohol, dissolved colors, suspended pigments, and perfume, Table 1 lists the typical composition of a lipstick.

Table 1. Typical Analysis of a Lipstick

solids, wt%		99.2
volatile compounds, wt %		0.8
Total		100.0
dyes and pigments, wt %		6.8
D & C Red No. 19	0.4	
D & C Red No. 21	1.2	
D & C Red No,. 5	0.8	
insoluble pigments	4.4	
oils wt %		78.2
mineral oil	3.8	
Castor oil	59.5	
oley aleohol	<0.1	
vegetable oil	12.8	
wexes, wt%		16.5
hydrocarbon waxes	6.7	
beeswax	3.8	
vegetable waxes		
carnauba wax	3.2	
hydrogenated coconut wax	0.5	
Castor wax	2.3	
Total		101.5

Methods of Analysis

In the analysis of lipsticks, first the insolûble materials dyes are separated from the fatty base material which in turn is separated into its components by liquid columm chromatogryphy. Separate methods deal with the determination of the individual dyes present.

Separation And Indentification

For the separation and identification of the components of a lipstick, two general schemes are utilized, the first employing an alumina, and the second a silica gel column.

The method employing an alumina column is relatively fast, and separates the oil and wax phases into gross fractions. A disadvantage of this method is that some unsaturated fatty acids will isomerize on the column. The procedure is detailed below

Table 2. Separation of Substanees Used in Cosmetics, on a Silica Gel Column

Solvent system	Elution after removal of ionies and inorganic substances	Additional compounds eluted if sample was not treated to remove ionics and inorganic substances
Chloroform	highly nonpolar compounds	
	hydrocarbon oils	
	petrolatum	
	long chain esters	
	Ianolin	
99:1 Chloroform-ethyl ether	triglycerides	
	long chain fattly acids	
	long chain fatty alcohols	
	lauric acid	
	oleic acid	
	isopropyl myristate	
	cetly alcohol	
	oleyl alcohol	
	stearyl alcohols	
1:1 Chloroform-ethyl ether	oil-soluble surfactants:	
	ethoxylated fatty acids and alkyl phenols (<4 EtO)	
	glyceryl monoesters	
	diethylene glycol	

	Sorbitan monoesters glycery di-and tristearate and oleate castor oil long chain hydroxy esters soap and fattly acid diethanolamide (Spreads to next fraction; to prevent this, use more solvent)	
1:1 Chloroform-acetone	surfactants with intermediate polarity (<11 EtO) Spans, Tweens fatty acid alcohol amide Tergitol (<11 EtO)	
9:1Chloroform-methanol	highly hydrophilie surfactants (>10 EtO) polyoxyethylene glycols with moderate mol wt (Carbowax, 600, 1000) Spans, Tweens	
2:1 Chloroform-methanol	most highly hydrophilie materials glycerol polyoxyethylene glycols with high mot wt (Carbowax 4000) Tergitol (high Eto)	alkyl ary sulfonate sulfates sulfonates
1;1 Chloroform-methanol	fatty acid diethanolamide	Quaternary compounds sulfates sulfonates dialkyl quaternary ammonium Chloride steary 1 dimethy benzyl ammonium chloride triethanolamine
methnol	glycerol propylene glycol proteins gums	

Procedures

Preliminary Separation. Disperse 5 g of sample in 100 ml of carbon disulfide on a steam bath. Filter the mixture through a sheet of tared Whatman No. 1 filter paper. Wash the residue on the filter paper with 100 ml of hot carbon disulfide and add the wash liquid to the filtrate. Retain the filtrate for the subsequent separation of the oils and waxes.

Dry the residue on the filter paper at 105°C for 10 min, then weigh. Pass 200 ml of hot 1:9 hydrochloric acid through the filter and acid-soluble pigments in a tared beaker. Pass 200 ml of 20% ammonium hydroxide through the filter and collect the alkai soluble dyes and pigments in a tared beaker. Pass 200 ml of 20% ammonium hydroxide through the filter and collect the alkali-soluble dyes and pigments in a tared beaker. Dry and weigh the residue consisting of oxides and fillers, such as titanium dioxide remaining on the filter paper. Evaporate the separate acid-soluble and alkali-soluble fractions, dry, and weigh.

Evaporate the filtrate containing the oils and waxes to dryness on a steam bath, then dissolve the residue in 150 ml of hot absolute ethanol and chill to approximately -35°C. Filter the waxes insoluble at low temperature on a filter paper, and wash the residue in the flask and on the paper with cold ethanol. Use the combined filtrate for the separation of the oils.

Separation Of Waxes. Slurry activated alumina, Woelm neutral grade or equivalent, with n-heptane and pour the slurry into a 12in. long,3/4 in. OD glass Column fitted with a Teflon stopecock and a small prewashed cotton plug.

Do not use stopcock grease on any ground-glass joints. Place a small prewashed cotton plug on the top of the column of alumina. Dissolve 1 g of the wax residue in 25 ml of hot n-heptane, hot carbon tetrachloride, hot chloroform, hot ethyl acetate, and hot absolute ethanol, using a flow rate of 10 ml/min. Collect each 400-ml elution in 600-ml tared beakers. Evaporate all fractions to dryness on a steam bath and then at 105°C for 10 min, weigh each fraction, and calculate the percentage of each in the original sample. The various waxes present will be distributed in the fractions as follows:

heptane solution	hydrocarbon waxes
carbon tetrachloride solution	solid lanolin esters, beeswax
chloroform solution	carnauba wax
ethyl acetate solution	hydrogenated coconut oil
ethanol solution	castor wax

Separation Of Oils. Evaporate the ethanolic filtrate reatined from the preceding work to dryness, then dissolve 1 g of the residue in 25 ml of n-heptane and carry out the separation of the dissolved oils in a way identical to that described above for waxes, except that the solvents used should be at room temperature. The components will be distributed in the fractions in the following way:

heptane solution	hydrocarbon oils, mineral oil
carbon tetrachloride solution	liquid lanolin esters
chloroform solution	castor oil derivatives
ethyl acetate solution	castor oil
ethanol solution	eastor and soybean oils

Each fraction should be examined for appearance, color, odor, and feel when rubbed between the fingers. The "feel" can provide useful clues, such as the tackiness and drag of lanolin. The individual fractions can be identified by the comparison of their IR spectra with the spectra of known substances. If necessary, additional tests should be carried out to aid in the identification of the fractions, eg, the determination of the melting point is useful for waxes, the Liebermann-Burchard test for lanolin.

The second method used for the separation of the components of lipsticks utilizes a silica gel column. This method is relatively slow but gives a much better separation of the components present. Usually, the sample is first freed of anionies or cationics by passage through a mixedbed ion exchange column; if inorganic components are present, the solid sample is extracted with chloroform. The chloroform solution is placed on top of a 14 × 3/4 in. silica gel column and eluted with a number of solvent combination. Table 2 is a listing of the compound types eluted with the various solvent systems, which should be used in the order given in the table.

The silica method is not restricted to the analysis of lipsticks but has a wide applicability for various types of cosmetic preparations.

Analysis of Dyes Present In Lipsticks

The dyes present in lipsticks can be separated and determined by thin-layer chromatography. Two convenient methods are described in the literature, both utilizing silica gel plates of 350-375 um thickness.

Cotsis utilised four solvents for development, as follows:

No.1: benzene

No.2: 65:30:4 benzene-methanol-concentrated ammonium hydroxide

No. 3: 65:30:5 benzene-n-amyl alcohol-concentrated hydrochloric acid

No. 4: 60:30:10 benzene -n-propanol-concentrated ammonium hydroxide

The lipstick is dissolved under reflux in 3:1 benzene-acetone (1g in 50), and the resulting solution spotted immediately on the TLC-plates. The analysis is considered finished when the solvent front travels 15 cm from the application line. Most dyes can be separated by using solvent No. 2, but some require the development with one or more additional developing solents. Table 3 lists the systems recommended for various dye mixtures.

Together with the sample, standard dye solutions should also be spotted on the plate and the components of the unknown mixture determined by comparing the R, values. Identity of the dyes should be confirmed also by fluorescence under UV light and, if necessary, by their absorption spectra (see below). It is critical that the chromatographic determination be carried out under constant and relatively low humidity conditions.

In the second method described for the analysis of dyes in lipsticks, the lipstick is applied directly, with very light pressure, to a warm, TLC plate (heated at 100°C for 3&5 min) in two or three overlapping streaks so that the total amount deposited should be about 5-8 mg on a 4×8 in. plate. The still warm plate is placed in a tank containing dichloromethane solvent and developed until the solvent reaches the top of the plate, then dried and redeveloped for a total of 2-4 developments. This treatment separates the oils and waxes and moves them to the top of the plate where they no longer interfere with the subsequent development of the dyes present. During this development, the unsulfonated dyes are also separated in the following order: D &C Red 36 and D & C Orange 17. After removal of these zones the plate should be developed in the same direction with 15:3:09:2.1 ethyl acetate-methanol-concentrated ammonium hydroxide-water. Usually a solvent front movement of 15-17 cm is enough; if the bands are not well resolved, the plate should be redeveloped after drying. This solvent system separates the following dyes in descending order: D & C Red 19, D & C Red 8 + 10, D&C Orange 4, D & C Red 27, D & C Red 3, D & C Red 21, D & C Orange 5, monobromofluoresecein, fluorescein, and FD & C Blue 1.

Table 3. Development Solvents Recommended for the Analysis of Dyes in Lipsticks

Dye mixture	Developing solvent	Approximate developing time
D & C Orange 17 D & C Red 30	benzene	10-15 min
D & C Red 36 D & C Red 30 D & C Red 34 D & C Yellow 5	developing solvent No. 2, then developing solvent No. 1	45 min + 10-15 min
D & C Red 9 D & C Red 10 D & C Red 13	developing solvent No. 3. multiple development is required: develop, dry, redevelop, and repeat until the separation is complete	

If the presence of D & C Red 7 is likely, a modification of the method is recommended. The plate is first spotted as a row of small overlapping drops with a pH 8.0 phosphate buffer prepared by mixing 5-3 ml of 0.1 M dispotassium hydrogen phosphate and 94.7 ml of potassium dihydrogen phosphate and diluting to 200 ml; both original phosphate solutions should contain a few drops of toluene as a preservative. The plate is then air-dried and the lipstick applied as given above, just below the buffer zone, and developed with dichloromethane. Then the plate is developed in the same direction with 20:4:3 *n*-butanol-95% ethanol-concentrted ammonium hydroxide until the solvent front travels-95% ethanol-concentrated ammonium hydroxide until the solvent front travels 5 cm. The plate is removed and dried under a jet of air and with gentle heat while the base of the plate is elevated slightly so that backflow of solvent and color into the D & C Red 7 zone, which remains near the origin, is prevented. The development is repeated once or twice, until a colorless zone, about 1/4 in. wide, has developed above the D & C Red 7 zone. Then this zone is scraped from the plate and the plate is developed with ethyl acetate-methanol-ammonium hydroxide water as in the basic method.

The individual zones are scraped from the plate and determined spectrophotometrically. Table 4 lists the solvent systems, absorption maxima, and absorbance values.

Table 4: Spectral Data of Dyes Used in Lipsticks

Dye	Solvent*	Absorption maximum, nm	Extinction coefficient*
FD&C Red 3	A	532	1240
D & C Red 7	B	515	540
D & C Red 9	B	487	380
D & C Red 10	B	497	630
D & C Red 19	B	555	2560
D & C Red 21	A	525	1720
D & C Red 27	A	550	1460
D & C Red 30	C	536	290
D & C Red 34	B	522	620
D & C Red 36	C	485	820
D & C Orange 4	B	483	530
D & C Orange 5 tribromofluorescein	A	518	1670
D & C Orange 5 dibromolfuorescein	A	513	1690
D & C Orange 17	C	477	770
FD & C Yellow 5	A	624	
FD & C Blue 1	A	430	460

"Solvent A=3:1 accetone-water containing 1% NH_4OH
Solvent B= *n*-amyl alcohol shaken with hydrochloric acid
Solvent C=3:1 benzene-acetone.
Extinction coefficient =$E^{1\%}$/cm = A/Ce where A=absorbance, C=% concentration, I=cell path length, in cm.

Quality Control of Lipsticks

For quick quality control, the lipsticks produced are compared to "standard lipsticks " concerning color, shade, and other physical characteristics. The standard lipsticks are prepared in the following way.

Procedure

Weigh 20 g of the mixture of selected organic dyes into a 150-ml beaker, add 20 g of castor oil, and stir until a smooth mixture is obtained. Grind on a roller mill three times, or until a reading of greater than 7 is obtained on the n.s. scale of a Hegeman gage. Collect the paste in a beaker.

Weigh 9.0 g of the paste into a 250-ml beaker, add 15.5 g of castor oil, and stir by hand, then add 76 g of molten lipstick base, place in a hot water bath, and stir with a stirring motor. While stirring, add 3.3 ml of a 1:1 mixture of polyethylene glycol 400 and propylene glycol.

Into a second 1250-ml beaker weigh 9.0 g of the paste, 19.4 g of a titamium dioxide paste containing a 1:1 mixture of titanium dioxide and castor oil, mixed and ground three times in a roller mill, an mix by hand. Add 76g of molten base, place in a hot water bath, and stir with a stirring motor; while stirring, add 3.3 ml of the polyethylene glyeol-propylene glycol mixture. Allow each sample to stir for 10 min and then remain in the water bath, without stirring, fpr 2-3 hr. Stir, and pour into lipstick molds.

Nail Enamels

Most nail enamels are mixtures of film formers, plasticizer, resin, and solvent, along with suspended pigment. The predominant film former is cellulose nitrate; dibutyl phthalate, tricresyl phosphate, and camphor are employed as plasticizers and aryl sulfonamide-formaldehyde polymers frequently are used as the resin. The sulfonamide resins contribute excellent depth, flow, adhesion, and good water resistance to the film.

Table 5. Typical Analysis of a Nail Enamel

solids, wt %		28.0
pigment	1.0	
cellulose nitrate	18.1	
plasticizer		
dibutyl phthalate +tricresyl phosphatew	3.2	
camphor	1.5	
resin	4.2	
solvent, wt %		70.5
ethanol	6.2	
ethyl acetate	23.3	
butyl acetate	24.5	
toluene	16.5	
Total		*98.5*

The pigments may be organic lakes, guanine, bismuth oxychloride, or titanium dioxide. The solvents are mixtures of butyl acetate, ethyl acetate, toluene, isopropyl alcohol, and ethanol. A typical nail enamel composition is given in Table 5.

Methods of Analysis

Solids (Nonvolatile Matter)

The amount of nonvolatile matter in nail enamels is determined by heating for 3-4 hr at 80°C. Heating should be discontinued immediately when the solvent odor disappears or when the odor of camphor, if present, becomes noticeable. As little camphor as possible should be removed because it is considered as part of the solids or non volatiles. a small evacuable oven is useful for periodically removing vapors as they accumulate; however, the use of vacuum is not recommended.

Composition of the Nonvolatile Matter. The nonvolatile matter is separated into its components by the utilization of various solvents. The separated individual components are identified by their infrared spectrum. The procedure is given below

Procedure

Disperse 5 g of sample in 25 ml of acetone in a Corex test tube, with the aid of a small magnet and magnetic stirrer, and centrifuge the mixture at 10,000 rpm for 10 min. The acetone-insoluble materials (pearl (guanine), pigments, some gelling agents) collect at the bottom of the tube and the gelling agents, such as bentonites, appear as a gel layer on top of the pigment layer. Decant the acetone into a tared beaker and save both layers. Repeat the acetone extraction of the pigments twice more with 25-ml portions of acetone. After the final centrifugation and decantation, if a gel layer is present, physically separate it from the pigment layer with the aid of a stream of acetone from a squeeze bottle. Dry the gel layer at 105°C, and identify it from the infrared spectrum. Dry the gel layer, and identify it from the infrared spectrum. Dry the pigment layer, and weigh.

Evaporate the composite acetone fraction in a tared beaker to dryness on the steam bath and weigh. Add 100 ml of benzene, disperse the residue with stirring and evaporate to about 20 ml on a steam bath. Repeat the addition of benzene and the evaporation two more times. On the final addition of benzene, warm the mixture on a steam bath and filter hot through a Whatman No. 1 filter paper, or equivalent, into tared beaker. Wash the cellulose nitrate residue on the filter paper with 50 ml of hot benzene, then dissolve the cellulose nitrate by pouring 100-200 ml of acetone through the filter, and collect in a tared beaker. Evaporate the acetone solution to dryness and weigh. Confirm the identification by comparing the IR spectrum with sepctra of known substanes.

Evaporate the retained benzene solution to dryness and dissolve in 80 ml of absolute methanol, then add 20 ml of water. Extract four times with 40 ml of petroleum ether. Combine the petroleum ether extracts in tared beaker, evaporate to dryness, weigh, and identify determine percent composition from the refractive index of the material as compared with calibration curves obtained from known binary mixture is present, determine perfect composition from the refractive index of the material as compared with calibration curves obtained from known binary mixtures.

Dilute the retained 80% methanol solution with 150 ml of water, acidify with hydrochloric acid extract twice with 150-ml portions of Chloroform. Combine the chloroform extracts, evaporate to dryness, weight, and identify the resin present from its IR spectrum.

Bismuth Oxychloride

Bismuth oxychloride, one of the important pigment substances, can be determined by a number of methods involving polarography or titrimetry. A titrimetric procedure utilizing EDTA is given below.

Procedure

Accurately weigh a sample containing approximately 150 -200 mg of bismuth oxychloride into a 100-ml beaker. Add 30 ml of acetone and swirl flask to disperse. With the aid of acetone, filter through a gooch crucible containing a tightly packed mat of asbestos, and then wash the beaker and crucible with ten rinses of acetone. Dry for 30 min at 105°C.

Place the crucible on a 500-ml suction flask, add 15 ml of concentrated nitric acid, and allow to stand for 10 min without vacuum. Start suction and then wash with five 10-ml portions of 1:1 nitric acid followed by five 10-l portions of water. Quantitatively transfer the contents of the flask to a 500-ml portion flask, cool to room temperature, and dilute to volume with water.

Transfer a 50-ml aliquot into a 150-ml beaker, add 4.0 ml of 0.0500 methylenediaminetetraacetic acid (EDTA) solution, and adjust to pH 3.0-4.0 with 20% w/v sodium hydroside solution ,using a pH meter.

Add, from aburet, 2.0 ml of standardized 0.05 M bismuth nitrate solution and approximately 0.2 g of hydroxylamine hydrochloride. Readjust to pH2.0-3.0 and add sufficient pyrocatechlol violet indicator prepared by mixing 100 mg of pyrocatechol violet powder and 5-6 g of sucrose, to impart a bright yellow color. Continue the titration with the 0.05 M bismuth nitrate solution while maintaining a pH of 2.5-3.0 with the addition of a 5% sodium hydroxide solution until there is a sharp color change form yellow to the blue end point.

$$\text{Bismuth oxychloride \%} = \frac{(V1M1 - V^2 1M2)}{w} \quad 260.5$$

where V_1 = Vol of EDTA solution added in ml (=4ml)]

M_1= molarity of the EDTA solution

V_2= vol of the bismuth nitrate solution used for titration, in ml

M_2= molarity of the bismuth nitrate solution

w = sample wt, in g

Free Formaldehyde

Free formaldehyde in nail enamels can be determined by polarography or by a colorimetric procedure The latter is given below.

Procedure

Accurately weigh 2-3 g of sample into a 40-ml centrifuge tube and add 25.0 of water. Stopper the tube and shake vigorously. Centrifuge the mixture and transfer 1.0 ml of the aqueous phase into a test tube. Add 9.0 ml of water and 10.0 ml of the acetylacetone reagent prepared by adding 150 g of ammonium acetate, 3 ml of glacial acetic acid, and 2 ml of acetylacetone into a 1-liter volumetric flask and diluting to volume with water. Shake and allow to stand for 40 min at 37°C. Read the absorbance of the solution in an ultraviolet spectrophotometer at 412 nm vs a reagent blank. Determine the amount of formaldehyde in the aliquot from a standard curve prepared by determining the absorbances of 1,2,3,4,5 8, and 10 ml of a form aldehyde solution with a concentration of 0.025 mg/ml.

Solvents

The components of the solvent used in nail enamels are separated and determined by gas chromatography. The sample is dispersed in isooctane (3 g in 8ml), filtered in a closed system, and the solution kept in a tube closed with a serum cap for analysis.

Table 6. Retention Time of Common Solvents Used in Nail Enamels

Compound	DC-200 silicone grease[a] 75°C	100°C	Carbowax 20m[a] 45°C
ethanol	2.1	1.25	2.5
isopropyl alcohol	2.5	1.50	2.5
acetone	2.5	1.50	1.3
Carbitol		2.00	
methyl ethyl ketone		2.50	
ethyl acetate	5.0	2.75	2.2
hexane		3.00	
chlorothene		3.75	
methyl Cellosolve		3.75	
benzene		4.00	
butanol		4.00	
cyclohexane		4.25	
heptane		5.25	
isooctane	10.0	5.25	1.5
ethyl Cellosolve		5.75	
methyl isobutyl ketone		6.25	
amyl alcohol		7.50	
toluene	16.5	8.10	5.0
amyl acetate		9.50	
butyl acetate	21.1	9.75	7.0
xylene		15.5	
butyl Cellosolve		19.8	

10ft x¼ in. OD, 5wt% stationary phase on acid-washed Chromosorb W60/80 mesh. Helium carrier gas at 60ml/min.

For the analysis, columns prepared with DC-200 silicone grease and Carbowax 20M are recommended; Table 6 lists the analytical conditions and the retention times obtained on these columns. If a thermal conductivity detector is used, a sample volume of about 5μl is recommended. If the determination of camphor by gas chromatography is needed, an analysis should be made on the DC-200 column at 180°C.

SHAMPOOS

Shampoos are preparations of surfactants which, when used properly, remove grease, dirt, and skin debris from the scal; and hair.

The surfactants used in shampoos can be divided into nonionic, anioic, and cationic surfactants. Ethoxylated lanolin alcoholos, polyethylene oxide, or silicone fluid are typical nonionic surfactants; soaps, alkyl sulfates as alkali metal, ammonium, or alkanolamine salts, alkyl aryl sulfates and sulfonates are typical anionic surfactants, whereas quaternary ammonium compound's and cationic protein are typical cationic surfactants. Other substances used in shampoo formulations include sequestering agents, mineral oil, lanolin, gums, and hexachlorophene. Inorganic salts may also be added.

Methods of Analysis

The analysis of a shampoo starts with the determination of its pH, in addition to the amount of nonvolatile matter ("Solids") and water present. If the sum of these two is less than 100%, the amount of alcohol present is determined also. For detailed analysis, the nonvolatile matter is separated in multistage processes into organic substance groups; certain elements and anions may be determined from the ash. The anionic, cationic, and nonionic surfactants present may be separated form each other and determined as a group. If the type of shampoo has been identified, detailed multistage separation processes permit the determination of individual substances or substance groups.

Composition Analysis

Nonvolatile Matter (Solids)

The amount of nonvolatile matter of shampoos is determined by drying a sample aliquot at 105°C for 2 hr.

Water

The water content of shampoos is determined by the Karl Fischer method by toluene distillation or by gas chromatography utilizing microporuus polymer beads, such as Porapak Q, as the column packing.

Alcohol

The determination of the ethanol content of the sample can conveniently be carried out by gas chromatographic analysis on a 6 ft x¼ in. OD column packed with Porapak Q microporous polymer beads, at 125°C. The measurement also permits the simultaneous determination of water.

Usually, a qualitative test is also carried out to check for the presence of propylene glycol. The test is performed from the aqueous phase obtained when the water content is determined by toluene distillation. Two procedures are given below.

Procedures

Catechol Test (13). To 3 ml of the aqueous phase, add 3 ml of freshly prepared 10% catechol solution and 6 ml of concentrated sulfuric acid. Heat in a boiling water bath for 30min. If the solution turns red and a precipitate forms, propylene glycol is present.

Iodoform Test To 5 ml of the aqueous phase, add 5 ml of a 0.2 M potassium periodate solution. After I min add an excess of a 5% sodium hydroxide solution followed by a o.1 N iodine solution. If a precipitate of iodoform forms immediately, propylene glycol is present.

If the test is positive, the amount of propylene glycol present can be determined by gas chromatography at 200°C, on the Porapak Q column specified for ethanol analysis.

Analysis Of The Nonvolatile Matter

Solubility in Ethanol

For the determination of the ethanol-soluble and nonsoluble parts, the dried nonvolatile matter is dissolved in hot ethanol (2g in 100 ml), and filtered. The residue is washed with not ethanol, then dissolved in hot water evaporated to dryness, and weighed.

Ash

The ethanol-insoluble residue is ignited and charred at a temperature as low as possibe to effect the combustion of carbon. After cooling in a desiccator, the ash is weighed. If desired, the ash may be tested for certain ions, according to the following procedures

Procedures

Borate. Add a few drops of sulfuric acid to a portion of the ash in a white procelain dish. Add several ml of methanol, stir well, and ignite in a darkened hood. A green flame indicates the presence of boron; note the first flash.

Sulfate Dissolve a portion of the ash in water, and add dropwise 0.3 M barium acetate solution. A white precipitate indicates the presence of sulfate.

Phosphate

Dissolve a portion of the ash in water, add 3 drops fo 6 N nitric acid, and then 6-8 drops of a N ammonium molybdate solution. On warming the mixture slightly, ammonium phosphomolybdate (yellow) gradually precipitates when phosphate is present.

Sodium and Potassium

Moisten a portion of the with hydrochloric acid. Scoop some of the mixture onto a previously ignited platinum loop and introduce into a Bunsen flame. A yellow flame persisting for several seconds indicates the presence of sodium. A reddish-violet flame confirms the presence of potassium. View the flame through blue cobalt glass to remove sodium flame interference.

Titanium

Heat a portion of the ash with 2-4 ml of cocentrated sulfurie acid and 1-2 g of sodium sulfate in a porcelain crucible. Cool and cautiously pour into 25 ml of cold water. Add 5 drops of 3% hydrogen peroxide to 5 drops of the above prepared mixture. A yellow color indicates the presence of titanium.

Organic Substances

Usually, tests are made for the presence of gums and proteins. Gums may be identified also from the original shampoo while the tests for proteins are performed from the water solution of the ethanol-insoluble matter.

Procedures

Gums

Precipitate the water-soluble gums by adding ethanol to the original shampoo or to the water solution of the ethanol-insoluble matter.

Separate the gum by centrifugation and decantation. Dissolve the gum in a small amount of water and reprecipitate by the addition of alcohol. Centrifuge and discard the decantate. Run an infrared spectrum on a cast film of the gum and compare with standard spectra to gums.

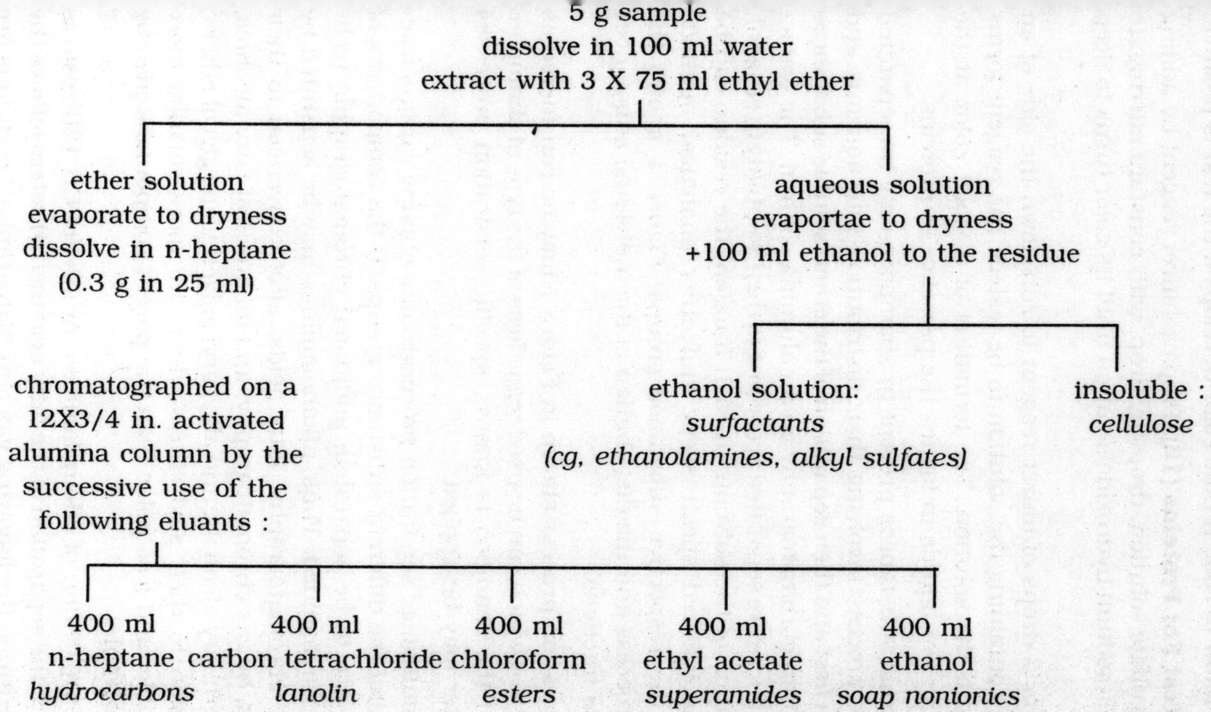

Fig. 1. Separation of the organic constituents of a shampoo.

Ninhydrin Test For Proteins (16)

To 5 ml of the solution to be tested, which must be almost neutral, add 0.5 ml of a 0.1% aqueous ninhydrin solution, heat to boiling for 1-2 min, and allow to cool. A blue color develops if the test is positive.

Biuret Test For Proteins (16). Prepare biuret reagent by adding a 1% copper sulfate solution, drops by drop, with constant stirring, to 50 ml of a 40% sodium hydroxide solution until its color turns to deep blue.

Allow 2 or 3 drops of biuret reagent to run down the side of an inclined tube containing the solution to be tested. The reagent forms a layer beneath the solution. The formation of a violet color at the interface of the two liquids indicates the presence of proteins.

The organic substances present in shampoos may be separated by multistage process involving their distribution into aqueous and ether solution first and then separation of the ether-soluble substances by liquid column chromatography on an alumina column. The water-soluble substances are separated according to their solubility in ethanol. After evaporation of the solvents in each fraction, the residue can be indentified by infrared spectroscopy and other analytical methods speicific for the respective substance groups. Figure 1 shows the separation proccess and the distribution of the individual substances in the various fractions.

The separation process shown in Figure 1 may be considered as a general method which can be used regardless of the type of shampoo. If the type of the shampoo is known, specific separation processes discussed later may be applied.

In the multistage separation processes one obtains various fractions combining the different substance groups. If the components of such groups are to be separated, additional chromatographic techniques are recommended. Thus, alkanolamines may be separated by ion exchange chromatography; fatty acids, after conversion to their methyl esters, by gas chromatography; and mixtures of fatty alcohols, ethoxylated primary alcohols, and alkyl aryl polyethylene glycol ethers, after conversion to their silyl ethers which are more volatile, more thermally stable, and less polar than the parent compounds, also by gas chromatography.

For the separation of alkanolamines, Amberlite CG 120 resin is recommended; the separation of the fatty acid methyl esters follows the general procedures; the following gas chromatographic conditions are recommended for the separation of the silyl ethers :

column	two 10 ft X 1/8 in. OD packed, used in the base line compensation mode
column packing	5 wt % SE-30 silicone gum rubber on silanized Chromosord W 80/100 mesh
temperature of	
injection port	240°C
column	programmed from 100°C to 300° C at 6°C/min
detector	300°C
carrier gas and flow rate	helium, 75 ml/min
sample volume	2 μl of the reaction mixture with the silylization reagent
dectector	dual flame ionization

Surfactants

In the shampoos, anionic, cationic, and nonionic surfactants are present. The nonionic surfactants are usually isolated during the separation process and the ionic surfactants are determined by direct titration. Methods for the determination of anionic and cationic surfactants are given below and procedures are outlined for their separation from the nonionic surfactants.

Aniomic Surfactants. The anionic surfactant in a sample is calculated from the volume of standard Hyamine 1622 solution required to titrate the sample.

Hyamine 1622 is the trade name, Philadelphia for benzyldimethy {2-[2-(p-1,1,3,3-tetramethylbuty phenoxy)ethoxy]ethyl} ammonium chloride

($C_{27}H_{42}ClNO_2H_2O$).

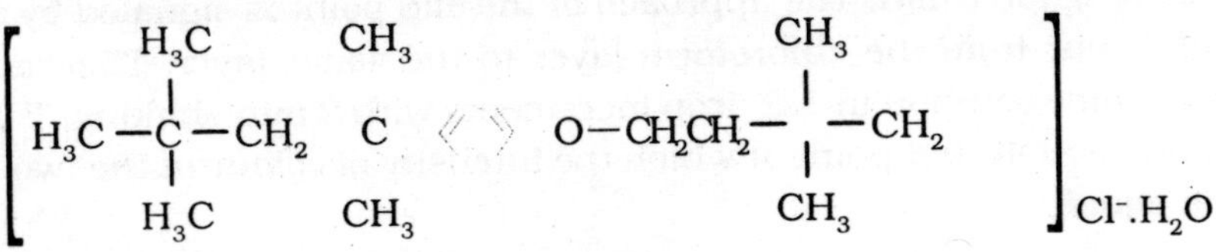

HYAMINE 1622

Procedure

Prepare a standard Hyamine solution by dissolving 1.50 g of Hyamine 1622 in 1 liter of water. Prepare a standard Aerosol OT solution by dissolving 3.00 g of 100% Aerosol OT, a product of American Cyanamid Co. (the S-sodium salt of sulfosuccinic acid bis (2-ethylhexyl)ester) in 1 litre of water. Prepare a standard methylene blue solution in the following way: dissolve 0.1 g of methylene blue in 100 ml of water, transfer 30 ml of this solution to a 1-liter volumetric flash, add 600 ml of water, 6.8 ml of concentrated sulfuric acid, and 50 g of sodium dihydrogen phosphate monohydrate, $NaH_2PO_4H_2O$. Swirl to disslove and dilute to volume with water.

Standardize the Hyamine solution in the following way: pipet 10 ml of the standard Aerosol OT solution, 25 ml of the standard methylene blue solution, and 15 ml of Chloroform into a 100-ml graduated Cylinder and proceed with the titration as described below.

$$F_H = \frac{W_A}{100V_H}$$

where F_H = aerosol equivalent of the Hyamine solution, in g/ml

W_H = amount of Hyamine presnet in 10 ml of standard solution, in g

V_A = vol of Hyamine solution used for titration, in ml

Weigh an amount of sample sufficient to give a titration of 15-25 ml as determined by a preliminary titration. Dissolve the sample in a beaker with about 50 ml of water, then transfer to a 100-ml volumetric flask and dilute to volume. Pipet 10 ml of this solution into a 100-ml graduated cylinder and add 25 ml of the standard methylene blue solution and 15 ml of chloroform. From a buret add quickly 90-95% of the standard Hyamine solution that will be required. Stopper the cylinder, shake for 30 see and allow the layers to separate. Continue addition of the Hyamine solution in small increments with vigorous shaking for 1 min. The approach of the end point is signaled by a shift of colour from the chloroform layer to the water layer. Then add the Hyamine solution in 1-2 drop increments with 2 min shaking. Take the end point at that point at which the intensity of colour in the two layers is equal.

$$\text{Anionic surfactants, wt \%} = \frac{(V_H)\ (F_H)\ (MW_S)\ (100)}{(W_S)\ (MW_A)}$$

where V_H = vol of standard Hyamine solution required for titration, in ml

F_H = aerosol equivalent of the Hyamine solution, in g/ml

MW_S = average molecular weight of the anionic surfactants present in the sample

MW_A = mol wt of Aerosol OT (=444.7)

W_S = sample wt, in g

Cationic Surfactants. The cationic surfactant in a sample is determined by titration with an anionic surfactant, such as Aerosol OT, in the presence of methy lene blue indicator. The procedure is actually the reverse of the procedure given for the determination of anionic surfactants.

Procedure

Prepare a standard Aerosol OT solution by dissolving 1.50 g of 100% Aerosol OT in 1 liter of water. Prepare a standard Hyamine solution by dissolving 3.00 g of Hyamine 1622 in 1 liter of water. Prepare a standard methylene blue solution in a way identical to that given above for anionic surfactants. Standardize the Aerosol OT solution in the following way: pipet 10 ml of the standard Hyamine solution, 25 ml of the standard methylene blue solution, and 15 ml of chloroform into a 100 ml granduated cylinder, and proceed with the titration as described below.

$$F_H = \frac{W_H}{100V_A}$$

where F_A = Hyamine equivalent of the Aerosol solution. in g/ml

W_H = amount of Hyamine present in 10 ml of standard solution, in g

V_A = vol of Aerosol solution used for titration, in ml

Weigh an amount of sample sufficient to give a titration of 15-25 ml as determine by a preliminiary titration. Dissolve the sample and carry out the titration as desribed for anionic surfactants with the exception of substituting the standard Aero-ol OT solution for the standard Hyamine solution.

$$\text{Cationic surfactants,wt \%} = \frac{(V_A)\ (F_A)\ (MW_8)\ (100)}{(W_S)\ (MW_H)}$$

where V_A = vol of standard Aerosol solution required for titration, in ml

F_A = Hyamine equivalent of the Aerosol solution, in g/ml

MW_S = average mol wt of the cationic surfactants present in the sample

MW_H = mol wt of Hyamine 1622 (=466.1)

W_S = sample wt, in g

Separation of Ionic and Nominic Surfactants. If necessary, nonionic and ionic surfactants can be separated with the help of ion exchange resins. In this process the ionic surfactants are retained by the resins and are then eluted by a multistage process outlined in Figure 2. The nonionic surfactants which are not retained by the resin are separated into petroleum ether soluble and insoluble fractions. Table 7 lists some of the nonionic surfactants according to their petroleum ether solubility.

Table 7. Petroleum Ether Solubility of Nonicate Surfactants[a]

Soluble	Insoluble
Triton X-100	Pluronic F-217
alkyl phenoxy polyethoxy ethanol	Myrj 53
Trycol LaL-4S	POL (50) stearate
ethylene oxide brached chain	Lipocol L-12
laury alcohol	POE (12) laury alcohol
Liposorb SQO	Tween 60 (dispersible-turbid)
sorbitan sesquioleate	POE (4) sorbitan monostearate
Lipocol S-2	Tween 61 (dispersible-turbid)
POE(2) cetyl ether	POE (20) sorbitan monosterate
Lipocol S-2	
POE (2) stearyl ether	
Brij 30	
POE (4) laury ether	
Brij 35	
POE (23) laury ether	

POE = Polyoxyethylene.

Procedures

Nonionic And Anionic Surfactants

Add 1-5 g of sample to 100 ml of water, swirl to dissolve and to minimize foam. Ethanol may be added to aid in solution, but its total volume should not exceed 30 ml. Add 20 g of Dowex 1-X4, 200-400 mesh anion exchange resin and stir for 4-5 hr. Filter the mixture and suspend the resin in 50 ml of 95% ethanol. Repeat the filtration and suspension of the resin twice more. Combine the filtrates and washings and adjust the alcohol-water balance to equal 1:1 95% ethanol-water. Wash the resin with 100 ml of petroleum ether and extract the combined ethanol-water solutions with the petroleum ether washing. Extract the solution twice more with 100-ml portions of pure petroleum ether. The combined extracts will contain the petroleum ether soluble nonionic surfactants whereas the aqueous alcohol solution the nonionic surfactants insoluble in petroleum ether.

Nonionic And Cationic Surfactants

Add 4-5 g of sample to 100 ml of water, swirl to dissolve and to minimize foam. If necessary, add 95% ethanol to aid in solution but do not allow the volume to exceed 30 ml.

Purify Dowex 50-X4 cation exchange resin in the following way. Slurry 20 g of the resin with 50 ml of methanol for 15 min, filter, and wash with 30 ml of methanol, then stir the resin with 50 ml of methanol for 15 min, filter, and wash with 30 ml of methanol. If necessary, continue the washing until the filterate is colorless.

Add the purified resin to the sample solution and add a few drops of congo red indicator. If it is not acidic, add enouth dilute hydrochloric acid, then stir the mixture for 4-5 hr testing occasionaly to ensure that it remians acidic to congo red. Filter and wash the resin by suspending 2-3 times in a total of 100 ml of 95% ethanol. Combine the filtrate and washing, neutralize to phenolphthalein with dilute sodium hydroxide, then evaportate to dryness. Extract the residue with 50 ml of acetone evaportae the acetone on a steam bath, then dry the residue at 105^{0}C for 15 min. The residue consists of the nonionic surfactants and carboxylic acids present in the shampoo.

Stir the resin with 50 ml of 10% diethylamine solution in benzene for 15 min filter, and wash with 25 ml of benzene. The combined filtrate contains the nonquaternary amines. Stir the resin with 25 ml of a 5% diethylamine solution in benzene for 15 min, filter, and wash with methanol. The combined filtrate and washing contains additional nonquaternary amines. Heat the resin with 50 ml of 1 : 1 concentrated hydrochloric acid-ethanol, filter, and wash with the same mixture.The combined filtrate and washing contains the quaternary ammonium compounds.

Analysis of Soap Shampoos

A soap shampoo can be identified by examination of its IR spectrum indicating the carboxyl groups of the fatty acids present. Another method of identification is to acidify the diluted shampoo; the formation of a fatty acid precipitate indicates the presence of a soap. Sudsing before and little or no sudsing after the addition of the acid indicates its presence if the amount is so small that no clear precipitate is formed.

If the shampoo is identified, it is separated in to chloroform-soluble and chloroform insoluble substances. The former consists of the fatty materials and the latter is comprised of alkanolamines and polyhydroxy compounds.

Fatty Acids (Chloroform Solubles)

Chloroform extraction of the shampoo will give the total amount of fatty materials. After evaporation of the solvent, the test is carried out for the presence of lanolin; also, the IR spectrum of the residue is compared with spectra of known substances.

Procedures

Chloroform Extraction

In a separatory funnel dissolve 2-3 g of sample in 50 ml of water, acidify with hydrochloric acid, and add a moderate excess of acid. Extract four times with 35-ml portions of chloroform. Combine the chloroform fractions, wash with 10 ml of water, and add the washing to the reserved extracted aqueous phase. Filter the chloroform soultion through a cotton plug into a tared beaker. Evaporate to dryness on a steam bath and dry at 105°C for 15 min. Weigh and express as chloroform extractables.

Lieberman burchard test for lanolin

Dissolve a small amount of the residue in 10 ml of chloroform, add 5 ml if acetic anhydride and 5-10 drops of concentrated sulfuric acid. After mixing, a characteristic green colour indicates the presence of lanolin.

Alkanolamines and Polyhydroxy Compounds

The water solution remaining after chloroform extraction contains the alkanolamines and polyhydroxy compounds. They are usually determined as a group, by diluting the water solution to 100 ml, and evaporating the water from an aliquot on a steam bath followed by drying at 105°C for 15 min. The residue is tested by IR spectroscopy to determine whether a polyhydroxy compound or an alkanolamine hydrochloride or both are present. Alkanolamines may be separated by ion exchange chromatography on Amberlite CG 120 resin, while glycerol can be identified by the procedure given below.

Procedure

Neutralize a 10 ml aliquot of the extracted aqueous solution to methyl red with carbon dioxide-free 0.1 N sodium hydroxide solution leaving the solution just barely yellow. Add 30 ml of 0.02 M potassium iodate solution and stir well. If the red color of methyl red appears immediately, glycerol is probably present.

Analysis of Alkyl Aryl Polyether Alcohol Shampoos

These are identified from the infrared spectrum of the nonvolatile matter and the ultraviolet spectrum of the ethanol solution of the sample. If the infrared spectrum indicates that the nonvolatile matter consists essentially of alkyl aryl poly ether alcohols, the percent solids may be taken as the percent of alkyl aryl polyether alcohol. The presence of alkyl aryl polyether alcohol also can be determined from the ultraviolet spectrum if no other ultraviolet absorbers are present.

Alkyl aryl polyether alcohols generally are used in conjunction with quaternary ammonium compounds which can be identified by the following procedure.

Procedure

Add a sample containing approximately 0.2 mg of quatermary compound to a separatory funnel. Add 2 ml of 10% sodium carbonate solution, 1 ml of 0.04% bromophenol blue solution, 50 ml of water, and 15 ml of chloroform, and shake for 1 min. A blue color in the chlorofrom layer indicates the presence of a quaternary ammonium compound.

Alkyaryl polyether shampoos also may contain polyoxyethylene-type surfactants which can be identified by the following procedure.

Procedure

Dissolve a sample containing approximately 20 mg of the polyoxyethylene compounds in 300 ml fo water; heat if necessary to achieve complete solution. Cool, then add 3 ml of concentrated hydrochloric acid and 10 ml of a 10%barium chloride solution. If any precipitate forms, filter and discard it. Slowly, with stirring, add 10 ml fo a 10% aqueous silicotungistic acid solution to the filtrate. A flocculent precipitate indicates the presence of a polyoxyethylene compound.

Analysis of Alkyl Sulfate Shampoos

In these shampoos, alkyl sulfates are used together with polyoxyethlene compounds, esters, soap, and fatty acid alkanolamines. After identification of the presence of the alkyl sulfate by IR spectroscopy, the individual components of the shampoo are separated after acid hydrolysis first into a chloroform phase containing the alcohols, fatty acids, and esters, and an aqueous phase containing the alkanolamine sulfates and ammonium sulfate. Further separation processes permit the isolation and determination of the individual compounds.

Procedures

Hydrolysis. Weigh 2-3 g of sample into an Erlenmeyer flask, add 50 ml of N hydrochloric acid and reflux for 1 hr. Extract the hydrolysis mixture with four 35 ml portions of chloroform. Combine the chloroform extracts, wash with 10 ml of water and add the washing to the extracted aqueous phase. Filter the chloroform extract through a cotton plug into a tared beaker and evaporate to dryness on a steam bath. Dry the residue at 105^{0} C for 15 min, weigh, and express as chloroform-extractable substances. In a like manner, evaporate the extracted aqueous phase to dryness and weigh.

Analysis of the Chloroform Extract. Examine the IR spectrum of the chloroform extract and continue the separation process based on the following finding :

Case A : the residue consists only of alcohols

Case B : the residue contains both alcohols and fatty acids

Case C : the residue consists of alcohols and esters

Case A. Assume an average mol wt of the laury (C_{12}) alcohol (MW = 186.34) and calculate the residue as lauryl sulfate (MW = 468.74).

Case B. Dissolve the residue in 1 : 3 ethanol-water containing 1% potassium hydroxide. Extract four times with 40-ml portions of ethyl ether and wash the combinded ether extract with three 20-ml portions of 1 : 3 ethanol-water. Shake gently during the first wash to avoid emulsification. The ethyl ether will extract the alcohols but not the fatty acids. Evaporate the solvents and weigh. If required, separate the individual components in each fraction, eg, by gas Chromatography.

Case C. Saponify the residue by refluxing for 2 hr with 25 ml of 95% ethanol, 1 g of potassium hydroxide, and 50 ml of benzene. Transfer the saponified mixture to a separatory funnel with a Teflon stopcock, add 50 ml of hot water, shake well, and draw off the aqueous layer. If an emulsion was formed, break it by partially submerging the separatory funnel in a steam bath and heating until the contents boil. Extract twice with 50-ml portions of benzene. Wash the combined benzene extracts with three 30-ml portions of 3 : 7 ethanol-water shaking gently during the first wash. Add the washings to the aqueous phase. Filter the benzene extract through a cotton plug into a tared beaker, evaporate to dryness on a steam bath, and dry at 105^0 C for 15 min. Weigh, express as unsaponified material, and retain for further analysis.

Acidify the combined aqueous phases with hydrochloric acid and extract with three 30-ml portions of chloroform. Run the IR spectrum of the aqueous phase and check for the presence of glycols (secondary C-OH bands at 8.8, 9.0, and 9.3 um) and polyoxyethylene compounds (7.4, 9.0, and 10.6 μm), and if necessary, analyze for these by the usual methods. Wash the combined chloroform extracts with water and filter through a cotton plug into tared beaker. Evaporate to dryness in a steam bath, dry at 105^{0}C for 15 min and weigh. Express the result as fatty acid. Determine the equivalent weight by titrating with 0.1 N sodium hydroxide to the phenolphthalein end point. Compare the IR spectrum of the residue with the spectra of known fatty acids, and if desired, determine the fatty acids present by gas chromatography, after transforming the mixture to the methyl esters.

Dissolve the unsaponified material in 50 ml of boiling heptane and cool the solution to room temperature. If there is any precipitated material, filter through filter paper, wash the residue with petroleum ether, and reserve the filtrate. Dissolve the residue on the filter paper in hot ehloroform and evaporate the chloroform solution to dryness on a steam bath. Dry the residue at 105^0 C for 15 min, weigh, and express as alcohols insoluble in heptane-petroleum ether.

Evaporate the reserved heptane-petroleum ether solution on a steam bath and dissolve the residue in 50 ml of petroleum ether. Transfer the solution, with the aid of 25 ml of petroleum ether, to a 9 in. X 3/

4 in. chromatographic column containing activated alumina (Alorco, grade F-20, 80/200 mesh), and allow the solution to flow through the column at 3-5 ml/min. collect the petroleum ether eluates in a tared 400-ml beaker. Pass an additional 175 ml of petroleum ether through the coloumn to remove the petroleum ether, then pass 125 ml of boiling ethanol through the column at a rate of 4-7 ml/min, with help of air pressure. Collect the ethanol fractions in separate tared beakers, then evaporate them to dryness on a steam bath, dissolve each in 10 ml of ehloroform and evaporate to dryness again. Dry the residue at 105^0 C for 15 min and weigh as alcohols soluble in heptane-petroleum ether.

Evaporate the combined petroleum ether eluates from the column to dryness on a steam bath, dry at 105^0 C for 10 min, and weigh. Express the results as hydrocarbons. Identify the components present from the IR spectrum.

Analysis of the Water Extract. Determine the amount, of ammonium sulfate in this solution by transforming it to sodium sulfate on an ion-exchange resin.

Prepare a 15 cm X 1.5 cm chromatographic column containing 20/50 mesh Dowex 50-X 8 ion exchange resin and wash it with water. Accurately weigh a sample containing approximately 10 mg of sulfate into a 100-ml volumetric flask and dilute to volume with water. Destroy any foam which may appear by adding a small amount of alcohol to the flask. Transfer a 5-ml aliquot to the column and collect the effluent in a 100- ml volumetric flask containing 20.0 ml fo a 0.05 M potassium acid phthalate buffer solution (pH4). Wash the column twice with 15-ml portions of water.

Remove the volumetric flask from the column, add 30 ml of ethanol and 0.3 g of barium chloranilate, and shake for 15 min. Dilute to volume with ethanol, mix well, and filter through Whatman No. 1 paper. Transfer a 40.0-ml aliquot of the filtrate to a 100-ml beaker and adjust to pH 4.00 $\pm$ 0.05 with dilute hydrochloric acid or dilute ammonium hydroxide. Transfer the solution to a 50-ml volumetric flask and dilute to volume with ethanol. Measure the absorbance at 530 nm vs a blank of 1 : 25 ethanol-water. Establish the amount of sodium sulfate with the help of a standard curve prepared by chromatographing solutions of sodium sulfate with known concentration through the same column. Regenerate the column after each analysis by passing 25 ml of 1:3 hydrochloric acid-water and then washing with water until the pH of the effluent is equal to the pH of the water.

$$\% \text{ ammonium sulfate} = 0.929\ (\% Na_2SO_4)$$

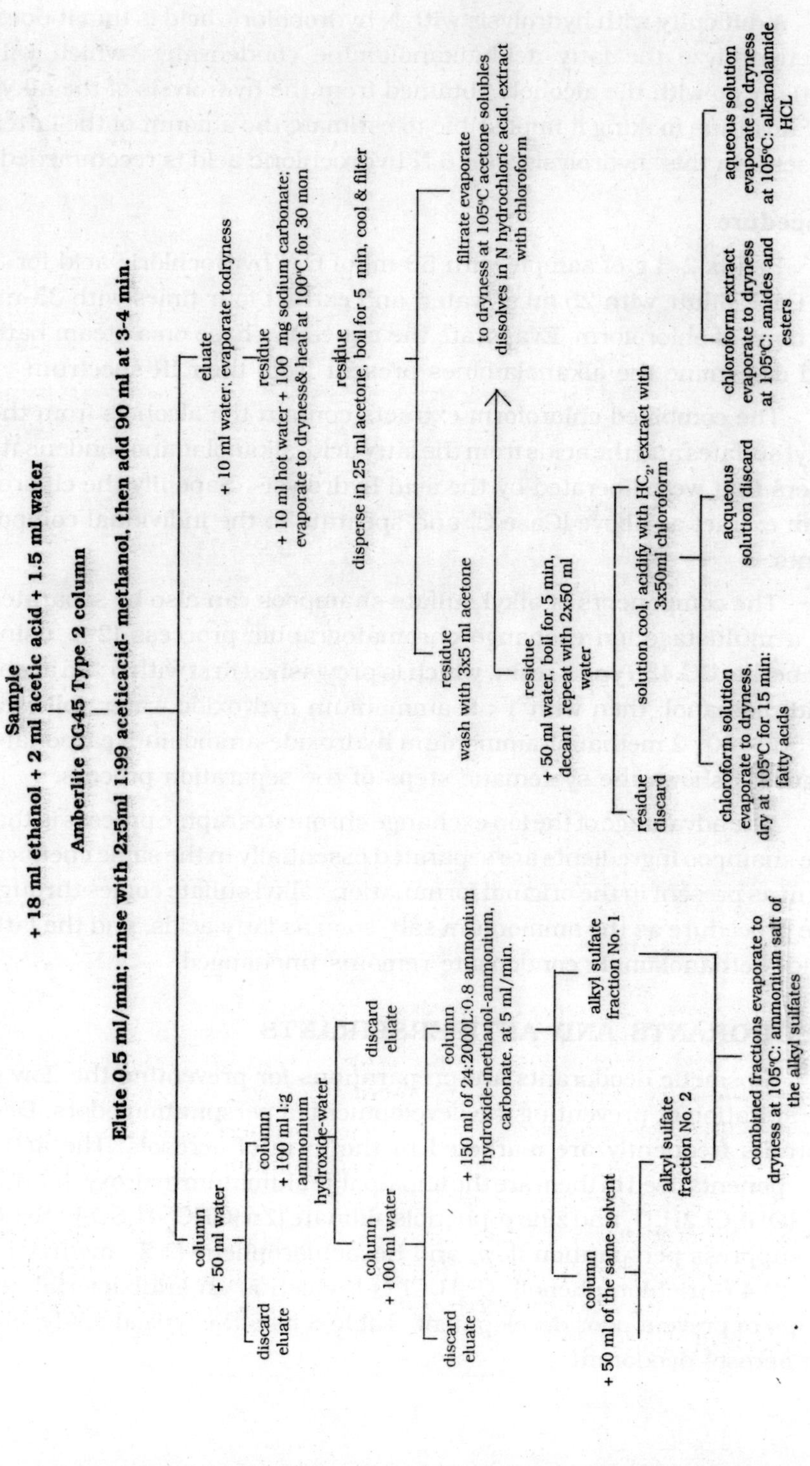

Fig. 3 : Ion Exchange chromatography of alkyl sulphate shampoos

A difficulty with hydrolysis with N hydrochloric acid is that it does not hydrolyze the fatty acid-alkanolamine condensates, which will partially go with the alcohols obtained from the hydrolysis of the alkyl sulfates thus making it impossible to estimate the amount of the latter present. In this, hydrolysis with 6 N hydrochloric acid is recommeded.

Procedure

Reflux 2-3 g of sample with 50 ml of 6 N hydrochloric acid for 3 hr. Cool, dilute with 25 ml of water, and extract four times with 35-ml portions of chloroform. Evaporate the aqueous phase on a steam bath and determine the alkanolamines present from their IR spectrum.

The combined chloroform extracts contain the alcohols from the alkyl sulfates and the acids from the fatty acid-alkanolamine condensate esters that were liberated by the acid hydrolysis. Saponify the chloroform extract as above (Case C) and spearate to the individual components.

The components of alkyl sulfate shampoos can also be separated by a multistage ion exchange chromatographic proccess (29), using Amberlite CG 45 Type 2 resin, which is prewashed first with 5 : 95 acetic acid-methanol, then with 1 : 9 ammonium hydroxide water, followed by 500 : 60 : 2 methanol-ammonium hydroxide-ammonium carbonate. Figure 3 shows the systematic steps of the separation process.

The advantage of the ion exchange chromatographic process is that the shampoo ingredients are separated essentially in the same chemical form as present in the original formulation : alkyl sulfate comes through the procedure as the ammonium salt, soap as fatty acids, and the fatty acid-diethanolamide condensate remains unchanged.

DEODORANTS AND ANTIPERSPIRANTS

Cosmetic deodorants are preparations for preventing the flow of perspiration or preventing the development of perspiration odors. Deodorants frequently are marketed in the form of aerosols. The active components used in them are the impalpable aluminum hydroxychloride, $Al_2 (OH)_5Cl.2H_2O_1$ and zine p-phenolsulfonate $(Zn (OHC_6-H_4SO_3)_2. SH_2O]$ to suppress perspiration flow, and hexachlorophene (2,2'- methylene-bis (3,4,6-trichlorophenol), $C_{13}H_6Cl_2O_2]$ which is an antibacterial and helps to prevent odor development. Table 8 lists the typical analysis of an aerosol deodorant.

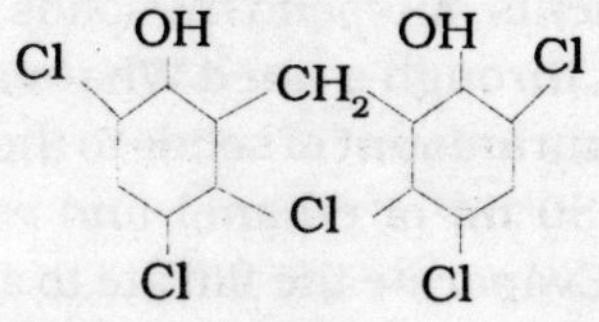

Table 8. Typical Analysis of an Aerosol deodorant

propellants, wt %		40.0
dichlorodifluoromethane[a]	24.8	
trichlorofluoromethane[b]	15.2	
ethanol, wt %		50.6
solids, wt %		10.2
isopropy myristate and isopropyl stearate	2.9	
talc	5.9	
alumimum hydroxychloride	1.2	
hexachlorophene	0.16	
Total		100.8

Methods of Analysis

The analysis of an aerosol deodorant starts by spraying some into the hand and observing the residue. If talc is present, it observed. Talc hides the aluminum hydroxychloride if present; otherwise it would appear as a fine powder or gritty material. Also, the infrared spectrum of the deodorant should be obtained by spraying some of the acrosol directly onto a salt plate.

In the systematic quantitative analysis, first the amount of propellants, ethanol, and propylene glycol are determined by gas chromatography. Subsequently, the amount of solids is determined and then it is separated into its components. The procedures are given below.

Procedures

Nonvolatile solids. Weigh and cool the can containing the aerosol deodorant in a dry ice-acetone bath, remove the value assembly and allow the propellants to evaporate as the can and contents warm to room temperature. When most of the propellant has evaporated, transfer the contents of the can to a tared beaker with the aid of some ethanol. Evaporate the mixture to dryness under a stream of dry air. weigh and express the result as air-dried solids.

Separation of Components. Suspend the solids in 100 ml of ethanol and mix intimately. Decant through a tared Whatman No. 1 filter paper while transferring a minimum amount of solids to the filter paper. Repeat the extraction twice with 50 ml of ethanol and collect the ethanolic filtrates in a tared beaker. Evaporate the filtrate to a volume of approximately 50 ml and retain for additional analysis. Dry the filter paper and the beaker which contains the residue, weigh, and express the result as alcohol-insoluble substances.

The alcoholic solution will contain the fatty acid esters, zinc phenolsulfonate, and hexachlorophene, whereas talc and aluminum hydroxyehloride are insoluble in ethanol.

Alcohol-Soluble Substances. Investigate the ultraviolet and infrared spectra of the alcoholic solution, and establish the presence of zinc phenolsulfonate and hexachlorophene from the spectrum as follows :

	Absorption maxima, nm	$E_{1\,cm}^{1\,\%}$
zinc phenolsulfonate	231	487
	274	45
hexachlorophene	295 shoulder	146
	300	160

If necessary, carry out the separation of the components present in the ethanolic solution by liquid-column chromatography on a silica gel or alumina column or by thin-layer chromatography using10:1 benzene-ammonium hydroxide as the solvent. The two tances also can be determined by the individual methods outlined below.

Zinc Phenolsulfonate. Accurately weigh a sample equivalent to 100 mg of zinc phenolsulfonate into a 250-ml Erlenmeyer flask, add 10 ml of concentrated hydrochloric acid, and approximately 50 ml of water. adjust to pH 10 $\pm$ 0.1 with concentrated ammonium hydroxide. Add 5 drops of a 0.1% ethanolic solution of Eriochrome Black T indicator solution and titrate with 0.05 *M* EDTA solution to a dirty blue (not clear blue) end point. Use a fluorescent light behind the beaker and a white background to facilitate seeing the end point.

$$\% \text{ zinc phenolsulfonate} = \frac{(V)\ (N)\ (5.55)}{W}$$

Where V= volume of EDTA solution used for titration, in ml

N = normality of EDTA solution

W = sample wt, in g

Herachlorophene

Accurately weigh a sample containing about 10 mg of hexachlorophene into a 125-ml separatory funnel containing 50 ml of benzene. Wash the benzene solution twice with 50 ml of water; discard the washings. Consequently, extract the benzene solution three times with 25,10 and 10 ml of N sodium hydroxide solution. Combine the alkaline extracts in a 125-ml separatory funnel, add 3 drops of a methyl orange indicator solution, and acidify with concentrated hydrochloric acid. Extract with two 30-ml portions of dichloromethane, combine the extracts, and concentrate to approximately 2 ml on a steam bath in a gentle stream of nitrogen. Transfer the residue with the aid of a Pasteur pipet into a silylation vial (available from Pierce Chemical Co., Rockford, Illinois, under catalog no. 13028-A), wash the evaporation flask and the pipet with two 1-ml portions of dichloromethane, add 1 ml of a 0.2% (w/v) methanolic dieyclohexylphthalate solution, and evaporate to dryness on a sand bath at 40-60°C in a gentle stream of nitrogen. After the methanol is evaporated close the vial with its cover and add 1 ml of Tri-Sil BSA [N,O-bis(trimethylsilyl) acetamide] solution (available from Pierce Chemical Co. under catalog no. 490107) with a hypodermic syringe through the septum of cover. The reaction commences immediately. Inject 2μl of the resulting solution into a gas chromatograph operated under the following conditions :

column	5ft x¼ in. OD, packed
column packing	5wt % SE-30 silicone gum rubber on acid-washed and silanized Chromosorb W 60/80 mesh
column temperature	programmed from 200°C to 300° C at 6° C/min
carrier gas and flow rate	helium, 60 ml/min
detector	flame ionization

If dichlorophene is also present, it will be separated from hexachlorophene and its amount can be determined separately from the chromatogram. Dicycolhexylphthalate, which was added to the sample, serves as the internal standard.

Prepare a standard containing appropriate amounts of hexachlorophene and dichlorophene if needed, and carry it through the procedure simultaneously.

The above procedure is of general use for cosmetic preparations. In case of samples containing solid particulate matter, apply the following modified procedure.

Accurately weigh a sample containing about 10 mg of hexachlorophene into a 150 ml beaker, add 50 ml of methanol, stir for ½ hr with a magnetic stirrer, then filter through a medium-porosity sintered glass filter in to another 150-ml beaker. Transfer the insolubles from the filter back to the original beaker, add 25 ml fo methanol, stir for ½hr, then filter again, and repeat the extraction and filtration once more.Concentrate the combined filtrates to less than 5 ml, but not to dryness, on a steam bath with a gentle stream of nitrogen, then transfer the concentrated solution to a 125-ml separatory funnel with 50 ml fo benzene and continue as given in the original procedure.

Alcohol-Insoluble Substances

Wash the residue with moderate speed with 50 ml of ice water using a suction flask to speed the filtration. Part of the aluminum hydroxychloride is water soluble; test the filtrate for aluminum and chloride.

Heat the residue with 50 ml of 0.1 N hydrochloric acid, decant through a Whatman No.1 filter paper and wash with 25 ml of 0.1 N hydrochloric acid. Test the filtrate for aluminum. If positive, impalpable aluminum hydroxychloride is indicatel.

Wash the residue twice with 25 ml of water, decant, and discard the washings. Evaporate the residue to dryness and obtain its IR spectrum. The resiude will consist mostly of talc.

HAIR SPRAYS

Hair sprays are intended primarily for the temporary setting or curling of the hair. This is achieved with the help of a tough, clear adhering film. Polyvinylpyrrolidone (PVP), polyvinylpyrrolidone-vinyl acetate copolymer (PVP-VA), ethyl cellulose, shellac, and dimethylhydantion formaldehyde (DMHF) are some of the resins commonly used for filmforming. Various plasticizers, such as lanolin and its derivatives, high molecular weight alcohols and esters, and silicones are added to plasticize the resin and increase its water repellancy. Other materials such as ultraviolet absorbers or proteins also may be present. Anhydrous ethanol is used as a vehicle and fluorinated hydrocarbons as the propellant.

Table 9. Typical Analysis of a Hair Spray

propellants, wt %		68.0
dichlorodifluoromethane	20.7	
trichlorofluoromethane	47.3	
ethanol, wt %		27.3
water, wt %		0.37
nonvolatiles, wt %		4.2
polyvinylpyrrolidone	3.8	
mineral oil	0.3	
diethyl phthalate	0.1	
Total		99.87

Methods of Analysis

The first step in the analysis of hair sprays is the analysis of the propellants and ethanol by gas chromatography. The following conditions are recommended :

column	15 ft x ¼ in. OD packed
column packing	20 wt % diethylhexyl sebacate or hexadecane on Chromosorb W 60/80 mesh
temperature of	
injection port	250°C
column	65°C
detector	250°C
carrier gas and flow rate	helium, 60 ml/min
sample size	5 µl
detector	thermal conductivity

The chromatogram is evaluated quantitatively by comparison with one obtained by analyzing a standard sample under identical conditions. The preparation of the standard is outlined below.

Procedure

Place approximately 8 ml of benzene into a tared heavy-duty centrifuge tube, close with a serum cap, and wind a stout rubber bank tightly around the meek of the serum cap. Accurately weigh the tube with the benzene. Introduce approximately 0.3 of each propellant or mixed propellants. Weigh. Add by hypodermic syringe approximately 0.3g of ethanol into the tube and weigh.

Water, if present, is determined after cooling the can at -25^0 C for 5 mn. A 6-in. long plastic tube is affixed to the valve stem and the other end of the tube is inserted through a hole in the cap of the Karl Fischer titration flask containing 30 ml of neutralized anhydrous methanol. The valve is actuated and approximately 20 g of hair spray is delivered into the methanol. The amount of sample is weighed by difference and then the water content is determined by the usual Karl fiseher method.

After the propellants, alcohol, and water have been determined, the aerosol can is cooled in a dry ice-acetone bath, opened, allowed to warm to room temperature and the propellants evaporated. Than, the concentrate mixture is transferred into a tared beaker, using ethanol to aid in the transfer, evaporated to dryness under a stream of dry air and weighed. The result is expressed as air-dried solids.

Qualitative tests are carried out from the air-dried solids to detect the presence of lanolin and proteins. The presence of silicone compounds may be established from the infrared spectrum and the ultraviolet absorption spectrum can be used to detect the presence of sunscreens, aromatic quaternary ammonium compounds, etc. If such compounds are present, separation and quantitation can be achieved by liquid-column chromatography and thin-layer chromatography.

For the determination of the resins and plasticizers present, the residue is moistened with a few ml of ethanol and macerated with a stirring rod. Than 150 ml of ethyl ether is added and filtered through a tared What man No.4 paper by allowing only a minimum amount of the residue to pass onto the paper. The procedure is repeated twice, then the resin is dried and weighed to obtain the amount of resin present. It can be identified from its infrared spectrum. The combined ether solutions are evaporated to dryness and weighed to obtain the amount of plasticizer present. Infrared spectroscopic analysis of the residue permits the determination of the type of plasticizer present.

SUNSCREENS

Sunscreens are usually solutions, lotions, or quick breaking foams. Their primary function is to absorb ultraviolet light in the 280-320 nm region. Table 10 lists some of the sunscreens in use.

Methods of Analysis

The first step in the analysis of a sunscreen is the determination of the water, ethanol, and propylene glycol content. If the product is an aerosol, the propellants are analyzed by gas chromatography. The amount of air-dried solid is determined, from 5-10 g of sample, and the residue is tested for lanolin, glycerine, propylene glycol, gums, and quaternary ammonium compounds.

The identification and determination of the active ingredient in the sunscreen are carried out from its ultraviolet spectrum. Table 10 lists the absorption maxima and the extinction coefficient values. If an identification cannot be made at this point, the sample first should be separated from some of the oils and other materials present, by dissolving it in 8:2 methanol-water and extracting with petroleum ether. The active sunscreen substance remains in the methanol layer.

If identification cannot be made from the ultraviolet and/or infrared spectra, thinlayer chromatography should be employed for separation of the sunscreen. Identification can be made from the R values and the spectra of the eluted spots.

The other substances present in sunscreens can be separated on an alumina column into hydrocarbons, esters, and vegetable oils and waxes using carbon tetrachloride, chloroform, and ethyl acetate as the eluants. If adequate separation is not achieved on the alumina column, the analysis has to be carried out on the silica gel column.

Testing for Effectiveness. The effectiveness of a sunscreen is expressed by the so-called K value measured at 297.5 and 310 nm. The first is a measure of the protection from burning of the skin whereas the second gives a measure of absorption of the tanning energy.

Procedure

Accurately weigh a 0.1-g sample into a 100-ml volumetric flask and dilute to volunte with ethanol. If necessary, carry out further dilution so that the absorbance of the final solution should be between 0.200 and 0.700 Measure the absorbance on an ultraviolet spectrophotometer at 297.5 and 310 nm against an ethanol blank.

$$\text{K value} = \frac{A}{(C)\ (L)\ (10)}$$

where A = absorbance measured

C = concentration of the sunscreen in the final solution, in wt %

L = cell path length, in cm

CREAMS AND LOTIONS

From the point of view of the analyst, creams and lotions are handled similarly. The basic ingredients necessary in these formulations are water, water-insoluble materials such as waxes, hydrocarbons, fatty acids, high molecular weigh alcohols, and isopropyl esters, and surfactants, such as polyoxyethylene compounds, alkylsulfates, and glycery monostearate. The formulations are termed either as oil-in-water (o/w) or water-in-oil (w/o) emulsions.

Type. In the analysis of creams or lotions, their type is first determined. If the product mixes readily with a mineral oil, it is a w/o emulsion, and if it mixes readily with water, it is an o/w emulsion. in case of the latter type, its pH is also measured from a 10% (w/v) aqueous mixture. Water-soluble or oil-soluble dye sprinkled on the surface of the emulsion will indicate whether it is o/w or w/o type.

Water. The water content of creams and lotions can be determined by the Karl Fischer method. The toluene distillation method is not recommended because of the codistillation of propylene glycol and glycerol.

Table 10. Active Substances Used in Sunscreens and Their Ultraviolet Absorption Data[a]

Sample	Absorption maximum, nm	$E_{1\,cm}^{1\,\%}$
benzyl salicy late	305	213
benzyl cinnamate	278	1030
cinnamic acid	272	1445
dipropylene glycol salicy late	304	206
Escalol 506		
(amyl-p-N,N-dimethy laminobenzoate)	310	1265
isobutyl salicy late	306	240
methyl cinnamate	276	1391
Uvinul D50	287	448
(2,2',4,4'-tetrahydroxy benzophenone)	348	640
Univul N35		
(substituted acrylonitules)	301	462
Uvinul N 539	303	348
Uvinul 490	282	465
(mixture of D49 and other phenones)	339	486

Propylene Glycol. The presence of propylene glycol can be checked by the qualitive tests. If the test is positive, its amount can be determined quantitatively.

Silicones. For checking the presence of silicones, 1 vol of the sample is shaken with 2 vol of 1:1 toluene-dioxane. The mixture is centrifuged and the top layer, consisting mostly of touene, is drawn off, the toluene evaporated, and the residue checked by IR spectroscopy for silicones.

Nonvolatile Material. The sample is heated for 2 hr at 105°C. After cooling in a desiccator, the residue is weighed. If a large amount of propylene glycol is present, it is advisable to run "air-dried solids" until constant weight is obtained. Infrared investigation of the residue can give information on the presence of alcohols, alkanolamines, amides, esters, hydrocarbons, fatty acids, polyhydroxy compounds, soaps, etc.

Ash. The sample is weighed into a crucible and heated first on a steam bath for 1 hr with the aid of a stream of air, then on a Bunsen burner until the sample is charred. Subsequently, it is transferred to a muffle furnace and ashing is completed at 600° C. After cooling in a desiccator, the ash is weighed. If desired, the ash may be tested for certain ions and substances.

Zinc Oxide. Dissolve a portion of the ash in water and filter. Ignite the filter paper in a crucible. A yellow color which fades on cooling indicates the presence of zinc oxide.

Esters of p-Hydroxybenzoic Acid. p-Hydroxybenzoic acid esters can be identified as a group by their ultraviolet spectrum. The procedure for sample preparation is given below.

Procedure

Weigh a 2-g sample into a 50-ml beaker, add 20 ml of boiling methanol, stir vigorously, cool, and filter. Add 10 ml of water and 1 drop of concentrated hydrochloric acid to the filtrate, them extract three times with 20-ml portions of petroleum ether, discarding the petroleum ether extracts. Diluter the extracted methanol solution to 100 ml with methanol and run the ultraviolet spectrum of the solution.

Alkyl Sulfates (Sulfonates). The presence of alkyl sulfates can be established with the help of the following procedure.

Procedure

Transfer an aliquot of the sample containing 0.1-0.4 mg of alkyl sulfate (sulfonate) into a separatory funnel. Dilute to approximately 20 ml with water, neutralize with hydrochloric acid, then add 3-5 drops in excess. Add 1 ml of a 0.1% aqueous methylene blue solution and mix thoroughly. Add 20 ml of chloroform shake gently for 1 min and let stand for 5 min. Drain the chloroform layer into a second separatory funnel, add 20 ml of water, shake gently for 1 min, and allow to stand for 5 min. A blue color in the chloroform layer indicates the presence of an alky sulfate (or sulfonate).

Quaternary Ammonium Compounds. The presence of quaternary ammonium compounds can be determined by the following procedure.

Procedure

Transfer an aliquot of the cream containing approximately 0.2 mg of quaternary ammonium compound into a separatory funnel, add 2 ml of a 10% sodium carbonate solution and 1 ml of a 0.04% bromphenol blue solution. Dilute with 50 ml of water, add 15 ml of chloroform, shake gently for 1 min, and then allow to stand for 5 min. A blue color in the chloroform layer indicates the presence of a quaternary ammonium compound.

Emulsifiers. The emulsifiers can be identified by the following procedures.

Procedures

Beeswax-Borax w/o Emulsion. Tests of the ash are positive for boron and sodium and the sample contains less than 35% water.

Beeswax-Borax o/w emulsion. Tests of the ash are positive for boron and sodium. The pH of a10% aqueous mixture is 8-9.

Soap o/w Emulsion. Tests of the ash for sodium and carbonate are positive, the pH of a 10% aqueous mixture is 8-9, the IR spectrum of the nonvolatile material shows a band at 6.5 μm, and tests for glycerol or other polyhydroxy compounds are usually positive. Sample contains greater than 70% water.

Triethanolamine - soap o/w Emulsion. The sample yields no ash and contains more than 70% water; the pH of a 10% aqueous mixture is 7-8; the IR spectrum of the nonvolatile material shows a band at 6.5 μm; tests for glycerol or other polyhydroxy compounds are usually positive; and triethanolamine is found in the aqueous solution after extraction with chloroform.

Glyceryl Monostearate-soap o/w Emulsion. The sample gives a positive test for combined glycerol, contains more than 60% water, and glycerol monostearate is detected in the IR spectrum of the chloroform extractable material.

Chloroform Extractable Material. The investigation of the substances which can be extracted with chloroform permits the identification and determination of the most important components present in creams and lotions. The procedure consists of successive extractions; it is outlined below. It is applicable only to sharp emulsions because other types of emulsifiers, such as alkyl sulfates, quaternary ammonium compounds, complex silicates, and polyoxyethylene-type surfactants may emulsify the chloroform.

Procedures

Weigh a 3-g sample into a 250-ml separatory funnel, add 50 ml of water acidify with concentrated hydrochloric acid, and extract four times with 35-ml portions of chloroform. Combine the chloroform extracts in a second separatory funnel and wash once with 10 ml of water. Add the washing to the extracted aqueous solution and save. Filter the chloroform extracts through a cotton plug into a tared 250-ml beaker, evaporate to dryness on a steam bath with the aid of a stream of air, dry for 10 min at 105°C, cool, weigh and express as chloroform extractable material. The chloroform extracts all fatty materials but not such substances as alkanolamines, inorganic salts, and polyhydroxy compounds.

Test the residue for lanolin by the Liebermann Burehard test (p.82). Also run an infrared spectrum of the extracted material for identification and compare with the spectrum of the nonvolatiles. Retain the chloroform extractable material for additional analysis.

Aqueous Extract. Transfer the aqueous extract from above to a 100-ml volumetric flask and dilute to volume with water. Pipet a 40-ml portion into a tared 100-ml beaker and evaporate to dryness on a steam bath with the aid of a stream of air. Dry for 10 min at 105°C, cool, weigh, and express as chloroform insoluble material. Run an IR spectrum of an aliquot of the residue for identification, test for the presence of polyhydroxy compounds and also for alkanolamine by the following: Add excess n- propanol to the residue in the beaker, boil to a small volume, chill, scratch the side of the beaker with a glass rod to induce crystallization, filter off the crystals, and dry. Run an infrared spectrum and identify the alkanolamine if present.

Chloroform Extract. To the extractable material, add 25 ml of 95% ethanol, 1 g of potassium hydroxide, and 50 ml of benzene, and saponify by standing for 2 hr on a steam bath. Transfer the entire mixture to a separatory funnel having a Teflon stopcock, add 50 ml of hot water, shake well, and draw off the aqueous layer into a second separatory funnel. Extract the aqueous solution twice with 50-ml portions of hot benzene. Reserve the extracted aqueous solution. Combine the benzene extracts, and wash three times with 30-ml portions of 3:7 ethanol-water. Shake very gently during the first washing to avoid emulsification. Add the washings to the reserved extracted aqueous solution. Filter the washed benzene extract through a cotton plug into a tared 250-ml beaker, evaporate to dryness on a steam bath with the aid of a stream of air,and dry for 10 min at 105°C. Cool, weight, and express as unsaponified material. Run an infrared spectrum and look for hydrocarbons and alcohols.

Dissolve a weighed portion of the unsaponified material in warm heptane and allow to cool to room temperature. If there is any precipitate, filter through a filter paper, washing the paper with heptane. Dissolve the residue on the filter paper by passing hot chloroform through the paper into a tared beaker. Evaporate to dryness, weigh, and express as heptane-insoluble alcohols. Separate the substances present in the heptane solution by coulmn chromatography, on an alumina column,under the subheading "separation of waxes." Acidify the reserved extracted aqueous solution with concentrated hydrochloric acid and extract with three 30-ml portions of chloroform. Test an aliquot of the extracted aqueous solution for glycerol. Carry out the test for polyoxyethylene compounds as outlined below from another aliquot of the extracted aqueous solution. Wash the combined chloroform extracts with water.Filter the washed chloroform extract through a cotton plug into a tared 250-ml beaker evaporate to dryness on a steam bath with the aid of a stream of air, and dry for 10 min at 105°C. Cool, weigh, and express the residue as fatty acids.

Test for Polyoxyethylene. Dissolve or disperse a sample containing 20-30 mg of polyoxyethylene compound, heating if necessary in 300 ml of water. Add 3 ml of concentrated hydrochloric acid and 10 ml of a10% aqueous barium chloride solution. If the resulting solution is not clear, filter, and discard the precipitate. To the clear solution, add slowly and with stirring, 10 ml of a 10% aqueous silicotungstic acid solution. A flocculent precipitate is considered as a positive test for polyoxyethylene.

Aerosols

Cosmetics or toiletries that have been formulated as aerosols include hair sprays, hair conditioners, shave creams, shampoos, colognes, perfumes, makeups, hand creams, depilatories, deodorants, sunscreens, nail enamel driers, various powders, etc. The propellants used usually are halogenated C_1 and C_2 hydrocarbons. Table 11 lists some of the commonly used propellents. In cosmetics, these usually are used as. mixtures; Table 12 enumerates some of them.

Table 11. The Most Frequently Used Propellants in Cosmetic Aerosol Preparations

Chemical name	Formula	Propellant No	Bp, °F	Vapor pressure at 70°F psig
propane	C_3H_8		-43.9	109
dichlorodifluoromethane	CCI_2F_2	12	-12.6	70
difluoroethane	$CH_2F\text{-}CH_2F$	152a	-11.2	63
vinyl chloride	$CH_2{=}CHCI$		-7.0	34
isobutane	$CH_3\text{-}CH(CH_3)\text{-}CH_3$		13.6	31
monochlorodifluoroethane	$CCIF_2\text{-}CH_3$	142b	15.1	30
octafluorocyclobutane	$CF_2CF_2CF_2CF_2$	C318	21.5	25
n-butane	$CH_3\text{-}CH_2\text{-}CH_2\text{-}CH_3$		31.1	16
dichlorotet rafluoroethane	$CCIF_2\text{-}CCIF_2$	114	38.8	13
trichloromonofluoromethane	CCI_3F	11	74.8	2.6
methylene chloride	CH_2CI_2		104.2	0

Table 12. Propellant Mixtures Used Most Frequently in Cosmetics

Propellants	Ratio wt/wt
12/11	60/40
12/114	20/80
12/142b/C318	12/22/66
12/vinyl chloride/methylene chloride	30/20/50
12/11/vinyl chloride	39/39/22
114/142b	30/70
12/11/isobutane	45/45/10
152a/isobutane/propane	25/63/12

Methods of Analysis

The analysis an aerosol product consists essentially of three steps. First, certain physical tests are performed; second, the composition of the propellant is determined and finally, the cosmetic formulation (ie, the concentrate) present in aerosol form is investigated. The latter is done by the already discussed methods, after the evaporation of the propellant and the vehicle present.

Physical Tests

The physical tests carried out with aerosols include the determination of the internal pressure, aerosol particle size, specific gravity of the propellants, net weight delivery, spray test, and container safety test.

Specific Gravity of the Propellant

The specific gravity of the propellant used in the acrosol cans is determined by using a Fisher-Porter pressure bottle as shown in Figure 4. The procedure is given below.

Procedure

Accurately weigh a clean, dry, Fisher-Porter bottle and place it in a thermostatically controlled water bath at 25^0 C. Pipet 20 ml of water at 25^0 C into the bottle, replace the seal and screw cap, and record the reading on the graduated scale to the nearest ½ division after reaching temperature equilibrium. Continue pipetting in additional 20-ml aliquots of water and recording the scale readings to a total volume of 160 ml of water. Plot a curve of volume of water vs scale reading

Attach a copper cooling coil to the discharge value of the propellant tank, and submerge the cooling coil into a dry ice-acetone bath. Open the discharge valve on the tank and waste approximately 50-100 ml of the propellant, than insert the end of the coil into the pressure bottle and collect the propellant until the bottle is approximately one-half full.

Immediately cap the pressure bottle to avoid the loss of propellant vapor as the liquid propellant warms up. Allow the propellant to warm to 25°C in a thermostatically controlled water bath. than read the volume on the graduated scale to the nearest ½ division. Accurately weigh the bottle and contents.

Specific gravity (25/25) = W/V

where w = weight of the propellant, in g

v = volume of the propellant established from the calibration curve, in ml

Net Weight Delivery

For the determination of the net weight delivery, a random sample of at least 10 packages is selected. After the removal of any dust cover or caps not required for dispensing the product, the gross weight of each package is determined and, after hand-shaking for 15 sec, the content of the lightest container is exhausted by holding the valve wide open for 35 min. Now, the exhausted container is weighed. The result is the so-called wet-tare weight and is equal to the weight of the container plus any product remaining after exhaustion.

Consequently, the regulation allowance is determined and subtracted from the wet-tare weight to obtain the corrected wet-tare weight. The regeneration allowance is defined as the difference between the weight of product which would be delivered through normal usage and the weight of product delivered by the present acclerated procedure; it is calculated by multiplying the label weight of the container by 0.02 and rounding the result to the next lowest 1/16 oz.

By subtracting the corrected wet-tare weight from the gross weight, the adjusted net weight of the package is obtained. If this is equal to or greater than the lable weight the lot is assumed to be satisfactory. However, if it is less than the label weight, the determination is repeated with each container in the lot and the average deviation is considered. If this is zero or positive, the lot is accepted; if it is negative, a larger lot has to be tested to determine whether the entire lot has a low fill. In this case, the lot is rejected.

Spray Test

During the filling operation of the containers, they are periodically checked qualitatively for defects such as "streamers" (solid or nearly solid stream of liquid), "drippers" (dripping valve), or no spraying.

Container Safety Test. For this test, random samples from each batch are heated at 140^{0}F for 1 hr in a hot-air oven. If any of the containers explode, the bottoms become convex, or the valves detach, they are classed as defecets and the batch is rejected.

Determination of Propellant Composition

The analysis of the propellant mixture in most aerosols is straightforward and can be carried out conveniently by gas chromatography (39). For sampling, a hypodermic needle is fitted to the valve of the aerosol can, and approximately 0.5 g of propellant is injected into a heavy-duty centrifuge tube closed with a serum cap, containing about 8 ml of benzene. After mixing, 5 ul samples are taken out from this tube with a microliter syringe and injected into the gas chromatograph.

Two 15ft×¼in. OD columns operated at 40^{0}C are recommended for the analysis containing 20 wt % hexadecane and diethylhexyl sebacate respectively on silanized Chromosorb W 60/80 mesh. The first column should be used mainly for initial screening and the second column for the confirmation and determination of the identified propellants. Table 13 lists the relative retention data of the most widely used propellants, together with some other fluorinated hydrocarbons and benzene used as the solvent, on the two columns.

Table 13. Relative Retention Data of Propellants at 40^{0}C^0

	Stationary phase	
	diethylhexyl sebacate	hexadecane
octafluorocyclobutane (C318)	0.214	0.122
1-chloro-1,2,2trifluoroethylene (1113)	0.268[a]	0.196
propane	0.275[a]	0.220[b]
1,2-difluoroethane (152a)	0.289[d]	0.141[c]
dichlorodifluoromethane (12)	0.296[d]	0.220[b]
1,2-dichloro-1,1,2,2- tetrafluoroethane (114)	0.345	0.290
isobutane	0.366	0.378
monochlorodifluoromethane (22)	0.368[a]	0.152[c]
1-chloro-1,1-difluoroethane (142b)	0.402	0.236[b]
n-butane	0.449	0.527
vinyl chloride	0.529	0.353
trichlorofluoromethane (11)	1.000	1.000
1,1,2-trichloro-1,2,2-trifluoroethane (113)	1.254	1.342
dichloromonofluoromethane (21)	1.354	0.515

1,2-dibromo-1,1,2,2-tetrafluoroethane (114B2)	1.634	1.363
methylene chloride	2.565	1.070
benzene	6.786	5.661

[a] Values marked with the same superscript cannot be separated on the column indicated.

HAIR DYES

There are many types of hair dyes; some of them result in temporary coloring and other provide a semipermanent coloring. The most important hair colorant products are those which result in a permanent coloring.

Permanent hair coloring preparations consist of dye intermediates, mostly aromatic amino and nitro compounds, usually in an aqueous solution of soap or synthetic detergent, such as alkanolamines or alkyl sulfates. Solubilizing agents, such as ethanol or propylene glycol, are also included. Besides these major components, the preparation also may contain some additional substances, such as glycerol or lanolin for hair conditioning and antioxidants to prevent premature oxidation of the dye intermediate.

Just prior to application, the hair coloring preparation is mixed with an oxidizing agent, usually a 6% aqueous hydrogen peroxide solution. The dye intermediates are oxidized in a multistage reaction to other intermediates, and coupling and condensation occurs between the intermediates forming substances with chromophoric bonds. During application, the basic substances pre ent in the preparation swell the hair, allowing the soluble dye intermediates to penetrate it, where the reaction is completed froming complexes with the hair keratin.

Methods of Analysis

The analysis of the base of the dye preparation is carried out according to the methods already discussed for shampoos. Besides these, special methods have been developed to determine the total and free ammonia present. The dye intermediates present are determined by thin-layer or gas chromatography. The preparations are also evaluated for coloring effect.

Determination of Total and Free Ammonia

This determination is carried out with the help of the Conway-O'Brink diffusion technique. for the determination, the so-called diffusion dishes are used which consist of three concentric compartments which will be referred to as inner, middle, and outer, and a cover which fits the outer compartment.

Procedures

Total Ammonia. Add by means of a 1-ml microburet 0.8000 ml of N sulfuric acid into the inner chamber. Add 2 ml of saturated aqueous potassium carbonate solution to each of the middle and outer compartments, and 1 drop of 0.025% of Tergitol NPX nonionic surfactant solution to the inner compartment.

Accurately weigh approximately 300 mg of sample into the middle chamber. Cover the dish immediately and swirl gently to evenly disperse the sample. Allow the dish to stand undisturbed on a level surface overnight. Carefully remove the cover making sure that none of the saturated potassium carbonate solution drops in the inner chamber. Add 1 drop of a mixed indicator solution consisting of the solution of 0.5 g of methy red and 0.75 g of bromocresol green in 1 liter of ethanol to the inner compartment and titrate the excess acid with N sodium hydroxide solution to a yellow green end point using a 1-ml buret.

$$\% \text{ ammonia} = \frac{(V_a N_a - V_b N_b) 1.70}{p}$$

Where V_a = volume of the sulfuric acid added to the inner chamber, in ml

N_a = normality of the sulfuric acid

V_b = volume of sodium hydroxide used for the titration, in ml

N_b = normality of the sodium hydroxide

w = sample wt, in g

Free Ammonia

Add by means of a 1-ml microburet 0.8000 ml of N sulfuric acid into the inner chamber. Add 2 ml of water to the middle compartment, 2 ml of saturated aqueous potassium carbonate solution to the outer compartment, and 1 drop of 0.025% Tergitol NPX nonionic surfactant to each of the inner and middle compartments.

Accurately weigh approximately 300 mg of sample into the middle chamber and continue the procedure as outlined above for total ammonia. Calculate % free ammonia given above.

Analysis of Dye Intermediates

Since most preparations contain a number of dye intermediates and these are present in low concentrations, their separation and determination are fairly difficult. Thin-layer ehromatography permits the most complete separation and, if the number of intermediates is limited. gas chromatography may also be applied. The base of the preparation appears to give little if any adverse effect upon the chromatogrphic analysis.

Table 14. Symbols Used in Figures 5 to Identify the Individual Substances

Res	resorcinol
Hy	hydroquinone
Cat	catechol
PDA	p-phenylenediamine
oPDA	o-phenylenediamine
mPDA	m-phenylenediamine
pAP	p-aminophenol
mAP	m-aminophenol
oAP	o-aminophenol
2,5TDA	2,5-diaminotoluene
2,4TDA	2,4-diaminotoluene
3,4TDA	3,4-diaminotoluene
pMAP	p-methlaminophenol
DAA	2,4-diaminoanisole
4No	4-nitro-ophenylenediamine
2Np	2-nitro-p-phenylenediamine
2A4	2-amino-4-nitrophenol
2A5	2-amino-5-nitrophenol

4A2	4-amino-2-nitrophenol
Pic	picramic acid
4Clo	4-chloro-o-phenylenediamine
4Clm	4-chloro-m-phenylenediamine
oAn	o-anisidine
pAn	p-anisidine
NPhen	N-phenyl-p-phenylenediamine
NNDM	N,N-dimethy-p-phenylenediamine
NNDE	N,N-diethy-p-phenylenediamine
1,5N	1,5-naphthalenediol
αN	α-naphthol
4,4'	4,4'-methylenebis (N,N-dimethylaniline)

Thin-Layer Chromatography

Most preparations require chromatography on a number of plates and in a number of systems.

Kotteman carried out the analysis on a 0.5-mm thick silica gel G plate employing two-dimensional chromatography. After spotting the sample and a standard solution on the plate, it was developed with Solution A in one direction until the solvent front reached a line drawn 15 cm above the base; then the plate was rotated 90^0, a new standard was applied, and the plate was developed with Solution B to a second line drawn 15 cm above the new base. The plate was then sprayed first with Spray Solution No.1, then with Spray Solution No.2. Figure 5 shows the developed plate with the spots of 30 dye intermediates; Table 14 identifies the individual substances.

The standard applied contained p-phenylenediamine, p-aminophenol, resorcinol, α-naphthol, 2-amino-4 nitrophenol, 2,5-toluenediamine, 3,4-toluenediamine, and 4-nitro-o-phenylenediamine in ethanol solution with a concentration of 2 mg/ml for each substance.

The hair dye sample was prepared for analysis by adding 2 ml of the preparation to 0.5 ml of a 5% sodium sulfite solution and diluted to 4 ml with ethanol. Below, the procedures for the preparation of the developing solution and spray reagents are given.

Table 15. TLC Plates Used for the Analysis of Oxidation Hair Dyes

silica gel G, 0.25 mm thick, dried at 110° C for 1 hr
aluminum oxide G, 0.25 mm thick, dried at 110° C for 1 hr
cellulose, precoated plates
cellulose, precoated plates, dipped in a 20% solution of formamide in acetone
celluose, precoated plates, dipped in a 5% solution of DC-555 silicone oil in ethyl ether
celluose, precoated plates, dipped in a 5% solutione of Carbowax 1000 in acetone
kieselguhr G, 0.25 mm thick, dried at 110° C for 1 hr, then dipped in a 5% solution of Carbowax 1000 in acetone

Table 16. Solvent Systems Used in the Thin-Layer Chromatography of Oxidation Hair Dyes

No	Solvents	Ratio
1	acetone-ethyl ether	2:98
2	acetone-ethyl ether	5:95
3	acetone-ethyl ether	30:70
4	methylisobutyl ketone-ethyl ether	5:95
5	Carbitol[a] ethyl ether	10:90
6	methanol-acetic acid-ethyl ether	10:2:88
7	butanol-acetic acid-ethyl ether	10:10:80
8	cyclohexane-ethyl ether	50:50
9	acetic acid-ethyl ether	50:50
10	acetic acid-ethyl ether	10:90
11	ethyl ether	
12	acetic acid-chloroform	20:80
13	acetone-acetic acid-chloroform	10:20:70
14	acetone-chloroform	30:70
15	methanol-chloroform	10:90

16	methanol-acetic acid-chloroform	30:6:64
17	diethy ether-chloroform	30:70
18	Cellosolve[b] - chloroform	5:95
19	Cellosolve[b] - chloroform	10:90
20	nitrobenzene-chloroform	2:98
21	methanol-chloroform	5:95
22	chloroform	
23	Pyridine-ethyl acetate-acetic acid-water	50:50:10:3
24	n-butanol-acetic acid-water	60:20:20
25	ethyl acetate-acetic acid-formic acid-water	18:3:1:4
26	n-butanol-ethanol-water-acetic acid-sodium earbonate	50:10:40:1:1
27	ethyl acetate[c] - benzene	50:50
28	ethyl acetate[c] - benzene	60:40
29	ethyl acetate - benzene	50:50
30	ethyl acetate - benzene	60:40
31	ethyl acetate[c]	
32	n- butanol[c]	
33	acetone-ethyl acetate[c]	20:80
34	acetone-benzyl alcohol-ethyl acetate[c]	20:5:75
35	isopropyl alcohol-water	70:30
36	isopropyl ether-formic acid-water	90:7:3
37	butanol-acetic acid-ethyl ether[c]	5:5:90

[a] Diethylene glycol monoethyl ether.
[b] 2- Ethoxyethanol.
[c] Saturated with water.

Procedures

Developing Solution A

To 65 ml of water add 20 ml of concentrated ammonium hydroxide and 2 ml of 50% hypophosphorous acid. Add this solution to a mixture of 50 ml of petroleum ether, 250 ml of chloroform, and 25 ml of n-butanol in a separatory funnel. Shake the mixture and allow to stand until the lower layer is clear; heat may be required to clear the lower layer. Use the lower layer as developing Solution A.

Developing Solution B

Mix 350 ml of chloroform, 60 ml of ethanol, 20 ml of glacial acetic acid, and 100 ml of ethyl acetate.

Spray reagent 2

Mix 14 ml of concentrated hydrochloric acid with 5 g of benzidine

Table 18. Rf Obtained on the Silica Gel G Plate

	Solvent systems																
	1	2	3	4	5	6	7	8	9	10	11	12	13	14	15	16	17
resorcinol	0.57	0.57	0.58	0.57	0.86	0.85	1.00	0.15	0.94	0.90	0.43	0.36	0.53	0.43	0.29	0.76	0.21
hydroquinone	0.60	0.57	0.59	0.60	0.88	0.81	1.00	0.18	0.84	0.90	0.44	0.36	0.52	0.49	0.30	0.74	0.26
pyrogallol	0.51	0.49	0.53	0.43	0.66	0.76	0.93	0.18	0.92	0.82	0.23	0.23	0.36	0.27	0.20	0.59	0.17
catechol	0.48	0.57	0.63	0.57	0.83	0.85	1.00	0.17	0.93	0.93	0.42	0.48	0.58	0.46	0.31	0.76	0.25
a-naphthol	0.74	0.76	0.76	0.81	0.93	0.94	1.00	0.43	0.95	0.96	0.62	0.82	0.77	0.68	0.46	0.85	0.58
1,5-naphthalenediol	0.67	0.70	0.72	0.74	0.93	0.83	1.00	0.29	0.95	1.00	0.56	0.60	0.68	0.63	0.34	0.79	0.42
p-phenylenediamine	0.10	0.17	0.28	0.11	0.28	0.13	0.06	0.02	0.07	0	0.06	0.02	0.03	0.23	0.28	0.32	0.06
o-phenylenediamine	0.17	0.41	0.53	0.16	0.38	0.54	0.46	0.03	0.45	0.31	0.08	0.25	0.23	0.45	0.34	0.62	0.09
m-phenylenediamine	0.14	0.25	0.36	0.18	0.36	0.45	0.28	0.03	0.22	0.13	0.11	0.06	0.09	0.29	0.30	0.48	0.11
2,5-diaminotoluene	0.12	0.21	0.32	0.12	0.39	0.14	0.06	0.02	0.05	0	0.07	0.05	0.06	0.26	0.35	0.40	007
2,4-diaminotoluene	0.15	0.24	0.37	0.16	0.31	0.44	0.19	0.02	0.10	0.05	0.010	0.07	0.06	0.24	0.34	0.50	0.08
3,4-diaminotoluene	0.18	0.20	0.31	0.13	0.11	0.52	0.35	0.02	0.10	0.21	0.08	0.22	0.19	0.33	0.35	0.63	0.08
2,4-diaminoanisole	0.10	0.20	0.30	0.12	0.29	0.30	0.08	0.02	0.05	0	0.06	0.04	0.04	0.21	0.33	0.46	0.06
o-anisidine	0.65	0.71	0.71	0.73	0.68	0.84	0.87	0.34	0.59	0.89	0.44	0.59	0.56	0.68	0.59	0.80	0.56
p-anisidine	0.39	0.49	0.54	0.46	0.59	0.70	0.39	0.14	0.41	0.25	0.26	0.28	0.25	0.51	0.49	0.71	0.28
N-phenyl-p-phenylenediamine	0.44	0.53	0.55	0.49	0.68	0.77	0.49	0.14	0.48	0.22	0.31	0.23	0.16	0.52	0.51	0.75	0.27
o-aminophenol	0.52	0.54	0.58	0.55	0.72	0.80	0.86	0.15	0.48	0.60	0.33	0.08	0.14	0.44	0.38	0.74	0.21
m-aminophenol	0.41	0.47	0.53	0.45	0.63	0.75	0.78	0.08	0.52	0.56	0.28	0.07	0.13	0.35	0.32	0.67	0.14
p-aminophenol	0.27	0.36	0.44	0.30	0.46	0.43	0.21	0.05	0.34	0.05	0.18	0.02	0.04	0.032	0.27	0.46	0.11
p-methylaminophenol	0.48	0.57	0.58	0.49	0.61	0.60	0.17	0.12	0.19	0.10	0.32	0.07	0.09	0.38	0.35	0.49	0.17
2,4-diaminophenol	0	0.06	0.14	0	0	0.04	0.03	0	0.04	0	0	0	0	0	0	0.16	0
4-nitro-o-phenylenediamine	0.30	0..40	0.52	0.32	0.42	0.75	0.87	0.04	0.85	0.68	0.18	0.42	0.61	0.38	0.32	0.68	0.10
4-nitro-m-phenylenediamine	0.37	0.45	0.55	0.41	0.50	0.75	0.89	0.05	0.85	0.71	0.25	0.40	0.51	0.43	0.34	0.69	0.15
2-nitro-p-phenylenediamine	0.35	0.42	0.50	0.48	0.53	0.72	0.72	0.07	0.04	0.47	0.22	0.15	0.21	0.43	0.38	0.68	0.15
2-amino-5-nitrophenol	0.56	0.59	0.60	0.61	0.77	0.85	1.00	0.16	0.93	0.90	0.33	0.45	0.61	0.45	0.39	0.77	0.28
4-amino-2-nitrophenol	0.53	0.57	0.60	0.57	0.75	0.84	0.95	0.16	0.85	0.82	0.38	0.60	0.52	0.67	0.50	0.77	0.30
2-amino-4nitrophenol	0.25	0.32	0.38	0.27	0.49	0.32	1.00	0.07	0.82	0.85	0.17	0.38	0.57	0.41	0.34	0.75	0.20
2-amino-4,6-dinitrophenol	0.03	0	0.04	0.05	0.04	0.60	0.94	0	0.94	0.86	0	0.71	0.64	0.03	0.08	0.66	0.02

and dilute to 1 liter with water. Shortly before use, mix this solution with equal volume of 10% aqueous sodium nitrite solution. The mixture is stable only for 2-3 hr.

Table 17. Spray Reagents and the Developed Color of the Spots

	Spray reagent[a]	Color
resorcinol	S	red
hydroquinone	AS	gray-black
pyrogallol	AS	dark black
catechol	AS	brown-gray
α-naphthol	AS	gray-black
1,5-naphthaienediol	AS	black
p-phenylenediamine	DAB	red
o-phenylenediamine	DAB	yellow to orange
m-phenylenediamine	DAB	orange yellow
2,5-diaminotoluene	DAB	orange
2,4-diaminotoluene	DAB	yellow
3,4-diaminoanisole	DAB	yellow to orange
2,4-diaminoanisole	DAB	orange
o-anisdine	DAB	yellow
p-anisidine	DAB	yellow
N-phenyl-p-phenylenediamine	DAB	dark orange to red
o-aminophenol	DAB	yellow
m-aminophenol	DAB	yellow
p-aminophenol	DAB	yellow
p-methyl aminophenol	DAB	lemon yellow
2,4-diaminophenol	DAB	dark brown to red
4-nitro-o-phenylenediamine	DAB	yellow
4-nitro-m-phenylenediamine	DAB	yellow
2-nitro-p-phenylenediamine	DAB	orange
2-amino-5-nitrophenol	DAB	orange
4-amino-2-nitrophenol	DAB	yellow
2-amino-4-nitrophenol	DAB	yellow
2-amino-4,6-dinitrophenol	DAB	orange to red

[a]Spray reagents:

S= 2 g of sucrose dissolved in 10 ml of concentrated hydrochloric acid and mixed with 9 ml of ethanol

AS= ammoniacal silver nitrate solution prepared in the following way:

Table 20. R_f Values Obtained on the TLC Plates Containing a Liquid Stationary Phase

	Cellulose plate				Cellulose plate					Cellulose plate	Kieselguhr plate
	formamide				DC-55 silicone oil					Carbowax 1000	Carbowax 1000
	solvent systems				solvent systems					solvent system	solvent system
	27	28	29	30	31	32	33	34	35	36	37
resorcinol	0.24	0.48	0.16	0.42	0.38	0.69	0.35	0.49	0.85	0.40	0.41
hydroquinone	0.13	0.37	0.08	0.21	0.40	0.69	0.35	0.40	0.91	0.36	0.44
pyrogallol	0.06	0.018	0.04	0.10	0.28	0.52	0.26	0.35	0.78	0.17	0.52
catechol	0.50	0.55	0.41	0.44	0.38	0.69	0.50	0.56	0.82	0.69	0.39
a-naphthol	0.74	0.70	0.71	0.68	0.54	0.69	0.65	0.56	0.85		
1,5-naphthalenediol	0.63	0.66	0.54	0.56	0.38	0.69	0.56	0.54	0.92	0.43	0.32
p-phenylenediamine	0.09	0.19	0.04	0.015	0.07	0.22	0.17	0.23	0.48	0	0.05
o-phenylenediamine	0.56	0.60	0.51	0.47	0.32	0.44	0.41	0.48	0.71	0	0.60
m-phenylenediamine	0.41	0.40	0.28	0.32	0.26	0.33	0.31	0.40	0.63	0	0.29
2,5-diaminotoluene	0.12	0.25	0.09	0.23	0.09	0.29	0.17	0.27	0.52	0	0.03
2,4-diaminotoluene	0.30	0.44	0.27	0.43	0.28	0.47	0.27	0.40	0.66	0	0.25
3,4-diaminotoluene	0.50	0.51	0.45	0.45	0.34	0.57	0.47	0.52	0.76	0	0.21
2,4-diaminoanisole	0.18	0.30	0.14	0.27	0.18	0.29	0.20	0.27	0.57	0	0.05
o-anisidine	0.96	0.94	0.89	0.88	0.52	0.65	0.59	0.65	0.84	0.42	0.64
p-anisidine	0.82	0.81	0.79	0.75	0.33	0.54	0.54	0.61	0.79	0	0.64
N-phenyl-p-phenylenediamine	0.78	0.86	0.83	0.93	0.43	0.68	0.39	0.51	0.79	0	0.64
o-aminophenol	0.34	0.49	0.28	0.45	0.37	0.65	0.33	0.46	0.77	0	0.69
m-aminophenol	0.22	0.36	0.18	0.33	0.34	0.58	0.32	0.41	0.74	0	0.40
p-aminophenol	0.13	0.25	0.10	0.18	0.23	0.52	0.32	0.36	0.69	0	0.10
p-methylaminophenol	0.50	0.42	0.44	0.36	0.31	0.68	0.39	0.44	0.74	0	0.28
2,4-diaminophenol	0.02	0.03	0	0.02	0.03	0.26	0.05	0.07	0.20	0	0
4-nitro-o-phenylenediamine	0.34	0.52	031	0.51	0.37	0.56	0.33	0.47	0.74	0.05	0.29
4-nitro-m-phenylenediamine	0.26	0.44	0.25	0.39	0.35	0.52	0.29	0.43	0.72	0.16	0.27
2-nitro-p-phenylenediamine	0.35	0.53	0.32	0.54	0.36	0.54	0.26	0.46	0.81	0	0.35
2-amino-5-nitrophenol	0.45	0.62	0.40	0.63	0.42	0.56	0.35	0.49	0.85	0.41	0.43
4-amino-2nitrophenol	0.59	0.74	0.58	0.64	0.43	0.67	0.39	0.50	0.77	0.15	0.70
2-amino-4-nitrophenol	0.51	0.61	0.40	0.48	0.35	0.54	0.48	0.49	0.85	0.21	0.62
2-amino-4,6-dinitrophenol	0.0	0.03	0	0	0.24	0.36	0.20	0.23	0.61	0.72	0.60

2 g of silver nitrate is dissolved in 100 ml of water, concentrated ammonium hydroxide solution is added until the precipitate which, concentrated ammonium hydroxide solution is added until the precipitate which forms initially just dissolves, then 1 ml is added in excess

DAB = 1 g of p-dimethylaminohenzaldehyde and 1 g of concentrated hydroxhloric acid is dissloved in 100 ml of ethanol

Table 19. R_f Values Obtained on the Alumina and Cellulose Plates

		Alumina plate				Cellulose plate			
		solvent systems				solvent systems			
	18	19	20	21	22	23	24	25	26
resorcinol	0.08	0.18	0.02	0.23	0.04	1.00	0.85	0.96	0.74
hydroquinone	0.09	0.17	0.03	0.28	0.03	1.00	0.85	0.92	0.75
pyrogallol	0	0	0	0	0	1.00	0.73	0.85	0.59
catechol	0.04	0.04	0	0	0	1.00	0.86	0.97	0.75
α-naphthol	0.61	0.76	0.64	0.74	0.54	1.00	0.96	1.00	0.84
1,5-naphthalenediol	0.33	0.49	0.09	0.27	0.02	1.00	0.90	0.99	0.78
p-phenylenediamine	0.83	0.87	0.64	0.74	0.49	0.56	0.57	0.25	0.45
o-phenylenediamine	0.70	0.83	0.41	0.61	0.36	0.97	0.73	0.59	0.57
m-phenylenediamine	0.86	0.96	0.57	0.71	0.47	0.89	0.63	0.37	0.46
2,5-diaminotoulene	0.80	1.00	0.65	0.82	0.63	0.64	0.62	0.36	0.45
2,4-diaminotoluene	0.80	0.92	0.65	0.84	0.56	0.90	0.65	0.44	0.45
3,4-diaminotoluene	0.55	0.69	0.45	0.62	0.34	1.00	0.74	0.65	0.53
2,4-diaminoanisole	0.82	0.94	0.58	0.84	0.56	0.78	0.63	0.40	0.45
o-anisidine	1.00	1.00	0.95	0.97	0.93	1.00	0.86	0.97	0.62
p-anisidine	0.92	1.00	0.79	0.89	0.76	1.00	0.77	0.74	0.57
N-phenyl-*p*-phenylenediamine	0.91	1.00	0.88	0.90	0.79	1.00	0.87	0.90	0.72
o-aminophenol	0.04	0.11	0.03	0.13	0.10	1.00	0.74	0.58	0.64
m-aminophenol	0.28	0.53	0.15	0.41	0.13	1.00	0.72	0.59	0.55
p-aminophenol	0.40	0.64	0.17	0.50	0.16	0.90	0.68	0.45	0.53
p-methylaminophenol	0.38	0.75	0.28	0.64	0.26	1.00	0.71	0.51	0.59
2,4-diaminophenol	0	0	0	0	0	0.42	0.47	0.21	0.25
4-nitro-o-phenylenediamine	0.42	0.60	0.41	0.59	0.37	1.00	0.79	1.00	0.57
4-nitro-m-phenylenediamine	0.47	0.67	0.48	0.59	0.45	1.00	0.77	1.00	0.57
2-nitro-p-phenylenediamine	0.77	0.88	0.68	0.79	0.62	1.00	0.67	0.64	0.45
2-amino-5-nitrophenol	0.03	0.19	0.04	0.41	0.12	1.00	0.86	1.00	0.70
4-amino-2-nitrophenol	0.83	1.00	0.74	0.83	0.69	1.00	0.81	0.64	0.54
2-amino-4-nitrophenol	0.06	0.08	0	0	0	1.00	0.84	0.98	0.55
2-amino-4,6-dinitrophenol	0	0	0	0	0	1.00	0.85	0.96	0.73

The most detailed investigation of the thin-layer chromatography of oxidation dye intermediates was reported by Goldstein, Kopf, and Feinland. They studied the separation on three plates by adsorption, and on four plates by partition chromatography, with a large number of developing solvents. Tables 15-17 contain information on the plates, developing solvents, and the spray reagents and colors. For the analysis, the hair dye preparations were diluted with equal volume of methanol prior to spotting them on the plates. Tables 18-20 list the R_f values obtained in the various systems. The best general systems were found to be silica gel G with solvent systems 1,2,6 and 12, alumina with solvent systems 18-20, and formamide-impregnated cellulose with solvent systems with solvent systems 29 and 30. Table 21 lists the best systems for the identification (separation from the rest) of specific intermcdiates.

Gas Chromatography. Goldstein, Kopf, and Feinland successfully analyzed hair dye preparations by gas chromatography, on a 6 ft X ¼ in. OD column containing 6% sodium hydroxide and 10% Ucon Oil 50-HB-5100 or Carbowax 20M on Chromosorb P 60/SO mesh. For the analysis, 1-4 g of the hair dye preparation was mixed with 1 ml of a 0.25% solution of N,N-diethyl-1-naphthylamine in isopropyl alcohol and diluted to 10 ml with isopropyl alcohol. The following intermediates could be determined with concentrations as low as a few hundreths of 1% by using flame ionization detector: o-phenyenediamine, p-phenylenediamine, 2,5-diaminotoluene 2,4-diaminotoluene,and 2,4-diaminoanisole.

Table 21. Best TLC-Systems for the identification of Specific Dye Intermediates

Intermediate	Best chromatographic systems (Tables 18-20)
resoreinol	21,27
hydroquinone	11,21,30
pyrogallol	13,15,25,30
catechol	12
a-naphthol	8,11,12,13,24,20
1,5-naphthalenediol	8,11,17,19
p-phenylenediamine	16,23,25,30
o-phenylenediamine	7,10,18,29
m-phenylenediamine	6,7,9
2,5-diaminotoluene	6,23
2,4-diaminotoluene	6,23

3,4-diaminotoluene	5,18
2,4-diaminoanisole	6,23
o-anisidine	2,3,4,8,17,22,27
p-anisidine	7,20,22,25,28,29,30
N-phenyl-p-phenylenediamine	7,10,20,22,27,28,29,30
o-aminophenol	10,19,21
m-aminophenol	18,19
p-aminophenol	9,20
p-methylaminophenol	20,22
2,4-diaminophenol	23
4-nitro-o-phenylenediamine	4,10
4-nitro-m-phenylenediamine	10,13,20
2-nitro-p-phenylenediamine	7,10
2-amino-5-nitrophenol	19,21
4-amino-2-nitrophenol	12,14,28,29
2-amino-4-nitrophenol	6,12,15
2-amino-4,6-dinitrophenol	12,36

Analysis of Dye Developer

Dye developers containing dilute hydrogen peroxide are analyzed for the peroxide content and for storage stability.

Hydrogen Peroxide Content. The peroxide content is determined by the following titrimetric procedure.

Procedure

Accurately weigh a 0.5-g sample into a 250-ml Erlenmeyer flask. Add 100 ml of water, shake, and allow to stand for 1 min. Add 5 ml of concentrated sulfuric acid and 6 drops of ferroin indicator (0.025 M solution of o-phenanthroline ferrous complex). Titrte with standardized 0.1 N ceric ammonium sulfate solution to a sharp blue-green end point.

$$\%\text{hydrogen peroxide} = \frac{(V)\ (N)\ (1.7)}{W}$$

where V = vol of ceric ammonium sulfate solution used for titration, in ml

N = normality of the ceric ammonium sulfate solution

W = sample wt, in g

Storage Stability

Two tests are used in practice. The first carries out the test for 20 hr at 100° C; it is generally accepted that hydrogen peroxide solutions which show a 93% or higher stability value under this condition will exhibit satisfactory shelf stability at room temperature for at least a year. The second test is carried out for seven days at 150° F (66°C); here, a 99% or higher stability value is necessary.

Procedure

Prior to the determination, clean the flasks to be used for the test in the following way.

Fill the flasks completely with 10% sodium hydroxide for a minimum of 1 hr and then rinse thoroughly with water. Fill the flasks completely with 1:9 nitric acid and allow to stand for 3 hr and rinse thoroughly with water. Cover loosely with aluminum foil and dry in oven at 105°C.

20 HR-100°c Test. Determine the hydrogen peroxide concentration of the sample, then place 50 ml of the sample in a 50-ml volumetric flask and weigh. Cover the mouth of the flask losely with aluminum foil to protect the sample from contamination and place it in a 100°C water bath for 20 hr. Immerse the flask in such a way that the water level is just at the 50-ml mark and the base of the flask is not resting on the bottom of the bath. At the end of the 20 hr remove the flask, cool to room temperature, and add enough water to obtain the original weight. If the upper portion has solidified, reheat until the sample is fluid, then mix thoroughly and determine the hydrogen peroxide concentration of the solution.

Seven days - 150°F Test. Determine the hydrogen peroxide concentration of the sample, then place 50 ml of the sample into a 50-ml volumetric flask and weigh. Cover the mouth of the flask loosely with aluminum foil and place in a 66°C (105°F) oil bath for 7 days. Immerse the flask so that the oil is just at the 50-ml mark and the base of the flask is not resting on the bottom of the bath. At the end of 7 days, remove the flask from the bath, cool to room temperature, and add enough water to obtain the original weigh. Mix well and determine the hydrogen peroxide concentration of the solution. If the upper portion has solidified, reheat until the sample is completely fluid, then mix well and analyze.

$$\% \text{ stability} = \frac{C_2 \ 100}{C_1}$$

where C_2 = H_2O_2 concentration after the test

C_1 = H_2O_2 concentration before the test

Hair Coloring Evaluation

The evaluation of hair coloring is done with human hair. Prior to the evaluation of the dye preparation, 16-in. tresses are constructed by fastening each tress ¼ in. from the top with one clip. A standard bleaching solution is prepared and applied to each tress, then are fully saturated with the bleach by immersing them in the bleaching tray. Do not allow the bleaching mixture to get on the metal clip. After a bleaching period of 90 min, the tresses are rinsed with warm water, shampoo, and again water, and combed and dried. The tresses are then divided into smaller parts. Just prior to the application, the tresses are wet, reshampooed with a 1% detergent solution, rinsed and towel-dried. The color preparation is mixed with the developer in the prescribed portion and applied to the hair. The excess dye is removed by light pressing, the hair is dried and mounted for observation and evaluation of the hair color.

The chromatogram is evaluated quantitatively by comparison with one obtained by analyzing a standard sample under identical conditions. The preparation of the standard is outlined below.

Procedure

Place approximately 8 ml of benzene into a tared heavy-duty centrifuge tube, close with a serum cap, and wind a stout rubber band tighty around the neck of the serum cap. Accurately weigh the tube with the benzene. Introduce approximately 0.3 g of each propellant by means of a hypodermic syrige fitted to the valve of an aerosol can of pure propellant or mixed propellants. Weigh. Add by hypodermic syringe approximately 0.3 g of ethanol into the tube and weigh.

Water, if present, is determined after cooling the can at- 25^0 C for 5 min. A 6-in long plastic tube is affixed to the valve stem and the other end of the tube is inserted through a hole in the cap of the Karl Fischer titration flask containing 30 ml of neutralized anhydrous methanol. The valve is actuated and approximately 20 g of hair spray is delivered into the methanol. The amount of sample is weighed by difference and then the water content is determined by the usual Karl Fischer method.

After the propellants, alcohol, and water have been determined, the aerosol can is cooled in a dry-ice-acetone bath, opened, allowed to warm to room temperature and the propellants evaporated. Then, the concentrate mixture is transferred into a tared beaker, using ethanol to aid in the transfer, evaporated to dryness under a stream of dry air and wieghed. The result is expressed as air-dried solids.

Qualitative tests are carried out from the air-dried solids to detect the presence of lanolin and proteins. The presence of silicone compounds may be established from the infrared spectrum and the ultraviolet absorption spectrum can be used to detect the presence of sunscreens, aromatic quaternary ammonium compounds, etc. if such compounds are present, separation and quantitation can be achieved by liquid-column chromatography and thin-layer chromatography.

For the determination of the resins and plasticizers present, the residue is moistened with a few ml of ethanol and macerated with a stirring rod. Then 150 ml of ethyl ether is added and filtered through a tared Whatman No. 4 paper by allowing only a minimum amount of the residue to pass onto the paper. The procedure is repeated twice, then the resin is dried and weighed to obtain the amount of resin present. It can be identified from its infrared specrtrum. The combined ether solutions are evaporated to dryness and weighed to obtain the amount of plasticizer present. Infrared spectroscopic analysis of the residue permits the determination of the type of plasticizer present.

SUNSCREENS

Sunscreens are usually solution, lotions, or quick breaking foams. Their primary function is to absorb ultraviloet light in the 280-320 nm region. Table 10 lists some of the sunscreens in use.

Methods of Analysis

The first step in the analysis of a sunscreen is the determination of the water, ethanol, and propylene glycol content. If the product is an aerosol, the propellants are analyzed by gas chromatography. The amount of air-dried solids is determined, from and withdrawing a 2-ml sample of air with a gas syringe. The gas sample is injected into a gas chromatograph equipped with a flame ionization detector. The method can be calibrated by weighing a small amount of the particular perfume oil or flavoring extract and diluting to a known volume with a solvent, injecting known volumes of the solution into a number of different 1-gal jars and analyzing the air in the jar under identical conditions. Selective permeation of specific fragrance compounds can be detected by comparison of chromatograms of nonpermeated us permented fragrance.

Testing Caps

To evaluate the behavior of caps during storage,six caps,smeared with product, are stored at 70^{0}F and six at 120^0 F and each is observed daily for one week and weekly for two months. If the product dries out, re-apply. The CPAS are observed for staining and discoloration and stress cracking. If no stress craking is observed, clean the cap off with a dry cloth and then put some ink on the cap with a felt pen. Rub the ink over the cap's surfaces with the fingers. Quite small stress cracks can be made visible in this manner. Some plastic caps appear opaque, but can be shown to transmit light if held up to a strong light. If a shield is placed around the cap so that only the transmitted light is seen, minor stress cracks can be observed.

In conjunction with the above tests, the liners in the caps are also observed for possible discoloration, delamination from the backing, fallout, seizure to the neck finish, and poor fit in the cap when mounted on bottles that are filled with product.

Testing Collapsible Tubes

Most of the tests on tubes are carried out in the same manner as described for bottles. Most tubes are received already capped, therefore, cap tightness as well as liner cleanliness must be checked.

The quality of the crimp is checked by observing stored samples for leakage. In addition, known pressures are applied to the closed tube, and the mean pressure required to open the crimp is calcuated as well as the 95% confidence limits.

The stored plastic tubes are evaluated for softening of the plastic by means of a hardness gage or subjective observations. Other tests are related to the compatibility of the tube's internal lining (coating), the permeation of the tubes, and the resistance of the coating to flexing.

Metal tubes are stored and checked for corrosion on the interior surface near the crimp as well as the general interior surface and also for resistance of the liner to cracking at a crease or bend.

Testing Labels. Labels are tested for adhesion stability and abrasion, as well as for compatibility with the formulation stored in the particular package on which the label is to be applied.

An accelerated test for storage stability of most combinations of labels and plastic containers may be carried out by heat-sealing the labels to the plastic and then heating for various periods of time. The oven temperature should be below the softening point of the plastic.

A temperature of 210^0 F for 5 hr or 175^0 F for 16 hr suffices for most label-plastic combinations. Labels that firmly adhere after the test should be satisfatory, under normal conditions, for one year.

To test the resistance against abrasion, two bottles, with applied labels, are rubbed together so that the labels are in contact and the labels are evaluated for ease of scuffing. Alternatively, one can use an abrasion machine which drags a weighted pad back and one that is not too low, but permits enough space for expansion of the product at higher temperatures.

For the determination, six bottles are selected, tared, filled to overflow with water, then reweighed.

$$\text{Overflow volume, fl oz} = \frac{\text{net wt of water, in g}}{29.57}$$

Subsequently, sufficient water is drawn out with a hypodermic syrings until the label content is reachedwhen the bottle with water is reweighed.

$$\text{label fill, fl oz} = \frac{\text{net wt of water, in g}}{29.57}$$

$$\text{\% free space} = \frac{\text{net wt of water at overlow--net wt of water at label fill}}{\text{net wt of water at overflow}} (100)$$

At this stage, the fill height is measured with a micrometer depth gage. This is the so-called low fill height. Then, enough water is added to the bottle to raise the fill height by 0.065 in. The bottle is reweighed and the % free space recalculated for this fill height ("high-fill height"). This second measurement is necessary because the variation of the filling machine is taken as $\pm$ 0.0325 in. =0.065 in.

Plastic Material

Sometimes the identification of the plastic used to produce the bottles may be of interest. This identifcation can be carried out by pyrolysis followed by subsequent investigation of the pyrolysis products by infrared spectroscopy or gas chromatography. Attenuated total reflectance (A.T.R.) spectrophotometry is a method which was successfully applied for this purpose . Since thick, stiff pieces of plastic, such as bottle walls, are sometimes difficult to clamp against the internal reflection plate without scratching it, a small section of plastic may be compressed between the flat jaws of a small vise that has been heated to 100^{0}C. The plastic section is then trimmed with a razor blade and clamped against the internal reflection plate.

The following relatively simple procedure is often quite satisfactory for sample pyrolysis and subsquent identification by IR spectroscopy.

Procedure

Place a 4×2 mm piece of the sample in a 4-in test tube. Hold the tube at a 20°angle and heat gently in a low Bunsen flame. When the sample pyrolzes, the tarry materials will condensate on the upper wall of the tube. Remove the tarry material with a glass stirring rod and rub gently onto a salt plate in the area of impingement of the infrared beam.

The methods for pyrolysis combined with the direct gas chromatographic analysis of the pyrolyzates are well established.

Permeation of Fragrances. Bottles as well as other packages are usually tested for possible permeation of the fragrances present in the cosmetic formulation inside the package. The simplest way is to smell the outside of the bottle after storage; a more quantitative method is provided by the use of gas chromatography. The filled bottle are placed into 1-gal glass jars equipped with a screw cap and stored at room temperature as well as at 120° F for 24 hr or longer if deemed necessary. Subsequently, the air around the test bottle is sampled by puncturing the metal cap with a small nail should test a minimum of 12-18 pieces of an item, representing all molds, at each of two temperatures, at 70°F and 120°F. Such samples should be representative of the sample population. Samples should be filled with the final product to normal fill heights and capped in the manner that will probably prevail during production. For plastic bottles the application torque should be slightly greater than the minium torque required to reach a stop position after all parts are assembled. The relationship between application torque and release may be established using a Owens-Illinois torque tester. For the application and release torques calculate the mean and 95% confidence limits. The control should approximate the sample in size, weight, and % headspace.

Storage. One group of samples is stored at 70° F and one group at 120° F. One third of the samples of each group should be stored in an inverted position. All samples are weighed before storage and after 24 hr. If a significant weight loss occurs after 24 hr, the samples are weighed daily for one week and then weekly for one month. Samples are observed weekly for any leakage, cracking of caps, loosening of caps, breakdown of product, or any other abnormalities. The containers are not opened at this stage unless the test is being terminated.

Table 22. Tests for the Evaluation of Cosmetic Packages

Gereral Tests
compatibility with the product
resistance of the finish to th product
weight loss during storage
%delivery and/or % retention
deliverability
behavior on cyeling the temerature between-40⁰ F and 120⁰F
light stability
permeation of fragrance
stress cracking
identification of the plastic material of the container
dry rub or scuff resistance of printed ink films on packaging materials
resistance of ink on printed packaging materials to fats, oils, and the product
fill height
accelerated ageing of films and foils
accelerated ageing of the package-product combination
capacity
dimensions of the package
antistatic test
metal containers: corrosion
glass containers: polaroscopic evalution
thermal shock test

Tests on Bottles
liquid expansion
balloning or collapse
ai leakage
bursting pressure
penetration of liquids into submerged bottles
leakage at closure
drop test

Tests on Caps
proper fit
application and removal torque of threaded closures
vacuum test for closure leakage
leak test (weight loss)
water vapor transmission
stress cracking of cap
liner: identification
adhesion to cap

compatability
seal
delamination
fit

Tests on Collapsible Tubes
ballooning or collapse
quality of crimp
leakage on cap threads
softening of plastic
metal tubes: corrosion
chemical composition

Tests on Labels and Decor
thickness and density of paper
effect of product on label
effect of product on label mounted on coutainer
dimensions
adhension and stripping strength of adhesives
pinholes in paper and laminated foil
resistance against abrasion
resistance against pinching
resistance against scratching with fingernail
wate repellancy
humidity resistance.

While samples are in storage they are examined for collapse of the walls, either concavity convexity. These are causes fo rejection.

Compatibility

At the end of one month, sooner if package failure is indicated, the samples are removed from storage, equilibrated to room temperature and weighed. The package is checked for dispensability. If the product has bodied-up, it is compared with the control in a glass bottle. If the product in the glass bottle has also bodied-up, it is compared with the control in a glass bottel. If the product and not an effect produced by the test package. Incompatibility of the package with the product is noted as any staining of the package. Incompatibility of the package with the product is noted as any staining of the package, discoloration, or breakdown of product that is caused by the package.

Seal

The test for seal is made by comparing the weight loss obtained over the period of the test. Weight loss obtained in this manner will include weight loss through the closure plus that due to permeation through the container wall. If weight loss is high, one can differentiate between the two routes by dipping some of the filled and capped bottles into molten high malting point wax so that the closure is covered and then stored in this form. In this manner, weight loss is restricted to the wall of the container. Table 23 lists typical weight loss values for various types of plastic bottles.

Leakage

Leakage refers to product that has migrated into the interface between the bottle neck and the cap inner wall, but does necessarily represent weight loss. For example, a cream or lotion might get into the interface, but would not evaporate. Leakage is therefore detected by carefully opening the package in an upright position and closely observing the neck finish for the slightest sign of product seepage.

After the above tests have been performed the samples are returned to storage, if they pass all tests, and are retested at monthly intervals for two more months. The room temperature samples are left on test for one year unless the tests are terminated earlier for any reason.

Accelerated Leakage Test. Twelve bottles are placed in a vacuum chamber (four bottles each in upright, horizontal, and inverted positions) under a vacuum of 29 in. of mercury and allowed to stand at room temperature for 16 hr, after which they are checked.

The horizontal and inverted samples are usually most useful for detecting leakage or weight loss by this test.

Table 23. Average Weight Loss of Plastic Bottles"

Content of Bottle	Polyvinyl chloride bottles, oz/yr	Polyethylene bottles, oz/yr	Polypropylene bottles, oz/yr
water	1	0.1	0.3
ethanol	1.3	0.2	0.4
shampoo	1	0.1	0.3
two-phase-product (water-ethanol)	1	0.2	0.3
liquid hair dressing	0.5	0.2	0.3
bath oil	0.1	0.8	0.4
empty bottle	0.08	0.03	0.05

" Based on four weeks' storage at 120^0 F 6-oz bottles.

Thermal Cycling

A separate group of packages, prepared in the same manner as those used for the compatibility test, are stored for 24 hr at 120^0 F, then removed, equilibrated to room temperature, and then stored at - 40^0 F for hr. The cycle is continued as long as is deemed necessary.

Each package is carefully observed daily for stress cracking or other abnormal effects. With components such as compacts, the closure and hinge action is observed. Acceptability of the adhesive used for compacts, mirrors is also tested in this manner.

Drop Test

A random selection of bottles are filled with water to normal fill heights and sealed. Dropping of bottles at 3 ft onto asphalt tile over concrete. Each bottle is successively dropped on its bottom corner, side, and flat bottom. The same bottles go through the same drops at 4,5 and 6 ft or until failure.

Rocking

Empty bottles and bottles that have been stored for compatibility testing are placed on a flat surface and are gently rocked. A bottle that has a bulged bottom and thus rocks easily, is rejectable.

Fill Characteristies. Capacity (overflow volume), label fill, % free space, and fill heights are the values determined on production mold bottles. Label fill is measured on a bottle to determine if its produces an "aesthetic fill."

EVALUATION OF PACKAGES

Package evaluation as used here, refers primarily to the testing of those packaging components which are or are likely to be in contact with the product, Bottles, caps valves, dip tubes, liners,labels, plugs, films, seals, and coatings are a few examples.

The task of the package evaluation laboratory in many companies is to assist package design and purchasing groups in selecting an acceptable package for the product in question. Determining whether a package is acceptable or not requires that a large number of characteristics be tested. Table 22 lists some of the tests that are run on almost every type of package, and on the four very common component types: bottles, caps collapsible tubes and labels.

The tests listed in Table 22 are sufficient to test the majority of components with few additions. for example, in testing plastic parts, such as compacts, it is useful to subject the part to thermal cycling. the compact is cycled between - 40⁰F and 120⁰ F for a period of days or weeks and then examined for proper closure and hinge action. Sometimes cycling is used to simulate extreme climatic conditions encountered during shipment or storage. Acute observation powers and ingenuity play an important role in devising a critical test program for a new previously untested packaging component.. In planning such a test program a large number of factors must be considered:

Compliance With City, State, and Federal Statules. Tests should be performed which will show noncompliance, if present. Flammability tests on aerosols and breakage tests on glass aerosols should be performed. Percent delivery of net contents of aerosols should be determined.

Accelerated and Nonaccelerated Tests. One usually employs accelerated as well as nonaccelerated tests in the evaluation of a component. The usual conditions are one month at 120⁰ F vs 1 yr at room temperature. If color stability is being checked, a carbon are Weather-O-Meter is used and usually 60 hr exposure is taken as being equivalent to 6 months "average" U.S.A. sunlight. To test for accelerated indoor exposure one can move the parts being tested very close to the illuminant for various periods of time and then calculate the time required to give equivalent exposure at the distances from lights that are normally encountered indoors.

Duration of Test. For compatability testing, the sample is stored for one month at 70⁰ F and 120⁰ F, and at the end of this period conclusions are made and reported. However the samples may be continued on test for up to two additional months at 120⁰ F and up to one year at 70⁰ F.

Controls. All tests are run parallel with the same product in glass controls. Thus, any product breakdown obtained in glass will not be attributed to the package that is on test.

Severity of Test. The severity of any test that is to be run has to be judged on the basis of the type of information that is to be obtained. If one is testing a package- product combination for its probable shelf life under normal environmental conditions, the conditions will be much less severe than, eg, if one has to evaluate which of two plastics has the greatest stress-crack resistance. Some of the more important tests are discussed briefly at next page.

Testing Bottles

Frequently, when one is developing a new package with a vendor, very few pieces are submitted during the early stages of evaluation. In such situtions, valuable conclusions can be drawn from test results on one to six items. However, ideally one forth across the lable. Here, the labels are evaluated by comparison of the number of passes required to give a certain amount of deterioration.

In other tests, the label is pinched to crease the printing or decoration and scratched at the crease with the fingernail using light to moderate pressure. The deterioraion or cracking of the label is observed and compared with standards or specified as acceptable lables.

For compatibility tests, the cosmetic formulation is smeared on half of the label and stored at 120°F. The label is observed after $^1/_2$,1,3,6,24, and 48 hr by wiping clean a portion of the label with a cloth and checking for blistering, penetration, discoloration and resistance to scratching.

Miscellaneous Tests

A few tests performed on metalized or lacquered components are outlined below.

Perspiration Test. The package is placed in a jar or desiccator and smeared with a "synthetic perspiration solution" using a cotton swab which is left in contact with the package. The jar or desiccator is closed and allowed to stand or 24 hr at room temperature (70°F). The sample passes the test if there is no breakdown, delamination of softening of the lacquer, or discoloration of the metal.

The synthetic perspiration solution is prepared by dissolving 3g of butyric acid, 3g of technical grade valeric acid, 5 gt of 70% acetic acid, and 5 g of sodium chloride in water and diluting to a total weight of 100 g.

Markol Test. This test determines the completeness of cure of the lacquer on the package. The package is immersed in Markol solution and stored for 24 hr at room temperature (70°F) then taken out, washed, and checked for decoloration or softening of the lacquer layer.

The Markol solution consists of a solution 14.1g of propylene glycol, 1`.2g of D&C Orange No.5, 1.2g of D&C Red No. 21, and 2.4g of D&C Red No. 27 inenough propylene glycol monolaurate to give a total weight of 100g.

Copper Sulfate Test. This test is carried out to evaluate gold stamping on packages. The packages are immersed for 15 min at room temperature (70°F) in a copper sulfate solution then rinsed with water and compared with an untreated package. The gold stamping must remain intact and show no discoloration, bare spots, or breakdown; the exposed metal surface will evolve hydrogen gas.

The copper sulfate solution for the test is prepared by dissolving 25 g of copper sulfate in water, adding 50 ml of concentrated hydrochloric acid and diluting with water 1500 ml.

Shampoos

Shampoos are preparations of surfactants which, when used properly, remove grease, dirt, and skin debris from the scalp and hair.

The surfactants used in shampoos can be divided into nonionic, anionic, and cationic surfactants. Ethoxylated lanolin alcohols, polyethylene oxide, or silicone fluid are typical nonionic surfactants; soaps, alkyl sulfates as alkali metal, ammonium, or alkanolaine salt, alkylaryl sulfates and sulfonates are typical anionic surfactants, whereas quarternary ammonium compounds and cationic protein are typical cationic sufractants. Other substances used in shampoo formulations include sequestering agents, mineral oil, lanolin, gums, and hexachlorophene. Inorganic salts may also be added.

Methods of Analysis

The analysis of shampoo starts with the determination of its pH, in addition to the amount of nonvolatile matter ("solids") and water present. If the sum of these two is less than 100%, the amount of alcohol present is determined also. For detailed analysis, the nonvolatile matter is separated in multistage processes into organic substance groups; certain elements and anions may be determined from the ash. The anionic, cationic, and nonionic surfactants present may be separated from each other and determined as a group. If the type of shampoo has been identified, detailed multistage separation processes permit the determination of individual substances or substance groups.

Composition Analysis

Nonvolatile Matter (Solids). The amount of nonvolatile matter of shampoos is determined by drying a sample aliquot at 105°C for 2 hr.

Water. The water content of shampoos is determined by the Karl Fischer method, by tolune distillation, or by gas chromatography utilizing microporous polymer beads, such as Porapak Q, as the column packing.

Alcohol. The determination of the *ethanol* content of the sample can conveniently be carried out by gas chromatographic analysis on a 6ft × 1/4 inOD column packed Porapak Qmicroporous polymer beads, at125°C. The measurement also permits the simultaneous determination of water.

Usually, a qualitative test is also carried out to check for the presence of *propylene glycol.* The test is performed from the aqueous phase obtained when the water content is determined by toluene distillation. The procedures are given below.

Procedures

Catechol Test (13). To 3 ml of the aqueous phase, add 3 ml of freshly prepared 10 catechol solution and 6 ml of concentrated sulfuric acd. Heat in a boiling water bathfor 30 min. If the solution turns red and a precipitate forms, propylene glycol is present.

Imdoform Test. To5 ml of the aqueous phase, add 5 ml of a 0.2 *M* potassium periodate solution. After 1 min add an excess of a 5% sodium hydroxide solution followed by a 0.1 *N* iodine solution. If a precipitate of iodoform forms are immediately, propylene glycol is present.

7

Analysis for Colour for Drugs and Cosmetics

Various materials are used to colour drugs and cosmetics. The list is enormous and includes synthetic organic materials like chemicals, vegetables, herbs, animal extracts as well as inorganic substances of both synthetic mineral origin.

Methods of Analysis

Identification

Any of the techniques used to identify dyes are applicable to certifiable colours. Physical properties such as solubility, crystal structure and crystal colour provides clue.

By far the best means of identification are infrared, ultraviolet, and visible absorption spectrometry(Figs. 1-18). Spectra in more than one solvent system can be very informative. It is rare that two colors will have the same spectrum in several different solvents. Useful solvents for water-soluble dyes are water, 1:100 ammonium hydroxide, 1:100 acetic acid, 1% Peregal O (a nonionic surfactant), and 95% sulfuric acid.

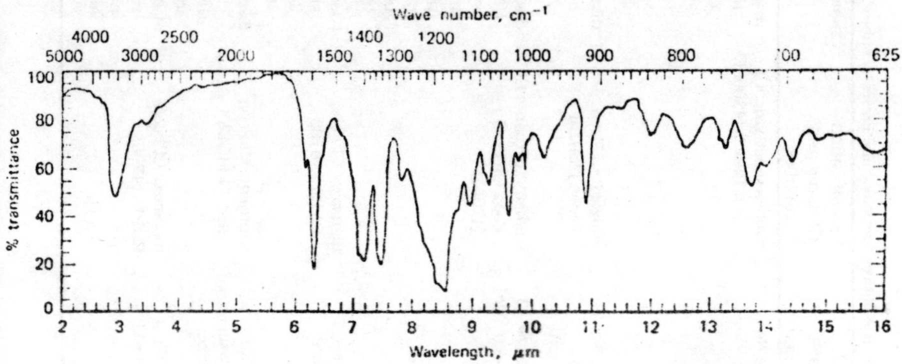

Fig. 1. Infrared spectrum of FD&C Blue No. 1. Courtesy Sadtler Research Laboratories, Inc.

Table 1. Colour Additives Previously and Presently subject to Certification by the FDA and Provisionally Listed for Food, drug and Cosmetic Use (FD&C Colors)

Official FDA name; trade name(s)	Classification CI name and number	Chemical name	Manufacturing process	Structural Formula	Molecular weight	Infra-red spectraum	Visible spectrum
FD&C Blue No. 1[a] (Brilliant Blue) (FCF)	triphenylmethane; CI Food Blue 2 (42090)	disodium salt of 4-[(4-4 (*N*-ethyl-*m*-suloben zylamino) phenyl] (2-sulfoniumphenyl)- -$\Lambda^{2,5}$methylene [1-(N-xyl)-$\Lambda^{2,3}$-cyclohexa-dicnimine	condensation of benzal-dehyde-*o*-sulfonic acid with a-(N-ethylani-lino)m-toluenesulfonie acid ("benzylethyl aniline sulfonic acid")		792.8	Fg. 1	Fig.2
FD&C Blue No. 2 (Indigotine, Indigotin IA)	indigoid: CI Food Blue : (73015)	disodium salt of 5,5'-indigotindisulfonic acid	sulfonation of indigo		466.4	Fig. 3	Fig. 4
FD&C Green No. 3 (Fast Green FCF)	triphenylmethane; CI Food Green 3 (42053)	disodium salt of 4-: [4-(*N*-ethyl-*m*-sulfoben sylamino) phenyl] (4-hydroxy-2-sulfonium phenyl)-methylene]-[1-(*N*-ethyl-*N*-*m*-sulfo-benzyl)-$\Lambda^{2,3}$-cyclo hexadienimine]	condensation of *p*-hydroxybenzaldehyde-*o*-slfonic acid wit *a*-(*N*-ethylailino)-*m*-toulenesulfonic acid		808.9	Fig. 5	Fig. 6
FD&C Red No. 2 (Amarnath)	monoazo: CI Food Red 9 : 16185	trisodium salt of 1-(4-sulfo-l-naphythylazo)-2-naphthol-3, 6-di-sulfonic acid	coupling of diazotized naphthionic acid with R salt		604.5	Fig. 7	Fig. 8
FD&C Red No.3[a] (Erhythrosine, Erythrosine Bluish)	xanthene: CI Food Red 14 (45430)	disodium salt of 9-*o*-carboxyphenyl-6 hydroxy-2,4,5,7-tetra iodo-3-isoxanthone	iodination of fluorescin (D&C Yellow No. 7)		879.9	Fig. 9	Fig. 10
FD&C Red No. 4 (Ponceau 8X)	monoazo: CI Food Red 1: 14700)	disodium salt of 2-(5-sulfo-2,4-xylylazo)-1-naphthol-4-sulfonic acid	coupling of diazotized I-amino-2, 4-dimethyl-benzene-5-sulfonic acid with 1-naphthol-4-sulfonic acid		480.4	Fig. 11	Fig. 12

Table 1 *(continued)*

Official FDA name; trade name(s)	Classification CI name and number	Chemical name	Manufacturing process	Structural Formula	Molecular weight	Infrared spectraum	Visible spectrum
FD&C Violet No. 1 (Wool Violet 5BN) or Acid Violet 6B)	triphenylimethane;CI Food Violent 2 (42640)	monosodium salt of 4-{[14-(V-ethyl-*m*-sulfobenzylamino)phenl]-[4-(*N*-ethyl-*m*-sulfonium-benzylamino) phenyl]-methylene}-(*N*,.*N*-dimethyl-D^{2,3}-cycloheadienimine)	condensation of *p*-dimethylaminobenzaldehyde with *a*-(*N*-ethylanilino)-*m*-toluenesulfonic acid and oxidation		733.9	Fig. 13	Fig. 14
FD&C Yellow No. 5[a] (Tartrazine)	pyrazolone; CI Food Yellow 4 (19140)	trisodium salt of 3-carboxy-5-hydroxy-1-*p*-sulfophenyl-4-*p*-sulfophenylazo-pyrazole	(a) condensation of phenylhydrazine-*p*-sul fonic acid with oxalacetic ester, coupling of the product with diazotized sulfanilie acid, then hydrolyzation of the ester with sodium hydroxide or (b) condensation of phenylhydrazine-*p*-sulfonic acid with dihydroxytartaric acid		534.4	Fig. 15	Fig. 16
FD&C Yellow No. 6 (sunset Yellow)	monoazo; CI Food Yellow 3 (15985)	disodium salt of 1-*p*-sulfophenylazo-2 naphthol-6-sulfonic acid	coupling of diazotized sulfanilie acid with 2-naphthol-6-sulfonic acid		452.4	Fig. 17	Fig. 18
FD&C lakes			extension of the AI or Ca salt corresponding to the FD&C color on alumina hydrate				

Colour additives for food use subect to certification

Table 1 *(continued)*

Official FDA name; trade name(s)	Classification CI name and number	Chemical name	Manufacturing process	Structural Formula	Molecular weight	Infra-red spectraum	Visible spectrum
Citrus Red No. 2 (for coloring orange skins only)	monoazo (13156)	1-(2,5-dimethoxyphenyl-azo)-2-naphthol	coupling of diazotized 2,5-dimethoxyamiline		590.5		
Orange B (for coloring sausage skins only)	pyrazolone	disodium salt of 1-(4-sulophenyl)-3-ethyl-carboxyl-4-(4-sulfo-naphthylazo)-5-hydroxyphrazole					

Table 2: Color Additives Previously and Presently subject to certification by the FDA and provisionally Listed for Drug and Cosmetic Use (D&C Colours)

Official FDA name; trade name(s)	Classification CI name and number	Chemical name	Manufacturing process	Structural Formula	Molecular weight
D&C Blue No. 4 (Alphazurine FG. (Erioglaucine)	triphenylmethane; (42090)	NH_4 salt corresponding to FD&C Blue No. 1	same as FD&C Blue No. 1		783.0
D&C Blue No. 6 (Indigo)	indigoid; CI Vat Blue 1 (73000)	indigotin			262.3
D&C Blue No. 9 (Carbanthrene BLue, Indanthrene Blue GCD)	anthrauinone vat; CI Vat Blue 6 (69825)	3,3'-dichloroindanthrene	chlorintation of indan-therene		511.3
D&C Green No. 5 (Alizarin Cyanine Green F. Alizarin Cyanine Green	anthraquinone; CI Acid Green 25 (61570)	disodium salt of 1,4-bis-(*o*-sulfo-*p*-toluino)-anthraquinone)	condensation ofleuco-quinizarin with *p*-toluidine and sulfo -nation		622.6

Table 2. contd......

Official FDA name; trade name(s)	Classification CI name and number	Chemical name	Manufacturing process	Structural Formula	Molecular weight
D&C Green No. 6 (Quinizarin Green SS)	anthraquinone; CI Solvent Green 3 (61565)	1,4-bis(*p*-toluino)-anthraquinone	condensation of leuco-quinizarin with *p*-toluidine		418.5
D&C Green No. 8 (Pyranine Concentrated	pyrene (59040)	trisodium salt of 10-hydroxy-3,5,8-pyrene trisulfonic acid	sulfonation of pyrene to tetrasulfonic acid, salting out with sodium chloride, hydrozyzation in sodium hydroxide solution, adding of formic acid, and salting out with sodium chloride		524.4
D&C Orange No. 4 (Orange II)	monoazo; CI acid Orange 7 (15510)	monosodium salt of 1-*p*-sulfophenylazo-2-naphthol 874	coupling of diazotized sulfanilic acid wit 2-naphthol		350.3
D&C Orange No. 5 (Diiodofluorescein)	fluoran	4,5-dibromo-3,6-fluoran-	bromination of fluores- (D&C Yellow No. 7)		490.1
D&C Orange No. 11 (Erhythrosine Yellowish Na, Erythrosine Yellowish)	xanthene	disodium salt of 9--*o*-carboxyphenyl-6-hydroxy-2-naphthol	conversion of D&C Orange No. 10 to the 2,4-dinitoaniline with		584.1
D&C Orange 17 (Permatone Orange of Permanent Orange)	monoazo (12075)	1-(2,4-dinitrophenylazo)-2-naphthol	coupling of diaotized 2,4-dinitroaniline with 2-naphthol		628.1
D&C Red No. 6	monoazo; CI Pigment	disodium salt of 4-(*o*-	coupling of diazotised 6-		338.1

Table 2. contd......

Official FDA name; trade name(s)	Classification CI name and number	Chemical name	Manufacturing process	Structural Formula	Molecular weight
(Lithol Robin B)	Red 57 (15850)	sulfo-*p*-tolyazo-3-hydroxy-2-naphthoic acid	amino-*m*-toluene-sulfonic acid with 3-hydroxy-2-natphthoie acid		
D & C Red No. 7 (Lithol Rubin B Ca)	monoazo; CI Pigment REd 57 (15850)	calcium salt corresponding-ing to D&C Red No. 6	heating of D&C Red No. 6with calcium chloride		424.5
D&C Red No. 8 (Lake Red C)	monoazo; CI Pigment Red 53 (15585)	monosodium salt of 1-(4-chloro-*o*-sulfo-5-tolyly-azo)-2-naphtol	coupling of diazotized 2-amino-5-chloro-*p*-toluenesulfonic acid with 2-naphthol		398.8
D&C Red No. 9 (Lake RedC Ba)	monoazo; CI Pigment Red 53 (15575)	Barium salt corresponding to D&C Red No. 8	Boiling of D&C Red no. 8 with Barium chloride		444.5
D&C Red No. 10 (Lithol Red, Lithol REd R)	monoazo; CI Pigment Red 49 (15630)	monosodium salt of 2-(2-hydroxy--1-naphthyl-azo)-1-naphthalene-sulfonic acid	coupling of diazoitiszed 2-naphthylamine-1-sulfonic acid (Tobias acid) with 2-naphthol		400.4
D&C Red No. 11 (Lithol Red Ca)	monoazo; CI Pigment Red 49 (15630)	calcium salt correspond-ing to D&C Red No. 11	heating of D&C REd No. 10 with calcium chloride	calcium salt of D&C Red No. 10	397.4
D&C Red No. 12 (Lithol Red Ba)	monoazo; CI Pigment Red 49 (15630)	barium salt corresponding to D&C Red No. 10	heating of D&C Red No. 10 with strontium chloride	barium salt of D&C.Red No. 10	446.1
D&C Red No. 13 (Lithol Red Sr.)	monoazo; CI Pigment Red 49 (156330)	strontium salt corre-sponding to D&C Red No.10	heating of D&C Red No. 10 with strontium chloride	strontium salt of D&C Red No. 10	421.2

Table 2. contd......

Official FDA name; trade name(s)	Classification CI name and number	Chemical name	Manufacturing process	Structural Formula	Molecular weight
D&C Red No. 17 (Toney Red, Sudan 111)	diazo: CI Solvent Red 23 (26100)	l-*p*-phenylazophenylazo-2-naphthol	coupling of diazotized aminoazobenzene with 2-naphthol		352.4
D&C Red No. 19 (Rhodamine B)	xanthene: CI Basic Violet 10 (451170)	3-ethochloride of 9-*o*-carboxyphenyl-6-diethylamino-3-ethyl imino-3-isoxanthene	(a) fusion of *m*-diethylaminophenol with phthalic anhydride and treatment of the base with dilutehydrochloric acid or (b) treatment of fluorescein chloride under pressure with diethylamine		479.0
D&C Red No. 21 (Tetrabromo-fluorescein)	fluoran: CI Solvent Red 43 (45380A)	2,4,5,7-tetrabromo-3,6-fl·· randiol	bromination of fluorecein *D&C Yellow No. 74	free acid of D&C Red No. 22	647.
D&C Red No. 22 (Eosin YS, Eosine G)	xanthene; CI Acid Red 87 (45380)	disodium salt of 2,4,5,7-tetrabromo-9-*o*-carboxyphenyl-6-hydroxy-3-isoxanthone	conversion of D& C Red No. 21 to the sodium salt		691.9
D&C Red No. 27 (Tetrachlorotetra bromofluorescein	fluoran: CI Solent Red 18 (45410A)	2,4,5,7-tetrabromo 12,13,14,15-tetrachloro-3,6-fluorandiol bromination	condensation of resorcinol with tetrachlorophthalic anhydride and	free acid of D&C Red No. 28	785.7

Table 2. contd......

Official FDA name; trade name(s)	Classification CI name and number	Chemical name	Manufacturing process	Structural Formula	Mole-cular weight
D&C Red No. 28 (Phloxine B)	xanthene; CI Acid Red 92 (45410)	disodium salt of 2,45,7-tetrabromo-9-(3,4,5,6-tetrachloro-o-carboxy phenyl)-6-hydroxy-3-isoxanthone	conversion of D&C Red No. 27 to the sodium salt		829.7
D&C Red No. 30 (HelindonePink) (CN)	indigold; CI Vat Red 1(73360)	6,6'-dchloro-4,4'-di methylthioindigo	(a) oxideation of 6-chloro-4-methylthioindoxyl or (b) chlorination of 4,4'-dimethylthio indigo		393.3
D&C Red No. 31 (Brilliant Lake) Red R)	monoazo: CI Pigment Red 64 (15800)	calcium salt of 4-hydroxy-4-phenylazo-2-naphthoic acid conversion to the calcium salt	coupling of diazotized aniline with 3-hydroxy 2-naphthoic acid and		311.3
D&C Red No. 33 (Acid Fuchsin D or Naphthalene Red B; Fast Acid Fuchsine B)	monoazo; CI Acid red 33 (17200)	disodium salt of 8-amino 2-phenylazo-1-naphthol-3,6--disulfonic naphthol-3,6-disulfonic solution	coupling of diazotized aniline with 8-amino-l-naphthol-3,6-disul-naphthol-3,6-disul-		467.4
D&C Red No.34 (Deep Maroon or Franchon Maroon;	monoazo; CI Pigment Red 63 (15880)	calcium salt of 4-(1-sulfo-2-naphthylazo)-3 hyxroxy-2-naphthoic	coupling of diazotized 2-naphthylamine-l-sulfonic acid with 3-		460.5

Table 2. contd......

Official FDA name; trade name(s)	Classification CI name and number	Chemical name	Manufacturing process	Structural Formula	Molecular weight
Lake Bordeaux B)		acid	hydroxy-2-naphthoic acid and conversion to the calcium salt		
D&C Red No. 36 (Flaming Red)	monoazo; CI Pigment Red 4 (12085)	1-(*O*-chloro-*p*-nitrophenyl-azo)-2-naphthol with2-naphthol	coupling of diazotized 2-chloro-1-nitroaniline		327.7
D&C Red No. 37 (RhodamineB-Stearate)	xanthene; CI Solvent Red 49 (45170B)	3-ethostearate of 9-*o*-carboxyphenyl-6-di-ethylamino-3-ethyl-imino-3-isoxanthene	same as for D&C Red No.19, except treatment of the base with stearic acid		727.0
D&C Violet No. 2 (D&C Blune No. 3 or Alizurol Purple SS)	anthraquinone;CI Solvent Violet 13 (60725)	1-hydroxy-1-*p*--toluino-anthraquinone	(a) condensation of quinizarin with *p*-toluidine or (b) condensation of 1-hydroxy-4-halogeno-anthraquinone with *p*-toluidine		
D&C Yellow No. 7 (fluorescein)	fluoran; CI Acid Yellow 73 (45350)	3,6-fluorandiol	condensation of resorcip not with phthalic anhydride in the presence of zinc chloride or sulfuric acid		332.3

Table 2. contd......

Official FDA name; trade name(s)	Classification CI name and number	Chemical name	Manufacturing process	Structural Formula	Molecular weight
D&C Yellow No. 8 (uranine)	xanthene; CI Acid Yellow 73 (45350)	disodium salt of 9-*o*-carboxyphenyl-6-	conversion of D&C Yellow No. 7 to the sodium salt	disodium salt of D&C Yellow No. 7	376.3
D & C Yellow No. 10 (Quinoline Yellow) WS, Quinoline Yellow)	quinoline; CI Acid Yellow 3 (47005)	disodium salt of disulfonic acid of D&C Yellow No. 11	sulfonation of D&C Yellow No. 11		
D&C Yellow No. 11 (Quinoline Yellow SS, Quinoline Yellow Spirit Soluble)	quinoline; CI Solvent Yellow 33 (47000)	2-(2-quinolyl)-1, 3-indandione	condensation of quinaldine with phthalic anhydride in the presence of zinc chloride		
D& C Lakes					

Table 3. Color Addtives Previously and Presently Subject to Certification by the FDA and Provisionally Listed for Use in Externally Applied Drugs and Cosmetics (Ext D&C Colors)

Official FDA name; trade name(s)	Classification CI name and number	Chemical name	Manufacturing process	Structural Formula	Molecular weight
Ext D&C Green No. 1 (Naphthol Green B)	nitroso; CI Acid Green 1 (10020)	ferric salt of 6-sosidum sulfo-1-isonitroso-1.2-naphthoquinone	treatment of I-naphthol-6-sulfonic acid with nitrous acid and conversion to the ferric sodium salt		878.5

Table 3. contd......

Official FDA name; trade name(s)	Classification CI name and number	Chemical name	Manufacturing process	Structural Formula	Molecular weight
Ext D&C Yellow No. 1 (Metanil Yellow)	monoazo; CI Acid Yellow 36 (13065)	monosodium salt of 4-*m*-sulfophenylazodiphenylamine	coupling of diazotized metanilic acid with diphenylamine in alcohol		375.4
Ext D&C Yellow No. 7 (Nphthol Yellow S)	nitro; CI Acid Yellow 1 (10316)	disodium salt of 2,4-diniro-1-naphthol-7-sulfonic acid	nitration of the di- or trisulfonic acids of 1-naphthol or the nitroso compound of the 2,7-disulfonic acid		358.2
Ext D&C Lakes					

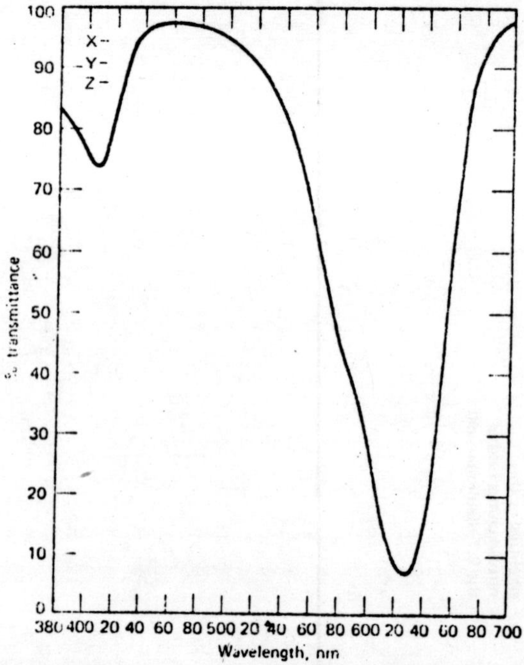

Fig. 2. Visible spectrum of FD&C Blue NO. 1 : Concentration, 8.0 ppm; cell thisckness, 1.0 cm; solvent, water; reference, water.

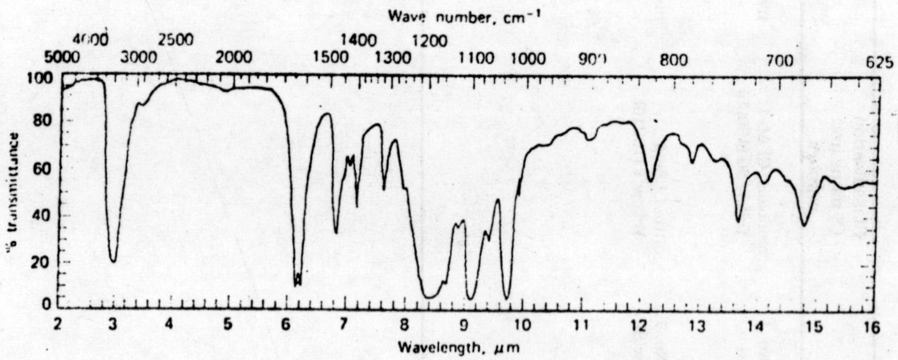

Fig. 3. Infrared spectrum of FD&C Blue No. 2, Courtesy Sadtler Reseach Laboratories, Inc.

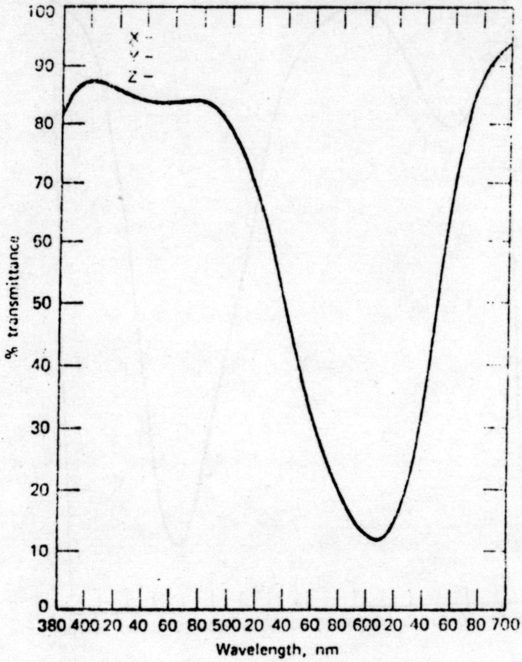

Fig. 4. Visible spectrum of FD&C Blue No. 2 : Concentration, 22.0 ppm; cell thisckness, 1.0 cm; solvent, water; reference, water.

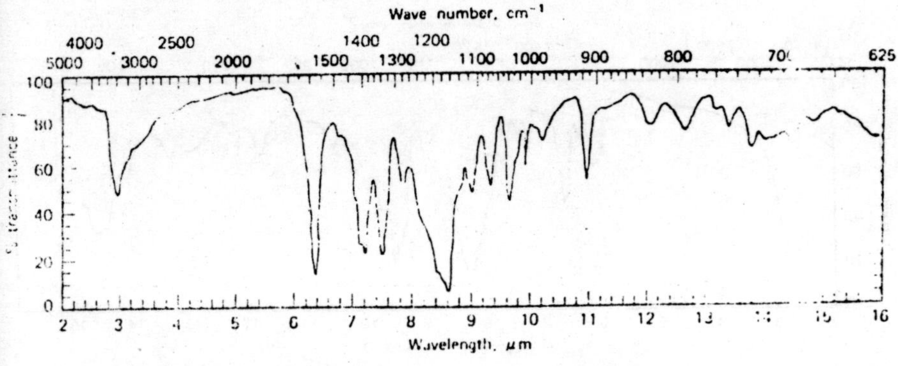

Fig. 5. Infrared spectrum of FD&C Blue No. 3, Courtesy Sadtler Reseach Laboratories, Inc.

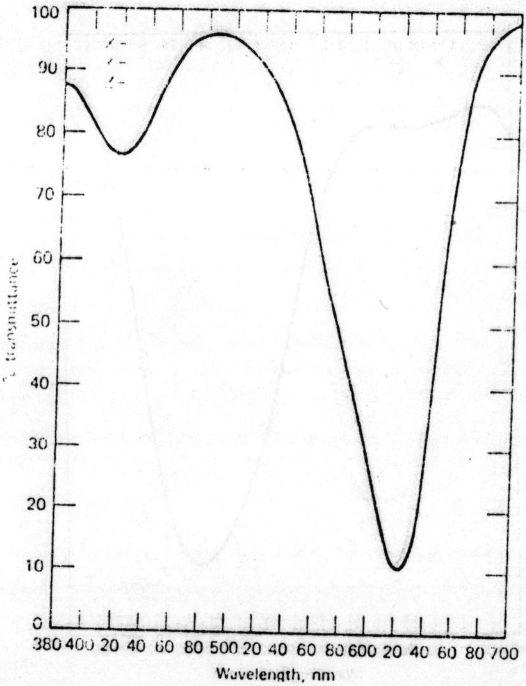

Fig. 6. Visible spectrum of FD&C Blue No. 3 : Concentration, 7.0 ppm; cell thickness, 1.0 cm; solvent, water; reference, water.

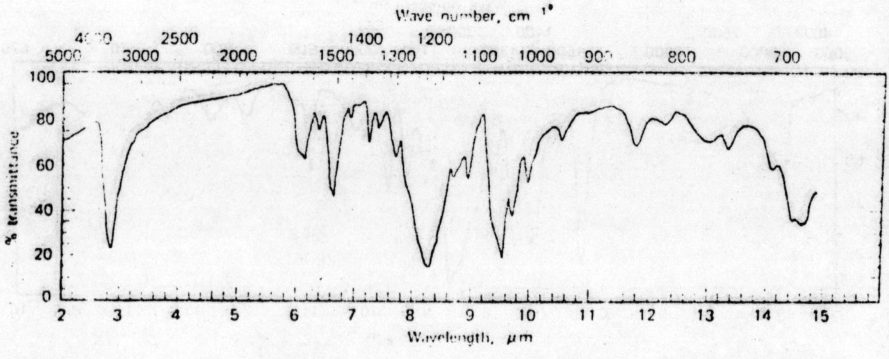

Fig. 7. Infrared spectrum of FD&C Blue No. 2, Courtesy Sadtler Reseach Laboratories, Inc.

Separation

When a single dye will not suffice to produce a desired shade, mixtures of dyes are frequently used. In many cases resolution of these mixtures is necessary in order to identify or quantify the individual colors. Solvent extraction is often used for this purpose. However, resolution of complicated mixtures usually requires more sophisticated techniques based on differential migration. Included in this category are chromatography, electrophoresis and counter recurrent distribution.

Chromatography

Chromatography is the most widely applied separation technique. Both ascending and descending paper chromatography are used quite effectively, as are thin-layer and centrifugal chromatography. Liquid column chromatography is favoured when quantitative data are needed.

Procedures

Paper Chromatography

Method for FD&C colours (3). Place 1 drop of fresh 1% aqueous sample solution on a 6×22 cm strip of Whatman No. 1 filter paper. The sample should be reasonably free of salt, sugar, starches etc. Allow it to dry. Suspend the strip in an airtight tank containing 0.5-1 cm of 2:3 waterethylene glycol monomethyl ether acetate (methyl Cellosolve acetate). Alternatively, 1:4 water-methyl Cellosolve acetate can be used. Develop 2-3 hr.

I all FD&C colors are present, ten colored zones may be observed. From the bottom up, the zones are as follows:

1. FD&C Yellow No. 5
2. FD&C Red No. 2
3. FD&C Blue No. 2
4. FD&C Red No. 1 plus FD&C Red No. 4
5. FD&C Yellow No. 6
6. FD&C Blue No.1 plus FD&C Green No. 2 plus FD&C Green No. 3
7. FD&C Yellow No. 1
8. FD&C Violet No. 1 plus FD&C Green No. 1
9. FD&C Orange No. 1
10. FD&C Red No. 3

FD&C Red No. 1, Green No. 2, Yellow No. 1, Green No. 1, and Orange No. 1 are no longer certifiable as FD&C colors.

Method for Anthraquinone Dyes (4). Spot a dimethylformamide solution of the sample on 8×8 in. Whatman No. 1 filter paper. Uniformaly im-

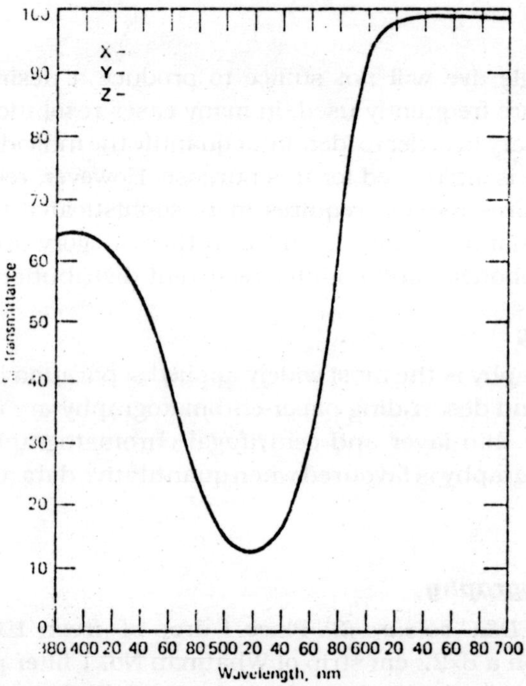

Fig. 8. Visible spectrum of FD&C Blue No. 2 : Concentration, 24.0 ppm; cell thickness, 1.0 cm; solvent, water; reference, water.

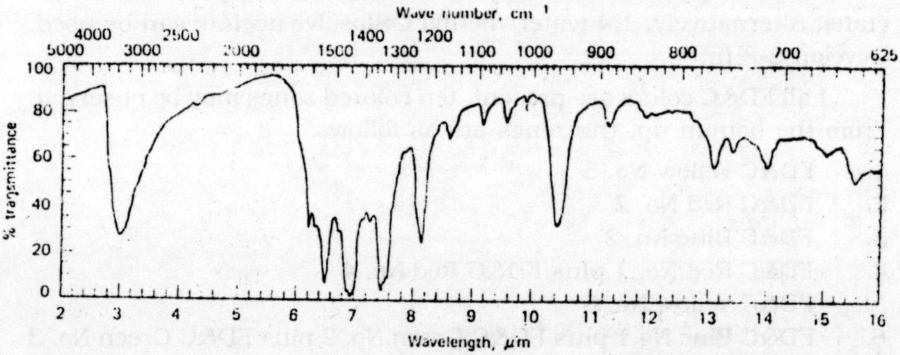

Fig. 9. Infrared spectrum of FD&C Blue No. 3, Courtesy Sadtler Reseach Laboratories, Inc.

pregnate the paper with 1:99 refined soybean oil-ethyl ether by rapidly spraying it from top to bottom in horizontal strips. Elute the sheet in a 12 × 25 × 25 cm glass tank with 4:1 methyl Cellosolve-water until the solvent front approaches the top of the paper (about 21/2 hr). Compare vs standards simultaneously prepared.

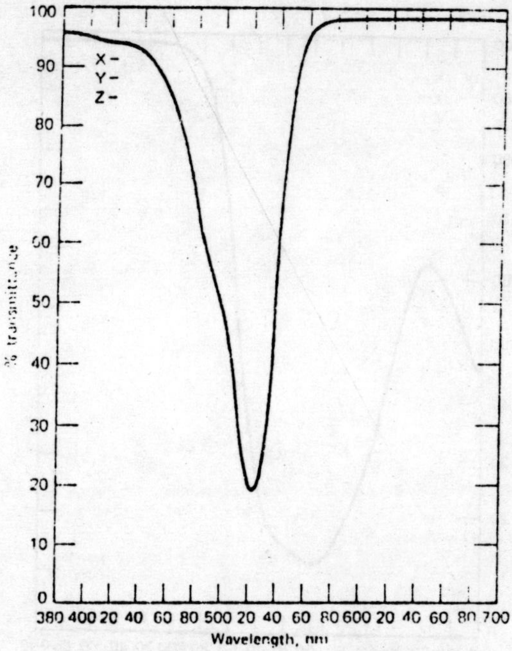

Fig. 10. Visible spectrum of FD&C Red No. 3 : Concentration, 7.5 ppm; cell thisckness, 1.0 cm; solvent, water; reference, water.

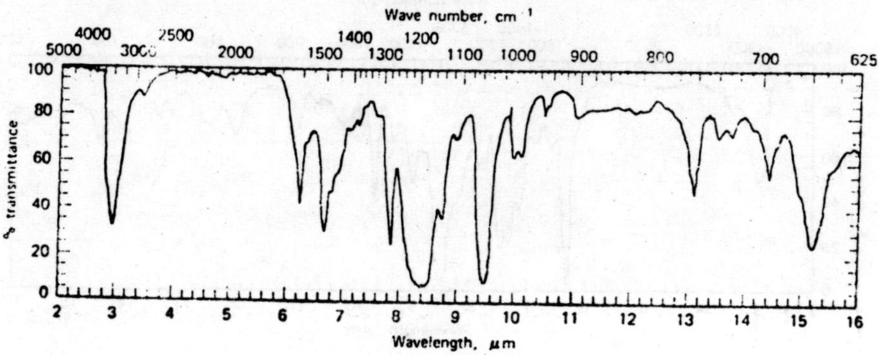

Fig. 11. Infrared spectrum of FD&C Red No. 4, Courtesy Sadtler Reseach Laboratories, Inc.

Color	R_f *approx.*
D&C Green NO. 5	0.98

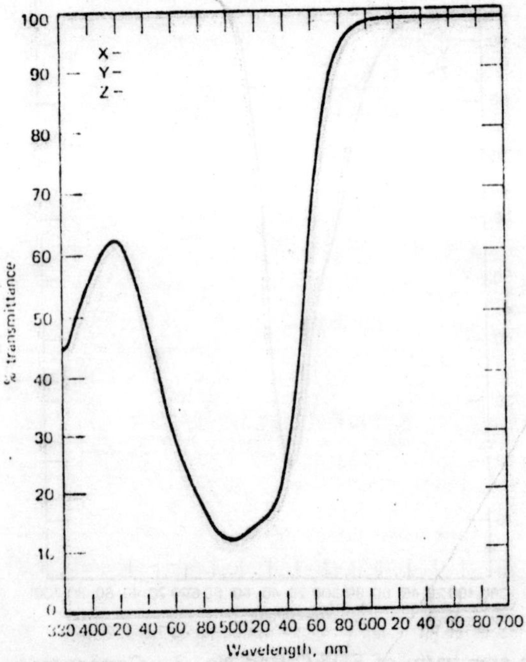

Fig. 12. Visible spectrum of FD&C Red No. 4 : Concentration, 20.0 ppm; cell thisckness, 1.0 cm; solvent, water; reference, water.

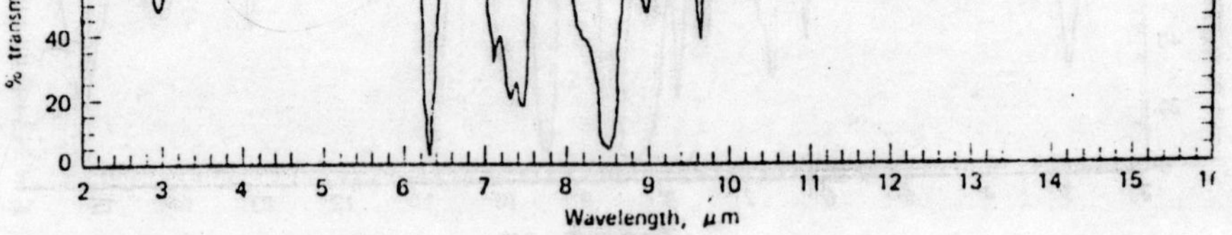

Fig. 13. Infrared spectrum of FD&C Voilet No. 1, Courtesy Sadtler Reseach Laboratories, Inc.

"monosulfonated" D&C Green No. 5	0.86
D&C Green No. 6	0.14
Ext D&C Violet No. 2	0.90
D&C Violet No. 2	0.24

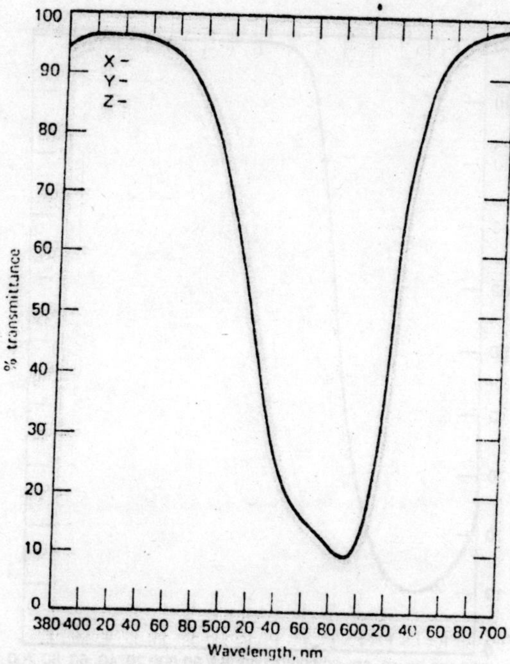

Fig. 14. Visible spectrum of FD&C Violet No. 1 : Concentration, 7.3 ppm; cell thickness, 1.0 cm; solvent, water; reference, water.

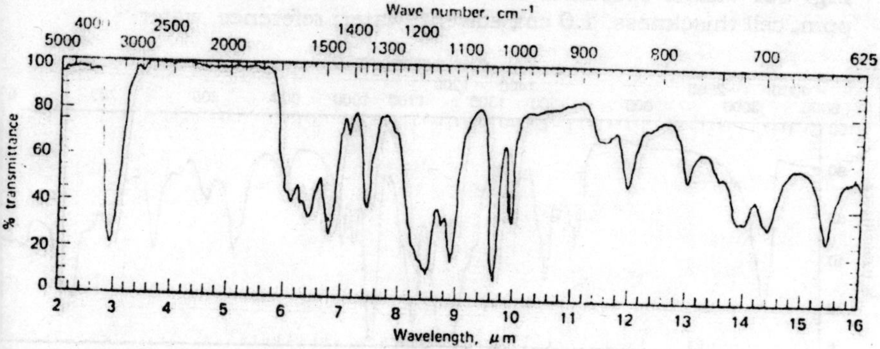

Fig. 15. Infrared spectrum of FD&C Yellow No. 5, Courtesy Sadtler Reseach Laboratories, Inc.

Liquid Chromatography

General Method for FD&C Colors (3). Prepare 30%, 25% and 20% solutions of sodium chloride.

To prepare solutions containing both ethyl alcohol and sodium chloride, mix the required reagents with water. For example, to prepare 20% ethyl alcohol plus 15% sodium chloride, mix 12 parts of 95% ethanol, 30 parts of 30% sodium chloride solution and 18 parts of water.

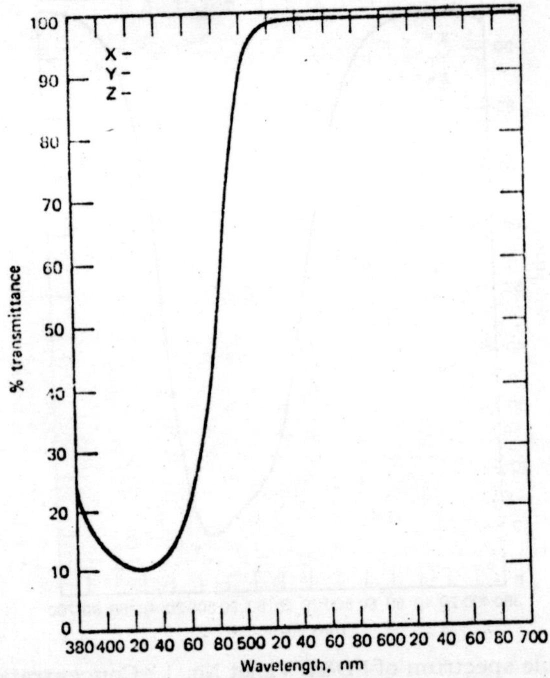

Fig. 16. Visible spectrum of FD&C Yellow No. 5 : Concentration, 20.0 ppm; cell thisckness, 1.0 cm; solvent, water; reference, water.

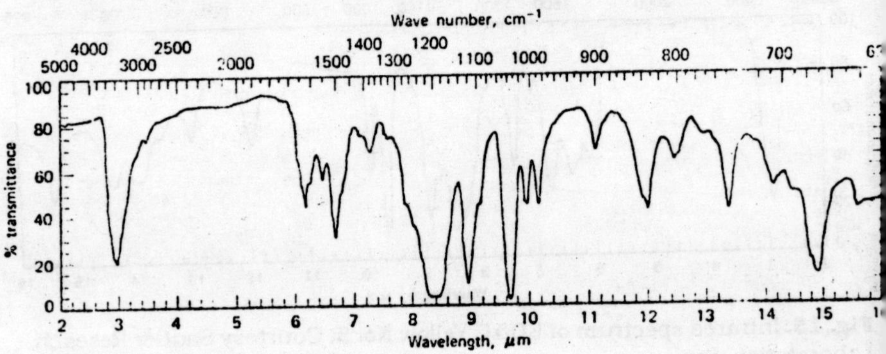

Fig. 17. **Infrared spectrum of FD&C Yellow No. 6, Courtesy Sadtler Reseach Laboratories, Inc.**

Slurry Solka-Floe BW-40 (manufactured by Grefco Inc., Dicalite Division, New York in water and pour the amount indicated into a 2.5 cm ID glass column. allow it to stand for 12 hr. Treat 0.5 of sample as directed in Table 6.

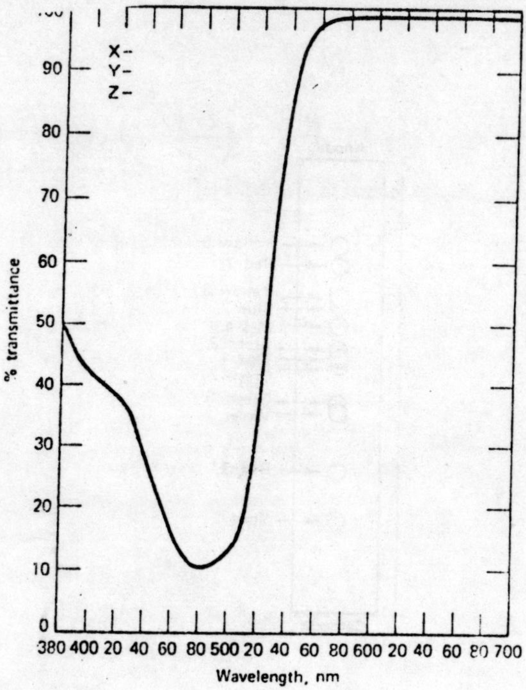

Fig. 18. Visible spectrum of FD&C Yellow No. 6 : Concentration, 8.0 ppm; cell thisckness, 1.0 cm; solvent, water; reference, water.

Method for Triphenylmethane Colors (5)

Slurry 80-200 mesh adsorption alumina (Fisher Scientific) in water and pack it into15.0 cm ´1.5 cm ID column to a height of 10 cm. Wash it with water until the eluate is clear.

Prepare an aqueous sample solution containing about 0.5 mg of each color. Adjust the solution to about 0.1 *N* with dilute acetic acid and pass it through the column. Wash the column with 50 l of water, then develop with 350 ml of 1.5% aqueous pyridine. The basic solvent alters the color of some triphenylmethane dyes. To observe the position of the colors after development pass 100 ml of water through the column followed by 100 ml of 1:100 acetic acid. The dyes then regain the original color.

Colors appear on the column as follows: FD&C Green No. 3, 20-28mm; FD&C Green No. 2, 22-34 mm; FD&C Violet No. 1,36-50mm;

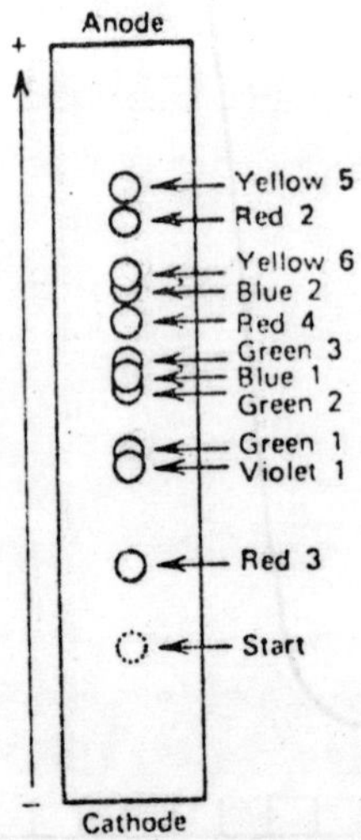

Fig. 19. Order of separation of dyes during electrophoresis.

FD&C Green No. 1, 55-75 mm; FD&C Blue No. 1, 56-72 mm (FD&C Green Nos. 1 and 2 are no longer certifiable).

Method for FD&C Red No. 2 and FD&C Yellow No. 5(6). Slurry alumina (Fisher Scientific adsorption alumina 80-200 mesh) in water and pack it into a 15 cm × 1.5cm ID column to a height of 7.5 cm. wash the column with water until the eluate is clear. Activate the column with 1:100 hydrochloric acid.

Dissolve a 0.010-g sample in 20 ml of 1:100 hydrochloric acid and pass it through the column. Wash the column with 100 ml of water. Colors are fixed on the top of the column as lakes. Elute FD&C Yellow No. 5 with 200-300 ml of 3.0% sodium acetate solution. Elute FD&C Red No. 2 with 100-200 ml of 0.4% sodium hydroxide.

Adjust the eluate fractions to pH 6.0 with hydrochloric acid and examine them spectrophotometrically.

Electrophoresis

The following method is given for separation of FD&C colors by electrophoresis.

Procedure

Thoroughly wet a cellulose acetate strip with a buffer solution consisting of equal parts of 0.1.1 sodium acetate and isopropyl alcohol adjusted to pH 4.6 with acetic acid. Blot between absorbent paper and spot a solution of the dye mixture on the strip. Separate by electrophoresis in the buffer solution using an applied voltage of 270V. Fading and oxidizing of riphenylmethane dyes can be minimized by conducting the separation in the dark under an inert atmsophere. See Figure 19: for order os' separation.

Table 6. General Method for FD&C Colors

Pass the following solutions through the columns in the order given, allowing as little mixing as possible between successive solutions	Collect the following bands as they separate and emerge from the tubes. Treat as indicated	Approx ml.
Column No. 1-50 g of Celluose		
1. 50 ml of 5% ethanol plus 15% sodium chloride (prewash)	water plus prewash (discard)	350
2. 0.5 g of sample dissolved in 50 ml of 20% sodium chloride		
3. 250 ml of 5% ethanol plus 1% sodium chloride	FD & C Green No. 3 plus FD&C Green No. 2[a] plus FD&C Blue No. 1	45
	tailing plus ethanol sodium plus ethanol solution (discard)	16
	FD&C Yellow No. 1[a] plus FD&C Yellow No. 5	55
	tailing plus ethanol solution (discard)	22
4. 250 ml of 0.5% sodium chloride	FD&C Blue No.2 plus FD&C Red No. 2 (separate on column No. 4)	132
	dilute tailing (discard)	55

5. sufficient water to remove remaining colors	remaining colors	112

Column No. 2 - 40 g of Cellulose

1. 50 ml of 20%ethanol plus 15% sodium chloride (prewash)	water plus prewash (discard)	394
2. solution of remaining colors from column No. 1 (in 112 ml) adjusted to 20% sodium chloride		
3. 250 ml of 20% ethanol plus 15% sodium chloride	FD&C Green No. 1[a] plus FD&C Violet No.1	96
	slight tailing of FD&C Violet No. 1 plus trace of FD&C Orange No. [a] (discard)	62
	FD&C Orange No. 1[a]	
4. 50 ml of 20% sodium chloride	ethanol solution (discard)	140
5. sufficient water to remove remaining colours	remaining colors	42

Column No. 3-30g of Cellulose

1. 50 ml of 20% sodium chloride (prewash)	water plus prewash (dicard)	
2. solution of remaining colors fom Column No.2 (in 42 ml) adjusted to 20% sodium chloride		
3. 200 ml of 1% sodium chloride plus 1% ammonium chloride	FD&C Red No. 4 (in basic form) ammonical solution (discard)	75

4. 50 ml of 20% sodium chloride plus 1% acetic acid	
5. 200 ml of 0.0625% sodium chloride	FD&C Red No. 1[a]
6. 50 l of water plus 1-2 drops of concentrated ammonium hydroxide	salt solution (discard)
7. sufficient water to remove the remaining color	FD&C Red No. 3

Column No. 4-30 g of Cellulose

1. 50 ml of 20% sodium chloride (prewash)	water plus prewash (discard)
2. solution of FD&C Blue No. 2 and FD&C Red No. 2 adjusted to 20% sodium chloride and from which the ethanol has been removed[6]	
3. 200 ml of 1% sodium chloride plus 1% amonium hydroxide	FD&C Red No. 2 (in bacis form) salt solution (discard)
4. sufficient water to remove remaining color	FD&C Blue No. 2

[a] These dyes are no longer certfiable as FD&C colors

[b] Add sufficient sodium chloride to the fraction to bring the concentration to 20%. Extract with an equal volume of peroxide-free ethyl ether. If the dye tends to pass it to the ether, add 0.5 ml of 10%, sodium hydroxide for each 100 ml of dye solution. Neutralise the acqueous phase, if necessary, and remove the ether by passing air through it.

Solvent Extraction

The method given below separates D&C Red No. 7 from D&C Red No. 10 by solvent extraction. This procedure is also applicable when D&C Red No. 6 is substituted for No. 7 and when D&C Red Nos. 11, 12, or 13 are present in place of D&C Red No. 10.

Procedure

Transfer a 0.25-g sample to a 250-ml Erlenmeyer flask. Add 100 ml of methyl Cellosolve and 5 ml of hydrocloric acid. Connect the flask to an air condenser and gently reflux the mix until it is in solution. Buffer the solution with 10 g of sodium bitartrate dissolved in 75 ml of boiling water and titrate with 0.1 *N* titanous chloride solution. Record the results as the combined titer for the two dyes, in ml.

Dissolve a second 0.25-g sample in 100 ml of methyl Cellosolve and transfer the solution to a 500-ml separatory funnel. Transfer any residual dyes with 10-ml portions of ethyl ether. Bring the ether volume to 150 ml, and add 250 ml of 10% sodium chloride solution. Withdraw the lower layer and extract it with a second 75-ml portion of ethyl ether. Withdraw and discard the lower layer. Combine the ether extracts and wash them with 30-ml portions of water until the washings are colorless; discard the washings. Transfer the ether layer to a 250-ml Eriecomeyer flask with two 10-ml portions of ethyl ether. Evaporate the solution to dryness, add 100 ml of methyl Cellosolve, and heat into solution. Buffer with 10g of sodium bitartrate in 75 ml of boiling water, heat to boiling, and titrate with 0.1 N titanous chloride solution. Calculate as D&C Red No. 10.

Subtract the ml. of titer for the D&C Red No. 10 from the ml of titer for the two dyes and calculate the difference as D&C Red No. 7.

Assay Methods

The pure dye content of certifiable colors is specified by the FDA as a means of controlling purity. The most widely used assay methods are titanous chloride titration and visible spectrometry. Spectrometry has the advantages of speed, simplicity, and specificity, and is rapidly supplanting titration with titanous chloride wherever possible.

Frequently the strength the consumer is interested in is the effective dye strength - the apparent strength of the dye when formulated into the finished product. This strength is generally some function of physical properties such as particle size of crystal form and does not always bear a direct relationship to the assay value.

Titration with Titanous Chloride

The method given below has several variations, depending on the nature of the color being tested. The appropriate variation for specific colors is indicated in Table 5. Table 7 gives the milliequivalent weight of many colors and the volume of 0.1*N* titanous chloride (in ml) needed for titration of 1g.

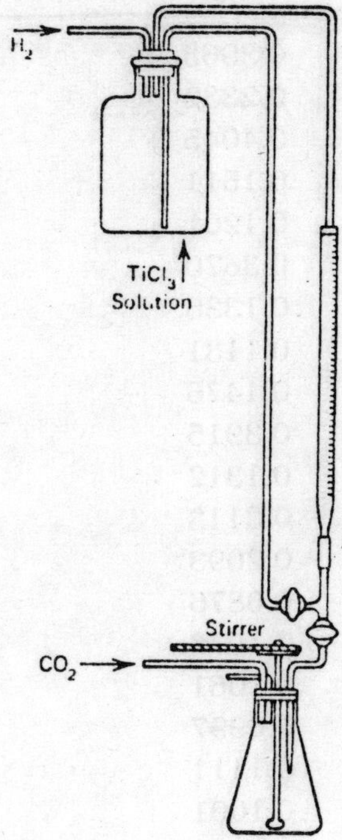

Fig. 20. Titanous chloride titration apparatus.

Procedure

Method A. Prepare a 1% aqueous sample solution. Pipet an amount equivalent to about 20 ml of 0.1 *N* titanous chloride solution into a 500-ml wide-mouth Erlenmeyer flask. Add 15 g of sodium citrate, and adjust the volume to 150-200 ml. with water. Using the apparatus shown in Figure 20 blanket the sample with nitrogen or carbon dioxide and, while boiling, titrate to the disappearance of color with standardized 0.1 *N* titanous chloride solution. If the end point is not sharp, add an excess of titanous chloride (not more than 0.3 ml of 0.1 *N* solution), and back titrate standardized 0.1 *N* ferrous ammonium sulfate solution.

Table 7. $TiCl_3$ Titration Factors

Color	Milliequivalent weight	ml of .1 *N* $TiCl_3$/g of color
FD&C Blue No. 1	0.3965	25.2
FD&C Blue No. 2	0.2332	42.9
FD&C Blue No. 3	0.4045	24.7
FD&C Red No. 2	0.1511	66.2
FD&C Red No. 4	0.1201	83.3
FD&C Violet No. 1	0.3670	27.3
FD&C Yellow No. 5	0.1336	74.9
FD&C Yellow No. 6	0.1131	88.4
Orange B	0.1476	67.8
D&C Blue No. 4	0.3915	25.5
D&C Blue No. 6	0.1312	76.3
D&C Green No. 5	0.3113	32.1
D&C Green No. 6	0.2093	47.8
D&C Orange No. 4	0.0876	114.2
D&C Red No. 6	0.1076	92.9
D&C Red No. 7	0.1061	94.2
D&C Red No. 8	0.0997	100.3
D&C Red No. 9	0.1111	90.0
D&C Red No. 10	0.1001	99.9
D&C Red No. 11	0.0994	100.6
D&C Red No. 12	0.1115	89.7
D&C Red No. 13	0.1053	95.0
D&C Red No. 17	0.0441	227.0
D&C Red No. 19	0.2395	41.8
D&C Red No. 30	0.1967	50.8
D&C Red No. 31	0.0778	128.5
D&C Red No. 33	0.1169	86.9
D&C Red No. 34	0.1151	86.9
D&C Red No. 36	0.0328	305.1
D&C Red No. 37	0.3633	27.5
D&C Yellow No. 7	0.1662	60.2
D&C Yellow No. 8	0.1882	53.2
Ext D&C Green No. 1	0.0732	136.6
Ext D&C Yellow No. 1	0.0939	106.6
Ext D&C Yellow No. 7	0.2909	335.0

Table 8. Absorptivity Factors (9)

	Solvent system	Absorption maximum, mm^2	Absorptivity liter $g\text{-}cm^6$
FD&C Blue No. 1	water	630	164
FD&C Blue No. 2	water	610	47.8
FD&C Green No. 3	water	625	156
FD&C Red No. 2	water	522	13.6
FD&C Red No. 3	water	527	110
FD&C Red No. 4	water	502	54.0
FD&C Violet No. 1	water	545	117
FD&C Violet No. 1	1:1 tehanol-water	595	154
FD&C Yellow No. 5	water	428	53
FD&C Yellow No. 6	water	484	55
Citrus Red No. 2	chloroform	515	70
Orange B	water	437	35.5
D&C Blue No. 4	water	630	170
D&C Blue No. 6	chloroform	603	79
D&C Green No. 5	water	610	21.3
D&C Green No. 6	chloroform	648	39.2
D&C Green No. 8	water $(OH)^-$	454	51
D&C Orange No. 4	water	484	65.3
D&C Orane No. 5	water (OH)–	503	163
D&C Orange No. 10	water $(OH)^-$	510	122
D&C Orange No. 17	chloroform	480	77
D&C Red No. 6	1:1 ethanol-water	511	61.5
D&C Red No. 7	1:1 ethanol-water	516	157.2
D&C Red No. 8	1:1 ethanol-water	486	52.2
D&C Red No. 9	1:1 ethanol-water	486	47
D&C Red No. 10	1:1 ethanol-water	494	68.5
D&C Red No. 11	1:1 ethanol-water	494	69
D&C Red No. 12	1:1 ethanol-water	494	59
D&C Red No. 13	1:1 ethanol-water	494	65.1
D&C Red No. 17	chloroform	514	94
D&C Red No. 19	water	554	236
D&C Red No. 21	water $(OH)^-$	518	150
D&C Red No. 22	water	518	140
D&C Red No. 27	water $(OH)^-$	537	129
D&C Red No. 28	water	537	122

D&C Red No. 30	chloroform	537	44
D&C Red No. 31	1:1 ethaqnol-water	518	80
D&C Red No. 33	water	530	66.2
D&C Red No. 34	1:1 ethanol-water	526	65.5
D&C Red No. 36	chloroform	490	84
D&C Red No. 37	water	545	154
D&C Violet No. 2	chloroform	588	36.3
D&C Yellow No. 7	water $(OH)^-$	489	247
D&C Yellow No. 8	water	489	228
D&C Yellow No. 10	water	413	92
D&C Yellow No. 11	chloroform	420	135
Ext. D&C Green No. 1	water	720	21.7
Ext. D&C Yellow No. 1	water	436	64
Ext. D&C Yellow No. 7	water	430	49

a. All neutral water systems are buffered with 0.01 N ammonium acetate
b. The absorption maximum and the absorptivity of a compound vary slightly depending upon the sample and the spectrophotometer used to determine them.Consequently the above data should be regarded as approximations only.

METHOD B: Prepare a 0.5% ethanolic sample solution. Proceed as in Method A substituting 50% ethanol for water.

METHOD C. Proceed as in Method A substituting 15g of sodium acid tartrate for sodium citrate.

METHOD D. Proceed as in Method C using about 10 mg of Light Green SF Yellowish, CI No. 42095 (formerly FD&C Green No. 2) as indicator. Make a blank determination and correct accordingly.

METHOD E. Prepare a 0.5% ethanolic sample solution. Proceed as in Method D substituting 50% ethanol for water.

Method F. Dissolve 0.2g of sample in 5 ml of sulfuric acid in a wide-mouth Erlenmeyer flask. Add 100 ml of ethanol. Heat and stir until all the dye is in solution. Dissolve 20g of sodium acid tartrate in 100 ml of boiling water, then add 20 ml of 30% sodium hydroxide solution. Stirring rapidly, add this solution to the sample solution. Using the apparatus shown in Figure 20, blanket the sample with nitrogen or carbon dioxide and titrate with standardized 0.1 *N* titanous chloride.

METHOD G. Place a sample equivalent to about 20 ml of 0.1 *N* titanous chloride in a 50-ml beaker. Pour 2 ml of fuming sulfuric acid down the side of the beaker. Mix; place on a steam bath for 30 min.

Pour the solution into a 500-ml wide-mouth Erlenmeyer flask containing 100g of ice. Add ice to the beaker and wash any remaining colour into the flask. Add 50 ml of ethanol and 20 g of sodium acid tartrate to the flask. Heat and titrate as in Method A.

Spectrophotometric Method

Generally, sample solutions are prepared in the solvent and absorbance is measured at the wavelength specified.

Other Assay Methods

Pure dye is determined gravimetrically and by elemental analysis in the few cases where spectrometry and titration are not applicable.

Procedures

Gravimetric Determination. *Method A*, Weight a 0.5-g sample and transfer it to a 400-ml beaker. Add 100 ml of ater. Heat to boiling. Add 25 ml of 1:49 hydrochloric acid and boil again. Wash down the sides of the beaker with distilled water and then cover. Keep the beaker on a steam bath for several hours or overnight. Cool to room temperature and transfer the precipitate to a tared Gooch crucible with 1:99 hydrochloric acid and wash with two 15-ml portions of water. Dry the crucible 3 hr at 135°C. Cool in a desiccator and weigh.

$$\%\text{ pure dye} = \frac{W(f)\,100}{w}$$

where W = weight of precipitate, in g
w = sample weight, in g
f = gravimetric conversion factors.
Several are listed below:

	f
FD&C Red No. 3 (disodium salt, monohydrate)	1.074
D&C Red No. 22 (disodium salt)	1.068
D&C Red No. 28 (disodium salt)	1.056

Method B. Transfer 0.500 g of a sample to a 400-ml beaker; add 50 ml of 0.1*N* sodium hydroxide. Swirl to dissolve. Add 50 ml of water and proceed as directed in Method A beginning with "Heat to boiling." No conversion factor is required since the colors for which this method is specified are acids.

Assay through Organic Sulfur Content: Weight 0.2 g of sample into a Parr peroxide bomb. Mix with about 14 g of sodium peroxide, 1 g of sugar, and 0.1 g of potassium chlorate, and ignite the bomb. Place the opened bomb in a beaker, cover with water, and heat at 50-60°C until the reaction ceases. Rinse the bomb into the beaker with water. Cool the solution and neutralize it with concentrated hydrochloric acid; then add 5 ml excess. Filter the solution into a second beaker, washing the filter paper with water. Heat the filtrate to boiling and while boiling add 25 ml of 10% barium chloride solution. Digest on a steam bath for 1-2 hr or allow the sample to stand in a warm place overnight. Filter through a tared Gooch crucible and wash the precipitate with water until it is chloride-free. Dry at 100°C for 20 min, then at 700°C for 20 min.

$$\% \text{ total sulfur} = \frac{W\,(0.1373)\,(100)}{w}$$

$$\% \text{ organic sulfur} = \% \text{ total sulfur} = \% \text{ inorganic sulfur}$$

$$\% \text{ pure dye} = \frac{(\% \text{ organic sulfur})\,(100)}{\text{theoretical } \% \text{ sulfur}}$$

where W = weight of barium sulfate precipitatem in g
w = sample weight, in g

Assay Through organic nitrogen content. *For Colors Requiring Reduction Prior to Digestion.* Weigh a quantity of sample containing 2 mg of nitrogen and transfer it to a 30-ml Kjedahl flask. Add 0.5 ml of a 9:1 mixture of 50% (w/v) hydriodic acid and 50% (w/v) hypophosphorous acid. Reflux 5-10 min turing the flask occasionally to ensure solution and reduction. Distill off most of the liquid. Remove the flask from the heater, cool, add 5 ml of 1:1 sulfuric acid, and evaporate to fumes. If considerable iodine remains, add 1-2 of water and again evaporate to fumes. Remove the flask from the heater, cool, and wash down the sides with 0.5 ml of water. Add 0.6 g of anyhydrous sodium sulfate and 0.5 ml of 20% mercuric acetate solution. Place on a heater and digest until the solution clears, then heat 1 hr more. If the dye contains ring nitrogen, heat for 2.5 hr after clearing and add more sulfuric acid if needed. Remove the flask, cool, and add 10-12 ml of water to dissolve the salts.

Transfer the sample to a micro-Kjedahl distilling apparatus using about 10 ml of water. set the electric controller of the steam generator to distill 20 ml in about 10 min. Add 5-6 ml of 50% sodium hydroxide solution and 3 ml of 21% sodium thiosulfate solution. Prepare an indicator solution by dissolving first 0.3g of methyl red in 60 ml of ethanol and diluting with water to 100 ml, then 0.2 g of methylene blue in 100 ml of 50% ethanol, and mixing the two solutions. Add 3 drops of the indicator solution to a 50-ml Erlenmeyer flask containing 5 ml of 2% boric acid solution. Position the flask so that the outlet from the condenser dips below the level of the liquid and steam distills for 5 min. Lower the receiving flask so that the condenser outlet is above the liquid in the flask and distilkl for 1-2 min to flush the condenser tube.

Titrate the solution in the receiving flask with standardized 0.02 *N* hydrochloric acid. Make a blank determination.

$$\% \text{ nitrogen} = \frac{(A - B)(0.014)(100)}{w}$$

where A = volume of titrant used for sample, in ml
B = volume of titrant used for blank, in ml
N = normality of titrant
w = sample weight, in g

$$\% \text{ pure dye} = \frac{\% \text{ nitrogen } (100)}{\text{theoretical } \% \text{ nitrogen}}$$

For Colors That Do Not Require Reduction Prior to Digestion. Weight and transfer a sample as descried above. Add 5 ml of 1:1 sulfuric acid and heat until thoroughly charred. Cool, then add 0.6 g of sodium sulfate and 0.5 ml of 20% mercuric acetate solution. Wash down the side of the flask with a minimum amount of water and proceed as described above starting with "Place on a heater and digest..."

Determination of Impurities

Insoluble Matter

The amount of insoluble matter in a colorant reflects the purity of the product and the practical problems the consumer will encounter. The solvent used to determine insolubles vary with individual colors; they are specified in Table 5.

Procedures

WATER-INSOLUBLE MATTER. Dissolve a 2-g sample in 200 l of hot water (about 90°C). Cool to room temperature. filter through a washed and tared Gooch crucible fitted with glass fiber filter paper. Wash the beaker and crucible with water until the filtrate is colorless. Dry to constant weight at 135°C.

TOLUENE-INSOLUBLE MATTER. *Method A.* Dissolve a 1-g sample in 150 ml of toluene. Stir and heat to boiling. Filter the hot solution through a washed and tared Gooch crucible fitted with glass fiber filter paper. Wash the beaker and crucible with 10-ml portions of toluene until the filtrate is colorless. Dry to constant weight at 100-105°C.

Method B. Fit a Gooch crucible with an asbestos mat and a cotton pad, then wash and tare it. Weigh 1 g of the sample into the crucible, placing the pad on top of the sample. Support the crucible in a Soxhlet extraction apparatus so that the bottom of the crucible is slightly above the top of the siphon tube. Extract with toluene until no more color is removed. Dry to a constant weight at 100-105°C. Cool in a desiccator and weigh.

ETHANOL-INSOLUBLE MATTER. Proceed as described in Method B above, substituting ethanol for toluene.

Xylene-insoluble matter. Proceed as described in Method B, substituting xylene for toluene.

ALKALINE-INSOLUBLE MATTER. Proceed as described for water-insoluble matter, substituting 1% sodium hydroxide solution or 1:14 ammonium hydroxide for water.

BENZENE-INSOLUBE MATTER. Proceed as descried in Method A, substituting benzene for toluene.

Extractables

Extraction with various solvents is a means of detecting impurities. These procedures, described below, are largerly empirical; their importance has greatly diminished with increased knowledge of the color additives and with the advent of more sophisticated analytical techniques such as chromatography.

Isopropyl Ether Extracts. Isopropyl ether tends to form highly explosive peroxide, especially when anhydrous. The addition of water or appropriate reducing agents will lessen the possibility of peroxide formation.

Procedures

For all the following methods, pretreat the isopropyl ether by washing 1 liter with two 100-ml portions of 0.5*N* sodium hydroxide followed by three 100-ml portions of water.

SOXHLET EXTRACTION METHOD. Extract a 5-g sample in a Soxhlet extractor for 2 hr with the treated isopropyl ether. Transfer the extract to a tared dish and allow to evaporate. Dry to constant weight over sulfuric acid. To determine a blank, extract the original sample for 2 hr more.

EXTRACTION WITH SEPARATION FUNNELS. *Neutral Ether Extracts.* Place 200 ml of a 5% aqueous sample solution in a separatory funnel and extract with two 100-ml portions of the washed isopropyl ether; shake for 1 min during each extraction. Decant the ether extracts into a second separatory funnel and wash them colorfree with 20-ml portions of water. Reserve the aqueous layer for the determination of alkaline ether extracts. Evaporate the washed ether extracts to dryness in a tared weighing dish on a steam bath; do not boil. Dry to constant weight in a desiccator.

Alkaine Ether Extracts. To the reserved aqueous layer add 2 ml of 10% sodium hydroxide solution and extract as described above. Wash the combined extracts colorfree with 0.1 *N* sodium hydroxide instead of water. Reserve the aqueous layer for the determinationof acid ether extracts. Dry and weight.

Acid Ether Extracts. To the reserved aqueous layer add 3 ml of 1:1 hydrochloric acid and extract as previously described. Wash the combined extracts colorfree with 1:199 hydochloric acid instead of water. Dry and weigh.

CONTINUOUS EXTRACTOR METHOD. Neutral Ether Extracts. Dissolve a 5-g sample in water and place it in a 250-ml continuous extractor. Extract for 5 hr with 100-ml of treated isopropyl ether. Transfer the extract to a separatory funnel, wash it colorfree, evaporate, and dry to constant weiht, as described in the previous method.

Alkaline Ether Extracts. To the aqueous solution in the extractor add 2 ml of 10% sodium hydroxide solution and extract as before. Wash the extract with 0.1 *N* sodium hydroxide instead of water.

Acid Ether Extracts. To the aqueous solution in the extractor add 3 ml of 1:1 hydrochloric acid and extract as before Wash the extract with 1:199 hydrochloric acid instead of water.

Extracts from Alkaline Solution. Dissolve a 5-g sample in 0.5 *N* sodium hydroxide. Place in a continuous extractor and proceed as described above under alkaline ether extracts.

Extraction with Other Solvents. The following procedures are given for the determination of impurities extractable with ethanol and chloroform.

Procedures

ETHANOLIC HYDROCHLORIC ACID EXTRACTS. Weight a 2-g sample into a 100-ml volumetric flask. Add 50 ml of ethanol and 0.1 ml of concentrated hydrochloric acid and shake for 2 min. Dilute to volume with ethanol, mix and filter. Evaporate 50 ml of filtrate in a tared dish on a steam bath. Dry at 98-100°C, and weigh.

CHLOROFORM EXTRACTS. Extract a 5-g sample with chloroform in a Soxhlet extractor for 16 hr. Transfer the extract to a separatory funnel and wash nearly with 0.05 *N sodium hydroxide, then add 0.002* N hydrochloric acid until the indicator is decolorised. Add 25 ml of ethanol and about 0.2 g of tetrahydroxyquinone indicator (THQ prepared sulfate indicator, Betz Laboratories, Inc., Trevase, Pa.) Titrate with 0.03 *N* barium chloride solution to a red end point. Make a blank determination.

$$\% \text{ sodium sulfate} = \frac{(A - B)(N)(0.07102)(195)(100)}{(w)(25)}$$

where *A* = volume of barium chloride solution required for sample, in ml

B = volume of barium chloride solution r equired for blank, in ml

N = normality of barium chloride solution

w = sample weight, in g

AOAC Method for Basic Dyes (14). Dissolve a 2-g sample and treat it with carbon as described in the AOAC method for sodium chloride in basic dyes. Place 25 ml of the filtrate obtained in a 125-ml Erlenmeyer flask, and continue as directed above fro sodium sulfate in acid dyes.

$$\% \text{ sodium sulfate} = \frac{(A - B)(N)(0.07102)(200)(100)}{(w)(25)}$$

General Gravimetric Method. Weight 5g of sample, dissolve it in 100 ml of warm water, and transfer to a 250-ml volumetric flask. Add 35 g of sulfate-free sodium chloride, stopper the flask, and let it stand for 1 hr. Swirl at frequent intervals. Dilute to volume with saturated sodium chloride solution and filter through dry filter paper. Precipitate the sulfate with barium chloride; filter, dry, and weigh the precipitate.

SODIUM ACETATE (16). Prepare silver toluene sulfonate by dissolving silver oxide or carbonate in a solution containing 10% excess *p*-toluenesulfonic acid, evaporating to dryness, and drying at 135°C for 8 hr.

Pre-treat *p*-toluenesulfonic acid by drying the monohydrate at 110°C overnight, then cooling and powdering the material.

To a 500-ml Erlenmeyer flask and 100 ml of water, 1 drop of *m*-cresol purple indicator, and sufficient 0.1*N* sodium hydroxie or 0.1*N* hydrochloric acid to a yellow-green end point.

Determine a blank by duplicating the above procedure without a sample, colorless with 30-ml portions of water. Extract the combined washings with 30 ml of chloroform, adding the chloroform layer to the main extract. Transfer the chloroform extract to a tared dish. Evaporate at room temperature. Dry to constnat weight in a desiccator.

Inorganic Salts. The inorganic salts present in certified colors are there either as a result of a step in the manufacturing process or because of deliberate addition by the manufacturer to meet the strength demands of the customer. The most common salts found are chlorides and sulfates of sodium.

Procedures

SODIUM CHLORIDE. *AOAC Method for Acid Dyes.* Dissolve 2g of the dye in 100 ml of waer and add 10g of activated carbon which is chloride and sulfate-free. Boil gently 2-3 min. Cool to room temperature, add 1 ml of 6 *N* nitric acid and stir. Dilute with water to 200 ml in a volumetric flask, then filter through dry paper. Repeat the treatment with 2-g portions of carbon until no apparent color rises when the filter paper is dipped into the filtrate.

Transfer 50 ml of filtrate to a 250-ml flask. Add 2 ml of 2:3 nitric acid, 5 ml of nitrobenzene, and 10 ml or more of standardized 0.1 *N* silver nitrate solution, depending on the chloride content. Shake the flask until the silver chloride coagulates. Prepare a saturated solution of ferric ammonium sulfate and add just enough concentrated nitric acid to discharge the red color; add 1ml of this solution to serve as the indicator. Titrate with 0.1 *N* ammonium thiocyanate solution which has been standardized against the silver nitrate solution until the color persists after shaking for 1 min.

$$\% \text{ sodium chloride} = \frac{(A)\,(N)\,(0.5844)\,(195)\,(100)}{(w)\,(50)}$$

where A = net volume of silver chloride solution required, in ml

N = normality of silver nitrate solution

w = sample weight, in g

Calculation is based on a 195-ml volume since 10g of carbon occupies 5 ml.

AOAC Method for Basic Dyes. Dissolve a 2-g sample in water and dilute to 200 ml in a volumetric flask. Add 10 g of carbon, stir for 1 min, and test for complete adsorption as described above. Repeat the carbon treatment if necessary. Filter through dry paper.

Evaporate a 50-ml aliquot to dryness, then heat to volatilize ammonium chloride. Transfer the residue to a 250-ml flask and determine sodium chloride as above.

$$\% \text{ sodium chloride} = \frac{(A)(N)(0.05844)\ (20)(100)}{(w)\ (50)}$$

General Potentiometric Method. Dissolve 0.5-1g of sample in 100 ml of water. Acidify with 5 ml of 1.5*N* nitric acid. Place a silver electrode in the sample solution and connect a calomel electrode to the solution with a saturated potassium sulfate bridge. (The bridge may be eliminated by using a glass electrode as the reference). Titrate the solution potentiometrically with 0.1 *N* silver nitrate solution; 1 ml of 0.1 *N* silver nitrate is equivalent to 0.05844 g of sodium chloride.

SODIUM SULFATE. *AOAC method for Acid Dyes* (14). Dissolve a 2g-sample and treat it with carbon as described in the AOAC method for sodium chloride in acid dyes. Place 25 l of the filtrate obtained in a 125-ml Erlenmeyer flask, and add 1 drop of a solution of 0.5% phenolphthalein in 50% ethanol. Make alkaline with 0.05 *N* sodium hydroxide, then add 0.002 *N* hydrochloric acid until the indicator is decolorized. Add 25 ml of ethanol and about 0.2 g of tetrahydroxyquinone indicator. (THQ prepared sulfate indicator, Bets Laboratories, Inc. Trevase, Pa.) Titrate with 0.03 *N* barium chlorid solution to a red end point. Make a blank determination.

$$\% \text{ sodium sulfate} = \frac{(A - B)(N)(0.07102)(195)(100)}{(w)(25)}$$

General Gravimetric Method. Weigh 5 g of sample, dissolve it in 100 ml of warm water, and transfer to a 250-ml volumetric flask. Add 35 g of sulfate-free sodium chloride, stopper the flask, and let it stand for 1 hr. Swirl at frequent intervals. Dilute to volume with saturated sodium chloride solution and filter through dry filter paper. Precipitate the sulfate ith barium chloride; filter, dry, and weight the precipitate.

SODIUM ACETATE (16). Prepare silver toluenesulfonate by dissolving silver oxide or carbonate in a solution containing 10% excess *p*-toluensulfonic acid, evaporating to dryness, and drying at 135° C for 8 hr.

Pretreat *p*-toluensulfonic acid by drying the monohydrate at 110°C overnight, then cooling and powdering the material.

To a 500ml Erlenmeyer flask add 100 ml of water, 1 drop of *m*-cresol purple indicator, and sufficient 0.1 *N* sodium hydroxide or 0.1 *N* hydrochloric acid to make the solution just yellow. Assemble the apparatus shown in Figure 21, and place the Erlenmeyer flask under the condenser.Place 30 ml of absolute ethanol in the distillation flask, then add through the powder funnel 5 g of sample, 1 g of silver toluenesulfonate, and 5 of *p*-toluenesulfonic acid. Wash the funnel and neck of the flask with 25 ml of absolute ethanol; shake the flask to mix the contents and attach it to the condenser.

Immerse the distillation flask in a beaker of hot water and boil the water. Collect about 25 ml of distillate, remove the heat, and slowly add 25 ml of absolute ehtnaol. Replace the heat source and collect an additional 25 ml of absolute ethanol. Replace the heat source and collect an additional 25 ml of distillate. Make a third addition of absolute ethanol and distill as before. Finally boil until the distillation rate s slow (about 30 min total distillation time from the beginning of the first distillation).

Wash down the condenser into the receiver with 50 ml of water. ADd 50.0 ml of standardized 0.1 *N* sodium hydroxide. Connect to a reflux condenser fitted with an absorption tube cntaining Ascarite; reflux for 10 min. cool to room temperature, add a few drops of *m*-cresol purple indicator, and titrate with 0.1 *N* hydrochloric acid to a yellow-green end point.

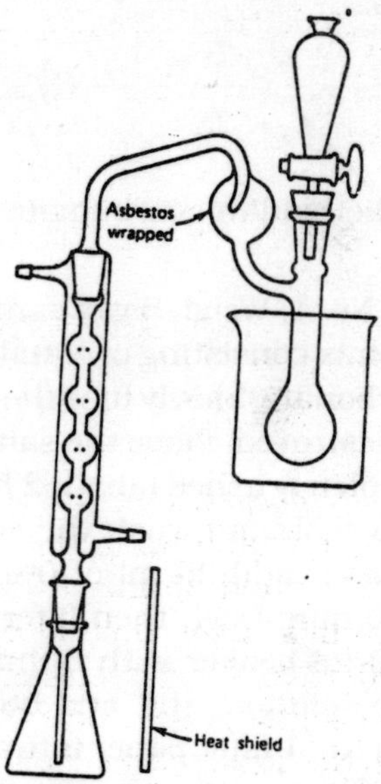

Fig. 21. Apparatus used in sodium acetate determination

Determine a blank by duplicating the above procedure without a sample.

SODIUM IODIDE. Prepare an eluant solution by dissolving 500g of ammonium sulfate in water and diluting to 2 liters, then mixing the solution with 200 ml of SDH No. 30 alcohol.

Weigh 0.5g of sample, transfer it to a 150-ml beaker, and dissolve it in 15 ml of water and 10 ml of alcohol. Wash 10g of Whatman Column Chromedia CF11 with the eluant solution. (Some lots of adsorbent contain an impurity with a spectrum similar to that of sodium iodide, which must be removed). Add the washed adsorbent and 15 ml of the eluant to the sample and mix. Then add 50g of the ammonium sulfate and mix well. Using 25 ml of eluant transfer the sample to a chromatographic column prepared and eluated as described in the general liquid chromatographic column prepared and eluted as described in the general liquid chromatographic method on. Record the ultraviolet spectra of the fractions as eluted. Usually sodium iodide cannot be detected in the first two fractions and is completely eluted in the first eight fractions. It is characterized by an absorption maximum near 222 nm.

Metallic Impurities

The following methods are used for the determination of metallic impurities in certified colors.

Procedures

Arsenic

Use either the silver diethyldithiocarbamate in method, or the arsine generation method.

CHROMIUM IN FD&C BLUE NO. 1. Weigh 5 g of sample into a platinum dish, Mix in 8.0 g of a fusion mix consisting of equal portions of sodium carbonate and potassium carbonate. Slowly fuse the sample over a flame until all organic material is destroyed. Place the sample in a 800-850°C muffle furnace until it is completely ashed (about 2 hr). Remove the dish from the furnace, allow it to cool, and wash the contents into a 150-ml beaker with 50 ml. of water. add 25 ml of 0% hydrogen peroxide solution, stir, and boil for 10 min. Cool, then filter through Whatman No. 1 filter paper into a 100-ml beaker with 50 ml. of water. Add 25 ml of 6% hydrogen peroxide solution, stir, and boil for 10 min. Cool, then filter through Whatman No. 1 filter paper into a 100-ml volumetric flask.Rinse the beaker and filter paper into the flask, then dilute to volume. Using a 5-cm cell determine the absorption spectrum from 450 to 310 nm vs water. Construct a baseline connecting the absorption min near 320 and 450 nm. Draw a line parallel to the absorbance axis and passing through the spectrum and the baseline at 370 nm. The absorbance at the intersection of this line with the sample spectrum equals A_1. The absorbance at the intersection of this line with the baseline equals A_2;

ppm chromium = $(A_1 - A_2)$ (50.4)

where 50.4 is the reciprocal of the slope of a least squares fit of the regression of *A* at 370 nm upon ppm of chromium determined by this method. This value is based on that reported in Reference 17.

Heavy Metals. See Vol. 8, p. 439. Use a 1-g sample and treat it as directed in Method 2.

Lead (18). This method is applicable to colors which do not contain calcium, strontium, or barium.

Prepare a 10% hydryxylamine hydrochloride solution in the following manner; Dissolve 10g of $NH_2OH.HCl$ in 20 ml of water and make slightly alkaline with ammonium hydroxide. Extract any lead with dithrizone (diphenylthiocarbazone). Remove excess dithizone with chloroform and boil off any chloroform remaining in the aqueous phase. Acifidy with hydrochloric acid and dilute to 100 ml.

Prepare a stripping reagent by adding 1 ml of glacial acetic acid to 20 ml of saturated sodium acetate solution and diluting to 100 ml.

Prepare a 0.5% starch solution in the following manner; Paste 1 g of soluble starch with several ml of cold water, pour into 200 ml of hot water, and while still hot, add two or three small crystals of mercuric iodide as a preservative.

Prepare a standardized sodium thiosulfate solution in the following way: To a 0.1 *N* sodium thiosulfate solution, add 5 ml of isoamyl alcohol per liter as a preservative. On the day the analysis is performed, dilute 1:100 or 1:20 with carbon dioxide-free water (depending on the lead concentration). Standardize against a lead solution prepared by dissolving 0.3197 g of lead nitrate in 100.0 ml of 1% nitric acid.

Transfer 5g of sample to a 500-ml Kjedahl flask. Add 10 ml of concentrated sulfuric acid and 10 ml of concentrated nitric acid and heat to sulfur trioxide fumes. Add 5 ml of concentrated nitric acid and again heat to sulfur trioxide fumes. Repeat the addition of nitric acid each time sulfur trioxide fumes appear until the dye is in solution and the digest is yellow. Then add 10 ml of a 1:1 mixture of concentrated nitric acid and 60-70% perchloric acid, and continue heating until the digest is colorless or pale yellow, and the bulk of the sulfuric acid is evaporated.

Cool the flask and neutralize with ammonium hydroxide. Add 20 ml of 50% citric acid solution and adjust to pH 8.5- with ammonium hydroxide using thymol blue indicator. Add 5 ml of 10% potassium cyanide solution and transfer the sample to a separatory funnel. Extract the lead with 20 ml of 0.002% solution of dithizone in chloroform.

Cool the flask and neutralise with ammonium hydroxide. Add 20 ml of 50% citric acid solution and adjust to pH 8.5-9 with ammonium hydroxide using thymol blue indicator. Add 5 ml of 10% potassium cyanide solution and transfer the sample to a separatory funnel. Extract the lead with with 20 ml of a 0.002% solution of dithizone in chloroform. (If there is enough iron present to cause excessive oxidation of the dithizone, as indicated by a yellow color in the chloform layer, add 10 ml of the 10% hydroxylamine hydrochloride solution to reduce the iron.) Let the chloroform layer settle; drain it into a second funnel. Repeat the extraction until the red lead dithizonate is completely removed.

Wash the combined chloroform extracts with 25 ml of water containing 1 drop of ammonium hydroxide. Drain the washed chloroform layer into a third funnel. Add 110 ml of 1:99 nitric acid and shake for 1 min. Drain and discard the chloroform layer and about 1 ml of the acid layer. Drain the acid layer through cotton, discarding the first 3 ml.Electrolyze a 100-ml aliquot as follows: Heat a latinum gause cylindrical anode to red heat in the oxidizing flame of a burner. Cool the anode and place it in the sample solution. Start the electrode rotating, heat the sample solution to 60-70°C, and add 0.1 of potassiumdichromate. Electrolyze 20 ml at 70-80°C, using 100 mA. Remove the heat and siphon the sample from the beaker while playing a stream of water directly on the anode; keep the level of liquid above the deposit at all times. The acid is entirely removed when the current falls to zero.

Dissolve the deposit from the anode with 4-5 ml of stripping reagent and 1 ml of freshly prepared 2% potassium iodide solution, contained in a flat-bottom vessel of such size that the solution just covers the anode. Add a few drops of the starch solution and titrate the liberated iodine with0.001 *N*sodium thiosulfate solution using the anode as a stirrer. Use a 0.005 *N* thiosulfate solution if the lead content is 1-5 mg. Similarly determine a blank.

MERCURY, *Ion Exchange Paper—X-Ray Emission Method.* Place a $1^1/_2$ in. in disc of ion exchange paper (Reeve Angel, Grade SB-2 Amberlite ion resin-loaded papers, anion exchanger, strong base-type, containing Amberlite IRA-400 resin, Chloroform) in the joint of a two-piece, $^3/4$ in. ID chromatographic column, joined by a threaded aluminum coupling and having a Teflon stopcock with fine adjustment control; tighten the joint. Using light suction draw water up through the paper. Wash the column and paper by passing 50 ml of 0.5 *N* hydrochloric acid through the colum at 1 ml/min. Leave several ml of solution in the column.

Dissolve the sample in dilute hydrochloric acid and adjust the acid concentration to 0.5 *N* hydrochloric acid. Filter through fine filter paper previously washed with 0.5 *N* hydrochloric acid. Divide the sample in two; add a known amount (1-5mg) of mercury to one portion. Carry a reagent blank and a standard, containing a known amount of mercury in 100 ml of 0.5 *N* hydrochloric acid, through the rest of the procedure.

Pass each solution through a column such as that described above at 1 ml/min. Follow the sample with 25 ml of 0.5 *N* hydrochloric acid, alsoat 1 ml/min. Drain the solution from the below the resin paper, remove the paper, and dry at room temperature.

Using a standard solution containing 1.354 mg/ml of mercuric chloride, set up the x-ray emission spectrograph, equipped with a molybdenum tube, lithium fluoride crystal, scintillation counter, and pulse height analyzer, on the mercury La line 2q = 36°. Mount the resin-loaded disc in the instrument holder. Using a least 16,000 counts determine the counts/sec at 2q = 35°, 2q = 36°, and 2q = 37.1°. For best reults take an average of four readings, rotating the sample 90° between readings.

Calculate as follow:

$$R_{36^\circ/35^\circ} = \frac{\text{counts/sec at } 2J = 36^\circ}{\text{counts/sec at } 2o = 35^\circ}$$

$$R_{37.1^\circ/35^\circ} = \frac{\text{counts/sec at } 2 = 37.1}{\text{counts/sec at } 2 = 35^\circ}$$

$R_{37.1^\circ/35^\circ}$ for blank, sample and standards should be equal if tungsten is absent. If tungsten is absent, calculate mg of mercury in the sample aliquot from as follows :

$$\mu g \text{ mercury} = \frac{(R_s - R_b)\,y}{R_{s+y} - R_s}$$

where R_s = calculated 36°/35° value for the sample aliquot

R_b = calculated 36°/35° value for the blank

R_{s+y} = calculated 36°/35° value for the sample aliquot to which Yμg of mercury has been added.

Y = µg of mercury added to the aliquot

Photometric Mercury vapor Method. Use the apparatus shown in Figure 22 (20). Preheat the furnace to 650°C and adjust the nitrogen flow to1 liter/min. Standardize the mercury vapor meter following the manufcturer's instructions. Adjust the attenuator so that the recorder scale is 200 mV.

Calibrate the meter by placing aliquots of mercuric chloride solution containing 0.01-0.03 mg of mercury on separate pieces of ignited asbestos in individual combustion boats. Cover the asbestos with 1-2 g of anhydrous sodium carbonate. Place the boats one at a time in the tube furnace and close the inlet. After 1 min start the nitrogen flow. Prepare a plot of response vs amount of mercury.

Treat 0.025 g of organic sample of 0.25g of inorganic sample in the same way. Iodine interferes with the determination.

Colorimetric Method. Use NF grade chloroform throughout this procedure. Prepare a 205 hydoxylamine hydrochloride solution. Remove heavy metals by shaking with 50-ml portions of 100 mg/liter dithizone in chloroform. Wash with several portions of chloroform to remove excess dithizone.

Prepare a 40% potassium bromide solution and remove heavy metals as described above. Make alkaline with 1-2 drops of 10% sodium hydroxide before storing.

Prepare a 50% ammonium acetate solution and remove heavy metals as described above.

Prepare a mercury standard solution and remove heavy metals as described above.

Prepare a dithizone solution containing 6 mg/liter of dithizone in chloroform, and use this throughout the portion of the procedure which follows.

Weigh a 1-g sample and transfer it to a two-neck, 500-ml digestion flask fitted with a Freidrichs condenser and a 50-ml dropping funnel. (If the sample is a triphenylmethane or oil-soluble dye, use a 0.5-g sample). Add 10 ml of 1:1:1 sulfuric acid-nitric acid-water and allow to stand for about 5 min. Heat gently for about 5 min, and 2 ml of 70% perchloric acid, and reflux for 2 hr (3 hr for triphenylmethane or oil-soluble dyes; 1 hr for lakes having a low dye content). Concurrently run two blanks containing all the reagents.

Allow the solution to cool. Wash the condenser and the funnel using sufficient water to bring the volume to about 100 ml. Add 10 ml of the 20% $NH_2OH.HCl$ solution and reflux for 10 min. Cool. Wash the condenser and funnel with 30 ml of water and transfer the sample to a 250-ml separatory funnel, filtering if necessary. Dilute to 200 ml. Add 20.0 ml of mercury standard solution to one blank; this is the standard. The second blank is the reagent blank.

Add 10 ml of the dithizone solution and shake vigorously for 1 min. Allow the chloroform layer to settle and transfer it to a second 250-ml funnel containing 50 ml of 0.25 *N* hydrochloric acid. Pass 5 ml of chloroform through mouth of the first funnel and add to the second. Repeat the extraction with 10-ml portions of dithizone solution untl the green color of the dithizone remains unchanged. Wash the contents of the first funnel with 10 ml of chloroform and add the wash to the dithizone extracts.

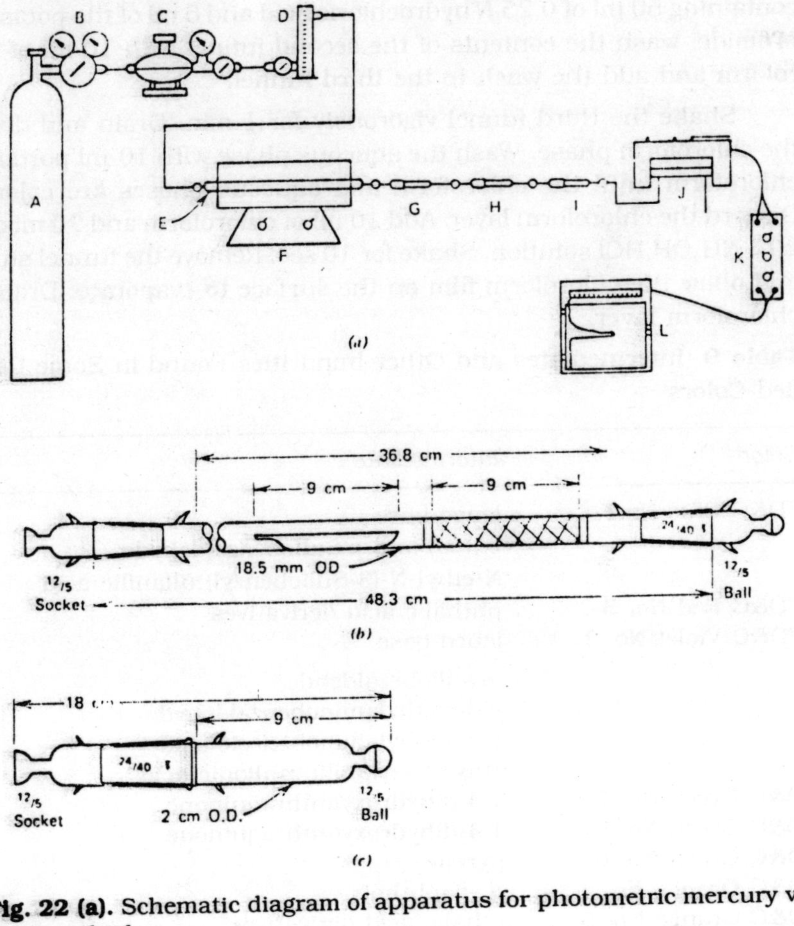

Fig. 22 (a). Schematic diagram of apparatus for photometric mercury vapour method

A. Tank of nitrogen
B. Two-stage pressure regulator
C. Low-pressure regulator
D. Flowmeter
E. Combustion tube
F. Comustion tube furnace
G. Dehydrite trap
H. Ascarite trap
I. Aluminum oxide trap
J. Mercury vapour meter
K. Attenuator
L. Recorder

(*b*) Quartz combustion tube with boat and copper oxide packing. (c) Schematic diagram of trap used to contai Ascarite, Dehydrite ana aluminum oxide

Shake the second funnel vigorously for 1 min. Allow the layers to settle and transfer the chloroform layer to a third 250-ml funnel containing 50 ml of 0.25 *N* hydrochloric acid and 5 ml of the potassium bromide. wash the contents of the second funnel with 10 ml of chloroform and add the wash to the third funnel.

Shake the third funnel vigorously for 1 min. Drain and discard the chloroform phase. Wash the aqueous phase with 10-ml portions of chloroform until the chloroform and aqueous phases are colorless. Discard the chloroform layer. Add 10 ml of chloroform and 20 ml of the 20% NH_2OH,HCl solution. Shake for 10 sec. Remove the funnel stopper and allow the chloroform film on the surface to evaporate. Drain the chloroform layer.

Table 9. Intermediates and Other Impurities Found in Some Certified Colors

Color	*Intermediate*
FD&C Blue No.1	leuco base
	o-, *m*-, and *p*-Sulfobenzaldehyde
	N-ethyl-N-(3-Sulfobenzyl) ulfanilic acid
FD&C Red No. 3	phthalic acid derivatives
FD&C Violet No. 1	leuco base
	m-sulfobezaldehde
	p-dimethylaminobenzaldehyde
	p-dimethylaminobenzoic acid
	ethylbenzylanilinesulfonic acid
D&C Green No. 5	1,4-dihydroxyanthraquinone
D&C Green No. 6	1,4-dihydroxyanthraquinone
D&C Green No. 8	pyrene
D&C Orange No. 4	β -naphthol
D&C Orange No. 5	pthalic acid derivatives°
D&C Orange No. 10	phthalic acid derivativess°

D&C Orange No. 11	phthalic acid derivatives[o]
D&C Orange No. 17	*β* -naphthol
	2,4-dinitroaniline
	phthalic acid derivatives[o]
D&C Red No. 8	Lake Red C Amine (2-chloro-5-aminoteluene-4-sulfonic acid)
D&C Red No. 9	Lake Red C Amine (2-chloro-5-aminotoluene 4-sulfonic acid)β-naphthol
D&C Red No. 17	minoazobenzene
	β-naphthol
D&C Red No. 19	*m*-diethylaminophenol
	o-(2hdryxy-4-diethylaminobenzoyl) benzoic acid
D&C Red No. 21	phthalic acid derivatives[o]
D&C Red No. 22	phthalic acid derivatives[o]
D&C Red No. 36	β-naphthol
D&C Red No. 37	*m*-diethylaminophenol
D&C Violet No. 2	1-hydroxy-4-*p*-toluinoanthroaquinone
D&C Yellow No. 7	phthalic acid derivatives[a]
D&C Yellow No. 8	phthalic acid derivatives[a]
D&C Yellow No. 10	phthalic acid derivatives[d]
D&C Yellow No. 11	phthalic acid derivatives[e]
Ext D&C Yellow No. 1	diphenylamine

[a] Determined by Method A on p. 505
[b] Determined by Method B on p. 505
[c] See specific procedure, p. 504
[d] Determined by Method C on p. 505
[e] Determined by Method D on p. 506

Add 10.0 ml of the dithizone solution; shake for 1 min. Drain the chloroform layer through absorbent cotton, discarding the first ml. Within 1 hr, determine the absorbances of the filtered chloroform solution of the sample, the blank, and the standard at 490 nm.

Intermediates

The percent of uncombined intermediates permitted in certified colors is very closely controlled. The amounts vary from color to color but generally no more than 0.2-0.4% of any one intermediate is tolerated. The intermediates encountered are usually the starting materials used in the manufacturing processes mentioned in Tables 1-3. Normally only one intermediate is found to any extent in a dye.

General Method The most frequently used method for determining intermediates is the liquid chromatographic procedure given below. With this method the intermediates usually separate from the dye but are not always isolated from each other. The analyst may have to depend on taking smaller cuts, the use of simultaneous equations, spectral shifts with change in pH, or some combination of these techniques in order to make quantitative determinations.

In addition to the expected intermediates, this method often resolves and detects degradation products, chance contaminants, and other undesirable impurities capable of causing the withholding of certification.

Procedure

Affix a short length of clean rubber tubing to the tip of the glass chromatographic column shown in Figure 23. Attach a pinchcock and place a glass wool plug in the constriction above the column tip. Slurry 60 g of Whatman Column Chromedia CF11 in 500 ml of the appropriate eluant, as given in Table 10. With the pinchcock open, pour the slurry into the column. Wash the column with 200 ml of eluant and let it drain until the liquid level is 2-3 ml above the level of the packed cellulose.

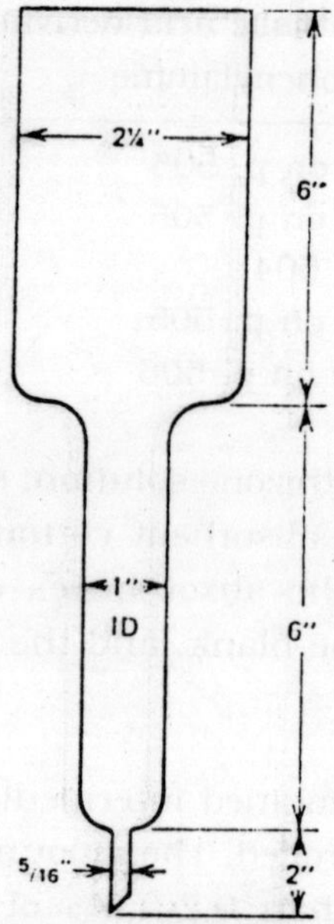

Fig. 23. Glass chromatographic column

Table 10. Solvents, Eluants and Treatment of Eluate Fractions for Individual Colors

Color	Solvent*	Eluant (w/v) solution	Treatment of fractions
FD&C Blue No. 1	25 ml water	35% ammonium	divide each fraction equally add 0.5 ml of concentrated hydrochloric acid to one portion and 0.5 ml of concentrated ammonium hydroxide to the other
FD&C Blue No. 2	25 ml water	25% ammonium sulfate containing 0.5% hydrochloric acid (v/v)	run as eluted
FD&C Green No. 3	25 ml water	35% ammonium sulfate	same as FD&C Blue No.
FD&C Red No. 2	25 ml water	35% ammonium sulfate	run as eluted
FD&C Red No. 3	5 ml ethanol and 25 ml water	25% ammonium sulfate containing 10% ethanol (v/v)	divide each fraction equally; add 0.5 ml of concentrated hydrochloric acid to one portion, run the other as is
FD&C Red No. 4	25 ml water	25% ammonium sulfate	add 1 ml of concentrated ammonium hydroxide to each fraction
FD&C Violet No. 1	25 ml water	12.5% ammonium sulfate	same as FD&C Blue 1
FD&C Yellow No. 5	2 drops concentrated hydrochloric acid in 25 ml of water	25% ammonium sulfate, containing 5% ethanol and 1% hydrochloric acid (v/v)	divide each fraction equally; add 1 ml of concentrated ammonium hydroxide to one portion, run the other as is
FD&C Yellow No. 6	25 ml of water	35% ammonium sulfate	run as eluted
Citrus Red No. 2	25 ml water	10% ammonium sulfate	run as eluted
Orange B	2 drops concentrated hydrochloric acid in 25 ml of water	50% ammonium sulfate containing 1% hydrochloric acid (v/v) for 600 ml, then 25% ammonium sulfate containing 1% hydrochloric acid (v/v) for remainder	same as FD&C Yellow 5
D&C Blue No. 4	25 ml water	35% ammonium sulfate	same as FD&C Blue 1
D&C Blue No. 6	slurried with 10 ml of ethanol then 10 ml of eluant added	10% ammonium sulfate	same as FD&c Red 3
D&C Blue No. 9	25 ml water	10% ammonium sulfate	run as eluted
D&C Green No. 5	25 ml water	25% ammonium sulfate	same as FD&C Red 4
D&C Green No. 6	slurried with 10 ml of ethanol then 10 ml of eluant added	10% ammonium sulfate	same as FD&C Red 4
D&C Green No. 8	25 ml water	40% ammonium sulfate	run as eluted
D&C Orange No. 4	25 ml water	25% ammonium sulfte	run as eluted
D&C Orange No. 5	dissolved in a minimum of concentrated ammonium hydroxide	25% ammonium sulfate	same as FD&C Blue 1

D&C Orange No. 10	dissolved in a minimum of concentrated ammonium hydroxide	25% ammonium sulfate	same as FD&C Red 3
D&C Orange No. 11	25 ml water	25% ammonium sulfate	same as FD&C Red 3
D&C Orange No. 17	slurried with 10 ml of ethanol	10% ammonium sulfate containing 10% ethanol (v/v)	run as eluted
D&C Red No. 6 D&C Red No. 7	slurried with 10 ml of ethanol, then 10 ml of eluant added	10% ammonium sulfate	divide each fraction equally; add 0.5 ml of concentrated hydrochloric acid to one portion, run the other as is
D&C Red No. 8 D&C Red No. 9	slurried with 10 ml of ethanol, then 10 ml of eluant added	10% ammonium sulfate	same as D&C Red 6
D&C Red No. 10 D&C Red No. 11 D&C Red No. 12 D&C Red No. 13	slurried with 10 ml of ethanol, then 10 ml of eluant added	10% ammonium sulfate	same as D&C Red 6
D&C Red No. 17	slurried with 10 ml of ethanol, then 10 ml of eluant added	10% ammonium sulfate containing 10% ethanol (v/v)	same as FD&C Blue 1
D&C Red No. 19	slurried with 5 ml of ethanol	35% ammonium hydroxide	same as FD&C Blue 1
D&C Red No. 21	dissolved in a minimum of concentrated ammonium hydroxide, and 5 ml of ethanol added	25% ammonium sulfate	same as FD&C Blue 1
D&C Red No. 22	slurried with 5 ml of ethanol	25% ammonium sulfate	same as FD&C Blue 1
D&C Red No. 27	dissolved in a minimum of concentrated ammonium hydroxide and 5 ml of ethanol added	30% ammonium sulfate containing 4% ammonium hydroxide (v/v)	same as FD&C Blue 1
D&C Red No. 28	slurried with 5 ml of ethanol	30% ammonium sulfate containing 4% ammonium hydroxide (v/v)	same as FD&C Blue 1
D&C Red No. 30	25 ml water	10% ammonium sulfate	run as eluted
D&C Red No. 31	slurried with 10 ml of ethanol and 10 ml of eluant	10% ammonium sulfate	same as F&DC Blue 1
D&C Red No. 33	25 ml water	Same 25% ammonium sulfate	as FD&C Blue 1
D&C Red No. 34	slurried with 10 ml of ethanol and then 10 ml of eluant added	10% ammonium sulfate	run as eluted
D&C Red No. 36	slurried with 10 ml of ethanol	10% ammonium sulfate	run as eluted
D&C Red No. 37	slurried with 10 ml of ethanol	35% ammonium sulfate	run as eluted

D&C Violet No. 2	slurried with 10 ml of ethanol	10% ammonium sulfate	same as FD&C Blue 1
D&C Yellow No. 7	25 ml of water	25% ammonium sulfate	same as FD&C Red 3
D&C Yellow No. 8	25 ml of water	40% ammonium sulfate	same as FD&C Red 3
D&C Yellow No. 10	25 ml water	40% ammonium sulfate	same as FD&C Blue 1
D&C Yellow No. 11	slurried with 5 ml of ethanol	10% ammonium sulfate	same as FD&C Blue 1
Ext D&C Green No. 1	25 ml water	saturated ammonium sulfate solution	run as eluted
Ext D&C Yellow No. 1	slurried with 10 ml of ethanol	500 ml of 10% ammonium sulfate containing 1.0% ammonium hydroxide (v/v) followed by 10% ammonium sulfate containing 1% hydrochloric acid (v/v) for remainder	same as FD&C Red 4
Ext D&C Yellow No. 7	25 ml water	35% ammonium sulfate	run as eluted

[a]The solvent indicated may not dissolve the dye but only leach it of impurities
[b]The eluant should be essentially free of iron and other ultraviolet-absorbing impurities.

Place 0.5 g of sample in a 150-ml beaker and add the solvent indicated in Table 10. The solvent does not necessarily dissolve the dye sample; it may extract the intermediates. Add 10g of Chromedia which has been previously washed with the appropriate eluant and mix. Add 50g of ammonium sulfate powder to salt out the dye and mix. Using 50 ml of eluant, transfer the mixture to the column. Let the column drain to the surface of the cellulose. Add eluant to the column at a rate equivalent to the rate of flow through the column. Collect as many 100 ± 1 ml fractions as can be obtained before the dye itself begins to emerge from the column. Similarly prepare and elute a blank column to which no sample has been added.

Treat the eluate fractions as directed in Table 4. Record the ultraviolet specra of the fractions vs blank (eluant plus reagents) and compare them with spectra of known compound - similarly prepared. For the ideal case in which there is no interference;

$$\%\ \text{intermediate} = \frac{(\sum A)\ (f + x)(100)}{(a)\,(b)\,(w)\,(1000)}$$

where ΣA = sum of the absorbances (corrected for column blank) of the sample fractions containing the intermediate

a = absorptivity in liter/g-em of the intermediate at the wavelength at which A is measured

b = absorption cell length, in cm

w = sample weight, in g

f = volume of the fraction collected, in ml

r = volume of reagnets added, in ml

*Determination of β-Naphthol.*β-Naphthol is extracted with an appropriate solvent, diazotized, and then determined, by titanous chloride titration or spectrophotometrically.

Procedures

TITRATIONS WITH TITANOUS CHLORIDE. Prepare a 0.5 *N* diazotized sulfanilic acid solution as follows: Dissolve 4.78g of sulfanilic acid in 500 ml of 1:9 hydrochloric acid. Dissolve 1.04g of sodium nitrite in 300 ml of water. Place 40 ml of the sulfanilic acid solutions in a 100-ml volumetric flask. Cool to 5°C, add 44 ml of the sodium nitrite solution, and allow it to diazotize. Test for excess nitrous acid with starch-iodide paper; destroy any excess with a few mg of sulfamic acid. Dilute to volume with water.

Weight a 10-g sample into a 1.5×8.0 cm extraction thimble, place it in a Soxhlet apparatus, and extract for 8 hr with petroleum ether (bp, 35-60°C).

Disconnect the extractor and add 15o ml of 1:10 hydrochloric acid to the flask. Gently boil off the ether on a hot plate and filter the solution through glass wool into a 250-ml volumetric flask. Rinse the extraction flask several times with small quantities of 1:10 hydrochloric acid, filtering the rinses through the glass wool and collecting them in the volumetric flask. Dilute to volume with water. Mix, then divide into two equal portions. Neutralize each portion with a dilute sodium hydroxide solution, using phenophthalein as an indicator.

Add 10g of sodium acetate trihydrate to one portion and cool to 5°C in an ice bath. Slowly add 25 ml of diazotized sulfanilic acid solution, stir 5 min, and test for excess reagent with alkaline β-naphthol solution on spot paper. If necessary add additional reagent until a positive test is obtained. Let stand 1hr or longer.

Heat on a water bath for 30 min to decompose any excess reagent. Test with b-naphthol solution on spot paper to determine that decomposition is complete. To both the coupled and uncoupled portions of solution add 10g of sodium bitartrate dissolved in 50 ml of hot water. Titrate the uncoupled blank with 0.1 *N* titanium chloride to a colorless end point. Titrate the coupled portion until the dye reduces and becomes yellow. Add 1-2 ml excess of titanium chloride solution and immediately back-titrate with standardized methylene blue solution or another suitable dye.

Subtract the volume of titrant required for the blank from the volume required for the coupled portion, and calculate % β-naphthol (1 ml of 0.1 *N* titanium chloride to a colorless end point. Titrate the uncoupled blank with 0.1 *N* titanium chloride to a colorless end point. Titrate the coupled portion until the dye reduces and becomes yellow. Add 1-2 ml excess of titanium chloride solution and immediately back titrate with standardized methylene blue solution or another suitable dye.

Subtract the volume of titrant required for the blank from the volume required for the coupled portion, and calculate % β-naphthol (1 ml of 0.1 *N* titanium chloride = 0.0036 g of β-naphthol).

SPECTROPHOTOMETRIC METHODS. *General Methods.* Prewash all isopropyl ether once with 0.1 *N* sodium hydroxide.

Prepare a *p*-nitrobenzenediazonium chloride solution in the following manner: Dissolve 0.02 g of *p*-nitroaniline in 2 ml of hydrochloride acid and dilute to 200 ml with water. Add 100 g of crushed ice and stir until the solution temperature is 5-10°C. Add 2 ml of 10% sodium nitrate solution and stir 10-15 min. Add small portions of 10% sulfamic acid solution until the reagent gives a negative test on starch-iodide paper.

For colors soluble in water: Dissolve 2g of sample in 250 ml of water. Acidify with 5ml of 6 *N* hydrochloric acid and extract with six 30-ml portions of prewashed isopropyl ether. Wash the combined ether extracts with 20 ml of 0.1 *N* hydrochloric acid and discard the aqueous layer. Extract with six 30-ml portions of 0.1 *N* sodium hydroxide.

Cool the combined sodium hydroxide extracts to 5-10°C with crushed ice and add the *p*-nitrobenzenediazonium chloride solution slowly with constant stirring. Stir the mixture for 15 min. Heat to 90°C on a steam bath, remove from the bath, and cool to room temperature. Extract with 20-ml portions of chloroform until the extracts are colorless. Wash the combined extracts with 30 ml of 0.1 *N* sodium hydroxide. Filter the chloroform layer through the cotton into a 500-ml flask. Dilute to volume with chloroform. Measure the absorbance of the sample solution at 490nm; determine the β–naphthol content by comparison with a standard solution prepared by dissolving 0.1g of 1-(4-nirophenylazo)-2-hydroxynaphthalene in 200 ml of chloroform, and diluting with chloroform to obtain a concentration of 5 or 10 mg/liter.

$$\% \text{ -naphthol} = \frac{(A)(c)(144)(0.05)}{(B)(w)(293)}$$

where A = absorbance of the sample solution
B = absorbance of the standard solution
c = concentration of the standard solution, in mg/liter
w = sample weight, in g

For colors soluble in isopropyl ether: Weigh a 2-g sample and add 250 ml of pre-washed isopropyl ether; warm into solution on a steam bath.Extract with six 30-ml portions of 0.1 *N*sodium hydroxide. Wash the combined extracts with 30 ml of prewashed isopropyl ether and proceed as above, beginning with "Cool the combined sodium hydroxide extracts..."

For colors insoluble in water or isopropyl ether: Extract a 10-g sample with prewashed isopropyl ether for 8-10 hr in a Soxhlet apparatus. Transfer the extract to a 1-liter separatory funnel. Rinse the Soxhlet extractor with two 20-ml prtions of the isopropyl ether and add the rinses to the separatory funnel. Extract with six 30-ml portions of 0.1 *N* sodium hydroxide and wash the combined extracts with 30ml of the isopropyl ether.. Dilute the sodium hydroxide extract to 500 ml with 0.1 *N* sodium hydroxide, place a 100-ml aliquot in a beaker, and proceed as above, beginning "Cool the combined sodium hydroxide extracts..."

Method for D&C Red No. 36. Prepare a *p*-nitrobenzendiazonium chloride solution in the following manner: dissolve 0.040 g of *p*-nitroaniline in 2ml of hydrochloric acid. Chill with 35 g of ice and 15 ml of water. Diazotize with 0.04 g of sodium nitrite, stir, and let stand for 5 min.

Stir 5 g of sample with 90 ml of ethanol and 10 ml of 10% sodium hydroxide for 30 min. Transfer the mixture to a 1-liter volumetric flask containing 600 ml of water, agitate, and dilute to volume.

Filter a 400-ml aliquot and buffer with 1 of sodium carbonate. Cool the solution with 100g of ice and add the *p*-nitrobenzenediazonium chloride solution. Let it stand for 10 min, stirring occasionally. Heat to 90°C, cool, and acidify with hydrochloric acid. Remove the coloring matter with 40-ml portions of chloroform continuing until the extracts are colorless. Wash the combined extracts with three 40-ml portions of water, then with 30 ml of 0.1*N* sodium hydroxide. Filter through absorbent cotton into a 50-ml volumetric flask. Dilute to volume with chloroform. Prepare a standard solution as described above and determine its absorbance and the absorbance of the sample at 490 nm. Calculate as above under colors soluble in water.

Determination of Phthalic Acid Derivatives. The following methods are given in Reference 26 for the determination of phthalic acid derivatives in color additives. Table 9 indicates which of the methods is applicable to individual colors requiring this test.

Procedures

Method A. Colors as Salts. Weigh a 2-g sample and transfer it to beaker with about 100 ml of water. Heat nearly to boiling and while stirrig, slowly add 1:9 hydro-chloric acid and dilute to about 160 ml.Digest on a steam bath for 1-2 hr. Cool and dilute with water in a 200-ml volumetric flask. Filter through dry paper.

Pipet 50 ml of filtrate into a 125-ml separatory funnel (do not great stopcocks) and extract with 30 ml of absolute ethyl acetate. Transfer the aqueous phase to a second funnel and extract with 25 ml of ethyl acetate. Transfer the aqueous phase to a third funnel and extract with 20 ml of ethyl acetate. Pass three successive 50-ml portions of water through the funnels in the same order that the extractions were made. Discard the ethyl acetate layers, combine the aqueous extracts, and evaporate to dryness.

Dissolve the residue in water and transfer to a 100-ml volumetric flask. Add 8.5 ml of 1:9 hydrochloric acid and dilute to volume. Filter through dry paper and measure the absorbance at 230 262 and 276 nm against 0.1 *N* hydrochloric acid as the blank. Also measure the absorbance of a standard solution prepared by dissolving 0.130-0.136 g of potassium acid phthalate in 500 ml c water, and diluting a 10-ml aliquot to 200 ml with 0.1 *N* hydrochloric acid.

Phthalic acid concentration, mg/100 ml = (mg of $KHC_8H_4O_4$) (0.00813).

Calculate Y for both sample and standard as follows:

$$Y = [A_{230} - (A_{230} - 0.7\,A_{27}) - A_{262}]$$

where A = absorbance of solution at the wavelength indicated

$$\%\ \text{phthalic acid} = \frac{(Y\ \text{sample} / Y\ \text{standard}(c)(0.4)}{w}$$

where c = phthalic acid concentration of standard solution, in mg/100 ml

n = sample weight, in g

Colors as Acids. To a 2-g sample add 6 ml of 10% sodium hyroxide and a few ml of water. Mix to dissolve. Dilute to about 100 ml and proceed as above beginning with "Heat nearly to boiling..."

METHOD B. Dissolve a 0.5-g sample in 20 ml of hot water. Cool and transfer to a 125-ml separatory funnel. Add 80 ml of chloroform and 2 ml of 10% sodium hydroxide and shake vigorously for 1 min. Drain the chloroform layer, and wash the aqueous phase Add 7 ml of 1:9 hydrochloric acid to the aqueous phase and then wash with two 30-ml portions of chloroform, discarding the chloroform. Transfer the aqueos solution to a beaker with water. Proceed as in Method A, beginning with "Dissolve the residue in water..."

METHOD C. Dissolve a 1-g sample in water and transfer it to a continuous extractor. Add 1 ml of 1:100 hydrochloric acid and extract for 8 hr with 250 ml of ethyl ether. Transfer the ether extract to a separatory funnel. Rinse the flask twice with ethyl ether and add the washings to the main extract. Wash the extract with four 10-ml portions of 1:19 hydrochloric acid. Back-extract the combined washings with 50 ml of ethyl ether and add the washings to the main ether extrct. Extract the combined ether layers with four 10-ml portions of 1% sodium hydroxide. Evaporate the alkaline extracts to dryness. Transfer the residue to a 200-ml volumetric flask with water, add 2ml of hydrochloric acid, and dilute to volume. Filter through dry paper. Measure the absorbance as described in Method A and calculae % phthalic acid in the same manner.

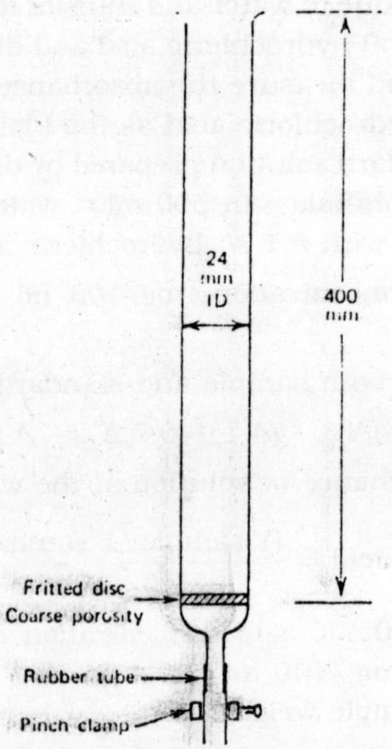

Fig. 24. Chromatographic tube.

Method D. Transfer a 0.5-g sampl to a 125-ml separatory funnel with 80 ml of chloroform. Add 20 ml of 1% sodium hydroxide and shake vigorously for 1 min. Drain the chloroform layer, wash the aqueous phase with two 30-ml portions of chloroform and discard the chloroform layers. Add 7 ml of 1:9 hydrochloric acid and wash wit two 30-ml portions of chloroform, discard the chloroform washings. Transfer the aqueous phase to a beaker and evaporate to dryness on a steam bath. Proceed as described in Method A beginning with "Dissolve the residue in water..."

Specific Methods for Other Intermediates. The following methods are given for the determination of various intermediates in specific certified colors.

Procedures

SULFOBENZALDEHYDES AND *N-ETHYL-N-*(3-SULFANILIC ACID IN FD&C BLUE No.1. Slurry 24 g of Whatman Column Chromedia (F11 in 1140 ml of eluant containing 400 g of ammonium sulfate per liter of water. Pour the slurry into a glass chromatographic tube shown in Figure 25. Let the eluant drain at rate of 5 ml/min or less until the liquid is 1-2 mm above the level of the packed cellulose.Close the pinch clamp.

Dissolve a 0.2-g sample in10 ml of water Add 2 g of the Chromedia and mix. Add 7 g of powdered ammonium sulfate and mix. Using 5 ml of the eluant, transfer the sample to the column. Drain until the flow nearly ceases. Eluate the column at a rate of 5 ml/min or less, collecting as many 10.0$\pm$0.05 ml fractions as necessary (about thirty) to remove the intermediates from the column. Record the ultraviolet spectra of the fractions vs eluant in a 1-cm cell. Compare these vs standard spectra obtained in the eluant.

o-Chlorobenzoic acid and *o*-sulfobenzoic acid elute just ahead of the sulfobenzaldehydes (SB) and may not be separated from them. They are identified by small maxima near 270 mm but are not estimated by this method. To calculate a fraction as SB, the ratio A_{252}/A_{274} must be 2.0 or greater.

o-m-And *p*-sulfobenzaldehydes elute together, generally in the fractions 7-15. They are calculated as total SB at 252 nm using an absorptivity of 51.6. This value is based on a mixture containing 92% *o*-sulfobenzaldehyde (*o*SB) and *m*-sulfobenzaldehyde (*m*SB) and 8% *p*-sulfobenzaldehyde (*p*SB). The isoabsorptive point of *o*SBand *m*SB is 252 nm.

N-Ethyl-*N*-(3-sulfobenzyl) sulfanilic acid generally elutes between fractions 15 an 30. It is calculated at the maximum near 274 mm, using absorptivity of 62.0.

m-SULFOBENZALDEHYE, *p*-DIMETHYLAMINOBENZALDEHYDE (*p*DMAB), *p*-DIMETHYLAMINOBENZOC ACID (*p*DMABA), AND ETHYLBENZYLANILINE-SULFONIC ACID (EBASA) IN FD&C VIOLET NO. 1. Affix a short length of clean rubber tubing to the tip of a 40.0 × 2.4 cm ID chromatographic tube with a sealed-in coarse fritted disc (Corning No. 38450, or equivalent). Attach a pinchcock. Slurry 30g of cellulose powder (Whatman Column Chromeda CF11) in 200 ml of 10% ammonium sulfate solution. With the pinchcock open, pour the slurry into the tube. Allow it to drain to the surface of the cellulose. Wash the column with 200 ml of 40% ammonium sulfate solution. Let the column drain until the liquid level is only 2-3 mm above the level of the packed cellulose. Close the pinchcock.

Place a 0.2-g sample in a 50-ml beaker, add 10 ml of water, and stir until dissolved. Add 2 g of cellulose and mix. Add 7g of ammonium sulfate and mix. Using about 5 ml of the 0% ammonium sulfate solution, transfer the mix to the column. Let the column drain just to the surface of the cellulose. Open the pinchcock and elute the column with 250 ml of 40% ammonium sulfate solution. Immediately begin collecting 0±1 ml fractions. As the last of the 40% solution passes into the column, add 15% ammonium sulfate solution and continue to collect fractions until color elutes (about 350 ml of this solution is required). Add 0.5 ml of concentrated ammonium hydroxide to each fraction and mix.

Prepare a blank column, elute it, and add ammonium hydroxide to the eluate, as descried above. The eluate should not have at any wavelength (400-220 nm) an absorbance greater than 0.4 when measured at a 5-cm path length vs water.

Record the ultraviolet spectra of fractions from 400 to 220 nm, using 1-cm cells. Read fractions 1-7 vs the 40% ammonium sulfate solution. Read the remaining fractions vs the 15% ammonium sulfate solution.

Examine the spectra to determine which compounds are present, *m*SB normally elutes in fractions 3-5. *pDMAB*, pDMABA, and EBASA elute together, normally in fractions 7-12.

$\%m\text{SB} = 0.477\ \Sigma(A_1 - A_2)_{248}$

where $\Sigma(A_1 - A_{2/248})$ = sum of the blank-corrected absorbances (also corrected for column blank where necessary) of the sample fractions containing *m*SB.

0.477 = (100/52.9) (3.96) (1)

100 = factor for conversion to %

3.96 = effective sample concentration, in g/liter
52.9 = absorptivity of *m*SB in liters/g-cm
1 = cell path length, in cm

$$\%pDMAB = 0.131\ \Sigma(A_1 - A_2)_{353}$$

$$\%p\mathrm{DMABA} = 0.248(A_1 - A_2)_{290} - 0.108\ \Sigma(A_1 - A_2)_{253} - 0.035\ \Sigma(A_1 - A_2)_{353}$$

$$\%\ \mathrm{EBASA} = 0.551\ \Sigma\ (A_1 - A_2)_{253} - 0.073\ \Sigma(A_1 - A_2)_{253} - 0.134\ \Sigma(A_1 - A_2)_{290}$$

where S $(A_1 - A_2)$ = sum of the blank-corrected absorbances at the indicated wavelengths (in mm) of the sample fractions containing a mixture of *p*DMAB, *p*DMABA, and EBASA

The values for % *p*DMAB, *p*DMABA and EBASA ae based on the use of simultaneous equations. Constants used to derive them are as follows:

Absorptivies, in 15% aqueous ammonium sulfate containing 1% NH_4OH_1 in liters/g-cm

	353 nm	*290 nm*	*253 nm*
*p*DMAB	194	17.0	30.0
pDMABA	0	99.0	24.0
EBASA	0	6.4	47.0

1,4-Dihydroxyanhraquinone in D&C Green no. 5. Dissolve a 0.5-g sample in 100 ml of 2% sodium hydroxide and transfer to a separatory funnel. Acidify with hydrochloric acid and extract with 100 ml of benzene. Transfer the aqueous layer to a second separatory funnel. Wash the benzene layer with 1% hydrochloric acid until the washings are colorless, adding the hydrochloric acid washings to the second funnel. Wash the combined aqueous layers with 30-ml portion of benzene until the benzene washings are colorless. Combine the benzene extracts and wash with 50-ml portions of 1% hydrochloric acid until the washings are colorless. Evaporate the benzene extracts to dryness. Dissolve the residue in ethanol and determine the 1,4-dihydroxyanthraquinone spectrophotometrically.

PYRENE IN D&C GREEN NO. 8. Determine water-insoluble matter as described on p. 489. Extract the insoluble residue with 50 ml of ethyl ether. Filter the extract into a tared dish. Evaporate the ethyl ether at 40-50°C; dry over sulfuric acid in a desiccator for 3 hr and weigh.

2,4-DINITROANILINE IN D&C ORANGE NO. 17. Paste a 1-g sample with 10 ml of concentrated sulfuric acid in a 500-ml beaker. Very slowly stir in 100 ml on a stream bath. Transfer to a 250-ml volumetric flask, cool, and dilute to volume with water. Filter 100 ml into a 500-ml separatory funnel. Add 30% sodium hydroxide until the sample solution is alkaline in litmus, cool, and extract with three 50-ml portions of ethyl ether. Wash the combined extracts with 20-ml portions of water. Transfer the ether solution into a beaker. Using 10 ml of ethyl ether, and evaporate to dryness on a steam bath. Dissolve the residue in warm 0.1 *N* ethanolic hydrochloric acid and transfer it to a 100-ml volumetric flask. Rinse the beaker into the flask with two 20-ml portions of ethanolic hydrochloric acid. Dilute to volume with the ethanolic hydrochloric acid and measure the absorbance at 290 nm, 335 nm, and 380 nm vs a standard solution of 0.01g/liter concentration.

$$\% \text{ 2,4-dinitroaniline} = \left[\frac{A_{335} - \dfrac{A_{380} + A_{290}}{2}}{B_{335} - \dfrac{B_{380} + B_{290}}{2}} \right]$$

where A = absorbance of sample at the wavelength specified

B = absorbance of the standard at the wavelength specified

Lake Red C Amine (2-chloro-5-aminotoluene-5-sulfonic acid) in D&C Red Nos, 8 and 9. Weigh a 1-g sample and transfer to a 500-ml beaker with 5 ml of acetone. Add 100 ml of 2% barium chloride solution. Boil for 10 min and filter the hot mixture through Whatman No. 12 paper into a separatory funnel. Return the filter paper and the dye to the original beaker and repeat the extraction and filtering twice more.

Cool the combined filtrates, acidify with 5 ml of 1:1 hydrochloric acid, and extract with three 20-ml portions of benzene. Wash the combined benzene extracts with 20 ml of water and add the wash to the aqueous layer. Filter the aqueous layer through cotton into a beaker. Boil for 15-20 min to remove benzene. Cool. Adjust the pH to about 8.0 with ammonium hydroxide and dilute with water to 500 ml in a volumetric flask.

Measure the absorbance of sample vs a standard solutions at 247 nm.

Aminoazobenzene in D&C red no. 17. Weight a 1-g sample and transfer to an Erienmeyer flask containing 100 ml of acetone. Heat to boiling on a steam bath. Slowly stir in 100-200 g of crushed ice and allow the mixture to stand for 15 min. Filter through a large fluted filter paper into a separatory funnel; wash the residue with 50 ml of 1:49 hydrochloric acid. Return the paper to the Erlenmeyer flask, add 100 ml of acetone, and heat to boiling on a steam bath. Repeat the precipitation and filtration. Make the combined filtrates alkaline to litmus with 30% sodium hydroxide and extract with 50-ml portions of petroleum ether until the extracts are colorless. Wash the combined petroleum ether extracts with 20 ml of 2% sodium hydroxide and then extract with 10-ml portions of 4 *N* hydrochloric acid unitl the acid extracts are colorless. Heat the combined acid extracts for 15 min on a steam bath, cool, and dilute to 250 ml with 4 *N* hydochloric acid. Determine amioazobenzene spectrophotometrically at 500 nm.

m-DIETHYLAMIOPHENOL IN D&C RED NO. 19. Prepare a *m*-diethylaminophenol standard solution in the following manner: Dissolve 0.2g of purified *m*-diethylaminophenol in 100 ml of 50% ethanol and dilute to 200 ml with water. Transfer a 20-ml aliquot to a 1-liter flask, add 100 ml of *N* sodium hydroxide, and dilute to volume with water.

Place 20g of potassium dihydrogen orthophosphate and 35g of sodium chloride in a 500-ml round-bottom flask. Weight a 2.5-g sample into a 200-ml beaker and paste with 50 ml of water. Add 50 ml of water and transfer the mixture to the round-bottom flask with several 10-ml portions of water. Dilute to 250 ml and adjust the pH to 6.6±0.2 with dilute sodiudm hydroxide. Fit the flask with a steam distillation trap and condenser and collect 175 ml of distillate.tansfer the distillate to a 250-ml volumetric flask, add 10 ml of 10% sodium hydroxide, and dilute to volume with water. Determine the absorbance of the sample solution and the standard solution at 295 nm.

m-DIETHYLAMINOPHENOL IN D&C RED NO. 37. Proceed as described for D&C Red No. 19, up to and including "... collect 175 ml of distillate." Transfer the distillate to a 500-ml round-bottom flask, rinse the receiver with several 10-ml portions of water, and add the washings to the flask. Add 30g of sodium chloride and 15g of potassium dihydrogen orthophosphate, and adjust the pH to 6.5-6.7 with 30% aqueos sodium hydroxide. Distill, collect about 175ml of distillate, and filter it into a 250-ml volumetric flask containing 10 ml of 10% sodium hydroxide. Wash the receiver with several 10-ml portions of water, filtering each wash, into the flask. Dilute to volume with water and measure the absorbance as described above.

o-(2-HYDROXY-4-*p*-TOLUINO-ANTHRAQUINONE IN D&C VIOLET NO. 2. Weigh 0.1g of sample and transfer to a 250-ml beaker. Add 100 ml of isopropyl ether, cover, and boil gently for 10 min. Cool, then transfer the solution to a 500-ml separatory funnel. If undissolved color remains in the beaker add 50 ml of isopropyl ether and boil again.

Extract the ether solution with 50 ml of 5% sodium hydroxide until no more purple is extracted. Wash the combined sodium hydroxide extracts with 25-ml portions of isopropyl ether until the ether washings are colorless. Acidify the sodium hydroxide solution with hydrochloric acid. Extract with 25ml of isoctane. Transfer the aqueous phase to a clean separatory funnel and extract with 10-ml potions of isooctane until the isooctane wash is colorless. Wash the combined isooctane extracts twice with 25 ml of water. Using fresh isooctane transfer the isooctane layer through an isooctane-washed cotton plug into a 100-ml volumetric flask. Dilute to volume with a isooctane; measure the absorbance at 249 nm.

DIPHENYLAMINE IN EXT D&C YELLOW NO. 1.Weight 2.5g of sample into a cellulose thimble and extract in Soxhlet extractor with ethyl ether for 4 hr. Transfer the extract to a 500-l separatory funnel, wash the extraction flask with two 10-ml portions of ethyl ether, and add the washings to the main extract. Shake the combined extract and washings with 30 ml of water made lakaline with sodium hydroxide. Transfer the ether layer to a beaker and evaporate nearly to dryness on a steam bath. Dissolve the residue in 20 ml of ethanol, transfer to a 100=ml vlumetric flask and dilute to volume with ethanol. Dilute 10 ml of this solution to 100 ml with ethanol. Determine the absorbance of the sample solution and a standard solution at 255, 285, and 315 nm.

$$\% \text{ diphenylamine} = \frac{(c)\left[(A_{285}) - \left(\frac{A_{225} + A_{315}}{2}\right)\right]}{(25)\left[(B_{285}) - \left(\frac{B_{225} + B_{315}}{2}\right)\right]}$$

where c = concentration of standard solution in g/liter

A = absorbance of sample solution at the indicated wave length

B = absorbance of standard solution at the indicated wavelength

LUECO CONENT OF TRIPHENYLMETHANE COLORS.Weigh a 0.5-g sample, tansfer to a 250-ml volumetric flask, and dilute to volume with water. Pipet a 10-ml aliquot of the solution into each of two 100-ml volumetric flasks. to the first flask, also add 15 ml of a freshly prepared solution consisting of 0.04 g of chloranil in 100 ml of *N,N*-dimethylformamide.

Place th flask in a boiling water bath for 60 min, cool, and dilute to a volume with water. dilute the aliquot in the second volumetric flask in volume with water. Pipet a 10-ml aliquot from each flask into separate 500-ml volumetric flasks, and dilute to volume with water. Measure the absorbance of each solution in a 1-cm cell at the absorption maximum.

$$\% \text{ leuco base} = \frac{(A - A_1)(100)}{(L)(c)(f)(a)}$$

where A = absorbance of the sample solution treated with chloranil

A_1 = absorbance of the untreated sample solution

L = length of cell path, in cm

e = effective sample concentration, in g/liter (= 0.004)

f = molecular weight of the color divided by the molecular weight of the leuco base

a = absorptivity of the color, liter/g-cm

Subsidiary and Isomeric Colors

Subsidiary colors are generally dyes which contain more than or less than the number of functional groups present in the parent compound eg, lower and higher sulfonated colors in FD&C Yellow No. 6, and lower iodinated colors in FD&C Red No. 3. Isomeric colors are those which have the same molecular weight as the parent dye but different molecular structures, eg. 2-(2-hydroxy-1-naphthylazo)-6-0 and -8-naphthalenesulfonic acids in D&C Red No. 11. Their presence or absence depends upon the quality of the intermediates used to prepare the dyes as well as the manufacturng process. Thus, they may be found in some samples of color and not in others. Subsidiary and isomeric colors usually have little practical effect on the apparent color of the dye but their amounts are controlled by the FDA. Too much or too many of them can prevent certification. The methods covered here reflect present analytical capabilities, rather than chief impurities found in certifiable colors.

FD&C Blues. FD&C Blue Nos. 1 and 2 may contain lower sulfonated compounds; in addition isatinsulfonic acid and 5,7'-disulfonated indigo may be found in FD&C Blue No. 2.

In the procedure which follows, lower sulfonated colors in FD&C Blue No. 1 are determined by spectrophotometric measurement after successive extractions.

Procedure

Prepare a salt-acetate solution by dissolving 125g of sodium chloride in water, adding 12 ml of glacial acetic acid and 100 ml of a 13.6% sodium acetate solution, and diluting to 500 ml.

Prepare a 0.1% aqueous sample solution. To a 10-ml aliquot add 40 ml of the salt-acetate solution and extract successively in three separatory funnels, each containing 100 ml of isoamyl alcohol. Wash the alcohol extracts with 100-ml portions of the salt-acetate solution until the washings are colorless. Pass each wash successively through the funnels in the same order as used above. Dilute the alcohol layers with one or more volumes of petroleum ether. Remove the dyes from the alcohol-ether mixtures by washing with several 10-ml portions of water. Pass each washing through the funnels as above. To the combined aqueous extracts add ammonium acetate to a concentration about 0.04 *N*. Determine the subsidiary colors present spectrophotometrically by comparison with the spectra of a standard solution of Guinea Green B_1 Cl No. 42085 (formerly FD&C Green No. 1).

The lower sulfonated colors may also be separated into fractions according to the degree of sulfonation. Two separation schemes are described in the literature (39). In the first scheme, the dye mixture is dissolved in water and the solution is made acidic. This solution is extracted with isoamyl alcohol which in turn is washed with several portions of 1:99 hydrochloric acid. The trisulfonated colors plus some of the disulfonated compounds pass into the aqueous solution as the mono-sulfonated and disulfonated compounds remain in the amyl alcohol. After dilution with petroleum ether the disulfonated compounds can be extracted with water.

If no trisulfonated compounds are present, another scheme can be applied. The dye mixture is first extracted with hot benzene; the unsulfonated compounds will be dissolved as the mono- and disulfonated substances remain in the residue. The disulfonated compounds (with traces of monosulfonated substances) can be extracted from the residue with hot water. The aqueous solution is acidified and extracted wth isoamyl alcohol, the alcohol extract is diluted with petroleum ether, and the disulfonated compounds are extracted with water. The monosulfonated colors remain in the alcohol-ether solution.

The isatinsulfonic acid, 5,7'-disulfonated indigo, and lower sulfonated compounds present in FD&C Blue No. 2 can be isolated by column chromatography and determined spectroscopically in the respective fractions. The recommended procedures follow.

Procedures

ISATINSULFONIC ACID. Prepare the eluant by dissolving 20g of potassium chloride in water, adding 10 ml of concentrated hydrochloric acid, and diluting with water to 100 ml. Slurry Solka-Floz BW-40 in the eluant and pack the slurry into a 40 × 2.5 cm column to a height of 6-8 in. Wash the column with 100 ml of eluant and drain the liquid to the top of the adsorbent.

Dissolve 0.01 g of sample in 10 ml of water. Add 1 ml of concentrated hydrochloric acid and 2 g of potassium chloride. Transfer the solution to the column with small portions of the eluant and elute with the eluant. Isatin moves rapidly down the column as a yellow band and can be seen at levels of 2% or more. Collect the fractions and determine the isatin spectrophotometrically at 250 nm.

5,7'-DISULFONATED INDIGO AND LOWER SULFONATED COLOR. Prepare a hydrocholoric acid-hydroxylamine hydrochoride solution by mixig 1 vol of concentrated hydrochloric acid ith 4 vol of 2.5% hydroxylamine hydrochloride solution. Just before use, wash 500 ml of a *n*-butanol with three 150-ml portions of 10% sodium hydroxide, and then with 1:49 hydrochloric acid until it becomes acidic. In a separatory funnel, mix 1 vol of the washed butanol with 2 vol of chloroform, and allow to settle. Use the lower layer as the mobile phase and the upper layer as the stationary phase.

Mix 5 ml of stationary phase with 8-9 g of Celite 545 previously dried for 12 hr at 135°C and pack the mixture in a 20×2.5 cm chromatographic column. Dissolve 0.005g of sample in 5ml of 1:4 hydrochloric acid, add 8-9 g of dried Celite, mix, and transfer the mixture to the top of the column.

Develop with the mobile phase. The lower sulfonated color elutes first and the isometric color elute ahead of the parent compound. Dilute the fraction containing the lower sulfonated color with an equal volume of chloroform and extract with two 10-ml portions of water. Combine the aqueous extracts and dilute to 25 ml with water. Similarly collect and extract 10-ml portions of water. Combine the aqueous extracts and dilute to 25 ml with water. Similarly collect and extract the fraction containing the isomeric color. Dilute necessary.

Determine each color spectrophotometrically. Compare the spectra of the lower sulfonated color with that of a standard solution of FD&C Blue No. 2.

FD&C Green No. 3. This dye may contain lower sulfonated compounds as impurities. They are determined by the procedure given for FD&C Blue No. 1.

FD&C Reds. FD&C Red No. 2 may contain the sodium salts of 1-(4-sulfo-1-naphthylazo-2-naphthol-6- and -8-monosulfonic, -6.8-disulfonic, and -3,68-trisulfonic acids, 1-naphthylazo)-2-naphthol-3,6-disulfonic acid, and 2-(4-sulfo-1-naphtylazo)-1-naphthylamine-4-sulfonic acid. By using the paper chromatographic method for FD&C Yellow No. 5, they can be separated as groups (isomeric, lower, and higher sulfonated compounds) from the parent compound (41). In addition, two methods employing column chromatography are given below; Method 1 is used to determine the disodium salts of four lower sulfonated compounds (9); Method 2 is used for the tetrasodium salt of the 3,8-trisulfonic acid (CI No. 16290) and the trisodium salt of the 6,8-disulfonic acid (CI No. 16255). A paper chromatographic method for mono- and disulfonic acids is also available.

Procedures

Method 1. Extract 150 ml of *n*-butanol with three 50-ml portions of 10% sodium hydroxide, and then wash the butanol with 50-ml portions of water until neutral. Mix 100 ml of the washed butanol with 100 ml of carbon tetrachloride in a separatory funnel, and add 100 ml of 1:19 hydrochloric acid containing 20 mg/ml hydroxylamine hydrochloride. Shake the mixture for 3 min, then allow the layers to separate. Use the upper layer as the stationary, and the lower layer as the mobile phase.

Mix 10g of Celite 545 with 5 ml of the stationary phase, and firmly pack the mixture into a 45 × 2.5 cm chromatographic column.

Dissolve 0.05 g of sample in 25 ml of the stationary phase, mix a 5-ml aliquot of this solution with 10g of Celite, and pack the mixture on the top of the column. Elute with the mobile phase, and collect the desired fractions. Dilute them to 25 ml with the mobile phase and determine the amount of color spectrophotometrically, using the disodium salt of 1-(4-slfo-1-naphthylazo)-2-naphthol-6-sulfonic acid as the standard.

Method 2. Fill a 90 × 2.5 cm chromatographic column to a height of about 60 cm with an aqueous slurry of Solka Floe BW-40, and wash the column with 200 ml of 55 aqueous sodium chloride.

Dissolve 0.5 g of sample in 100 ml of 5% aqueous sodium chloride solution, transfer a 5-ml aliquot to the column, and elute with 5% sodium chloride solution. The tetrasodium salt elutes first followed by the trisodium salt.

Collect each fraction separately, and determine the colors specterophotometrically.

The separation and determination of lower iodinated substances in FD&C Red No. 3 is possible with paper and column chromatography.

Procedures

PAPER CHROMATOGRAPHY. Mix 400 ml of methyl ethyl ketone, 100 ml of acetone, 100 ml of water, and 1 ml of concentrated ammonium hydroxide; use this mixture as the eluant. Place two 3-in wide blotting-paper drapes in a 18 × 6 in. tank, one on each side, add the eluant in the tank and allow time to equilibrate.

Prepare a 0.1% sample solution in 2:98 ammonium hydroxide. Apply a 0.1-ml aliquot in a 0.5 × 2.5 in. band to a 3-in. wide Schleicher & Schuell No. 2043 chromatographic paper, 1.5 in from the bottom of the strip. Suspend the strip in the tank so that the lower edge dips 0.5 in. into the eluant. Develop for 6 hr protected from light. Remove the strip and dry in the dark. Extract each spot from the chromatogram with small amounts of 1:199 ammonium hydroxide. Dilute as needed, filter, and determine the individual colors spectrophotometrically. The order of elution, absorption maxima, and approximate absorptivities of the disodium salts are listed below:

Order of elution	Color	Absorption maximum, nm	Absorptivity of disodium salts
1	2,4,5,7-tetraoidofluorescein	527-530	108 (for monohydrate)
2	2,4,7-triiodofluorscein	517-520	140
3	2,4,5-triiodofluorescein	516-519	116
4	2,7-diiodofluorescein	511-513	179
	2,5-diiodofluorescein	509-511	145
5	4,5-diiodofluorescei	507-509	122
6	2-iodofluorescein	501-503	193
7	4-iodofluorescein	497-500	154
8	fluorescein	491-493	228

COLUMN CHROMATOGRAPHY. Prepare ethanol wash solution by diluting 75 ml of 95% ethanol to 100 ml with water. Prepare 1 liter of each of the following eluants:

eluant No. 1: 25% aqueos sodium chloride solution containing 5 ml of concentrated ammonium hydroxide per liter.

eluant No. 2: 2% aqueous sodium sulfate solution containing 5 ml of concentrated ammonium hydroxide per liter.
eluant No. 3 1% aqueous sodium sulfate solution containing 5 ml of concentrated ammonium hydroxide per liter
eluant No. 4 1:199 ammonium hydroxide
eluant No. 5 add 5 ml of concentrated ammonium hydroxide to 000 ml of 95% ethanol and dilute with water to 1 liter.

Use a glass chromatographic column equipped at the top with the eluant distribution system as shown in Figure 25. Fill the tube with 3 in. of water; add 0.5g of dry Whatman Column Chromedia CF11 and allow to settle. Add a slurry of 16g of Solka Floe BW-100 in 150 ml of water to the column. Open the outlet and drain the liquid nearly to the top of the packing. Add 100 ml of eluant No. 1 washing the cellulose from the sides of the tube and keeping a level surface on the column. Drain the liquid to about 1 in. above the column packing. Wrap the 1-in diameter section of the column with aluminum foil to protect the sample from light.

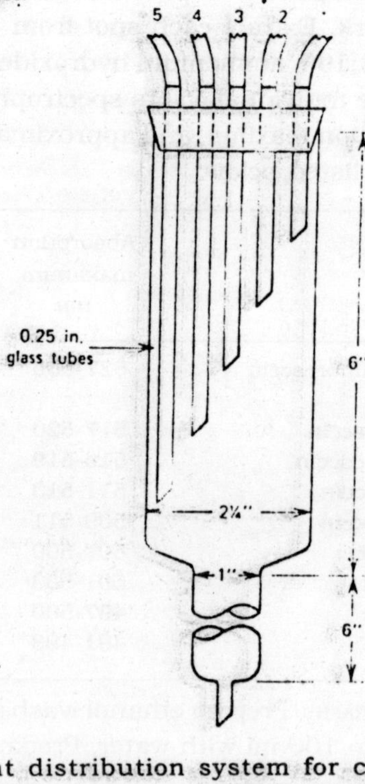

Fig. 25. Eluant distribution system for column chromatographic determiknation of the imparities of FD&C Red No. 3.The numbers above the inlet tubes refer to the serial number of the respective eluant

Dissolve a 0.1-g sample in 100 ml of 1:199 ammonium hydroxide. Pipet tml of the sample solution onto the column, mixing it with the eluant present and taking care not to disturb the surface of the packing. Drain the solution just to the packing surface. Carefully wash down the sides of the tube with eluant No. 1 and draininto the column. Add 20 ml of eluant No. and about 3 g of the Chromedia to the column. When the cellulose has settled to form a protective cap over the surface, fill the column with eluant No. 1. Place the remaining eluant No. 1 in a flask and connect to tube No. 1. Place eluants Nos. 2-5 in suitable flasks and connect to the appropriate tubes. Elute the column successively with eluants Nos. 1-5. Collect the individual bands eluted and determine the individual colors spectrophotometrically. The order of elution and the identity of the subsidiary colors are as follows:

eluant No. 1	band 1	unidentified color
	band 2	fluorescein
eluant No. 2	band 3	mixture of 2 and 4-monoiodofluoresceins
	band 4	mixture of 2,4-, 2,5-, and 2,7-diiiodofluoresceins
eluant No. 3	band 5	mixture of 4,5-diiodofluorescein and 2,4,7-triiodofluorescein
	band 6	2,4,5-triiodofluorescein
eluant No. 4	band 7	2,4,5,7-tetraiodofluorescein
eluant No. 5	band 8	undentified color

The amount of the individual colors can be estimated with reasonable accuracy if it is assumed that their absorptivities equal that of FD&C Red No. 3.

FD&C Red No. 4 may contain 2-(2,4-xylyazo)-1-naphthol-4-sulfonic acid and 2-(5-sulfo-2,4-xylylazo)-1-naphthol, which are lower sulfonated colors. These can be separated from the main color by paper chromatography using the procedure on p. 518 for FD&C Yellow No. 6) or by the following modification of Method 1 given for FD&C Red No. 2.

Procedure

Using the procedure given in Method 1 for FD&C Red No. 2, substituting 1:40 hydrochloric acid for 1:19 hydrochloric acid prepare and elute the column and collect the colored leading edge of the mobile phase.

If the eluate is red, dilute it to 25 ml with the mobile phase and determine the color spectrophotometrically vs a standard solution of 2-(2-(2,4-xylyazo)-1-naphthol-4-sulfonic acid. If the eluate is yellow, transfer it to a separatory funnel and add an equal volume of chloroform. Wash the two 10-ml portions of 10% ammonium sulfate solution. Add a second volume of chloroform and extract it with two 10-ml potions of 10% ammonium sulfate solution containing 10 mg/ml of sodium hydroxide. Adjust the aqueous extract to 25 ml with the extracting solution and determine the color spectrophotometrically vs a standard solution of 2-(5-sulfo-2,4-xylylazo)-1-naphthol.

In addition to the lower sulfonated colors, 2-(4-sulfo-1-naphthylazo)-1-naphthol-, 2-(3-sulfo-2,6-xylylazo)-1-naphthol-, and 2-(6-sulfo-2,4-xylylazo)-1-naphthol-4-sulfonic acids may be present in FD&C Red No. 4. These three subsidiary colors can be separated from the main color by the procedures given below. The last compound can also be separated from FD&C Red No. 4 by paper chromatography using 200:88:2:40 butanol-water-ammonium hydroxide-ethanol or 300:150:5:80 butanol-water-acetic acid-ethanol as the eluant.

Procedures

2-(4-SULFO-2-NAPHTHYLAZO)-1-NAPHTHOL-4-SULFONIC ACID. Prepare the eluant by dissolving 50g of sodium chloride in water containing 0.5 ml of concentrated ammonium hydroxide and diluting to 1 liter. Slurry Solka Floc BW-40 in water, pack two 1-in, chromatographic columns 12 in. high with the slurry, and wash each with 50 ml of the eluant.

Dissolve 0.025 of sample in 10 ml of water and add it to the first column. When the color settles on the column, wash it with the eluant until most of the FD&C Red No. 4 is eluted. Strip the remaining color from the column with water and collect. Add 20 g of solid sodium chloride to each 100 ml of the color solution and transfer it to the second column. Elute the FD&C Red NO. 4 with the eluant, then elute the subidiay color with water and determmine it spectrophotometrically.

2-(3-SULFO-2,6-XYLYLAZO)-1-NAPHTHOL-4-SULFONIC ACID. Prepare the eluant by dissolving 800 g of anyhydrous sodium sulfate in 5 litres of 0.2*M* hydochloride acid. Slurry powdered cellulose (Whatman Column Chromedia CF 11 or quivalent) in the eluant, pour sufficient slurry into a 24 × 2 in. chromatographic column to make a 15 in. bed, and wash the column with 100 ml of the eluant.

Prepare a 0.5% aqueous sample solution and pipet a 20-ml aliquot onto the column. Elute the column with the eluant; collect the fractions containing the subsidiary color, which elutes before FD&C Red No. 4 Saturate these fractions with sodium sulfate and pass the resulting solution through a 1-in diameter columnpacked with a 3-in bed of cellulose. Elute the color with 100 ml of water and determine it spectrophotometrically vs a standard solution.

2(6-SULFO-2,4-XYLYLAZO)-1-NAPHTHOL-4-SULFONIC ACID. Slurry Solka Floe BW-40 in water, pack a 1-in. diameter chromatographic column 12-in. high with the slurry, and wash it ith 50 ml of a 20% sodium sulfate solution. Prepare a 0.5% aqueous sample solution, pipet a 10-ml aliquot ono the column. Elute with 20% sodium sulfate solution. FD&C Red No. 4 is quantitatively adsorbed. Collect the fractions and determine the color spectrophotometrically vs a standard solution.

FD&C Violet No. 1. The subsidiary dyes in this color consist of lower and higher sulfonated compounds. They may be determined by the method given below.

Procedure

Prepare a 0.20% aqueous sample solution. Take a 5-ml aliquot and add 45 ml of 1:99 hydrochloric acid. Extract is successively in three separatory funnels, each containing 50 ml of isoamyl alcohol. Wash the alcohol extract with 50-ml portions of 1:99 hydrochloric acid until the washings are colorless. Pass each wash portion successively through the funnels as above. Combine the original hydrochloric acid solution and any colored washings.

Dilute the isoamyl alcohol layer with two volumes of petroleum ether. Wash this mixture with 20-ml portions of water until the washings are colorless. Combine the alcohol ether layer and evaporate them on a steam bath to 50 ml.

Immediately determine the higher sulfonated colors in the hydrochloric acid solution, and the lower sulfonated colors in the condensed alcohol-ether layers spectrophotometrically, against a standard solution of FD&C Violet No. 1.

FD&C Yellows. The subsidiary dyes which may be present in FD&C Yellow No. 5 include the disodium salts of 3-carboxy-5-hydroxy-1-*p*-sulfophenylazopyrazole and 3-carboxy-5-hydroxy-1-*p*-sulfophenyl-4-phenylzophyrazole, lower sulfonated compounds, and the ethyl ester of the parent color. The lower sulfonated compounds can be separated from the parent color either by extraction or column chromatography; the latter method is a modification of Method 1 described for FD&C Red No. 2. The lower sulfonated colors and the ethyl ester of the parent compound can be separated from the parent compound by paper chromatography. In neither procedure are the two lower sulfonated compounds separated from each other. The three methods at next page.

Extraction Method. Dissolve 0.2g of sample in 100 ml of water; heat on a steam bath if necessary. To 50 ml of this solution and 1 ml of concentrated hydrochloric acid and extract the solution successively in three separatory funnels,each containing 50ml of amyl alcohol. Wash the alcohol extacts by shaking successively with 30-ml portions of 0.25*N* hyrochloric acid until the washings are practically colorless. Pass each acid portion through the funnels in the order used for the original alcohol extraction. Dilute the alcohol extracts in each funnel with 1-2 vol of petroleum ether and extract the lower sulfonated colors by washing with several 10-20 ml portions of water. Pass each portions through the funnels in reverse order to that previosly followed. Transfer the water solution to a 100-ml volumetric flask, add about 1 g of solid ammonium acetate, and dilute to a volume with water. Determine the compounds present spectrophotometrically at 434 nm vs a standard.

Column Chromatographic Method. Using the procedure given in Method 1 for FD&C Red No. 2, prepare and elute the desired fraction from the column. Dilute the eluate with 2 vol of chloroform and extract it with two 10-ml portions of water. Add 1 ml of 1:39 hydrochloric cid to the combined aqueous extracts, adjust the volume to25 ml with water, and determine the color spectrophotometrically vs a standard.

Paper Chromatographic Method. Prepare a eluant by mixing 70 vol of methylethy ketone, 30 vol of acetone, and 30 vol of water. Use a tank suitable for ascending chromatography and saturate its atmosphere with the eluant. Prepare a 1% aqueous sample solution and apply 0.1ml within a 18cm × 0.7cm rectangle, 2.5 cm from the bottom of a 20 × 20 cm sheet of Whatman No. 1 chromatographic paper. Allow the paper to dry at or below 50°C. Mount the sheet in the tank so that the eluant is 1 cm below the baseline of the sheet. Elute to a height of 17.5 cm or until the separation is satisfactory. Visually compare the chromatogram with known similarly prepared or extract the colors from the paper and make a spectrophotometric determination.

The subsidiary dyes present in FD&C Yellow No. 6 are lower or higher sulfonated compounds of similar structure. The disodium salts of 1-(4-sulfophenylazo)-2-naphthol and 1-(phenylazo)-2-naphthol-6-sulfonic acid belong to the former category; the trisodiumsalts of 1-(4-sulfophenylazo)-2-naphthol-3,6- and -6,8-disulfonic acids belong to the latter. The lower sulfonic acids can be separated from the parent compound by Method 1 given for FD&C Red No. 2 (usng 1:49 hydrochloric acid) or by an extraction method (1). The higher sulfonated compounds can be separated from the parent compound by extraction or chromatographic procedures. Neither of these methods separates the impurities from each other. The three procedures are given below.

Procedures

LOWER SULFONATED COLORS—EXTRACTION METHOD. Dissolve 0.2g of sample in 20 ml of water, add 1 ml of concentrated hydrochloric acid, and dilute to 50 ml. Extract by shaking the solution successively in three separatory funnels, each containing 50 ml of amyl alcohol. Wash the alcohol extracts with 50-ml portions of 5% aqueous sodium chloride solution until the washings are colorless. Dilute each alcohol layer with 100 ml of petroleum ether and extract the lower sulfonated dye with several 10-ml portions of water. Pass each portion through the funnels in the reverse order to that previously followed. Combine the aqueous extracts in a 100-ml volumetric flask, add 1 ml of 2 *N* ammonium acetate solution and dilute to volume with water. Determine the lower sulfonated colors present spectrophotometrically at 485 nm vs a standard solution of D&C Orange No. 4.

HIGHER SULFONATED COLORS—EXTRACTION METHOD. Dissolve 0.1g of sample in 100 ml of 1:25 hydrochloric acid. Dilute 10 ml of this solution with 40 ml of 1:25 hydrochloric acid. Extract by shaking the solution successively in five separatory funnels, each containing 50 ml of isoamyl alcohol. Transfer the acid layer to a 100-ml volumetric flask. Wash the alcohol extracts with two 25-ml portions of 1:25 hyrochloric acid passing each portions through the funnels in the same order used for the original extraction. Add the washing to the acid layer in the flask and dilute to 100ml with water. Determine the higher fulfonated colors spectrophotometrically vs a standard.

HIGHER SULFONATED COLORS—CHROMATOGRAPHIC METHOD. In a separatory funnel, mix 100 ml of *n*-butanol and 100 ml of carbon tetrachloride. Add 100 ml of 1:4 hydrochloric acid, shake for 3 min and allow to settle. Use the lower layer as the stationary and the upper layer as the mobile phase. Prepare silane-treated Celite by adding 25 ml of General Electric GS-77 Dri Film to the bottom of an empty desiccator, placing a dish containing 200g of Celite 545 into the desiccator, and leaving it covered for least 3 hr. Test completion of the silanization by mixing a small amount of the treated Celite with water: the Celite should not be wetted.

Mix 15 g of the treated Celite with 7.5 ml of the stationary phase and pack the mixture into a 45 2.5 cm chromatographic column. Dissolve 0.05g of sample in 25 ml of the mobile phase. Transfer a 5-ml aliquot of this solution to the top of the column and elute with the mobile phase. the higher sulfonated colors will elute as one band before the parent compound. Determine their content in the fractions spectrophotometrically against a standard.

The lower and higher sulfonated compounds can be determined in one step by paper chromatography according to the method given in FD&C Yellow No. 5 except that a mixture of 350 vol of methyl ethyl ketone, 150 vol of acetone, 150 vol of water, and 1 vol of concentrated ammonium hydroxide is used as the eluant. The higher sulfonated compounds are separated from each other, but the lower sulfonated compounds are not.

*D&C Blue No. 4.*This color is analyzed for lower sulfonated colors. The method recommended is identical to the one given on p. 511 for FD&C Blue No. 1.

D&C Green No. 5. This color is analyzed for monosulfonated compounds by bromide-bromate titration after a preliminary separation by extraction.

Procedures

Weight 10g of sample and transfer to a 250-ml Erlenmeyer flask. Add 50 ml of a 10:2:1 glacial acetic acid-concentrated hydrochloric acid water mixture and 10 ml of a stannous chloride solution in concentrated hydrochloric acid with a stannous chloride concentration of 0.5g/ml.

Boil gently until the volume is reduced to about 25 ml, then dilute the hot mixture with 100 ml of water. Transfer to a 500-ml volumetric flask and dilute to volume with water. Filter a 100-ml aliquot into a 500-ml extraction funnel; make it alkaline with 25ml of 50% sodium hydroxide solution, cooling the funnel during the addition. Extract the liberated amine with two 100-ml portions of water. Extract the amine with five 25-ml portions of 0.3N hydrochloric acid and transfer the washings to an iodination flask.

Boil to expel the dissolved ether, concentrate to 100 ml, then cool. Add 25 ml of 0.3 *N* hydrochloric acid and about 100 g of crushed ice. Add 0.05 *N* potassium bromide-bromate to the agitating solution until it remains yellow for at least 30 sec, then add 5 ml of in excess. Stopper the flask and let is stand in an ice bath for 10 min.Add 2-3 g of potassium iodide and titrate while cold with 0.05 *N* sodium thiosulfate to a starch end point. Perform a blank determination. Calculate the result as *p*-toluidine; 1 ml of 0.05 *N* potassium bromide-bromate is equivalent to 1.34 mg of *p*-toluidine. Calculate the amount of monosulfonated dye present in the sample as follows:

$$\text{Monosulfonated dye, wt \%} = \frac{(W)(4.858)(100)}{w}$$

Where W = amount of *p*-toluidine, in mg
w = sample weight, in mg

D&C Oranges. D&C Orange No. 4 is analyzed for a lower sulfonated compound, possibly 1-(phenylazo)-2-naphthol, by column chromatography. The procedure is identical to Method 2 given for FD&C Red No. 2 except for some modifications in the two phases; 100 ml of the washed *n*-utanol is mixed with 100 ml of carbon tetrachloride and 100 ml of water; after separation, the upper layer is used as the stationary phase and the lower layer as the mobile phase.

The subsidiary colors present i D&C Orange No. 5 consist of related bromofluoresceins. They can be separated and determined by the following two-dimensional paper chromatographic procedure. Figure 26 shows the chromatogram obtained.

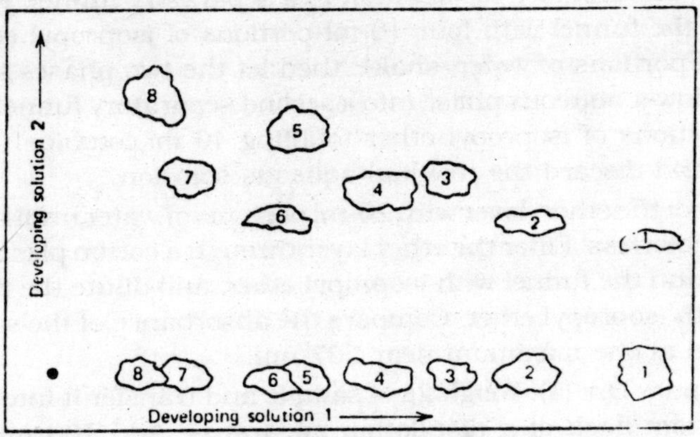

Fig. 26. Paper chromatographic separation of fluorescein and nine bromofluoresceins. 1. Fluorescein. 2. 2-Bromofluorescein and 4-bromofluorescein. 3. 2,7-Dibromfluorescein. 4. 2,4-Dibromofluorescein and 2,5-dibromofluorescein. 5. 2,4,7-Tribromofluorescein. 6. 4,5-Dibromofluorescein. 7. 2,4,5-Tribromofluorescein. 8. 2,4,5,7-Tetrabromofluorescein. The black dot in the lower left corner shows the initial spot fo the sample containg 0.033 mg of each compound.

Procedure

Prepare a 1% ammonical sample solution and spot 5 µl on a 18 × 22 in Whatman No. 1 chromatographic paper, about 1 in. from the edges. Immerse the 18 in. edge of the paper in an eluant composed of 1 g of sodium chooride and 1 ml of concentrated ammonium hydroxide dissolved in 100 ml of water (solution 1). Develop for 24hr. Remove the sheet from the tank, air dry it in the dark, then rotate it 90° and develop for an additional 48 hr inaneluant composed of 100 ml of solution 1,300 ml of *n*-butanol, and 70 ml of ethanol. Leach the spots from the paper with1:99 ammonium hydroxide and determine the individual compounds spectrophotometrically.

D&C Reds. Some of the D&C Red colors have a similar structure; thus the methods of analysis for subsidiary and isomeric dyes are identical in a number of cases.

4-Toluene-azo-2-naphthol-3-carboxylic acid and a subsidiary dye inD&C Reds No. 6 and 7 maybe determined as follows:

Procedures

4-TOLUENE-AZO-2-NAPHTHOL-3-CARBOXYLIC ACID. Place 0.25 g of sample in a 125-ml acetylation flask. Add 80 l of methyl Cellosolve and 5 ml of concentrated hydrochloric acid, attach an air condenser, and eflux for 15-20 min. Transfer the solution to a separatory funnel. Rinse the flask into the funnel with four 10-ml portions of isopropyl ether and two 75-ml portions of water, shake, then let the two phases separate. Drain the lower aqueous phase into a second separatory funnel, extract it with portions of isopropyl ether totalling 40 ml,combine the ether extracts, and discard the residual aqueous solution.

Extract the ether layer with 20-ml portions of water until the water extract is colorless. Filter the ether layer through a cotton pledget, rinse the coton and the funnel with isopropyl ether, and dilute the filtrate to 100 ml with isopropyl ether. Compare the absorbance of the sample vs a standard at the maximum near 507 nm.

SUBSIDIARY DYE (1). Weigh 2g of sample and transfer it into a q-liter round bottom flask of a distillation apparatus. Add 100 ml of 10% sodium hydroxide solution. 25 ml of methyl Cellosolve, and 10g of sodium hydrosulfite. Attach an adapter to the condenser and add 25 ml of 1:4 hydrochloric acid to the receiving flask. Start distillation. After aout 50 ml of distillate is collected slowly add 150 ml of water to the flask, at a rate equal to the distillation, then continue the distillation until the total volume is 300 ml. Transfer this solution to a 500-ml iodine flask and concentrate to 100 ml. Cool, then add 20 ml of hydrochloric acid and 100 g of crushed ice. Continue the procedure as given on p. 519 for D&C Green No. 5 starting with "Add 0.05 *N* potassium bromide-bromate...;" 1 ml of 0.05 potassium bromide-bromate is equivalent to 4.10mg of the subidiary dye.

A subsidiary dye frequently present in D&C Reds No. 8 and 9 is 4-(4-chloro-2-sulfo-5-tolylazo)-1-naphthol. It is determined by the following procedure:

Procedure

Transfer a 0.1-g sample to a 600-ml beaker. Add 100 ml of ethanol, 20 ml of 10% sodium hydroxide solution, and 80 ml of water. Cover, then boil gently for 5 min. Remove from the heat and add dropwise hydrochloric acid until the solution is acidic. Then, make it basic by the dropwise addition of a 2% ethanolamine solution and add 2 ml in excess. Evaporate to 100 ml on a hot plate, then add 100 ml of a 2% ethanolamine solution, bring to a boil, cool and filter.

Return the filter paper with the precipitate to the beaker and leach with a stream of 5:1 ethanol-10% sodium hydroxide solution. Add 80 ml of water, then dilute to 200 ml with the 5:1 ethanol-10% sodium hydroxide solution. Boil, adjust the pH, and filter as above. Combine the filtrates.

Transfer the filtrates to a 500-ml separatory funnel and acidify with about 15 ml of hydrochloric acid. Extract the dye with 75 ml of isoamyl alcohol and discard the aqueous layer. Wash the alcohol layer twice by shaking it with 50-ml portions of a 5% sodium chloride solution. Add 50 ml of isooctane to the alcohol layer and extract it with 50 ml of aqueous solution containing 1g of ethanolamine and 2.5g of sodium chloride. Repeat with 25-ml portions of the same solution until no more color is extracted. Combine the extracts in a 250-ml volumetric flask and dilute to volume with a solution of 2% ethanolamine in 5% sodium chloride. Determne the amount of dye present spectrophotometrically by comparison with a standard.

D&C Reds Nos. 10-13 may contain the subidiary dye 1-(naphthylazo)-2-naphthol, and the isomeric compounds 2-(2-hydroxyl-1-naphthylazo)-6- and -8-naphthalene-sulfonic acids. Methods for their determination follow. The two isomeric compounds are determined jointly.

Procedures

1-(NAPHTHYLAZO)-2-NAPHTHOL. Extract 0.1 g of the sample in a Soxhlet extractor with 100 ml of benzene until the leachings are practically colorless. Evaporate the extract to dryness. Dissolve the residue in ethanol and determine the color spectrophotometrically by comparison with a standard.

ISOMERIC COMPOUNDS Reflux0.25g of sample for 3 hr with 50 ml of acetic acid and 25 ml of 8 *N* hydrochloric acid, then cool to room temperature. Using small portions of ethyl ether, transfer the mixture to a 500-ml separatory funnel. Add 100 ml of ethyl and shake. Add 200 ml of water to separate the partially miscible solution into two layers.

Transfer the lower layer to a second separatory funnel and shake with 100 ml of ethyl ether. Transfer the lower layer to a third funnel and extract with 40 ml of isoamyl alcohol. Discard the lower acidic layer and reserve the alcohol extract.

Wash the ether extracts (the upper layers in the original extraction) colorless with portions of water totalling 40 ml using the same rotation for washings as used for the original extraction. Combine the aqueous washings and extract the dye with the retained 40 ml of isoamyl alcohol solution. Wash the alcohol extract twice with 30-ml portions of water, transfe the clored solution to a beaker, rinsing the funnel into the beaker with 5ml of isoamyl alcohol, and place on a steam bath to remove the dissolved ether. Filter the solution through cotton and dilute it to 50 ml with isoamyl alcohol. Determine the combined isomeric compounds spectro-photometrically at 495nm by comparison with a standard solution.

D&C Red No. 17 contains as impurities 1-(phenylazo)-2-naphthol (PAN) and an unidentified red substance; a thin-layer chromatographic procedure is recommended. PAN is also present in D&C Red No. 31, and can be separated by extraction.

Procedures

For D&C Red No. 17. Prepare a 2.5% solution of the sample in chloroform and apply a 0.2 ml aliquot across a 20 cm × 20 cm glass plate coated with a silica gel G layer, 0.375 mm thick. Develop the plate with toluene in a lined chromatographic tank until the solvent front reaches the top of the plate. Remove the plate and air dry. If the orange-yellow line of PAN is not adquately resolved from the D&C Red No. 17, repeat the elution. If PAN is separated from the D&C Red No. 17 but mixed with an unknown, scrape the commingled colors from the plate leach with chloroform, evaporate to 0.1-0.2 ml, and apply this solution to a 10cm × 10cm silica gel G plate, 0.375 mm thick. Develop the plate with methylene chloride. Leach the compounds from the plate with chloroform and determine spectrophotometrically, by comparison with a standard.

For D&C Red No,. 31. Extract 0.1g of sample in a Soxhlet extractor with 100 ml of benzene until the leachings are colorless or have a slight persistent bleed. Transfer the extract to a separatory funnel and wash with 1% sodium hydroxide solution until the washings are colorless. Wash the benzene layer alkali-free with 50-ml portions of water then evaporate the benzene solution to dryness. Dissolve the residue in ethanol, adjust the volume of the solution and determine the PAN spectrophotometrically by comparison with a standard.

D&C Red No. 19 may contain triethylrhodamine and a number of other subsidiarydyes present in small quantities. They are separated from the parent compound by column chromatography. Nine distinct bands are separated, triethylrhodamine elutes just before the parent compound

Procedure

Prepare silane-treated Celite as described in the procedure FD&C Yellow No. 6. Slurry 20g of the treated Celite with 18 ml of n-decanol which has been equilibrated with 1:99 ammonium hydroxide, then pack the slurry tightly into a 1-in diameter chromatographic column.

Dissolve 0.05 g of sample in 5 ml of water, add 1 drop of concentrated ammonium hydroxide, and add the solution to the column. Dilute with 1:99 ammonium hydroxide and collect 20-ml fractions. Determine the amount of triethylrhodamine in the specified fraction spectrophotometrically, at 540 nm, against a standard solution.

D&C Red No. 21 may contain a number of lower brominated compounds of similar structure. They are separated from the parent compound by paper chromatography.

Procedure

Weigh 2 g of sample and transfer it to a 100-ml volumetric flask. Add 50 ml of a solvent prepared by mixing 50 ml of No. 1 ethanol, 35 ml of water, and 15 ml of concentrated ammonium hydroxide. Shake, and warm if necessary. After solution, dilute to volume with the solvent. Apply 0.1 ml of sample solution to a 3 × 16 in. Schleicher & Schuell No. 2043 chromatographic paper and let it dry in the dark. Suspend the srip in a 18 in. × 6 in. ID glass tank, and develop in the dark for 24-48 hr by the ascendig technique using 100:44:1:22.5 *n*-butanol-water-ammonium hydrosixe-ethanol. Remove the strip and dry in the dark. Wash each colored zone into separate volumetric flasks using 1:199 ammonium hydroxide, filter of centrifuge if necessary, and determine the individual substances spectrophotometrically. Their absorption maxima and approximate absorptivities are listed below:

	Asborption maximum, nm	Absorptivity, liter/g-cm
fluorescein	492	258
4-monobromofluorescein	498	206
2,4-and 2,5-dibromofluorescein	506	188
4,5-di-bromofluorescein	504	163
2,4,5-tribromofluorescein	512	157
2,4,57-tetrabromofluorescein	518	149

D&C Red No. 22 may contain uranine (D&C Yellow No. 8) as an impurity; D&C Red No. 33 may have Chromotrope 2R and an unidentified blue color. These impurities are determined by column chromatography according to the procedures given at the next page.

Procedures

FOR D&C RED NO. 22. Slurry 20g of Solka Floc SW-40-A in 800 ml of water, pack it in a 120 × 2.2 cm chromatographic column, and wash the column with 50 ml of 5% sodium sulfate solution. Prepare a 0.3% aqueous sample solution and pipet a 5-l aliquot into a beaker. Add 0.1 ml of 10% sodium hydroxide solution and 1g of anhydrous sodium sulfate, dilute to 20 ml with water, and then add, with stirring, 0.5g of Sola Flc. Transfer the mixture to the top of the column with small portions of 5% sodium sulfate solution, and elute the uranine with this solution. Make the eluate alkaline,with sodium hydroxide and determine the uranine spectrophotometrically at 490 nm.

FOR D&C RED NO. 33.Prepare a Solka Floc slurry as above, pack it in a 100x2 cm chromatographic column to a settled height of 50cm, then wash the column with a 20% sodium chloride solution. Prepare a 0.1% aqueous sample solution. To a 5-ml aliquot, add 20 ml of a 20% sodium chloride solution; transfer it to the column with the sodium chloride solution. Elute the column with 10% sodium chloride solution containing 1% ammonium hydroxide. Chromotrope 2R elutes first followed by the parent compound; the blue dye remains at the top of the column. When the Chromotrope band is separated by about 10 cm from the main band, change the eluant t a 5% sodium chloride solution cntaining 1% ammonium hydroxide. Neutralise the fractions with acetic acid and determine the individual dyes spectrophotometrically by comparison with standard solutions.

D&C YELLOW NO. 10. This color may contain the following higher sulfonated and isomeric compounds: 2-(2-quinolyl-6-sulfonic acid)-1, 3-indandione-5-sulfonic acid, 2-2-quinolyl-S-sulfonic acid)-1,3-indandione--sulfonic acid, 2-(2-quinolyl-6,8-disulfonic acid)-1,3-indandione-5-sulfonic acid, 2-(2-quinolyl-6,8-disulfonic acid)-1,3-indandione, 2-(2-quinolyl-6-sulfonic acid)-1,3-indandione and 2-(2-quinolyl-8-sulfonic acid)-1,3-indandione. These colors are separated from each other and the parent compounded by column chromatography, using a 2.5% solution of tri-isooctylamine in *n*-butanol as the stationery phase, and 1:9 hydrochloric acid equilibrated with the stationary phase s the mobile phase.Silanized Celite 545, which has been dried in a desiccator over dichlorodimethylsilane for 24 hr, is used as the support material. The individual compounds emerge in the order given above and they are determined in the respective fractions by their ultraviolet spectra.

Determination in Mixtures

Colors in Foods and Drug. The following liquid chromatographic method is used for all FD&C color. Recovery is high (about 90%) except FD&C Blue No. 2.

Procedures

REAGENTS. *Resin-Hexane.* Dissolve 50 ml of Rohm and Haas Aberlite LA-resin in 950 ml of *n*-hexane. Shake the solution with 200 ml of 1:4 acetic acid. Discard the lower phase.

Resin-Butanol. Dissolve 100 ml of Amberlite LA-2resin in 900 ml of butanol. Shake the solution with 400 ml of 1:4 acetic acid and 15ml of water saturated with amonium sulfate. Discard the lower phase.

pH 7.5 buffer. Mix 75 ml of 0.1 *M* citric acid with 925 ml of 0.2 *M* Na_2HPO_4.

Resin-Butanol, pH 7.5. Dissolve 50ml of Amberlite LA-2 resin in 950 ml of butanol and 3.0 ml of glacial acetic acid. Shake the solution with 400 ml of the pH 7.5 buffer. The pH of the lower phase should be 7.3-7.7. If it is not, repeat the preparation adjusting the amount of acetic acid. Discard the lower phase.

pH 3.0 buffer. Mix 11.5 ml of 0.2 *N* hydrochloric cid and 250 ml of 0.2 *M* potassium acid phthalate solution. Dilute to 1 liter.

Resin-Butanol, pH 3.0. Mix 50 ml of Amberlite LA-2 resin, 950 ml of butanol, and 8.0 of concentrated hydrochloric acid. Shake the mixture with three successive 200-ml portions of the pH 3.0 bufer. the pH of the aqueous phase should be 2.8-3.2. If it is not, repeat the preparation adjusting the amount of hydrochloric acid used.

SAMPLE PREPARATION. Weight 5 g of sample into a tissue blender. The sample should contain 0.2 mg or more of each color but no more than 5 mg of total color. Add 25 ml of 1:4 acetic acid and blend into a fine mixture. Transfer the suspensions to a mortar and grind in about 5g of Celite. Add more Celite as necessary to give the proper texture for the particular sample. The mixture should be wet enough to pack under pressure but dry enough to crumble when disturbed. With many samples the entire sample preparation can be done in a mortar.

CHROMATOGRAPHIC SEPARATION. Mix 20 g of Celite and 8 ml of 1:4 acetic acid. Pack about 15 g of the mixture into a 5.2 cm ID x 20.0 cm glass chromatographic column. Transfer the sample onto the column and pack. Flush the mortar with the remaining Celite-acid mixture, transfer it to the column, and pack. Cover the surface with a porous disc. Elute fats and chloroform-souble colors from the column with 100 ml of chloroform followed by 50 ml of hexane. Elute FD&C Red No. 2 FD&C Red No. 4, FD&C Yellow No. 5, and FD&C Yellow No.6 from the column with 200 ml of the resin-hexane solution. Next, elute FD&C Blue No. 1, FD&C Green No. 2, FD&C Green No. 3 and FD&C Violet No. 1 from the column with the first resin-butanol solution.

Alternate Method A. Grind the sample and pack the column as described above except use pH 7.5 buffer in phase 1:4 acetic acid. Elute fats and chloform soluble colors with chloroform. Elute FD&C Blue No. 2 and FD&C Red No. 3 with pH 7.5 resin-butanol.

Alternate Method B. Grind the sample and pack the column as described above except use pH 3.0 buffer in place of 1:4 acetic acid. Elute fats and chloroform-soluble colors with chloroform. Eliminate the chloroform was if FD&C Red No. 3 is to be determined. Elute colors with the pH 3.0 resin-butanol solution.

ISOLATION OF COLORS FROM THE RESIN SOLUTIONS. *From Resin-Hexane.* Wash 200 ml of extract with three 100-ml portions of water. Add 30 ml of water. Add concentrated ammonium hydroxide dropwise until the sample is alkaline, as indicated by the extraction of color into the aqueous phase. Extract all the color with 10-ml portions of dilute ammonium hydroxide. Quickly wash the combined aqueous extracts with 20 ml of chloroform, discard the chloroform, and acidify the aqueous layer with acetic acid.

From Resin-Butanol and Resin-Butanol at pH 3.0. Dilute 100 ml of extract with 200 ml of hexane. Discard the aqueous layer which separates. Then extract as described above.

From Resin-Butanol at pH 7.5. Wash the organic layer with several portions of dilute ammonium hydroxide. Acidify the aqueous layer, and extract with ethyl ether. Extract the ether solution with dilute ammonium hydroxide to isolate FD&C Red No. 3 from other FD&C colors.

The methods included below are applied to specific types of dyes in foods.

Procedures

ACID COAL TAR DYES. *Water-Solube Colors.* Dissolve or disperse the sample in water, or extract the color with water. Neutralize the solution or dispersion, and add sodium chloride so that the content is 20-25%. Extract any flavoring oils or alcohol present with ethyl ether. Wash the ether with water and add the wash to the salt solution. Chromatograph as described after Color Extracted with 80% Ethanol.

Oil-Soluble Colors. Dissolve or disperse the sample in an organic solvent such as petroleum ether or ethyl ether, or extract the color from the sample with solvent. Chromatograph on aluminum oxide, silicic acid, or other adsorbent. Identify the colors spectrophotometrically.

Colors Exracted with 80% Ethanol (Water-Soluble, with or without Oil-Soluble Colors). Place the sample in blender, add four or five times its weight of 80% ethanol, and gind until all the material is finely divided. Allow insolubles to settle and decant the liquid through glass wool. Stir the residue with about 30 ml of 80% ethanol, allow the slurry to settle, and filter as before. If the color has not been completely extracted, repeat the procedure using 80% ethanol containing 1% ammonium hydroxide. If natural colors make complete extraction difficult to observe extract the sample twice with 80% ethanol and twice with 80% ethanol containing 1% ammonium hydroxide.

Extract the ethanol solution with petroleum ether until no more color is extracted. Concentrate the ether layer on a steam bath, chromatograph on aluminium oxide, silicic acid, or other adsorbent, and identify the oil-soluble colors spectrophotometrically.

To the ethanol solution add 1/10 its volume of 20% sodium chloride-1% sodium hydroxide solution. Extract with three portions of ethyl ether, each portion equal in volume to that of the solution being extracted. Reserve the aqueous salt phase. Wash the combined ethanol-ether layer with four or five small portions of 20% sodium chloride 1% sodium hydroxide solution and add the washes to the aqueous salt phase. All the water-soluble color is now in the aqueous salt solution except erythrosine, some of which may still be in the ethanol-ether layer. To recover erythrosine, first remove any ethanol from the the layer with four 0.1 *N* aqueous acid washes, each about half the original volume of the 80% ethanol employed. Extract the erythrosine from the ether with 0.1*N* sodium hydroxide.

The aqueous salt solution containing the water-soluble acid colors is usually opaque at this point due to the presence of suspended matter from food products. To purify, neutralize the solution and chromatograph as follows:

Prepare a thin aqueous slurry with 30g of powdered cellulose, such as Solka Floc BW-40. Pour the slurry into a 1× 40 in. column and allow the liquid to drain almost to the top of the adsorbent bed. Wash the column with 20% sodium chloride solution. Add 2-3 g of cellulose to the sample solution and stir until dispersed. Pass the mixture into the column; follow it with a wash of 50 ml of 20% sodium chloride to remove all or most of the material derived from the food. The dye remains adsorbed at the top of the column.

To concentrate the color, wash with water. To purify the color, wash with sodium chloride of such concentration that the color moves down the column at a moderate rate. Collect he color and rechromomatograph to concentrate it if necessary. To separate colors add successive 25-50 ml portions of sodium chloride solution, each solution being one half the concentration of the preceding portion until a concentration is found which moves one color out ahead of others. Continue the wash at this concentration until the color is eluted.

Some color mixtures require variations in the development procedure. Salt-acid, salt-ammonium hydroxide, salt-alcohol, sodium sulfate, potassium sulfate, and dilute acid solutions may be necessary in some cases.

Identify the colors spectrophotometrically.

WATER-SOLULBLE BEDS. Macerate about 2 g of sample in 25 ml of cold water to leach the color. Filter the sample through Whatman No. 1 filter paper into a separatory funnel. Add 2 ml of hydrochloric acid and 2 ml of *n*- amyl alcohol for each 5 ml of filtrate. Shake well; discard the aqueous layer. Evaporate alcohol layer to dryness on a steam bath and dissolve the residue in 1 drop of water.

Spot 2µl of the aqueous test solution on chromatographic paper and resolve using two-dimensional chromatogrphy. Develop about 35 min in each of the following eluants: *eluant No. 1* containing 0.125g of sodium chloride and 1.0 ml of concentrated ammonium hydroxide diluted to 100 nil; *eluant No. 2* containing 4.00 g of sodium citrate and 9.60 ml of concentrated ammonium hydroxide diluted to 100 ml.

Color	R_1 *eluant No. 1*	*eluant No. 2*
Ext D&C Red No. 15 (formerly FD&C Red No. 1)	0.14	0.10
FD&C Red No. 2	0.33	0.37
FD&C Red NO. 3	0.05	0.03
FD&C Red No. 40	0.43	0.31

Acid and Basic Colors.Extract basic colors with chloroform. To extract acid colors adjust a sample to pH 9 with sodium carbonate and shake for 10 min with 10 ml of chloroform. Centrifuge and separate the chloroform layer containing basic colors. Mix the aqueous phase (plus any precipitate) with a large excess of 0.1% cetyleyclohexyl-dimethylammonium bromide. Shake with chloroform. Centrifuge and evaporate the chloroform layer at a low temperature. Dissolve the residue in 0.5 ml o chloroform and chromatograph onpaper impregnated with aluminum oxide. Develop 24 hr by descending elution using 10:5:5 ethanol-water-ammonium hydroxide.

The following methods are used to determine dyes found in specific foods.

Procedures

Colors in Oranges. Using 250 ml of chloroform, wash the color from ten oranges. (Surface waxes, oil, and some natural pigments also wash off.) Combine the washings and dilute to 250 ml. Evaporate a 50-ml aliquot o a steam bath and dissolve the residue in about 25 ml of petroleum ether.

Fill a 2.5 × 10 cm glass column with petroleum ether. Sift adsorbent alumina (Fisher *N*-540) into the column to a height of about 4 cm.

Pass the petroleum ether solution of the sample into the column.Wash with 50 ml of petroleum ether followed by 200 ml of carbon tetrachloride. Discard the washing. Elute the coloring matter with ethanol. Evaporate the eluate to dryness on a steam bath.

Dip a 7 × $22^1/_2$ in. strip of Whatman 3MM paper into 5% (w/v) light mineral oil in ethyl ether. Air dry. Dissolve the eluted sample in a few drops of chloroform and spot as a 6 in. band $2^1/_2$ in. from the bottom of the paper. Develop 3 hr by descending chromatrography using 6:4 acetone-water as an eluant. Examine the chromatogram for coal tar colors.

Dry the chromatogram and extract the individual colors from the paper with ethanol. Examine each specrophotometrically vs standards.

COLORS IN SOFT DRINKS AND CORDIALS. Dilute the sample with water and pour the mixture onto an acidic (aninotropic) aluminum oxide column. Wash con-comitant substances such as sugars from the column with 70% ethanol. Elute the color with 10 ml of 70% ethanol, to which 1 ml of 10% ammonium hydroxide has been added. Evaporate the eluate to 1-2 ml and resolve the colors by paper chromatography.

COLORS IN MACARONI. Mix 10g of finely ground sample for 10 min with 25 ml of 50% ethanol. Centrifuge the mixture for 10 min. at 5000 rpm. Acidify the clear solution with 8-10 drops of 2% tartaric acid. Pour onto a column 1 cm in diameter, containing a 1-cm layer of dry, ground gluten. Add 10 drops of 1.5% (v/v) ammonium hydroxide and elute. Transfer the eluate to chromatographic paper and eluate with 2:1:1 butanol-ethanol-water.

Colors in Drugs and Cosmetics. The following methods are used to determine D&C colors in specific types of mixtures.

Procedures

Colours in Oils. *Liquid Chromatographic Method.* Prepare the following columns using 20mm ID × 300 mm glass tubes;

(a) Florisil column–add 1.5 ml of water to 100g of 60-80 mesh Florisil (manufactured by Floridin Co., 570 Sylvan Ave., Englewood Cliffs, N.J.), activated at 650°C and stored at 130°C. Shake to mix; let stand overnight. Pack the column 4 in. high and wash with petroleum ether.

(b) Alumina column—heat 80 200 mesh alumina 1 hr at 400°C. Add 50 ml of petroleum ether to the tube which has been closed off . Add 18g of alumina, mix, and drain the ether to the top of the column.

(c) Magnesia column-mix equal weights of Sea Sorb-43 and Celite 515. Pack 9g of the mixture as described above for the alumina column. Compress with slight air pressure.

(d) Silicic acid column — add 4 in. a mixture of equal weights of 100-mesh silicic acid and Celite 545. Wash with *n*-hexane, using pressure.

Dilute 10 ml of sample with 10 ml of petroleum ether and place on the Florisil column. Elute with petroleum ether, collecting the colored zone (eluate No. 1). Elute with ether, collecting the colored zone (eluate No. 2). Elute with 1:3 ethanaol-ethyl ether, collecting each resolved color separately; usually the natural base-oil color, which is discarded, is followed by D&C Violet No. 2, then D&C Yellow No. 11. Elute with acetonitrile and collect any D&C Red No. 35.

Evaporate the individual ethanol-ethyl ether and acetonitrile eluates to dryness, dissolve the residues in chloroform, and determine their visible spectra.

Evaporate eluate No. 2 to dryness. Add eluate No. 1 to the residue and evaporate to about 15 ml. Transfer the solution to the alumina column and wash with 50 ml of petroleum ether; discard the eluate. Add two 10-ml portions of chloroform. If the chloroform eluate is green or blue, add it to the next eluant. Elute the column with 1:3 ethanol-chloroform until the eluate is colorless. Evaporate the eluate; dissolve any residue in petroleum ether.

Add the above solution to the magnesia column. Wash with 25 ml of petroleum ether, discarding the eluate. Elute the chloroform collecting the individual colored zones. The first fractions contains D&C Green No. 5 and Ext D&C Blue No. 5. The second fraction contains Ext D&C Orange No. 4 and Ext D&C Red No. 14. Elute with 1:3 ethanol-chloroform collecting the individual colored zones. They are D&C Red No. 18, Ext D&C Yellow Nos. 9 and 10, and D&C Red No. 17. Evaporate the individual fractions to dryness and compare the visible spectra of the residues in chloroform with standards.

If the spectrum of the blue-greenportion does not conform to a known color, evaporate the chloroform and dissolve the residue in *n*-hexane. Transfer it to the silcic acid column and elute with 1:1 *n*-hexane-benzene. Collect the eluate until it is colorless. Elute with benzene and collect the eluate until it is colorless. Evaporate the individual fractions to dryness and compare the visible spetra of the residues in chloroform with standards.

If the spectrum for D&C Red No. 17 has a minimum at 385 nm, Ext D&C Yellow Nos. 9 and 10 may be present. To resolve, evaporate the chloroform, dissolve the residue in a minimum volume of petroleum ether and transfer it to the magnesia column. Elute with 1:3 ethanol-chloroform and collect the individual colored fractions. Evaporate each fraction to dryness and compare the visible spectra of the residues in chloroform with standards.

Extraction method. Dissolve 10g of sample in 50 ml of petroleum ether. Filter, if necessary, into a separatory funnel. Extract with three 20-ml portions of *N, N*-dimethylformamide (DMF); discard the ether layer. Combine the DMF solution and extract with four 25-ml portions of petroleum ether, back-extracting each time with 5ml of DMF. Discard the ether extracts. Dilute the combined DMF solution with an equal volume of water and extract with 30 ml, then 10 ml of chloroform. Discard the aqueous DMF layer. Combine the chloroform extracts and wash them with water to remove any dissolved DMF. Evaporate the chloroform solution to dryness under vacuum at room temperature. Dissolve the residue in 25 ml of DMF and transfer it to a separatory funnel. Add 25 ml of water extract the solution with three to five 25-ml portions ether. Discard the aqueous DMF layer and wash the combined ether layers with water. Evaporate the ether solution under vacuum at room temperature. Examine the residue chromatographically or spectrophotometrically.

COLORS IN LIPSTICKS (71). Prepare the following reagents: *Buffer solution*—prepare a 0.1 *M* K_2HPO_4 solution and add a few drops of toluene as a preservative. Prepare a 0.1 *M*KH_2PO_4 solution and add a few drops of toluene. Mix 5.3 ml of the first solution with 94.7 ml of the second solution. Dilute to 200 ml with water. *Solvent A* mix 20 ml of 1-butanol, 4 ml of ethanol, and 3 ml of concentrated ammonium hydroxide. *Solvent B*—mix 15 ml of ethyl acetate, 3 ml of methanol, and 3 ml of 3:7 ammonium hydroxide. Prepare fresh.

Apply 0.2 ml of buffer solution in a $^1/_4$ in band 2 cm from the bottom of a 4× 8in silica gel G 375 μm thick glass plate. Air dry for about 20 min. Remove the shiny surface from the rounded end of the lipstick sample with tissue, and streak 5-8 mg of it just below the buffered zone of the warmed plate.

Line a No. 11 museum jar with paper and saturate it with dichloromethane. Allow the tank to equilibrate for a few minutes. Place the warm plate in the tank and develop it in the dark until the solvent reaches the top of the plate. Remove and dry the plate. Redevelop two to four more ties to remove oils and waxes to the top of the plate. Unsulfonated pigments colors separate in zones in the following descending order: D&C Red No. 36, D&C Orange No. 17, D&C Red No. 35. Scrape colored zones from the plate, leach with chloroform, and determine visible spectra vs standards.

Place the same plate in a covered, unlined Desaga tank containing 189 ml of Solvent A. Develop to a height of 5 cm. Dry the plate with heat and air. Repeat development once or twice until a 1/4 in. zone appears above the D&C Red No. 7. The D&C Red No. 7 remains close to the baseline while other colors present move through the buffer. Scrape the zone containing D&C NO. 7 from the plate, leach with 30% acetic acid, and determine the visible spectrum vs a standard.

Line three sides of a Desaga tank with paper. Pour 315 ml of Solvent B over the lining and equilibrate for 10 min. Place the plate in the tank. With adsorbent layer facing the liner. Add glass beads to the tank until the solvent reaches the edge of the continuous coated portion of the plate. Develop to a height of 15-17 cm. If necessary, dry the plate and redevelop. Remaining colors separate in the following descending order: D&C Red No. 19, D&C Red No. 8 plus D&C Red No. 10, D&C Orange No. 4, D&C Red No. 27, D&C Red No. 3, D&C Red No. 21, tribromofluorescein, D&C Orange No. 5, monobromofluorescein, fluorescein, FD&C Blue No. 1. Scrape colored zones from the lates and leach as follows: D&C Red No. 8 plus D&C Red No. 10 in ethanol D&C Red No. 1 in 30% (v.v) acetic acid; halogenated fluoresceins in 1:9 ammonium hydroxide. Determine the visible spectra vs. known standards.

If the sample contains no D&C Red No. 7, it is not necessary to treat the plate with buffer or to develop it in Solvent A. To detect D&C Red No. 7 develop a 2 × 4 in. plate in a covered 500-ml tall-form beaker. Develop twice in dichloromethane, then once in 42 ml of Solvent B. The appearance of multiple bands which darken upon drying to a dull, nonfluorescent, deep red color and which overlap other colors suggest the presence of D&C Red No. 7. A dark red zone at the baseline also indicates its presence. This color is frequently found in dark red zone at the baseline also indicates its presence. This color is frequently found in dark red or purple lipsticks.

8

Analysis of Ayurvedic Medicines

GENERAL SCHEME OF ANALYSIS

I. Materials and solutions employed in tests (list)

II. A. Solutions used in Volumetric Determinations (list)
  B. Indicators (list)

III. Determination of pH

IV. Determination of
  A. Refractive index
  B. Specific Gravity.

V. Determination of Fineness of particles

VI. A. Disintegration Tests for Tablets/Pills
  B. Uniformity of weight of tablets

VII. Determination of
  A. Ash
  B. Acid insoluble ash
  C. Water soluble ash
  D. Water soluble extractive
  E. Alcohol soluble extractive
  F. Loss on drying
  G. Alcohol
  H. Water

VIII. Determination of Foreign inorganic & organic matter

IX. Determination of:
  A. Fat content
  B. Volatile oil content
  C. Acid value
  D. Saponification value
  E. Iodine value

X. Tests for detection of adulterants in oils/fats
  A. Test for the absence of Vanaspati in Ghee
  B. Test for detection of Arachis oil in sesame oil
  C. Test for Detection of Cotton seed oil in other oils

XI. Qualitative reactions for:

1. Aluminium
2. Arsenic
3. Borate
4. Calcium
5. Carbonates
6. Chlorides
7. Copper
8. Gold
9. Iron
10. Lead
11. Magnesium
12. Mercury
13. Phosphate
14. Potassium
15. Silicon
16. Silver
17. Sodium
18. Sulphur
19. Sulphate
20. Tin
21. Alkaloid

XII. Quantitative Estimations

Determination of:

1. Aluminium
2. Arsenic
3. Borate
4. Calcium
5. Camphor
6. Chloride
7. Copper
8. Iron
9. Gold
10. Lead
11. Magnesium

12. Mercury
13. Phosphate
14. Silica
15. Silver
16. Sulphur free and total
17. Tin
18. Potassium and Sodium

XIII. Determination of total sugars & Reducing sugars as invert sugar

A. Sucrose

B. Table

XIV. Determination of Resin content.

I. Material and Solutions Employed in Tests

Acetic acid	:	Of the Indian Pharmacopoeia (approximately 33 per cent w/w of $C_2H_4O_2$)
Acetic acid, glacial	:	Of the Indian Pharmacopoeia (approximately) 99 per cent w/w of $C_2H_4O_2$)
Alcohol (95 per cent)	:	Of the Indian Pharmacopoeia
Alcohol (90 per cent)	:	Of the Indian Pharmacopoeia
Alcohol (70 per cent)	:	Of the Indian Pharmacopoeia
Ammonia solution dilute	:	Of the Indian Pharmacopoeia (approximately 10 per cent w/w of NH_3)
Ammonia solution strong	:	Of the Indian Pharmacopoeia (approximately 28.5 per cent w/w of NH_3)
Ammonium acetate $CH_3\ CO_2NH_4$	:	Of the Indian Pharmacopoeia appendix
Ammonium acetate solution	:	Dissolve sufficient *Ammonium acetate* in water to produce a solution containing 61.5 per cent w/w of CH_3CO2NH_4
Ammonium carbonate	:	Of the Indian Pharmacopoeia appendix.
Ammonium carbonate solution	:	Dissolve 5 g of *Ammonium carbonate* in a mixture of 7.5 ml of *dilute*

		Ammonia solution and 50 ml. of water, add sufficient water to produce 100 ml., and filter if necessary.
Ammonium chloride	:	Of the Indian Pharmacopoeia
Ammonium chloride solution	:	a 10.0 per cent w/w solution of *Ammonium chloride* in water.
Ammonium oxalate $(CO_2NH_4)_2.H_2O$	:	Of the Indian Pharmacopoeia appendix.
Ammonium oxalate solution	:	a 2.5 per cent solution of ammonium oxalate in water
Ammonium phosphate solution	:	a 10.0 per cent w/v solution of *Ammonium phosphate* in water.
Ammonium polysulphide solution	:	Dissolve a sufficient quantity of *Sublimed sulphur* in *Ammonium sulphide solution* to produce a deep yellow solution.
Ammonium sulphide solution (yellow)	:	Saturate 120 ml of *dilute Ammonia solution* with washed *hydrogen sulphide*, add 80 ml of dilute ammonia solution. *Ammonium sulphide solution* must be recently prepared.
Ammonium thiocynate NH_4SCN_S	:	Of the Indian Pharmacopoeia: appendix.
Ammonium thiocyanate solution	:	10.0 per cent w/w solution of *Ammonium thiocyanate* in water.
Amyl alcohol $C_5H_{11}OH$	:	Of the Indian Pharmacopoeia appendix.
Barium chloride $BaCl_2$, $2H_2O$	:	Of the Indian Pharmacopoeia appendix.
Barium chloride solution	:	a 10.0 per cent w/w solution of *Barium chloride* in water.
Boric acid solution	:	Of the Indian Pharmacopoeia
Bomine, Br_2		Of the Indian Pharmacopeia appendix.
Carbon disulphide CS_2	:	Of the Indian Pharmacopoeia appendix.

Carbon tetrachloride CCl_4	:	Of the Indian Pharmacopoeia appendix.
Ceric ammonium sulphate $Ce(SO_4)\ 2(NH_4)_2\ SO_4\ 2H_2O$	:	Of the Indian Pharmacopoeia appendix.
Chloral hydrate	:	Of the Indian Pharmacopoeia.
Chloral hydrate solution	:	Dissolve 50 g of *Chloral hydrate* in 20 ml of water.
Chlorine Cl_2	:	Of the Indian Pharmacopoeia appendix.
Chloroform	:	Of the Indian Pharmacopoeia.
Chloroform water	:	Of the Indian Pharmacopoeia.
Ether solvent	:	Of the Indian Pharmacopoeia.
Ferric ammonium sulphate $Fe(NH_4)(SO_4)_2\ 2H_2O$	:	Of the Indian Pharmacopeia appendix.
Ferric ammonium sulphate solution acid	:	Dissolve 0.2 g of *Ferric Ammonium sulphate* in 50 ml of water and add 6 ml. dilute of *nitric acid* and sufficient water to produce 100 ml.
Ferrous sulphate	:	Of the Indian Pharmacopoeia.
Formaldehyde solution	:	Of the Indian Pharmacopoeia.
Glycerol, Glycerin	:	Of the Indian Pharmacopoeia.
Hydrochloric acid	:	Of the Indian Pharmacopoeia appendix.
Hydrochloric acid dilute	:	Of the Indian Pharmacopoeia appendix.
Hydrogen peroxide solution	:	Of the Indian Pharmacopoeia appendix. (Approximately 6 per cent w/w of H_2O_2).
Hydrogen sulphide H_2S	:	Of the Indian Pharmacopoeia appendix.
Iodine	:	Of the Indian Pharmacopoeia.
Iodine trichloride ICl_3	:	Of the Indian Pharmacopoeia appendix.
Lead acetate	:	Of the Indian Pharmacopoeia.
Lead acetate solution	:	a 10.0 per cent w/w solution of *Lead acetate in Carbon dioxide* free water.

Lycopodium	:	Of the Indian Pharmacopoeia.
Manganese dioxide MnO_2	:	Of the Indian Pharmacopoeia appendix.
Nitric acid HNO_3	:	Of the Indian Pharmacopoeia.
Nitric acid, dilute	:	Mix 106 ml. of *Nitric acid* with sufficient water to produce 1000 ml. (approximately 10 per cent w/w of HNO_3).
Oxalic acid $(CO_2H)_2$ $2H_2O$	:	Of the Indian Pharmacopoeia appendix.
Perchloric acid (60% w/w)	:	Of the Indian Pharmacopoeia appendix.
Petroleum, light	:	Of the Indian Pharmacopoeia appendix.
O-Phenanthroline 1, : 10–Phenanthroline, $C_{12}H_{18}$–N_2H_2O	:	Of the Indian Pharmacopoeia appendix.
O-Phenanthroline ferrous complex solution	:	Dissolve 0.7 g of *Ferrous sulphate* in about 70 ml of water add 1.5 g. of *Ophenanthroline* and sufficient water to produce 100 ml.
Phloroglucinol, 1:3:5–Trihydroxybenzene C_6H_3 $(OH)_3$, $2H_2O$	:	Of the Indian Pharmacopoeia.
Phloroglucinol solution	:	a 1.0 per cent w/w solution of *phloroglucinol* in *Alcohol* (90 per cent).
Phosphoric acid	:	Of the Indian Pharmacopoeia (approximately 89 per cent w/w of H_3FO_4).
Potassium antimonate KSb O_3 $3H_2O$	:	Of the Indian Pharmacopoeia appendix.
Potassium antimonate solution	:	Boil 2 g of *Potassium Antimonate* with 95 ml of water until dissolved cool rapidly and add 50 ml of KOH solution and 5 ml of N/1 Nacl. Allow to stand for 24 hours; filter and add sufficient water to produce 150 ml.
Potassium chromate $K_2Cr_2O_4$	:	Of the Indian Pharmacopoeia appendix.

Potassium chromate solution	:	5.0 per cent w/w solution of *Potassium chromate* in water.
Potassium cyanide KCN	:	Of the Indian Pharmacopoeia appendix.
Potassium dichromate $K_2Cr_2O_7$	:	Of the Indian Pharmacopoeia appendix.
Potassium ferrocyanide $K_3Fe(CN)_6$	:	Of the Indian Pharmacopoeia appendix.
Potassium ferrocyanide solution	:	Wash about 1 g. of *potassium ferricyanide*, crystals, with a little water and dissolve the washed crystals in 100 ml of water.
Potassium ferrocyanide $K_4Fe(CN)_6\ 3H_2O$	:	Of the Indian Pharmacopoeia appendix.
Potassium ferocyanide	:	a 5.0 per cent w/w solution potassium ferrocyanide in water.
Potassium hydroxide	:	Of the Indian Pharmacopoeia.
Potassium Hydroxide solution	:	Approximately 5 per cent w/w of KOH.
Potassium Iodide	:	Of the Indian Pharmacopoeia.
Potassium Iodide solution	:	a 10.0 per cent w/w solution of *Potassium Iodide* in water.
Potassium permanganate	:	Of the Indian Pharmacopoeia.
Potassium cyanide solution	:	a 10.0 per cent w/v solution of *Potassium cyanide* in water.
Potassium permanganate solution	:	a 1.0 per cent w/w solution of *Potassium permanganate* in water.
Potassium thiocyanate KCNS	:	Of the Indian Pharmacopoeia appendix.
Pumice powder	:	The particles of *Pumice* of commerce powdered and sifted, which pass through a No.22 sieve but are retained by a No. 60 sieve.
Pyridine C_5H_5N	:	Of the Indian Pharmacopoeia appendix.
Silver nitrate	:	Of the Indian Pharmacopoeia.
Silver nitrate solution	:	a 5.0 per cent w/v solution of *Silver nitrate* in water.

Sodium bicarbonate	: Of the Indian Pharmacopoeia.
Sodium bicarbonate solution	: A 5.0 per cent w/v solution of *Sodium bicarbonated* in water.
Sodium carbonate	: Of the Indian Pharmacopoeia.
Sodium chloride	: Of the Indian Pharmacopoeia.
Sodium chloride solution Brine	: A saturated solution of *Sodium Chloride* in water.
Sodium cobaltinitrate $Na_3\ CO\ (NO_2)_6$	: Of the Indian Pharmacopoeia appendix.
Sodium cobaltinitrate solution	: a 30.0 per cent w/v solution of *Sodium cobaltinitrate* in water.
Sodium acetate	: Of the Indian Pharmacopoeia appendix.
Sodium hydroxide	: Of the Indian Pharmacopoeia.
Sodium hydroxide solution	: a 20.0 per cent w/w solution of *Sodium Hydroxide* in water.
Sodium phosphate	: Of the Indian Pharmacopoeia.
Sodium phosphate solution	: a 10.0 per cent w/v solution of *Sodium Phosphate* in water.
Sodium potassium Tartrate	: Of the Indian Pharmacopoeia appendix.
Sodium sulphate (anhydrous)	: Of the Indian Pharmacopoeia.
Sodium sulphate	: Of the Indian Pharmacopoeia.
Sodium thiosulphite	: Of the Indian Pharmacopoeia appendix.
Stannous chloride solution $Sn\ Cl_2.\ 2H_2O$	: Of the Indian Pharmacopoeia appendix.
Stannous chloride solution	: Dissolve 330 h. of *Stannous Chloride* in 100 ml of *Hydrochloric* acid and sufficient water to produce 1000 ml.
Starch	: Of the Indian Pharmacopoeia.
Starch, soluble	: Of the Indian Pharmacopoeia appendix.
Sucrose	: Of the Indian Pharmacopoeia.

Sulphur, Precipitated	:	Of the Indian Pharmacopoeia.
Sulphuric acid (conc.) H_2SO_4	:	Of the Indian Pharmacopoeia appendix.
Sulphuric acid, dilute	:	Mix 104 g. of *Sulphuric acid* and 896 g. of water and cool.
Toluene	:	Of the Indian Pharmacopoeia appendix.
Turmeric	:	Of the Indian Pharmacopoeia appendix.
Turmeric paper	:	Made by impregnating unglazed white paper with *Turmeric tincture.*
Turmeric tincture	:	Macerate10 g. of bruised turmeric in 60 ml. of alcohol (90 per cent) for one week; filter.
Uranyl zinc acetate solution	:	Dissolve 10 g of *Uranyl acetate* by heating with 50 ml. of water of 5 ml. of acetic acid, dissolve 30 g. of Zinc *acetate* by heating with 30 ml of water and 3 ml of *Acetic acid,* mix the two solution, allow to cool, filter.
Water	:	Purified water of the Indian Pharmacopoeia.
Xylene	:	Of the Indian Pharmacopoeia appendix.
Zinc acetate	:	Of the Indian Pharmacopoeia appendix.

II. *A.* solutions Used in Volumetric Determinations

Ammonium Thiocyanate, N/10

Ammonium Thiocyanate dissolved in water in contain in 1000 ml. 7.612 g. Of NH_4SCN

Ceric Ammonium Sulphate, N/10

Ceric Ammonium sulphate dissolved in a mixture of *Sulphuric acid* and water to contain in 1000 ml 33.26 g. of $Ce(SO_4)_2$, $2(NH_4)_2SO_4$, $2H_2O$.

To 750 ml. of the cold mixture prepared by diluting 136 ml of sulphuric acid to 1000 ml with water, add 74 g. of ceric ammonium sulphate. shake at intervals until solution is complete, and add, sufficient of the diluted sulphuric acid to produce 1000 ml. Ascertain its exact strength by titrating it against N/10 ferrous sulphate, using *O-Phenanthroline*-ferrous complex solution as indicator.

Ferrous Sulphate, N/10

Ferrous sulphate dissolved in water to contain in 1000 ml. ferrous iron equivalent to 5.585 g. of Fe.

Hydrochloric acid, N/1, N/2,N/10.

Hydrochloric acid diluted with water to contain in 1000 ml. the following quantities of HCl.

N/1 : 36.47 g. HCl

N/2 : 18.23 g. HCl

N/10 : 3.647 g. HCl

Iodine, N/10

Iodine and *Potassium Iodide* dissolved in water to contain in 1000 ml., 12.69 g. 1 and 18.0 g. KI.

Potassium Dichromate, N/10

Potassium dichromate dissolved in water contain in 1000 ml. 49.04 g. $K_2CR_2O_7$.

Potassium Hydroxide, Alcoholic, .5 N, N/2

Potassium hydroxide dissolved in alcohol (95 per cent) to contain in 1000 ml. the following quantities of KOH

for 1.5 N	... 84.16 g. KOH
for N/2	... 28.05 g. KOH

Potassium Hydroxide aqueous, N/10

Potassium hydroxide dissolved in water in contain in 1000 ml. 5.611 g. KOH.

Potassium permanganate, N/10

Potassium permanganate dissolved in water to contain in 1000 ml. 3.161 g. $KMnO_4$.

Silver Nitrate, N/10.

Silver nitrate dissolved in water to contain in 1000 ml., 16.99 g. $AgNO_3$.

Sodium Acetate, N/10

Sodium acetate dissolved in water to contain in 1000 ml. 18.61 g. CH_3COO_8Na.

Sodium Hydroxider, N/1,N/2, N/10

Sodium hydroxide dissolved in water to contain in 1000 ml. the following quantities of NaOH.

for N/1 ... 40.00 g. NaOH

for N/2 ... 20.00 g. NaOH

for N/10 ... 4.000 g. NaOH

When *Carbonate*—free solutions are required they may be prepared by the following method.

Dissolve *Sodium hydroxide* in water to produce a 4 to 60 per cent w/v solution and allow to stand. Taking precautions to avoid absorption of *Carbon dioxide*, siphon off the clear supernatant liquid and dilute with Carbon Dioxide free water to give the required normality.

Sodium Hydroxide, Alcoholic, N/10

Sodium hydroxide dissolve in alcohol (95 per cent) to contain in 1000 ml. 4.000 g. of NaOH.

Sodium Thiosulphate, N/10

Sodium thiosulphate dissolved in water to contain in 1000 ml. 24.28 g. $Na_2S_2O_3$, $5H_2O$.

Sulphuric acid, N/1, N/2, N/10

Sulphuric acid dissolved in water to contain in 1000 ml., the following quantities of H_2SO_4.

for N/1 ... 49.04 g. H_2SO_4

for N/2 ... 24.52 g. H2SO_4

for N/10 ... 4.904 g. H_2SO_4

B. Indicators

Ferric ammonium solution	:	A 10 per cent w/v solution of *Ferric ammonium Sulphate* in water.
Methyl orange	:	*Sodium 4—dimethyl aminoazo benzene—4—sulphonate.*
Methyl Orange solution	:	a 0.04 per cent w/v solution of *Methyl orange* in *Alcohol* (20 per cent).
Methyl red	:	4—Dimethyl aminoaze—2—carboxylic acid.
Methyl red solution	:	Warm 25 mg. of *Methyl red* with

		0.95 ml of N/20 *Sodium hydroxide* and 5 ml. of *Alcohol* (90 per cent) after solution is effected, add sufficient *Alcohol* (50 per cent) to produce 250 ml.
Phenolphthalein	:	Of the Indian Pharmacopoeia appendix.
Phenolphthalein solution	:	a 1.0 per cent w/v solution of phenolphthalein in alcohol (95 per cent).
Solochrome Black WDFA	:	The sodium salt of 2—*hydroxy*—5—*nitro*—4—*sulpho*—2—*naph* thaleneaze—() - naphthol. Gives a red colour with Calcium, Magnesium, zinc and many other metal ions. When metal ions are absent, for example, in the presence of an excess of *Sodium acetate*, the solution is blue.
Solochrome Black Mixture	:	A mixture of 0.2 part of soloschrome black WDFA with 100 parts of *Sodium chloride*.

Starch mucilage

Triturate 0.5 g. *Starch*, or 0.5 g. of *soluble starch*, with 5 ml. of water and add this, with constant stirring, to sufficient water to produce about 100 ml. Boil for a few minutes cool and filter.

Starch mucilage must be recently prepared.

III. Determination of pH

(*Asaras, aristas, arka, dravaka, avaleha, ksara, lavana*).

The pH value of an aqueous liquid may be defined as the common logarithm of the reciprocal of the hydrogen ion concentration expressed in grammes.

The pH value of a liquid is determined potentionmetrically by means of a glass electrode and a suitable pH meter.

Method

Operate the pH meter and electrode system according to the manufacture's instructions.

Standardise the meter and electrodes, if necessary, with *M/20 Potassium hydrogenpthalate (pH 4.00)* when measuring an alkaline solution.

Preparation of test solution

Asavas, arisrtas, arkas and dravakas

The sample may be used as such, filtered through a dry filter, if necessary.

Avaleha: a 10 per cent w/v suspension in water thoroughly mixed is centrifuged and the supernatant liquid is used.

Ksara and Lavana : A 10 per cent w/v solution in water, tiltered through a dry filter, is used.

IV. Determination of

A. Refractive Index

(*Ghrta, taila, paka*)

The refractive index (n) of a substance is the ratio of the velocity of light in a vaccum to its velocity in the substance. It varies with the wave length of the light used in the measurement.

It may also be defined as the ratio of the sine of the angle of incidence to the sine of the angle of refraction.

Refraction indices are stated in terms of sodium light of wave length 9893A at a temperature of 20° unless otherwise specified.

Refractometers

Commercial instruments are normally constructed for use with white light but are calibrated to give the refractive index in terms of the sodium D wave length.

The maker's instruction relating to a suitable light source should be followed.

Temperature control : A suitable device should be used for circulating water at the required temperature through the refractometer.

Preparation of sample

Ghtra, paka : The fat is extracted from an aliquot of the sample in a continuous extraction apparatus using light petroleum as solvent. The extract is filtered, the solvent is completely removed by distillation/evaporation and the residual fat is used.

Taila : The sample is filtered through a dry filter.

Procedure : Circulate water through the instrument at the required temperature. Place a drop of the liquid between the prisms, and take the reading after half a minute.

B. Specific gravity (*Aristas, asavas, dravakas*)

The specific gravity of a liquid is the weight of given volume of the liquid at the specific temperature compared with the weight of an equal volume of water at the same temperature, all weighings being taken in air.

Procedure : A pycnometer of 25 ml. capacity is cleaned, dried and weighed. It is filled up to the mark with water at the required temperature and weighed. The pycnometer is next filled up to the mark with the sample, filtered if necessary, at the same temperature and weighed. The specific gravity is determined by dividing the weight of the sample expressed in grammes by the weight of the water, expressed in grammes.

V. Determination of Fineness of particles (*Lepa, bhasma, sindura, pisti, Curna*).

The degree of coarseness of fineness of a powder is differentiated and expressed by the size of the mesh of the sieve through which the particle is able to pass.

The following terms are used in the description of powders.

Coarse powder (10/44) A powder of which all the particles pass through a *No. 10 Sieve* and not more than 40.0 per cent through *No. 44 Sieve.*

Moderately coarse powder (22/60) A powder of which all the particles pass through a No. 22 sieve and not more than 40.0 per cent through a *No. 60 sieve.*

Moderately fine powder (44/85) A powder of which all the particles pass through a *No. 55 sieve* and not more than 40.0 per cent through a *No. 85 sieve.*

Fine Powder (85) A power of which all the particles pass through a No. 85 sieve.

Very fine powder: A powder of which all the particles pass through a silk sieve in which not less than 120 meshes are included in a length of 2.54 cm. in each transverse direction parallel to the threads.

Sieves: The wire sieves used in sifting powdered drugs are distinguished by numbers which indicate the number of meshes are included in a length of 2.54 cm in each transverse direction parallel to the wires.

Procedure : A suitable quantity of the sample is weighed and transferred to the set of sieves from No. 10 to No. 85. The sieves are shaken in a sieve shaker for about 30 minutes and the residue on each sieve is weighed separately.

For "very fine powder" a silk sieve No. 120 is used.

VI. A Disintegration test for tablets/pills (*Mandura, lauha, vatigutika and varti*)

Apparatus

A glass or plastic tube 80 to 100 mm long with an internal diameter of about 28 mm., and an external diameter 30 to 31 mm fitted at the lower and with a disc of rust proof wire gauge complying with the requirements for a NO. 10 sieve, is suspended in a volume of water having a depth of not less than 15 cm and at a temperature between 35° and 39°, in such a way that it can be raised and lowered repeatedly in a uniform manner through a distance of 75 mm., at the highest position of the tube, the gauge first breaks the surface of the water and at the lowest position, the upper rim of the tube remains clear of the water. The tube may be manipulated by hand or mechanically.

Method

Place 5 tablets in the tube and raise and lower the tube in such a manner that the complete up and down movement is repeated thirty times a minute. The tablets are disintegrated when no particle remains above the gauge which would not readily pass through it. The time required for the five tablets to disintegrate in the manner described is not more than 15 minutes. If the tablets fail to comply, repeat the test on a further five tablets using a guided disc, as described below, inserted above the tablets in the tube. The tablets must then comply with the test.

The guided disc consists of a disc a suitable plastic material, about 20 cm in diameter and 2 mm, thick, the lower surface is flat and the upper surface has three holes equally spaced and 10 mm from the centre. In each hole a stainless steel wire of No. 22 Standard *Wire Gauge* is secured at a right-angle to the plan of the disc and the end of each wire is turned out radially and secured to a guide ring, 27 mm in diameter, made of similar material. The guide ring is coaxial with the disc in a parallel plane at a distance of 15 mm from the upper surface of the disc. The difference between the diameter of the disc and the internal diameter of the tube is not more than 2 mm. The total weight of the guided disc is not less than 1.9 g. and not more than 2.1 g.

B. Uniformity of weight of tablets

The average weight is determined by weighing 20 tablets. The tablets are also weighed singly. The deviation from the average weight in each case is calculated and expressed as a percentage. Not more than two of the tablets deviate from the average weight by a greater percentage than that shown in Table-I; and no tablet deviates by more than double that percentage.

If 20 tablets are not available, 10 may be used for the determination; not more than one then deviate from the average weight by a greater percentage than that shown in Table-I, and no tablet deviates by more than double that percentage.

Table—I

Average weight	Percentage deviation
0.12 g. or less	I 10 per cent
More than 0.12 g. and	I 7.5 per cent
Less than 0.3 g.	
0.3 g.or more	I 5 per cent

VII. A. Determination of Ash

(Ghrta, Taila, Guggulu, Lepa, Bhasma, Sindura, Pisti, Kvath curna, Curna, Vati-gutika, Rasa-yoga, Varti, Satva, Mandura, Lauha)

Method

Incinerate about 2 to 3 g., accurately weighed, of the prepared sample in a tared platinumor silica dish at a low temperature until free from carbon, cool and weigh. If a carbon-free ash can not be obtained in this way extract the charred mass with hot water, collect the residue on an ashless filter paper, incinerate the residue and filter paper add the filtrate, evaporate to dryness and ignite to constant weight at a low temperature.

Calculate the percentage of ash with reference to the moisture free drug.

B. Acid insoluble ash

Boil the ash for 5 minutes with 25 ml of *dilute-hydrochloric acid* (6N) collect the insoluble matter in a Gooch crucible, or on an ashless filter paper, wash with hot water and ignite to constant weight at a low temperature. Calculate the percentage of acid-insoluble ash with reference to the moisture free drug.

C. Water soluble ash

Boil the ash for 5 minutes with 25 ml of water; collect the insoluble matter in a Gooch crucible, or on an ashless filter paper, wash with hot water, and ignite to constant weight at a low temperature. Subtract the weight of the insoluble matter from the weight of the ash; the difference in weight represents the water soluble ash. Calculate the percentage of water-soluble ash with reference to the moisture free drug.

D. Determination of Water Soluble Extractive

(Lepa, Curna Satva)

Macerate 5 g. of the drug in coarse powder, with 100 ml of *chloroform water,* in a closed flask for twenty four hours, shaking frequently during six hours and allowing to stand for eighteen hours. Filter rapidly, taking precautions against loss of solvent, evaporate 25 ml of the filterate to dryness in a tared-shallow bottomed dish, and dry at 100°C to constant weight.

Calculate the percentage of water-soluble extractive with reference to the moisture-free drug.

E. Determination of Alcohol-Soluble Extractive

(Lepa, Curna, Satva)

Proceed as directed for the *determination of water soluble extractive,* using *alcohol* of the specified strength instead of *chloroform water.*

F. Loss on Drying

(Asava, arista, avaleha)

Note

The B.P. method of drying at 105° is not recommended for these preparations as they contain reducing sugar, the Laevulose moiety of which is decomposed at this temperature. The vaccum oven method is to be used. In this method of sample is spread on pure sand and dried in vacuo at 60-70°C.

Method

Digest pure quartz sand that passes through No. 40 but not No. 60 seive with hydrochloric acid, wash-acid-free, dry and ignite. Preserve in stoppered bottle.

Place 25-30 g. of prepared sand and a short glass rod in a nickel or stainless steel dish, about 55 mm in diameter and 40 mm deep, fitted with a cover. Dry thoroughly, cover dish, cool in desiccator.

Pipette out a quantity of asava--arista to yield about 1 g. of dry matter. In the case of avaleha weigh sufficient quantity of the sample to yield about 1 g. of dry matter in a dish, mix with a few ml. of water and transfer quantitatively to the dish containing prepared sand with the aid of water. Mix the sample thoroughly with the sand.

Dry at a temperature not more than 70°C under pressure not more than 50mm. Hg., making trial weighings at 2 hours intervals towards end of drying period until successive weightings do not differ by more than 2 mg Calculate the total solids from the loss of weight on drying.

Note:

As dry sand, as well as dried sample, absorbs appreciable quantity of moisture on standing over most desiccating agents, make all weighings as quickly as possible after cooling in desiccator.

G. Determination of Alcohol content

(Asavas and Aristas)

Note

The B.P. method of quadruple bulk distillation is not suitable for preparations containing low percentages of alcohol as the alcohol percentage of the quadruple bulk distillate will be only ¼ that of the original preparations. Specific gravity determinations of such dilute alcohol solution are likely to lead to inaccurate results.

It is preferable to us a method (e.g. *A.O.A.C.* method) in which the distillate is of the same strength as the original preparations. The alcohol tablets given in the A.O.A.C. should be used to obtain the alcohol content.

Method I (in the absence of volatile oils)

Measure 100 ml. of the preparation in a graduated flask at 20°C (The flask may be immersed in ice water contained in a Dewar vessel, the temperature being maintained at 20°C by adding water or ice). Transfer to a flask of 500 to 800 ml. capacity, wash the graduated flask with 50 ml of water, add the washings to the contents of the larger flask, and add a little pumice power. Neutralise, if necessary, with sodium hyroxide solution. (This may be conveniently done by titrating an aliquot of the sample, after dilution, with N/10 sodium hydroxide using phenolphthalein solution as indicator, calculating the volume necessary to neutralise 100 ml and adding this amount of sodium hydroxide to the sample in the flask. Connect the flask to a condenser by means of a duitable still-head and distil at least 90 ml. into a 100 ml. with water at the same temperature. Determine the specific gravity at 20°C, read off percentage of ethyl alcohol corresponding to the specific gravity from the appended table.

Method II (in the presence of volatile oils)

Measure 100 ml of the sample in a graduated flask at 20°C. Transfer to a separator, wash the graduated flask with about 25 ml of water, add the washings to the contents of the separator, and add sufficient powdered sodium chloride to saturate the liquid. Add about 100 ml of light petroleum (boiling point 40°C to 60°C), and shake vigorously for two to three minutes. Allow the mixture to stand for fifteen to thirty minutes and run the lower layer into a distillation flask. Wash the light petroleum in the separator by shaking vigorously with about 25 ml of sodium chloride solution, allow to stand, and run the wash liquor into the first brine solution. Make the mixed solutions just alkaline with N/1 Sodium hydroxide using solid phenolphthalein as indicator, add a little pumice powder and 100 ml. of water, distil 90 ml. and determine the amount of ethyl alcohol by Method I.

Table : Percentage by vol. at 15.56°C of ethyl alcohol corresponding to apparent specific gravity at 20°C/20°C

Apparent Specifc gravity	Percentage of alcohol V/V	Apparent Sp. gavity	Percent alcohol V/V
1.0000	0.00	0.9961	2.64
0.9997	0.20	0.9958	2.84
0.9994	0.40	0.9955	3.05
0.9991	0.60	0.9952	3.26
0.9988	0.80	0.9950	3.40
0.9985	1.00	0.9947	3.61

0.9982	1.20	0.9944	3.83
0.9979	1.41	0.9941	4.04
0.9976	1.61	0.9938	4.26
0.9973	1.81	0.9936	4.40
0.9970	2.02	0.9934	4.55
0.9967	2.22	0.9932	4.69
0.9964	2.43	0.9930	4.84
0.9928	4.98	0.9852	11.03
0.9926	5.13	0.9850	11.12
0.9924	5.28	0.9848	11.36
0.9922	5.43	0.9846	11.53
0.9920	5.58	0.9844	11.70
0.9918	5.73	0.9842	11.87
0.9196	5.88	0.9810	12.04
0.9914	6.03	0.9838	12.21
0.9912	6.18	0.9836	12.38
0.9910	6.34	0.9834	12.55
0.9908	6.49	0.9832	12.73
0.9906	6.65	0.9830	12.90
0.9904	6.80	0.9828	13.07
0.9902	6.96	0.9826	13.25
0.9900	7.12	0.9824	13.43
0.9898	7.27	0.9822	13.60
0.9896	7.43	0.9820	13.77
0.9894	7.59	0.9818	13.95
0.9892	7.75	0.9816	14.13
0.9890	7.90	0.9814	14.30
0.9888	8.06	0.9812	14.48
0.9886	8.23	0.9810	14.66
0.9884	8.39	0.9808	14.84
0.9882	8.55	0.9806	15.02
0.9880	8.71	0.9804	15.20
0.9878	8.88	0.9802	15.37
0.9876	9.04	0.9800	15.55
0.9874	9.21	0.9898	15.73
0.9872	9.38	0.9796	15.91
0.9870	9.54	0.9795	16.00
0.9868	9.70	0.9860	10.36
0.9866	9.87	0.9858	10.53
0.9864	10.03	0.9856	10.69
0.9862	10.20	0.9854	10.86

H. Determination of water

A 500 ml flask of connected by means of trap to a reflex condenser (Leibig type) by ground glass joints. The trap leads into a graduated receiver. The source of heat is an electric heating mantle. For most efficient working the upper portion of the flask and the connecting tube may be insulated with asbestos. A small tube containing a drying agent such as anhydrous calcium chloride may be fitted to the top of the condenser to prevent atmospheric moisture condensing inside apparatus.

When any evidence of greasiness appears e.g. if there is difficulty in the separation of the water and the entraining liquid, the condenser and receiver should be cleaned with chromic acid cleaning mixture, thoroughly rinsed with water and dried in an oven.

Entraining liquid: This may vary, but in most cases xylene or toluene is satisfactory. If the liquid is not known to be anhydrous it can be made so by distilling in the apparatus before use and using the liquid remaining in the flask.

Determination: Weigh in to the flask, which should be half filled with the entraining liquid, sufficient sample to yields 2-4 ml water if necessary, add a little porous porcelain in bits or a few glass beads to prevent bumping. Connect the apparatus and fill the receiver (if not already filled) with the entraining liquid, poured through the top of the condenser. Heat the flask gently until the liquid begins to boil and then more vigorously until there is not further increase in the volume of water in the receiver (usually about half to one hour). Rinse the inside of the condenser with a further quantity of the entraining liquid (20-30 ml is usually sufficient) which in this case should always be free from water, continue the distillation for a further 10 minutes. Allow the receiver to cool to room temperature and if any drops of water adhere to the sides of the receiver dislodge them with a piece of wire. When water and entraining liquid have separated completely, read the volume of water and from it calculate the percentage present in the sample.

Note : The results obtained will be slightly low due to some water being dissolved in the entraining liquid above the water in the receiver. In the case of xylene and toluene, the amount is negligible for normal design of apparatus, providing the receiver used, is not much too large for the volume of water collected. If an entraining liquid is used in which the solubility of water is appreciable the liquid should be saturated with water and distilled in the apparatus before the sample is added. The volume of water in the sample is then read by difference.

VIII. Determination of Foreign Organic and Inorganic Matter

Tests for foreign inorganic matter

The detection of elements/their compounds in the ash of the sample gives the test for foreign inorganic matter.

Tests for foreign Organic matter

Weigh 25-50 gm. of the drug sample, spread it out in a thin layer, and separate the foreign organic matter by hand as completely as possible. Weigh it and determine the percentage of foreign organic matter and calculate from the weight of the drug taken. Use the maximum quantity of sample for coarse or bulky drugs.

Determination of foreign organic matter

The drug should be in fine powder, the identity of the foreign matter is first established and then the number, length or area of the characteristic particles per mg., is found as follows:–

1. Determine the loss on drying at 100°C.

2. Mix a weighed amount of the air-dry material with weighed amount of lycopodium, using about 100 mg of the powder and 50 mg. of lycopodium and mixing them with a small flexible spatula on a glass plate.

3. Incorporate with the mixed powders a quantity of suspending fluid, such as an oil or a mixture of two volumes of glycerol, one volume of nucilage of tragacanth and two volumes of water, by thoroughly mixing with the spatula for about 10 minute till a smooth paste results. Transfer the suspension to a small corked tube by draining it off from a corner of the place. Then rub down a little more of the suspending fluid with the residue on the plate and transfer to the tube, continuing the process until and the powder is in the tube and adjust the final volume so that, when the drop is mounted under a cover glass and viewed under the microscope with a 4 mm objective, about 10 to 20 spores are present in the field of view. (Generally about 4 ml of suspending agent is required for 50 mg. of lycopodium).

4. Oscillate the corked tube gently until the suspension is uniform, avoiding the formation of air-bubbles, and using a dry glass tube having an internal diameter of about 2 mm. Place one drop of the suspension upon each drop with a needle of a thin glass rod over an area slightly less than that of the cover-glass. Apply the cover-glass and set aside for a short time in a level place to allow the powder to settle evenly. It is advisable to prepare two additional slides at this stage, in case, a repetition of the determination is required.

5. Select 25 fields on one slide. According to the scheme represented in the diagram, count the characteristic particles of the foreign organic matter and also the spores present in the 25 fields; make a second similar count, using a second slide.

6. Prepare a second similar suspension and repeat the whole operation.

7. From the mean of four results, which should not differ by more than 10 per cent for the two suspensions, and the percentage of moisture present. Calculate; with reference to the powder dried at 110°C the number of characteristic per mg. of the powder.

8. The number of characteristic particles per mg. of the pure foreign matter is next determined in a similar way and is calculated with reference to the material dried at 110°C. If this number can be obtained from the literature a special experiment is unnecessary.

9. Calculate the percentage of foreign organic matter from the formula:—

$$\text{Percentage of Foreign organic matter: } \frac{94{,}000 \times 100 \times n \times w}{s \times m \times p}$$

Where n = number of characteristic particles in 25 fields.

s = number of spores in the same fields.

w = Weight in mg. of lycopodium taken.

m = Weight in mg. of the sample, calculated on the sample dried at 110°C.

p = number of characteristic particles per mg. of the pure foreign matter calculated on the material dried at 110°C.

94,000=number of spores per mg of lycopodium.

(Note : The specified fields are brought into view by using a mechanical stage or by using a counting field finder).

B. For particles which are rod-shaped:—

Trace the length of the pieces by a camera lucida at a definite magnification and measure them on the drawing.

C. For measurement of the area:—

Trace the particles carefully in outline, using a camera lucida. Cut out of the tracing and calculate the area form the total weight of the pieces of the paper and adjust the volume in a corked tube. Staining with solution of safranine followed by dilute acid is to be preferred to the use of phloroglucinol in some instances, as for the staining of nux vomica trichomes.

(*Note:*—When the amount of foreign matter is a small proportion such as 2 per cent, a much larger number of fields must be counted. For the purpose, about 40 sq. mm. is used by counting nine strips across the counting square (see diagram), each strip having a width equal to the diameter of the field of view).

It is also desirable for critical work to determine a special constant by using a mixture prepared from authentic materials, of approximately the same composition as the sample to be examined. Such a constant is nearly always slightly different from that obtained with pure foreign matter, because certain particles of one powder may be mistaken for those of another ingredient. The errors thus made in finding the constant will eliminate the similar errors that will be made when examining the sample.

IX. Determination of:—

A. Fat content: *(Avaleha, Ghrta)*

Transfer a weighed quantity of the well-mixed sample to an extraction thimble. Extract with anhydrous ether (petroleum ether, b.p. 4060°C may be used if the fat is not to be used for any subsequent determinations: if fat values are to be determined, ether should be used) in a continuous extraction apparatus for 6 hours. Filter the extract into a clean, dry weighed flask, wash the extraction flask with small quantities of ether, filter the washings into the weighed flask. Evaporate the solvent and dry to constant weight at 100°C.

B. Volatilic oil content : ***(Arka, ghrta, taila, guggulu, vati-gutika, and rasa-yoga, varti).***

The determination is made by distilling the drug with water, collecting the distillate in a graduated tube in which the aqueous portion of the distillate is automatically separated and returned to the distilling flask, and measuring the volume of the oil. The constant of volatile oil is expressed as a percentage v/w.

Apparatus

The apparatus consists of the following parts

a) Distilling flask: a spherical flask of 1000 ml capacity with a ground neck (standard joint B34, British Standard); taper of ground socket 1 in 10, internal diameter of larger end 34.35 to 34.65 mm.

b) Still-head, condenser, graduated measuring tube and return-flow tube made in one piece, in accordance with the following specification:

Group Joint accurately fitting a ground neck of flask taper 1 in 10, external diameter of smaller end 31.0 to 31.2 mm. minimum length of ground zone 34 mm.

Tube AC

Length 190 to 210 mm.

Internal diameter 13 to 15 mm.

Tube CDE

Length CD 145 to 155 mm.

Internal diameter 7 to 8 mm.

Condenser FG

Length, 145 to 155 mm.

Internal diameter 14to 15 mm.

Internal diameter at constructions 9 to 10 mm.

Stopper K and tubulure K

Taper 1 in 10

nominal internal diameter of larger and end of ground socket 7.5

mm nominal external diameter of smaller end of ground cane 5.7 mm. angle GHK 30° to 40°C.

Tube GH

Internal diameter 7 to 8 mm.

Measuring tube JL

Length of graduated portion 145 to 155 mm capacity 4 ml. sub divided into 0.05 ml.

Diagram showing the position of the fields selected for counting the characteristic and spores. The numbers indicate the distances in mm. of the positions on the fields from the centre of the cover glass.

For clearing a powder, having a characteristic epidermis etc. Mix the lycopodium and powder with 3 to 3.5 ml of solution of chloral hydrate as described above for the other suspending agents. Transfer to a small specimen tube and heat by suspending it inside a boiling tube which is immersed in a water bath. When the particles are cleaned and nearly colourless, cool and add sufficient of the glycerol and tragacanth suspending agent to produce the required volume.

For stating lignified particles, rub the mixed lycopodium and powder phloroglucinol solution. Allow it to become nearly dry and mix it with about 1 ml. of hydrocholoric acid. Then incorporate the suspending fluid and any chloral hydrate which may be necessary.

Tube HJ

Length HJ 30 to 40 mm.

Tube BL

Internal diameter 7 to 8 mm

Vertical height of junction B below to be graduation mark J 20 to 2 mm.

Distance between vertical axis 100 to 110 mm.

c) Burner : a luminous Argand–type burner with a chimney and sensitive regulating cap.

d) Stand : a retort stand with asbesios covered ring and clamp carrying a piece of metal tubing N connected by a short length of rubber tubing, with the water inlet tube of the condenser jacket.

For stating lignified particles, rub the mixed lycopodium and powder phloroglucinol solution. Allow it to become nearly dry and mix it with about 1 ml. of hydrocholoric acid. Then incorporate the suspending fluid and any chloral hydrate which may be necessary.

Tube HJ

Length HJ 30 to 40 mm.

Tube BL

Internal diameter 7 to 8 mm

Vertical height of junction B below to be graduation mark J 20 to 2 mm.

Distance between vertical axis 100 to 110 mm.

c) Burner : a luminous Argand–type burner with a chimney and sensitive regulating cap.

d) Stand : a retort stand with asbesios covered ring and clamp carrying a piece of metal tubing N connected by a short length of rubber tubing, with the water inlet tube of the condenser jacket.

The whole apparatus is effectively screened for draughts. The glass apparatus is cleaned before each distillation by washing successively with acetone and water, then filling it to stand and finally rinsing with water.

When fully assembled the apparatus is totally enclosed. When an air-bent is required it should be arranged at the stopper K'.

Method : Proceed by method I or II.

Method-I Mix a suitable quantity of the sample, accurately weighed or measured (solids should be reduced to powder form), with 30 ml of water and a few small pieces of porous earthern-ware in the distilling flask. Connect the flask to the still head remove the stopper K', and run water into the tubulure K until it overflows at B.

Heat the flask, with frequent agitation, until abolition commences and continue. The distillation at a rate that leaves the lower part of the condenser cold at the point G. Rotate the flask occasionally to wash down any material adhering to the upper part of the walls. At the end of 4 hours, discountine heating and after five minutes read off the volume of volatile oil in the graduated portion of the tube.

Continue the distillation for a further period of one hour and again read off the volume of the oil. Repeat if unnecessary, until successive reading do not differ. The measured yield of volatile oil is taken to be the content of volatile oil in the drug.

Method-11- Connect the distilling flask, Containing 300 ml of water and a few piece of porous earthenware to the still-head. Remove the stopper K' and run water into the tubular K until it overflows at B. Introduce 1 ml of xylene at K by means of a pipette, the tip of which is inserted into the lower part of the tubular K. Heat the flask until ebulliton commences and continue the distillation at a rate that leaves the lower part of the condenser cold at the point G. After thirty minutes read off the volume in the graduated portion of the tube.

Introduce the sample into the flask and carry out the distillation as described under method-1.

Subtract the volume of xylene previously observed from the volume of the oily layer; the remainder is taken to be the content of volatile oil in the dry sample.

(C) Acid value: *(ghrta, taila, paka)*

Note : This determination should be carried out on the fat/oil extracted from the sample by continuous extraction with ether.

The acid value of an oil fat is defined as the number of milligrams of potassium hydroxide required to neutralise the free acid in 1 gramme of the sample.

Method: Mix 25 ml ether with 25 ml alcohol (95 percent) and 1 ml of 1% phenolphthalein solution and neutralise with N/10 alkali (few drops). Dissolve about 5g of the fat or oil, accurately weighed, in the mixed neutral solvent, and titrate with N/10 potassium (or sodium) hydroxide, shaking constantly until a pink colour which persists for fifteen seconds is obtained.

(Alternatively, boiling neutral alcohol can be employed as solvent and the free fatty acids titrated while the liquid is still hot).

The titration should preferably not exceed about 10 ml.

$$\text{Acid value} = \frac{\text{No. of ml. of N / 10 alkali used} \times 5.61}{\text{weight of sample in g.}}$$

The free fatty acid content is also express as F.F. A., calculated as oleic acid %(1 ml N/10) alkali = 0.028 g. oleic acid)

(D) *Saponification Value:* (taila, ghrta, paka)

Note: This determination should be carried out on the fat/oil extracted from the sample by continuous extraction with ether.

reflux condenser and heat the flask in boiling water for one hour, shaking frequently. Add 1 ml of phenolphtanleim (1%) solution and titrate the excess alkali with N/2 hydro chloric acid (tritration=a ml) carry out a blank at the same time (titraton = b ml)

$$\text{Saponification value} = \frac{(b - a) \times 561}{\text{wt. in g. of sample}}$$

E) *Iodine value* (Taila, ghrta, paka)

The *iodine value* of an oil or fat is the weight of iodine absorbed by 10 parts by weight of the sample, when determined by one of the following methods.

Method I (Iodine Monochloride Method((Wij's method)

Place the sample, accurately weighed, in a dry iodine flask of 250 ml capacity, add 10 ml of carbon tetrachloride, and dissolve. (The approximate weight, in g. of the sample to be taken may be calculated by dividing 20 by the highest expected iodine value). Add 10 ml of chloroform and 20 ml. of iodine monochloride solution, insert the stopper, previously moistened with potassium iodine solution and allow to stand in a dark place at a temperature of about 17°C for thirty minutes. Add 15 ml. of potassium iodine solution and 100 ml of water; shake and titrate with N/10 sodium thiosulphate using starch mucilage as indicator. Note the number of ml. required (a). At the same time carry out the operation in exactly the same manner, but with the sample being tested, and note the number of ml. N/10 sodium thiosulphate required (b).

Calculate the iodine value from the formula

$$\text{Iodine value} = \frac{(b - a) \times 0.01269 \times 100}{\text{wt. of sample (in g.)}}$$

If (b-a) is greater than b/2 the test must be repeated using smaller quantity of the sample.

Method II (Iodine monobromide method) (Hanus method):

Iodobromide solutions: Dissolve 13.2 g. of idoine in 1000 ml of glacial acetic acid with the aid of gentle heat, if necessary cool the solution to 75° and determine the iodine content in 20 ml. by titration with N/10 sodium thiosulphate. Add to the remainder of the solution a quantity of bromide equivalent to that of the iodine present. Store in glass containers, protected from light.

Place the sample, accurately weighed in a 250 ml iodine flask, add 10 ml of chloroform and dissolve (The approximate weight in g. of the sample to be taken may be calculated by dividing 20 by the highest expected Iodine number. Add 25 ml of iodobromide solutions stopper the flask, and allow it to stand for 30 minutes protected from light. Then add in the order named 1330 ml of potassium iodine solution, (16.5 per cent w/v) and 100 ml of water, and titrate the liberated iodine with N/10 sodium thiosulphate using starch mucilage as indicator. Note the number of ml required (a). At the same time, carry out the operation inexactly the same manner, but without the sample being tested, and note the No. of ml. of *N-10 sodium thiosulphate required* (b).

Calculate the iodine value from the formula.

$$\text{Iodine value} = \frac{(b - a) \times 0.01269 \times 100}{\text{wt. (in g.) of sample}}$$

It (b-a) is greater than b/2 the test must be repeated using a smaller quantity of the sample.

Test for the absence of Vanaspati in ghee

The test is based on the presence of sesame oil Vanaspati. Vanaspati manufactured in India is statutorily required to contain 5% of sesame oil. As the Baudouin's test described below is capable of detecting 0.5% or less of sesame oil in other oil/fats, it is used indirectly by identification of vanaspati in ghee.

Shake 2 ml of the fat or oil with 1 ml of hydrochloric acid containing 1% percent w/v of sucrose and allow to stand for 5 minutes, the acid layer acquires a pink colour.

Note: The test should be carried out on the oil or fat extracted from ghtra and paka with ethyl ether.

Test for the detection of Arachis oil in sesame oil

Boil 1 ml of the oil with 5ml of 1.5 N alcoholic potash (8.416 per cent KOH in 95% alcohol) in a small flask fitted with a long air condenser for ten minutes. Add 50 ml of alcohol (50% v/v) and 0.8 ml of hydrochloric acid (specific gravity 1.16) and warm do dissolve any precipitate which may have formed, cool, stirring continuously with thermometer in the liquid, so that the temperature falls at the rate of about 1°C per minute.

The clouding points of sesame oil is 15°C and that of arachis oil 39-40°C. A figure significantly above 15°C test for the detection of cotton seed oil in other oils may be taken as evidence of the presence of arachis oil in sesame oil.

X. Qualitative Reactions

1. Aluminium

1. While gelatinous precipitate of aluminium hydroxide Al $(OH)_3$, is formed on addition of ammonia solution. It is slightly soluble in excess of the reagent. When freshly precipitated, it dissolves readily in strong acids and bases, but after boiling it becomes difficultly soluble.
2. Addition of sodium phosphate solution white gelatinous precipitate of aluminium phosphate $AlPO_4$ is formed, which is insoluble in acetic acid, but soluble in mineral acids and in solutions of caustic alkalis.
3. "Aluminon" dyestuff is strongly absorbed by aluminium hydroxide giving a bright red adsorption complex of "lake". The test is applied to the precipitate of aluminium hydroxide obtained in the usual course of analysis, since certain other elements interfere. Dissolve the aluminium hydroxide precipitate in 2 ml. of M hydrochloric acid, add 2 ml. of 3 m ammonium acetate solution and 2 ml of 0.1 percent aqueous solution of the reagent. Shake, allow to stand for 5 minutes and add excess of ammoniacal ammonium carbonate solution to decolourise the excess of the dyestuff and also lakes due to traces of chromic hydroxide and silica. A bright red precipitate (or coloration), persisting in the alkaline solution is obtained.

2. Arsenic

1. Arsenious salts; neutral solutions react with silver nitrate to form yellow precipitate of silver arsenite—soluble in ammonia solution and in nitric acid.

2. Arsenious salts in neutral solutions react with solution of copper sulphate to form green-precipitate (Scheele's green) which on boiling gives a red precipitate of cuprous oxide.

3. Arsenic salts in neutral solutions react with siliver nitrate to form brownish red precipitate of silver arsenate soluble in acids and in ammonia but insoluble in acetic acid.

4. When nitric acid and excess ammonium molybdate solutions added to the solution of arsenic salts a crystalline yellow precipitate is obtained on boiling (Distinction from arsenites which give no precipitate and from phosphates which give precipitate in cold or upon gentle warming).

5. Arsenic salts in neutral or ammonical solutions react with magnesia mixture (a solution containing $MgCl_2$, NH_4Cl and a little NH_3) to give a white precipitate which forms red silver arsenate upon treating with silver nitrate solution containing a few drops of acetic acid (Distinction from phosphate).

3. Borate

The mixture obtained by the addition of sulphuric acid and alcohol (95%) to a borate when ignited, burns with a flame tinged with green.

4. Calcium

1. Solutions of calcium salts, when treated with ammonium carbonate solution, yield a white precipitate which after boiling and cooling the mixture, is insoluble in ammonium chloride solution.

2. Solutions of calcium salts, when treated with ammonium oxalate solution, yield a white precipitate which is soluble in hydrochloric acid and isoluble in acetic acid.

3. Calcium salts, when moistened with hydrochloric acid and introduced on a platinum wire into the flame of a Bunsen burner, give a brick red colour to the flame.

5. Carbonates

1. Carbonates, when treated with dilute acids, effervescence, liberating carbon dioxide which is colourless and produces a white precipitate in calcium hydroxide solution.

2. Solutions of carbonates, when treated with magnesium sulphate solution, yield a white precipitate at room temperature.

6. Chlorides

1. Chlorides when heated with sulphuric acid and manganese dioxide, evolve chlorine, recognisable by its odour and by its giving blue colour with potassium iodide and starch solution.
2. Solutions of chlorides, when treated with silver nitrate solution, yield a white curdy precipitate which is insoluble in nitric acid, but soluble after being well washed with water, in dilute ammonia solution, from which it is reprecipitated by the addition of nitric acid.

7. Copper (USP)

1. An excess of ammonia TS, added to a solution of a cupric salt, produces first a bluish precipitate and then a deep blue coloured solution.
2. With potassium ferroocyanide TS, solution of cupric salts yield a reddish brown precipitate insoluble in diluted acids.

8. Gold

1. Metallic gold is soluble in a mixture of three volume of hydrochloric acid and one volume of nitric acid, yielding a solution of chloroauric acid, and is insoluble in concentrated mineral acids.
2. Solutions of gold compounds, yield with hydrogen sulphide a black precipitate insoluble in dilute hyrochloric acid, but soluble in ammonium polysulphide solution, from which it is reprecipitated on the addition of dilute hydrochloric acid.
3. Auric compounds in neutral or weakly acid solution yield with stannous chloride solution, a purple colour and with hydrogen peroxide solution and sodium hydroxide solution, a precipitate which appears brownish black by reflected light and bluish green by transmitted light.

9. Iron

(a) Ferric

1. Solutions of ferric salts, when acidified with dilute hydrochloric acid and treated with ammonium thiocyanate solution, yield a blood red colour which is extracted by solvent ether or armyl alcohol and is discharged on the addition of mercuric chloride test solution or phosphoric acid.
2. Solution of ferric salts, when treated with hydrochloric acid and ammonium nitrosophenyldroxylamine solution, yield a reddish brown precipitate which is soluble in solvent ether.

3. Solutions of ferric salts, when treated with potassium ferricyanide solution, yield a reddish brown colour but no precipitate.
4. Solutions of ferric salts, when treated with potassium ferrocyanide solution; yield an intense blue precipitate which is insoluble in dilute hyrochloric acid.
5. Solutions of ferric salts, when strongly acidified with acetic acid and treated with a 0.2 % W/V solution of hydroxy 7-iodoquinoline- 5- sulpuric acid, yield a stable green colour.

(b) Ferrous

1. Solutions of ferrous salts, in dilute hyrochloric acid when treated with sufficient potassium permanganate solution to produce a faint pink colour, yield with ammonium thiocyanate solution a blood red colour which is extracted by solvent ether or amyl alcohol and is discharged on the addition of mercuric chloride test solution or of phosphoric acid.
2. Solutions of ferrous salts, when treated with potassium ferricyanide solution; yield a dark blue precipitate which is insoluble in dilute hydrochloric acid and is decomposed by sodium hyroxide solution.
3. Solutions of ferrous slats, when treated with potassium ferrocyanide solution, yield a white precipitate which rapidly becomes blue and is insoluble in dilute hydrochloric acid.

10. Lead

1. Strong solutions of lead salts, when treated with hydrochloric acid, yield a white precipitate which is soluble in boiling water and is re-deposited as crystals when the solution is cooled.
2. Solutions of lead salts, in the absence of very strong acid yield with hydrogen sulphide a black precipitate which is insoluble in dilute hydrochloric acid and in ammonium sulphide solution but is soluble in hot dilute nitric acid.
3. Solutions of lead salts, when treated with dilute sulphuric acid, yield a white precipitate which is almost insoluble in water, more nearly insoluble in dilute acetate solution.
4. Solutions of lead salts, when treated with potassium idodide solution, yield a yellow precipitate which dissolves when the mixture is boiled and is reprecipitated as glistening plates when the solution is cooled.

5. Solutions of lead salts, when treated with potassium chromate solution, yield a yellow precipitate which is readily soluble in sodium hydroxide solution and in not nitric acid, sparingly soluble in dilute nitric acid, and insoluble in acetic acid.
6. Solutions of lead salts, when treated with potassium cyanide solution, made alkaline with dilute ammonia solution, and shaken with diphenyl thiocarbazone solution, yield a brick red coloured lower layer.

11. Magnesium

1. Solutions of magnesium salts, when treated with ammonium carbonate solution and boiled, yield a white precipitate but yield not precipitate in the presence of ammonium chloride solution.
2. Solutions of magnesium salts, when treated with sodium phosphate solution in the presence of ammonium salts and dilute ammonia solution, yield a white crystalline precipitate.
3. Solutions of magnesium salts when treated with sodium hydroxide solution, yield a white precipitate which is isoluble in an excess of the reagent, but soluble in ammonium chloride solutions.
4. Solutions of magnesium salts, when treated with sodium hydroxide solution and diphenylcarbazide solution, yield a pink precipitate.

12. Mercury

1. Solutions of mercuric salts yield with hydrogen sulphide a black precipitate which is insoluble in ammonium sulphide solution and in boiling dilute nitric acid.
2. Solution of mercuric salts which are free from an excess of nitric acid, deposit a coating of mercury on bright copper foil, the deposit becomes bright when it is rubbed and may be volatised from the foil by heat and obtained in globules.
3. Solutions of mercuric salts, when treated with stannous chloride solution, yield a white precipitate which rapidly becomes gray with an excess of the reagent.
4. Neutral solutions of mercuric salts, when treated with potassium iodide solution, yield a scarlet precipitate which is soluble in excess of the reagent and in a considerable excess of the solution of the mercuric salt.

5. Solutions of mercuric salts, when treated with sodium hydroxide solutions, yield a yellow precipitate.

13. Phosphate

1. Solutions of phosphate when treated with silver nitrate solution yield yellow precipitate of normal silver orthophosphate Ag_3PO_4 (distinction from meta and pyro-phosphate) soluble in dilute ammonia solution and dilute nitric acid.
2. Solutions of phosphate yield a white crystalline precipitate of magnesium ammonium phosphate Mg (NH_4) PO_4 $6H_2O$ with magnesia mixture; it is soluble in acetic acid and in mineral acids, but practically insoluble in 2.5 percent ammonia solution.
3. Addition of a large excess (2-3 ml) of ammonium molybdate reagent to a small volume (0.5 ml) of a phosphate solution produces a yellow crystalline precipitate of ammonium phosphomolybdate.
4. Place a drop of the acid solution of phosphate upon quantitative filter paper; add a drop of the molybdate reagent, followed by a drop of the benzidine reagent. Hold the paper over ammonia vapour. A blue stain is formed when most of the mineral acid has been neutralised.

14. Potassium

1. Potassium compounds when moistened with hydrochloric acid and introduced on platinum wire into the flame of a Bunsen burner give a lilac colour of the flame, when viewed through suitable blue glass, the flame is reddish purple.
2. Moderately strong solutions of potassium salts which have been previously ignited to remove ammonium salts, when treated with platinic chloride solution in the presence of hydrochloric acid, yield a yellow crystalline precipitated which on ignition leaves a residue of potassium chloride and platinum.
3. Moderately strong solutions of potassium salts, which have been previously ignited to remove ammonium salts, when treated with perchloric acid (60%) yield a white crystalline precipitate.
4. Solutions of potassium salts, which have been previously ignited to remove ammonium salts when treated with sodium cobaltinitrate solution and acetic acid, yield a yellow precipitate.

15. Silicon

(1) *Silicon tetraflouride test*

This test depends upon the fact that when silica (isolated from a silicate by treatment with ammonium chloride solution or with hydrochloric acid, etc.) is heated with calcium fluoride and concentrated sulphuric acid, silicon tetrafluoride is evolved. The latter is identified by its action upon a drop of water held in a loop of platinum wire, when a turbidity (due to silicic acid) is produced.

(2) *Ammonium molybdate-benzidine test*

Silicates react with molybdates in acid solution to form the complex zilico-molybdic acid H_4 $(SiMO_{12}O_{40})$, of which the ammonium salt, unlike the analogous phosphoric acid and arsenic acid compounds, is soluble in water and acids to give a yellow solution. The test depends upon the reaction between silicomolybdic acid and benzidine in acetic acid solution whereby "Molybdenum blue" and a blue quinonoid oxidation compound of benzidine are produced.

Place a drop of the test solution and of the molybdate reagent upon drop reaction paper, and warm gently over a wire gauze. Add a drop of the benzidine reagent and hold the paper over ammonia vapour. A blue coloration results.

16. Silver

1. Solutions of silver salts, when treated with hydrochloric acid or with solutions of chlorides, yield a white curdy precipitate which is insoluble in nitric acid but soluble, after being well washed with water in dilute ammonia solution, from which it is reprecipated by the addition of nitric acid.
2. Solutions of silver salts, when treated with potassium chromate solution, yield a red precipitate which is insoluble in nitric acid.
3. Solutions of silver salts, when made slightly alkaline with dilute ammonia solution and then distinctly acid with acetic acid, and shaken with a 0.025% w/v solution of p-dimethylaminobenzyli-demerhodamine in amyl alcohol, yield a red precipitate which collects at the interface of the two layers.
4. Solutions of silver salts, when treated with potassium iodide solution yield a cream-coloured precipitate which is insoluble in dilute ammonia solution and in nitric acid.

17. Sodium

1. Sodium compounds when moistened with hydrochloric acid and introduced on a platinum wire into the flame of a Bunsen burner, give a yellow colour of the flame.
2. Solutions of sodium salts, when acidified with dilute acetic acid, filtered if necessary, and treated with uranyl zinc acetate solution, yield a yellow crystalline precipitate.
3. Solutions of sodium salts, when treated with about an equal volume of potassium antimonate solution, slowly yield a white crystalline precipitate.

18. Sulphur (Free Sulphur)

Extract a suitable quantity of the sample with carbon disulphide. Filter the carbon disulphide solution and evaporate off the solvent. To the residue add 10 ml of 10% alcoholic potash and boil until the sulphur has dissolved. Dilute with water, oxidise by adding hydrogen peroxide solution in excess and heat on a water bath for 1/2 hour. Acidity with hyrochloric acid, filter and to the filtrate add barium chloride solution. White precipitate of $BaSO_4$ shows the presence of sulphur.

19. Sulphates

1. Solutions of sulphates, when treated with barium chloride solution, yield a white precipitate which is insoluble in hydrochloric acid.
2. Solutions of sulphates, when treated with lead acetate solution, yield a white precipitate which is insoluble in ammonium acetate solution and in sodium hydroxide solution.

20. Tin

If organic matter is present, wet oxidise with sulphuric and nitric acid, remove nitric acid by heating until white fumes are given off, dilute with water and pass H_2S gas. A yellow precipitate is produced if tin is present. Filter off the precipitate, dissolve it in sodium hydroxide solution containing a little ammonium sulphide, acidify with acetic acid. Tin sulphide is reprecipitated.

Alkaloids

1. To a distinctly acidic solution of the substance and Dragendorff's (Potassium bismuth iodide) reagent, a red precipitate is formed.

2. Add Mayer's reagent (Potassium mercuric idoide), light yellow precipitate soluble in excess of the reagent and ethanol, is formed.

XI. Quantitative estimations

Determination of

1. Aluminium

Prepare a 2 per cent solution of (A.R.) 8-hydroxyquinoline in 2N acetic acid, add ammonia solution (1:1) until a permanent precipitate is just produced, and re-dissolve this by warming.

20 ml of the sample solution is pippetted out (preparation of the solution—refer total sulphur) and a 20% excess of the oxine solution (1 ml. will precipitate 0.001 g of Al) is added when the complex Al $(C_9H_6ON)_3$ will be formed. Complete the precipitation by the addition of a solution of 4.0 g of ammonium acetate in the minimum quantity of water, stir the mixture and allow to cool. Filter the granular precipitate through a sintered glass crucible of porosity No. 4 (or through a porcelain filtering crucible) and wash with warm water. Dissolve the complex in warm concentrated hydrochloric acid, collect the solution in a 250 ml. reagent bottle, add a few drops of indicator (0.1% solution of the sodium salt of methyl red or 0.1% methyl orange solution) and 0.5–1 g. of pure potassium bromide. Titrate slowly with standard 0.1 N (i.w., M/60) potassium bromate until the colour becomes pure yellow (with either indicator). The exact end point is not easy to detect, and it is better to add a slight excess of standard bromate solution (free bromine is thus present, and is tested for by removing a drop of the liquid on to potassium iodide starch paper), dilute the solution considerably with 2N hydrochloric acid (to prevent the precipitation of 5, 7-dibromo-8-hydroxy quinoline during the titration), then add (after 5 minutes) 10 ml. of 10% potassium iodide solution, and titrate the liberated iodine with standard 0.1 N sodium thiosulphate, using starch as indicator. Repeat the titration with two other 25.0 ml. portions of the aluminium solution.

Calculate the percent of aluminium by the relation.

1 ml. of N $KBrO_3$ = 0.002249 g. Al

2. Arsenic

In the presence of organic matter

Wet oxidise a suitable quantity of the material in the special 300 ml Kjeldahl flask (fitted with a B24 joint) by heating first with 10 ml of concentrated nitric acid. When the initial vigorous reaction has ceased, cool, add 120 ml of conc. sulphuric acid and continue the heating with further additions of nitric acid immediately the liquid darken. Heat until white fumes appear and the liquid is colourless begins to if a pale yellow colour persists, head the liquid further with a few drops of 30% hydrogen peroxide. Cool, add 15 ml of saturated ammonium oxalate solution and heat again until white fumes appear. Cool, add 7 ml of water, 5 g. of the chloride-hydrozing-bromide agent (mix together 100 g. of potassium bromide) and 10 ml of cone. HCl. Fit the condenser on the flask and distil into an extremely cooled mixture of 2 ml of conc. nitric acid and 10 ml of water. The exit end of the condenser must dip below the surface of the liquid.

Continue distilling until the liquid in the Kjeldahl flask is reduced to about half or until five minutes after the condenser is full of steam. Evaporate the distillate to dryness in a 100 ml beaker on the water bath and then evaporate twice more after the addition of 5 ml of water each time to remove nitric acid. Dissolve the residue in 3 ml of conc, sulphuric acid and dilute to 50 ml with water.

Determination

(1) If the quantity of arsenic present in the solution is sufficient the solution may be titrated with M/20 iodate.

1 ml of M/20 iodate=0.009895 g. As_2O_3. Or the iodine oxidation method may be employed.

Add 2 g. of sodium bicarbonate to the acid solutions and titrate with N/10 iodine.

1 ml of N/10 iodine=0.004945 g As_2O_3.

(2) If the quantity of arsenic is small, add 0.1 g of sodium sulphate to the prepared solution, and boil down to 25 ml to remove the sulphur dioxide. Add 8 ml of stannated hydrochloric acid and make up to 60 ml with water. Determine by the Gutzeit method.

3. Borate

Weigh out accurately 2 g of the material and extract with distilled water exhaustively. Made up the water extract in a 250 ml volumetric flask. Pipette out 25 ml of the solution and titrate with standard 0.1 N HCl using methyl orange as indicator.

To another 25 ml. of the solution, add the quantity of standard hydrocholoric acid determined in the previous titration. Cover the beaker or conical flask with a clock glass or Fisher "sppedyvap" beaker cover, heat to simmering temperature for 10 minutes to expel carbon dioxide (prolonged vigorous boiling may cause loss of boric acid which is volatile in steam), cool the solution to room temperature, and add just sufficient standard sodium hydroxide solution to restore the transition colour of original indicator. Then introduce about 2 g of mannitol and shake until dissolved; add a few drops of phenolphthalein and titrate with standard 0.1 N carbonate-free sodium hydroxide to the first permanent faint-pink colour. Add a further 0.5 g. of mannitol; if the solution becomes colourless, add more standard sodium hydroxide until the pink colour reappers. Repeat the process until the addition of mannitol has no effect upon the end point.

Calculate the percentage of $Na_2B_4O_7$ in the sample from the results of both the titrations.

4. Calcium

Preparation of sample for analysis

(I) In the absence of organic matter

An aliquot of the sample is dissolved in dilute hyrochloric acid. The solution is filtered and the filtered is made up to volume in a volumetric flask.

(2) In the presence or organic matter

Ignite a suitable quantity of the sample, accurately weighed, in a porcelain crucible at 500-550 C until the residue is white or nearly so. Moisten with 510 ml hydrochloric acid, boil for two minutes, evaporate to dryness and heat on steam bath for 3 hours to render S_iO_2 insoluble. Moisten the residue with 5 ml of hydrochloric acid, boil for two minutes, add 50 ml of water, heat on the water bath for a few minutes, filter and wash thoroughly. (The residue maybe reserved of necessary for the determination of Sio_2)

5. Camphor

1. The solution of camphor in aldehyde free alcohol gives an orange red precipitate of 2, 4- dinitrophenyl hydrozone when a solution of 2, 4 dinitrophenyl hydrazine is added with constant stirring followed by heating.

2. The light absorption, in the range 230 to 250 mm, of a 2 cm layer of a 0.25% (w/v) solution in ethanol (96%) exhibits a maximum only at 289 nm.

Determination

Transfer an aliquot of the solution prepared as above to a 250 ml beaker, add water if necessary to make to 50 ml heat to boiling, and add 10 ml of saturated ammonium oxalate solution and one drop of methyl red indicator. Almost neutralise with NH_4OH and boil until precipitate is coarsely granular. Cool, add NH_4OH (1+4) until colour is faint pink (PH 5.0) and let stand for at least 4 hours. Filter and wash with water at room temperature until filtrate is oxalate-- free. Break point of filter with a platinum wire, and wash precipitate into beaker in which the Ca was precipitated, using stream of hot water. Add about 10 ml of H_2SO_4 (1+4) heat to about 90.C, add about 50 ml of water and titration with N/10 potassium permanganate solution. Finally and filter paper to solution and complete the titration. 1 ml N/10= 0.0020 g. Ca.

6. Chloride

Preparation of sample for analysis

(1). In the absence of organic matter:

Extract an aliquot of the sample with hot water, filter and wash. Dissolve any residue remaining in nitric acid (1+4), filter, wash thoroughly and add the filtrate to the water extract.

(2). In the presence of organic matter:

Moisten a suitable quantity of the sample, accurately weighed in a platinum dish with 20 ml of 5 per cent sodium carbonate solution, evaporate to dryness and ignite as thoroughly as possible as a temperature not exceeding 500.C. Extract with hot water, filter and wash. Return the residue to the platinum dish, and ignite to ash; 10v dissolve in nitric acid (2+4), filter, wash, thoroughly and add this.solution to the water extract.

Determination

To the prepared solution, add a known volume of N/10 silver nitrate solution in slight excess. Stir well, filter, water the silver chloride precipitate thoroughly. To the combined filtrate and washings add 5 ml of ferric alum indicator (saturated solution of ferric ammonium alum) and a few of nitric acid and titrate the excess of silver with N/10 ammonium or potassium thiocyanate to permanent light brown. From the number of ml of N/10 silver nitrate solution, calculate quantity of Cl

1 ml of N/10 silver nitrate= 0.00355 g of Cl.

7. Copper

Method- 1 In the absence of arsenic, antimony and iron.

Preparation of sample for analysis.

(1) *In the absence of organic matter:*

An aliquot of the sample is dissolved in dilute hyrochloric acid. The solution is filtered and the filtrate is made up to volume in a volumetric flask.

(2) *In the presence of organic matter:*

Ignite a suitable quantity of the sample, accurately weighed in a porcelain crucible at 500-550 until the residue is white or nearly so. Moisten with 5-10 ml. hydrochloric, acid boil for two minutes, evaporate to dryness add heat on steam bath for 3 hours to render SiO2 insoluble. Moisten the residue with 5 ml of hydrochloric acid boil for tow minutes add 50 ml of water, heat on the water bath for a few minutes, filter and wash thoroughly. Make up the filtrate to a known volume in a volumetric flask. (The residue may be reserved, if necessary for the determination of Sio_2).

Determination

To an aliquot of the solution (containing the equivalent of 0.10 g of Cu), add a slight excess of sodium carbonate and acidify with 5 ml of acetic acid. Add 3 g of potassium iodide and titrate with N/10 sodium thiosulphate until nearly all the iodine has been removed; add mucilage of starch and one drop of N/10 silver nitrate (to make the disappearance of the blue starch iodide colour sharper) and complete the titration.

1 ml of N/10 thiosulphate= 0.006354 g Cu.

Method 11: In the presence of arsenic, antimony or iron, reparation of sample for analysis.

If the sample is free from organic matter transfer an aliquot of the sample containing about 0.1 g Cu to a 300 ml flask, add 5 ml of nitric acid and 7 ml of sulphuric acid. Digest on hot plate to white fumes, cool add about 30 ml of water, boil for one minute, cool and filter. Wash filter and residue six times with small portions of hot water.

If organic matter is present, transfer an aliquot containing about 0.1 g of Cu to a 300 ml Kjedahl flask, add 10 ml of nitric acid and heat gently at first and then more thoroughly. Add more nitric acid at intervals and continue the digestion until the solution is no longer dark. Continue heating until white fumes appear. Cool, add a small quantity of water and heat again to white fumes. Dilute with about 50 ml of water, filter and wash residue with small portions of water.

Method: To the filterate obtained as above add a slight excess of sodium carbonate, followed by acetic acid in slight excess. To prevent arsenic and antimony from reacting with potassium iodide, buffer the solution to a pH of about 3.7 by adding 25 ml of 6N acetic acid and 12 ml of 6N ammonia. To prevent interference from iron, add 1 g of sodium fluoride for every 0.1 g. of iron (which converts iron to complex fluoride immediately before titration).

After this treatment carry out the titration as in Method I.

8. Iron

Total Iron

Preparation of sample for analysis

1. In the absence of organic matter

To an aliquot of the sample add 5-10 ml of hydrochloric acid, boil for two minutes, evaporate to dryness on a steam bath to render S_iO_2 insoluble. Moisten residue with 5 ml of hydrochloric acid, boil for two minutes, add 30 ml of water, heat on the water bath for few minutes, filter and wash thoroughly. (Reserve residue, if necessary for determination of sand and silicious matter). Make up to volume in a volumetric flask.

2. In the presence of organic matter

Ignite a suitable quantity of the sample, accurately weighed, in a porcelain crucible in a muffle furnace at 500-500°C until the residue is free from organic matter. Moisten with 510 ml of hydrochloric acid, boil for two minutes and proceed as above.

Determination

To an aliquot of the sample, add 12 ml of hydrogen peroxide solution (6 per cent) to oxidise the iron. Boil off the excess of hydrogen peroxide.

Add sufficient hydrochloric or water to adjust the concentration of hydrochloric acid to approximately 3 N. Add 2 g. of potassium iodide, set aside for 3 minutes and titrate with 1 ml of N/10 thiosulphate=0.00585 g. of Fe.

Ferrous Iron

Applicable only to mineral products free from organic matter

To a suitable quantity of the sample, accurately weighed, add 20 ml of dilute hydrochloric acid. Filter, if necessary, and wash with water acidified with sulphuric acid. Titrate the filtrate with N/10 potassium permanganate. Each ml of N/10 permangante=0.005585 g. of Fe (as ferrous iron).

Ferric iron

Applicable only to mineral products free from organic matter

To a suitable quantity of the sample, accurately weighed, add 20 ml of dilute hydrochloric acid (1+3), heat, if necessary to dissolve the iron, and filter. Wash the filterate with water acidified with hydrochloric acid. Add sufficient hydrochloric acid to adjust the concentration to approximately 3 N. Add 2 g of potassium iodide, set aside for 3 minutes and filtrate with N/10 sodium thiosulphate 1 ml of N/10 thiosulphate=0.005585 g. of Fe (as ferric iron).

9. Gold

About 1 g. of the powered sample is treated with aqua regia and the mixture refluxed until the sample has completely dissolved. The solution is then evaporated to dryness on a waterbath 20 ml of hyodrochloric acid is added to the mass which is again evaporated to dryness until free from nitric acid.

5 ml of hydrochloric acid and 50 ml of water are added to this stage and the resulting solution heated to boiling. An excess of 5% aqueous hydroquinone solution (50 ml) is added to the solution and boiling continued for a further 20 minutes. It is allowed to cool, filtered through whatman 42 filter paper and the residue washed thoroughly with hot water. Any gold particles adhering to the sides of the beaker are transferred with the aid of ashless filter paper strips. The filter paper with residue and the filter aids are transferred to a previously weighed silica crucible and ignited to constant weight. From the weight of the residue consisting of pure gold, the percentage of gold in the sample is calculated.

10. Lead

Dissolve 1 g. of the sample in HNO_3 (1:1) by refluxing and filter through No. 41 filter paper. Wash well with H_2O containing few drops of HNO_3 and make upto 250 ml. Reserve the filtrate for the estimation of lead. Pipette out 50 ml of the made up solution into a clean 250 ml beaker and dilute to about 100 ml. with H_2O. Add NH_4OH solution to slight precipitation and then HNO_3 (1+1) in slight excess to redissolve the precipitate. Heat the solution to boiling and add 20-30 ml of hot potassium chromate (10% w/v) solution stirring constantly. Allow the precipitate to settle. Filter by decantation through a weighed sinter (G_4) which was previously heated to 100-110°C. Wash several times with boiling water until washings are colourless. Dry the precipitate of lead chromate at 140-150°C to constant weight. From the weight of lead chromate the percentage of lead is calculated using the factor 0.6411.

11. Magnesium

In the absence of organic

To an aliquot of the sample add 5-10 ml of hydrochloric acid, boil for two minutes, evaporate to dryness on a steam bath to render SiO_2 insoluble. Moisten residue with 5 ml of hydrochloric acid, boil for two minutes, filter and wash thoroughly. (Reserve residue, if necessary for the determination of sand and siliceous matter). Make up to volume in a volumetric flask. Precipitate calcium as given under "Determination of Calcium" and use the combined filtrate and washings from the calcium determination.

2. In the presence of organic matter

Ignite a suitable quantity of the sample, accurately weighed in a porcelain crucible muffle furnace at 500-550°C until the residue is free from organic matter. Moisten with 5-10 ml of hydrochloric acid, boil for two minutes and proceed as above.

Determination

To the combined filtrate and washings from the Ca determination, concentrated by evaporation if necessary add 30 ml HNO_3 and evaporate to the dryness to decompose ammonium salts. Takeup with 5 ml HCl and dilute to about 100 ml with water. Add 5 ml of 10% sodium citrate solution and 10 ml of 10% $(NH_4)_2HPO_4$ solution is faintly alkaline and precipitate forms; then add 25 ml ammonia solution, stir vigorously until precipitate is granular and keep in cool place overnight. Filter, and wash free from chloride with cold ammonia solution (1+10). Ignite in muffle at 500-550°C until all carbon is oxidised, then at 900-950° for about 4 hours to form $Mg_2P_2O_7$. Cool, and wash as $Mg_2P_2O_7$.

The precipitate of magnesium ammonium phosphate may be filtered washed in sintered glass crucible (G_4) successively with small quantities of alcohol and ether, dried by suction, desiccated and weighed as $MgNH_4PO_4$, $6H_2O$ (%).

12. Mercury present as sulphide

In the presence of the organic matter

Transfer an aliquot of the well mixed sample expected to contain 0.1 to 0.15 gms. of mercury to a kjeldahl standard joint flask of 300 ml. capacity, and 7 ml conc. HNO_3 and 15 ml conc. H_2SO_4, attached to a standard joint condenser and heat under reflux gently at first and then more strongly for about 30 minutes so that all the organic matter is dissolved. Cool, add 12 ml of conc. HNO_3 and boil. Continue the addition of HNO_3 and boiling until the liquid is colourless or pale yellow on continued boiling. Cool, wash down the condenser with 100 ml water remove the flask, and 1% potassium permanganate solution drop by drop until a pink colour persists. Add one drop of 6% hydrogen peroxide solution to remove excess of permanganate followed by 3 ml of conc. HNO_3 and titrate with N/10 ammonium thiocyanate using ferric alum as indicator.

1 ml of N/10 thicoyanate=0.01003 gms mercury.

13. Phosphate

To a neutral or weakly acid solution (50-100 ml) of the phosphate, containing note more than 0.10 g. of P_2O_5, and 3 ml. of conc. hydrochloric acid and a few drops of methyl red indicator. Introduce 25 ml of magnesia mixture followed by pure concentrated ammonia solution slowly whilst stirring the solution vigorously until the indicator turns yellow.

Avoid scratching the sides of the beaker with the stirring rod for wherever there is contact, an adhering crystalline deposit forms quickly. Continue to stir the solution for 5 minutes adding ammonia solution dropwise to keep the solution yellow, and finally add 5 ml. of concentrated ammonia solution in excess. Allow the solution to stand in a cool place for at least 4 hours or preferably overnight. Filter through a weighed sintered glass or porcelain filtered crucible which has been washed with alcohol and ether. Wash with small portion of dilute ammonia solution (1:19; ca 0.8 M) until a few ml. of the filtrate, when acidified with dilute nitric acid and tested with silver nitrate solution, gives no test for chloride. Now wash with three 10 ml. portions of rectified spirit (95 per cent ethyl alcohol), draining well after each washing; this serves to remove most of the adhering water. Finally, wash with five 5 ml. portions of anhydrous ether, draining after each washing. Then draw air through the crucible for 10 minutes, wipe the outside of the cold crucible with a clean line cloth and allow to stand in the air or in desiccator for 20 minutes. Weigh as $MgNH_4PO_4\ 6H_2O$.

14. Silica

The residue obtained after treating the substance with bromine and nitric acid and then subsequent treatment with con. HCl is taken in a platinum dish and ignited to constant weight. Then moisten it with 1 ml. of water, add 2 or 3 drops of con. sulphuric acid and about 5 ml. of the purest available (A.R.) hydrofluric acid. Place the crucible in a radiator or air bath and evaporate the hydrofluric acid in a fume cupboard (hood) with a small flame until the acid is completely expelled; the liquid should not be boiled. (The crucible may also be directly heated with a small non-luminous flame). Then increase the heat to volatilize the sulphuric acid, and finally heat with a Meker-type burner for 15 minutes. Allow to cool in a desiccator and weigh. Re-heat to constant weight. The loss in weight represents the weight of the silica.

15. Silver

Preparation of sample

1. In the absence of organic matter

To an aliquot of the sample, add 5 ml of nitric acid and 30 ml of water, heat to boiling, coal, filter, and wash thoroughly. Make up filtrate to volume in a volumetric flask.

2. In the presence of organic matter

Ignite a suitable quantity of the sample, accurately weighed, in a porcelain crucible in a muffle furnance at 500-550°C until the residue is free from organic matter. Cool the residue and prepare solution as above.

Determination

Transfer an aliquot of the solution to a 400 ml beaker add 3 ml of nitric acid and sufficient water to produce 250 ml Protect the solution from light. Heat to about 70°C and add N/5 hydrochloric acid dropwise until precipitation is complete and 2 or 3 drops of the acid are present in excess. Keep the solution hot until the precipitation is complete and 2 or 3 drops of the acid are present in excess. Keep the solution hot until the precipitation is completely coagulated, stirring frequently. Allow to cool and set aside in the dark for several hours. Transfer the precipitate to a sintered glass crucible (Grade 4, maximum pore size, 5 to 15) with the aid of N/100 hydrochloric acid and then twice with water, and dry to constant weight at 160°C. Each g. of residue is equivalent to 1.185 g. of $AgNO_3$.

16. Sulphur

I. Total Sulphur

Transfer a weighed quantity of the well mixed sample of a long-necked flask of 250 ml capacity, (A kjeldahl flask may be used). Add 1 ml of saturated solution of bromine in carbon tetrachloride, cover, and let stand for about 30 minutes, stirring several times. Add 15 ml of concentrated nitric acid, cover and let stand for about 30 minutes, stirring several times. Heat over a low flame, adding small quantities of concentrated nitric acid from time to time, until the solution is clear and does not darken on standing. Transfer the solution quantitatively to a 250 ml beaker with the aid of water. Evaporation on a hot plate to about 5 ml. Complete the determination as given under "Free Sulphur".

II. Free Sulphur

Extract a suitable quantity of the sample, accurately weighed, with carbon disulphide in a Soxhlet extraction apparatus, letting the extraction thimble drain at least 12 times. Transfer the extract to a 250 ml beaker. Evaporate the carbon disulphide in a draugh at room temperature. Add 10 ml of saturated solution of bromine in carbon tetrachloride, cover and let stand for about 30 minutes, stirring several times. Add 15 ml of concentrated nitric acid, cover and let stand for about 30 minutes, stirring several times. Evaporate on a hot plate to about 5 ml. Add about 50 ml of water, filter and wash with 2 per cent hydrochloric acid.

Add 2 drops of bromophenol blue (0.1 g + 1.5 ml N/10 NaOH in 25 ml of water) and then ammonia to first colour change. Add HCl dropwise until distinctly acid, then add 5 drops in excess. Dilute to 150 ml with water, heat to boiling and add 10% barium chloride solution dropwise until 50% excess is present. Cover beaker and digest on steam bath for one hour. Cool to room temperature, filter through quantitative filter paper, (Whatman No. 42) was 10 times with hot water, Ignite residue in a weighed porcelain Silica Crucible at 500°C, cool in a desiccator and weigh as $BaSO_4$.

17. Tin

Preparation of sample for analysis

(1) In the absence of organic matter

To a suitable quantity of the sample, accurately weighted, add 5 ml of hydrochloric acid (1+3) 100 and 100 ml of water. Heat to boiling, cool, filter and wash with hot water. Use filterate.

(2) In the presence of organic matter

Transfer a weighed quantity of the sample to a 300 ml Kjeldahl flask. Add 25 ml of conc. nitric acid. Allow initial reaction to subside. Then add cautiously 10-20 ml of conc. sulphuric acid. When reaction has quietened, heat cautiously avoiding foaming. Rotate flask occasionally to prevent caking of sample upon glass exposed to flame. Maintain oxidizing conditions throughout the digestion by adding small quantities of nitric acid whenever mixture turns brown or darkens. Continue digestion until organic matter is destroyed and SO_3 fumes are copiously evolved. Cool slightly, and add 75 ml of water and 25 ml of saturated ammonium oxalate, solution to assist in expelling oxides of nitrogen. Evaporate again until white fumes appear. Cool, and dilute with water to 200 ml in volumetric flask.

Tin (Gravimetric)

Reagents: 1. Wash solution—mix 100 ml of saturated ammonium alkali solution with 50 ml of glacial acid and 850 ml of water.

2. Ammonium polysulphide solution—Pass H_2S gas into 200 ml of ammonia solution in bottle immerses in ice water until gas has no longer absorbed and 200 ml ammonia and dilute with water to 1 litre. Digest this solution with 25 g. flowers of sulphur several hours and filter.

Procedure

If organic matter is absent the solution prepared as above is used.

If the solution has been prepared by wet oxidation an aliquot of the solution prepared as above is used. Add ammonia until just alkaline, them 5 ml of HCl (1+3). Dilute with 100 ml of water. Heat the solution (which should be about 100 ml in volume) to about 95°C and pass in a slow stream of H_2S. Digest for 1 hr. at 95°C and let stand 30 minutes longer.

Filter and wash precipitate of SnS alternatively with 3 portions each of the wash solution and hot H_2O. Transfer filter and precipitate to 100 ml beaker, add 10-20 ml of the ammonium polysulphide solution, heat to boiling and filter. Treat contents of the beaker with 2 additional portions of hot ammonium polysulphide solution and wash, filter with hot water.

Acidify combined filterate and washings with dil. acetic acid (1+), digest on hot plate for 1 hr., let stand overnight, and filter through double 11 cm paper. Wash 2 alternately with 2 portions each of the wash solution and hot water and dry thoroughly in weighed procelain crucible. Ignite over Bunsen flame, very gently at first to burn off paper and convert the sulphide to oxide, then cover the crucible and heat strongly to mettalic tin using factor 0.7877.

18. Determination of sodium and potassium by means of the flame Photometer

In this instrument the solution under test is passed under carefully controlled conditions as a very fine spray in the air supply to a burner. In the flame the solution evaporates and the salt dissociates to give neutral atoms. Some of these, though only a very small proportion, move into a higher energy state. It is the light emitted when these excited atoms fall back to the ground state which is used in flame photometry of this type emission flame photometry. Light of characteristic wave lengths is emitted and passed through a suitable filter, grating or prism on to a selenium cell or other photosensitive element, and the amount of current thus produced is measured. This varies with the concentration of sodium, for example, in the solution which is being tested. Using solutions of known sodium content, a calibration curve can be constructed and this used for reading the sodium content of the fluids examined.

The spray is formed by passing compressed air through an atomizer, into which the liquid which is being tested is drawn either by suction, or gravity, and then enters the burner in its air supply.

The light produced is first passed through a lens to focus it and then through suitable filters (both gelatin and interference filters are used a diffractions grating or prism before it falls on to the photosensitive element. For determining sodium an orange filter can be used, the intensity of the D line (589 m) being read. Potassium emits light at 404–4 and 766.5 mm. For the latter a deep red filter is used.

The detector may be a barrier larger cell (Solenium cells sensitive well into the infrared are available so that 766.5 mm. can be used for potassium) a photo tube or photomultiplier. The amount of current produced is read on a suitable galvanometer.

The most satisfactory dilution to use should be established experimentally. For sodium this may be 1 in 100, 1 in 2100, even 1 in 500; for potassium, it is usually lower, often 1 in 50, but it is possible by varying the sensitivity to use the same dilution for both. In determining the amount of any element present, possible interference of other elements also present has to be taken into account. This is of two kinds spectral, which occurs when two bands are near enough together to overlap, and may also arise from the general background of the itself, and ionic due to the fact that in the presence of each other two elements each emit more light than they would separately. (Forter and 1959).

Standard solutions

Standards should be put through each time determinations are done. Prepare suitable solutions as follows–

A) Stock sodium solution 1000 milii equivalents per litre, 58.5 gms of sodium chloride per litre of solution.

B) Stock potassium solution 10 milli equivalents per litre, 7.46 gms of potassium chloride per litre of solution.

A) Series of stock standard solutions can be prepared from these as follows. For sodium:

m Eq. Na/Litre		120	130	140	150	160
ml stock solutions	(A)	60	65	70	75	80
" "	(B)	25	25	25	25	25

made upto 500 ml with water.

For the potassium the following:

m Eq. K/litre		3	4	5	6	8
ml stock solutions	(A)	15	20	25	30	40
" "	(b)	70	70	70	70	70

made upto 500 ml with water.

When carrying out series of determinations, insert an appropriate standard solutions at frequent intervals to ensure that constancy of reading is being obtained.

XII. Determination of total sugars and Reducing sugar as invert sugar

Preparation of solution for analysis

Alcohol must be removed from spirituous preparation prior to the determination of sugars. At the same time the loss of laevulose which decomposes at higher temperature should be avoided. The following method is recommended for the preparation of the sample analysis.

Neutralise a suitable volume of the sample, accurately measured with sodium hydroxide solution, and evaporate to half the volume to remove alcohol. Cool the solution add 10 ml of clarifying solution I followed by 10 ml of solution II (see below) mix, make up to volume and filter through a dry filter paper. Use the filtrate for analysis.

If the sample is free from alcohol, weigh a suitable quantity, transfer to a volumetric flask, dilute with water, neutralise with sodium hodroxide solution, clarify with zinc ferrocyanide and proceed as above.

Reagents

Fehling's solution

A)Dissolve 69.278 g. of $CuSO_4$, $5H_2O$ in water and make upto 1 litre.

B)Dissolve 100 g of sodium hydroxide and 340 g of sodium potassium tartrate in water and make up to 1 litre.

Mix equal volumes of A and B before the experiment.

Clarifying Agent

Solution I Dissolve 21.9 g of zinc acetate and 3 ml of glacial acetic acid in water and make upto 100 ml.

Solution II Dissolve 10.6 g. of potassium ferrocyanide in water and make upto 100 ml.

Determination

Reducing sugars

Prepare a solution of the sugar of such concentration that not less than 15 ml and not more than 50 ml will be required to reduce the copper (0.15 to 0.25 g of invert sugar per 100 ml for ml Fehling's solution).

For preliminary titration: measure accurately 10 ml of Fehling's solution into a conical flask of about 300 ml capacity. From a burette add 15 ml of the sugar solution and heat to boiling over an asbestos covers wire gauge. Continue adding the sugar solution in fairly large portions at 15 seconds intervals until the colour of the mixture of copper appears to be nearly reduced then boil for a minute or two, add 3 to 5 drops of 1% methylene blue solution and continue the titration until the blue colour is discharged.

Accurate titration: Repeat the titration, adding before heating almost the full amount of sugar solution required to reduce all the copper. After boilings has commenced, maintain a moderate degree of ebullition two minutes, and, without removing the flame, add 3 to 5 drops of indicator and continue the titration so that it is just complete in a total boiling time of exactly three minutes. The end point is clearly indicated by the disappearance of the blue colour, the solution becoming orange. The flask must not be removed from the gauge at any stage of the titration.

The proportions of invert sugar, equivalent to 10 ml of Fehling's solution, are given in the Table. Calculate the reducing sugar, invert sugar.

Sucrose

Pipette an aliquot of the clarified solution into a 300 ml beaker, add 15 ml of N.HCl dilute to 150 ml with water, cover with clock glass and heat to boiling point. Continue to boil for two minutes, cool, add phenolphthalein, just neutralise with sodium hydroxide solution (10%), transfer to a 200 ml graduated flask and dilute to 200 ml.

Carry out the determination of invert sugar as given under "Reducing sugars". By reference to the Table calculate the percentage of total sugar expressed as invert sugar.

The difference between the percentage of total sugar (as invest sugar) and reducing sugar (as invert sugar) multiplied by 0.95 gives the percentage of sucrose.

Invert Sugar Table Por 10 ml. Fehling Solution

Ml. of sugar solution required	No sucrose		1 g. sucrose per 100 ml.		5 g. sucrose per 100 ml.		10 g. sucrose per 100 ml.		25 g. sucrose per 100 ml.	
			Solution containing besides invert sugar							
	Invert sugar factor	Mg. invert sugar per 100 ml.	Invert sugar sugar factor	Mg. invert sugar per 100 ml.	Invert sugar factor	Mg. invert sugar per 100 ml.	Invert sugar factor	Mg. invert sugar per 100 ml.	Invert sugar factor	Mg. invert sugar per 100 ml
1	2	3	4	5	6	7	8	9	10	11
15	50.5	336	49.9	333	47.6	317	46.1	307	43.4	289
16	50.6	316	50.0	312	47.6	297	46.1	288	434	271
17	50.7	298	50.1	295	47.6	280	46.1	271	43.4	255
18	50.8	282	50.1	278	47.6	264	46.1	256	43.3	240
19	50.8	267	40.2	264	47.6	250	46.1	243	43.3	227
20	50.9	254.5	50.2	251.0	47.6	238.0	46.1	230.5	43.2	216

21	51.0	542.9	50.2	239.0	47.6	226.7	46.1	219.5	43.2	206
22	51.0	231.8	50.3	228.2	47.6	216.4	46.1	209.5	43.1	196
23	51.1	222.2	50.3	218.7	47.6	207.0	46.1	200.4	43.0	187
24	51.2	213.3	50.3	209.8	47.6	198.3	46.1	192.1	42.9	179
25	51.2	204.8	50.4	201.6	47.6	190.4	46.0	184.0	42.8	171
26	51.3	197.4	50.4	193.8	47.6	183.1	46.0	176.9	42.8	164
27	51.4	190.4	50.4	186.7	47.6	176.4	46.0	170.4	42.7	158
28	51.4	183.7	50.5	180.2	47.7	170.3	46.0	164.3	42.7	152
29	51.5	177.6	50.5	174.1	47.7	164.5	46.0	158.6	42.6	147
30	51.5	171.7	50.5	168.3	47.7	159.0	46.0	153.3	42.5	142
31	51.6	166.3	50.6	163.1	47.7	153.9	45.9	148.1	45.5	137
32	51.6	161.2	50.6	158.1	47.7	149.1	45.9	143.4	42.4	132
33	51.7	156.6	50.6	153.3	47.7	144.5	45.9	139.1	42.3	128
34	51.7	152.2	50.6	148.9	47.7	140.3	45.8	134.9	42.2	124
35	51.8	147.9	50.7	144.7	47.7	136.2	45.8	130.8	42.2	121
36	518	143.9	50.7	140.7	47.7	132.5	45.8	127.1	42.1	117
37	51.9	140.2	50.7	137.0	47.7	128.9	45.7	123.5	42.0	114
38	51.9	136.6	50.7	133.5	47.7	125.5	45.7	120.3	42.0	111
39	52.0	133.3	50.8	130.2	47.7	122.3	45.7	117.1	41.9	107
40	52.0	130.1	50.8	127.0	47.7	119.2	45.6	114.1	41.8	104
41	52.1	127.1	50.8	123.9	47.7	116.3	45.6	111.2	41.8	102
42	52.1	124.2	50.8	121.0	47.7	113.5	45.6	108.5	41.7	99
43	52.2	121.4	50.8	118.2	47.7	110.9	45.5	105.8	41.6	97
44	52.2	118.7	50.9	115.6	47.7	108.4	45.5	103.4	41.5	94
45	52.3	116.1	50.9	113.1	47.7	106.0	45.4	101.0	41.4	92
46	52.3	113.7	50.9	110.6	47.7	103.7	45.4	98.7	41.4	90
47	52.4	111.4	50.9	108.2	47.7	101.5	45.3	96.4	41.3	88
48	52.4	109.2	50.9	106.0	47.7	99.4	45.3	94.3	41.2	86
49	52.5	107.1	51.0	104.0	47.7	97.4	45.2	92.3	41.4	84
50	52.5	105.1	51.0	102.0	47.7	95.4	45.2	90.4	41.0	82

XIII : Estimation of Resin

A known weight of sample is thoroughly extracted with ether. The ether extract is washed successively with (a) 1% Aqueous ammonium carbonate (b) 1% aqueous Sodium carbonate and (c) 0.1 to 1.0% aqueous Potassium hydroxide. These washings are combined, treated with mineral and acid to reprecipitate resin acids and extracted with ether.

The solvent is removed and weighed to give Resin acids. The aqueous portion is reserved for volatile oil determination.

Combined Acids (Resin esters)

The aqueous liquid remaining after determination of volatile matter's extracted with ether. The ether is removed and the residue is saponified with alc. potassium hydroxide. The solution is diluted with water for the experiment below. The aqueous solution is acidified and extracted with ether. The solvent is removed and the residue is weighed. This gives the value of combined acids in the resin.

Resin alcohols and Resins

The extract reserved from the previous determination is distilled and the residue dried and weighed to give the above values.

The amount of resin present in a sample may be given separately under different categories as above or as a total of all the values.

9

Ayurvedic Medicines

Ayur means 'life' and Veda means 'knowledge'. So Ayurdeva means 'Science of life'. It is considered divine in origin and is also known as 'Upa Veda' to 'Atharvaveda'. There are many references to health, diseases, treatments, description of medicinal plants etc., in 'Atharvaveda'. Ayurveda originated from this Veda.

Ayurveda has eight specialized branches :

1. Kayachikitsa (Internal medicine)
2. Balachikitsa (Paediatrics) (Kaumarabhritya)
3. Graha Chikitsa (Psychological medicine)
4. Shalakya Tantra (Ear, nose and throat disorders and opthalmology)
5. Shalya Tantra (Surgery)
6. Agada Tantra (Toxicology)
7. Rasayana Tantra (Geriatrics)
8. Vajikarana Tantra (Engenies and Aphrodisiacs)

The theory of 'Tridosha' consitituting Vata (air-motion), Pitta (fire-energy) and Kapha (liquid gelinertia) and Sapta Dhatus (seven tissues), Rasa (body fluids-prime element out of digestion), Ratta (blood), Mamsa (muscular tissue), Meda (adipose tissue), Asthi (bone tissue). Majja (nerve tissue and bone marrow) and Shukra (reproductive-generative tissue) and waste products. Three Malas are the three founders of this Sharira (body). All the physiological and pathological processes involve these constituents and are responsible for health and ill health in a person.

Vata, Pitta and Kapha are basic biological elements and control all the functions and activities of the body. Sapta Dhatus (Seven tissues) support the body and also each one of the tissues has a metabolic capability which helps it to digest the respective food and manufactures its associated higher tissues. In this process 'malas' emerge as waste products. Stool, urine, sweat, hair nail etc. are few malas. Health (Swasth) depends upon the equibalance condition of these three qualitatively and quantitatively.

Ayurveda strongly emphasizes on Prevention, Promotion, Cure and Rehabilitation. For this, it advocates to follow the principles of health, observation of principles; daily regimen (dinacharya). Seasonal regimen (Ritu Charya), Rathri Charya (Night routine), Sadvritta (ethical moral activities), ahara (food), nidra (sleep) and brahmacharya (regulated actions).

Ayurveda considers human beings as a whole. It believes that imbalance in the Doshas, Dhatus and malas generate diseases and the restoration of balance in these eliminates diseases. The aim of treatment is not only to cure and disease but to root out the cause so that it may not take place in future. The aim of the treatment is also to improve the vitality and to strengthen thee immune system. In Ayurveda, the diagnostic procedures are very critical in nature and the physician has to apply his deep knowledge and experience before starting the therapy.

The Ayurvedic treatment firstly insists on removing the causative factors. They practice and use single or compound herbal preparations, herb-mineral preparations and suitable dietary advices, daily activities etc. In chronic disorders, they advice Panchakarma therapy, which has special identity in Ayurveda. These Five Karmas (procedures) are aimed to cleanse the whole body and prepare the body in a way that it could not get the problems again and again. This can also be used for rejuvenation (Rasayana Therapy).

Unani Medicines

The Unani system of medicine originated from Greece. It as developed as a medical system by the Arabs. This system is also known as Ionian Medicine, Arab Medicine, Islamic Medicine, Greek-Arab Medicine and is widely practiced in countries like Egypt, Syria, Iraq, Persia, Pakistan, India, China and other Middle Eastern and Far Eastern countries. The Unani system of Medicine is based on the 'Hippocrates' four humour theory-blood (dam), phlegm (Balgham), yellow bile (Safra) and black bile (Sauda) in the body. Depending upon these four body humours and their consistency, the temperaments of persons are identified.

The humours are reassigned temperaments i.e. blood is hot and moist, phlegm is cold and moist, yellow bile is hot and dry; and black bile is cold and dry. The temperaments are known and identified as sanguine, phlegmatic, choleric and melancholic. These temperaments have an important role in Unani Medicine and form the basic for pathology, diagnosis and treatments. A little change in these temperaments invites a change in the person's state of health. Herbs, medicines or drugs also have temperaments. If a drug is said to be hot then it means that when it enters the body and interacts with bodily organs, it produces a temperament which is hot. The medicines used in this system of medicine help to restore hormonal balance and thus retains the health of the individual.

Diagnosis is generally made by reading the Nabz (Pulse), a rhythmic expansion of blood flow in the arteries which is felt by fingers. The physicians also use other methods of diagnosis like (Baul) Urine, (Baraz) Stool etc. along with modern diagnostic procedures. In Unani Medicine various types of treatments are practiced such as Illaj bit-tadbeer (regimental theory), Illaj bil-ghiza (dietotherapy), Illaj bid-Dawa (Pharmacotherapy) and Jarahat (Surgery). Generally single drugs or their combinations are used in treatments. The Pharmacopoeia consists of natural herbal drugs, animal, mineral and marine products. These are used in the form of decoctions, infusions, tablets, powders, syrups, confections and aquas. Since in this system, stress is laid on the particular temperament of the individual, the medicines generally prescribed and administered are such as to go well with the temperament of the patient without any side effects.

Siddha medicines

Siddha medicine, originally is a part of Ayurveda Rasashastra (alchemy) which was further developed by the Dravidians of South India. Later they transformed it into a separate system of medicine. The Siddha system of medicine deals with therapeutic procedures mainly. They are also known as Rasa Vaidyas. Mercury preparations, Arsenic preparations etc., generally dominate the therapeutic practice. Siddha physicians also use metallic and non metallic mercurial combinations, minerals, oils and vegetable poisons. There are good treatments for psoriasis, leprosy and other skin afflications and other chronic disorders. This system of medicine is widely practised in Srilanka, Malaysia, Mauritius, Singapore, etc. In the Southern part of India, specially Tamil Nadu there are a number of Siddha hospitals, dispensaries, colleges and practitioners.

Homoepathic medicines

Homoepathy is developed by Dr. Samuel Hahnemann but it is widely practised in India due to its low-cost and is used in acute and chronic conditions. It is developed from the natural law 'like is cured by like'. That is, a substance which causes groups of symptoms, whether physical, mental or emotional or behavioural in the healthy, can cure similar symptoms when they appear as a deviation from the normal in sick persons. Dr. Hahnemann took the 'Peruvian bark', the treatment for 'malaria' at that time, which produced malaria fever when he took inside the body.

Dr. Hahnemann presented the system based on some laws and principles . They are

1. The law of similars
2. The law of direction of cure
3. The law of single remedy
4. The law of minimum dose

In homoepathy, disease is regarded as a process and not a 'thing'. The homeopaths regard symptoms as a reaction to the underlying problems. He will concentrate on self healing. The homoeopathy aims at interpretation and matching of symptom picture of the patient with the correct drug for remedy. Diagnosis involves finding out what changes from the normal has a patient experienced. These changes may be physical, mental emotional sensory or even moral. Diagnosis in homeopathy is expressed not in the name of a disease but it the name of the remedy which corresponds to it.

In acute cases the remedy may be any one of the hundreds and the homeopath is guided to it by the individual version of disease produced by the patient. In chronic cases, the remedy will usually be what is called the 'constitutional', since it is indicated by the individuality of the patient and not the individuality of the disease.

Homoeopaths give one remedy at a time. They observe the changes in the patient produced by the remedy. A temporary aggravation of the symptom indicates that a curative process has begun and is a good sign. The medicines are prepared by grinding plant materials in alcohol to give 'mother tincture'. Minerals and insoluble materials are finely ground with lactose. Dilutions are then prepared by mixing with solvents and dropping the bottle on to a hard rubber slab or by trituration with more lactose.

Homoepathy can be successful in all diseases though not all patients. It is especially applicable in acute conditions where the patient has the vital energy to effect a cure, but relief is needed from distressing symptoms. Since homoeopathy stimulates the organism to the natural activity-healing, there are no risks involved. There is some initial aggravation, which is for a short span of time, depending on the condition of the patient.

- Sodium Benzoate
- Sodium Bicarbonate From Soda Ash
- Sodium Carboxy Methyl Cellulose
- Sodium Hexa Meta Phosphate
- Sodium Hypo Chlorite From Waste Chlorine Gas
- Sodium Hypochloride (Bleaching Powder)
- Sodium Meta Bi Sulphite
- Sodium Meta-Silicate
- Sodium Silicate From Rice/Paddy Husk
- Sodium Silicate From Silica And Soda Ash
- Sodium Sulphate (Anhydrous)
- Sodium Sulphide From Barium Compound
- Sodium Sulphide From Sulfur Caustic Soda
- Sodium Sulphite
- Sodium Tripoly Phosphate
- Softner (Cationic, Anionic & Nomiric)
- Solder Fluxes
- Solid Fuel Cake
- Solvent Extraction & Refining Plant
- Solvent Extraction And Refining Of Soyabeen Plant
- Solvent Extraction Plant
- Stearic Acid
- Strontium Carbonate
- Sulphur Milling Plant
- Sulphuric Acid
- Super Phosphate & Mixed Fertiliser (Npk)
- Synthetic Iron Oxide (Yellow)
- Tartaric Acid From Maleic An-Hydride
- Tartaric Acid From Tamarind
- Tartaric Acid From Tarmind Powder
- Tartaric Acid, Food Colour, Crude Pectine, Tamarind Oil
- Titanium Dioxide
- Tri Basic Lead Sulphate
- Ultra Marine Blue (5 Mt/Day)
- Urea Formaldehyde
- Urea Formeldehyde Resin
- Water Proofing Compound (Liquid & Powder)
- Water Proofing Compound (Liquid & Solid)
- Water Treatment Chemicals
- X-Ray Photography Developers & Fixer
- Zeolite - A
- Zinc & Copper Sulphate From Brass Ash
- Zinc Brightner
- Zinc Chloride
- Zinc Oxide
- Zinc Oxide (Chemical Process)
- Zinc Phosphate
- Zinc Stearate
- Zinc Sulfate 21% Agricultural Grade From Waste Ash
- Zinc Sulphate
- Zinc Sulphate Micro Nutrients Or Fertilizer
- Zinc Sulphate Micro-Nutrient Mixture
- Zinc-Metal From Zinc Ash
- Zircon

Computer Products

- Call Centre (Domestic)
- Call Centre (International)
- Compact Disc
- Computer Assembly (Hardware)
- Computer Education Institute
- Computer Monitor (Monochrome Monitor)
- Computer Ribbon (For Printer)
- Computer Ribbon Refilling/Reinking
- Computer Software (EOU)
- Cybercafe
- E-Commerce
- Floppy Disks
- Internet Servicd Provider(Isp)
- Laptop Computers
- Medical Transcription Centre
- Online Shopping Mall Portal
- Plastic Flopy Storage Box
- Portal

Cosmetics, Perfumes, Flavours & Essential Oils

- Aerosol Spray [Rose Flavour , Night Qeen, Jasmin]
- After Shave Lotion
- Agar Oil From Black Agar Wood
- Agarbatti Synthetic Perfumery Compound
- Air Freshner & Purifiers
- Air Freshners (Odonil Type)
- Aromatic Perfumery Compounds
- Bindi
- Bindiya (Shilpa Type)
- Car Shampoo
- Cosmetic Industries
- Detol Type Antiseptic Lotion
- Dhoop Batti Sticks
- Essences For Biscuit, Confectionery Items (Non-Essential Flavour)
- Essential Oil From Flowers
- Essential Oils From Jawa Citronella Oil
- Essentical Oil Form Lily, Mogra, Nishigandha
- Eucalyptus Oil
- Extraction Of Essential Oil & Packaging
- Extraction Of Oil (Jeera, Ajowon, Ginger, Cardamom Oil Etc.)
- Formulation Of Flavours
- Fractional Distillation Of Essencial Oil And Medicinal Plant
- Garlic Oilginger Oil
- Ginger Oil (Super Critical Co2 Process)
- Hair Dye (Godrej Type)
- Hair Dye Powder
- Hair Shampoo
- Herbal Cosmatic
- Herbal Hair Oil (Banphool Type)
- Herbal Natural Essential Oil
- Herbal Natural Essential Oil (Steam Distillation Process)
- Lamon Grass Oil
- Lily Essence
- Menthol Crystal Bold From Menthol Oil
- Menthol Crystals
- Menthol Crystals & Menthol Oil menthol Oil
- Nail Polish
- Non-Alcoholic Flavours
- Oleo-Resin & Capsisin Product Extraction Plant
- Oleoresin & Essential Oil Mfg
- Palmrosa Grass Oil
- Peppermint Oil
- Perfumery Chemicals Synthetic And Natural
- Red (Lal) Tooth Powder
- Rose Oil (Essential Oil From Flowers)
- Rose Plantation & Rose Oil Extraction (Rose Essential Oil)
- Sandal Wood Oil & Powder
- Scent & Perfumes
- Shampoo & Creams
- Shampoo & Creams (Cold Cream, All Purpose Cream & Varnishing Cream) Shaving Cream
- Shaving Cream & Shaving Soap
- Spice Oil Or Oleoresins (Extraction Of Essential Oil From Spices)
- Synthetic Purfumery Compound
- Talcum Powder (Face & Toilet Powder)
- Tejpatta Oil From Tejpatta
- Telcum Powder
- Tobacco Based Tooth Powder
- Tooth Paste
- Tooth Paste (Gel Type)
- Yara Yara (Perfumes For Soap, Detergent & Agarbatti Etc.)

Dyes & Dye Intermediates

- Acetonaphthone
- Azo Die Stuffs
- Beta Napthol (100 Eou)
- Coumarin
- Dye Fixing Agent (By Cold Process)
- Dye Intermediates
- Dye Intermediates - Indigo Blue
- Dyes & Dye Intermediates
- Fast Colour Base
- Leather Auxiliaries
- Metal Naphthenates
- Naphthalene Balls
- Naphthnol Astr
- Natural Coloured Oil (Turmeric Colour & Oil)
- Phthalo Cyanine Blue And Green
- Re-Active Dyes (Red, Orange, Yellow Colour) Used B-Napthol
- Textile Dyeing Auxiliaries
- Textile Printing Pigment Binder
- Ultra Marine Blue

Electrical & Electronic Industries

- Air Conditioner (A/C) Car & Room Servicing
- Air Conditioners (Window Type)
- All Aluminium Alloy Conductor (Aaac)
- Alternator (1 To 75 Kva)
- Aluminium Power Cables
- Aluminium/Copper Cable Lugs
- Arial Bunched Cable
- Armoured Cables
- Audio Cassette Assembling & Recording Unit
- Audio Cassette Manufacturing & Recording
- Audio Cassettes Manufacturing
- Audio Magnetic Tape
- Audio Stereo Cassette

Recorder Players
- Audio Video Assembling Unit
- Audio Video Cassette Assembling
- Auto Bulb/Lamp
- Auto Lamps (Auto Tail Lights)
- Battery (Ups, Invertor, Solar System, & Automobile Battery)
- Battery Plates & Assembly
- Button Cell (Miniature Watch Battry)
- Cable Creeping Lungs, Socket & Cable Creeping Tools
- Calculator, Torch & Alarm
- Capacitors
- Cardless Telephone
- Cassette Tape Recorder
- Ceiling Fan
- Chocke And Patti For Fluorescent Tube
- Choke & Starter For Fluorescent Tube
- Clay Plate For Electric Heater
- Colour Television (T.V.)
- Commutators
- Compact Disc Rom (Cd-Rom)
- Compact Disk Player
- Compact Fluorescent Lamps
- Compressor For Ac (Hermetic)
- Computerised Washing Machine
- Cooling Coils (For Airconditioners)
- Copper Clad Laminated Sheet Used For Making P.C.B.
- Ct/Pt Epoxy Casting Transformers
- Diesel Generator (20-200 Kva) Dg Set
- Dish Antenna And Satellite Network Equipment
- Distribution Transformer (250kva) Repairing
- Distribution Transformers
- Domestic Refrigeration
- Dry Cell Battery Manufacturing Unit
- Dry Cell Manufacturing
- Dry Cells, Rechargeable Cells
- Electric & Ordinary Detonators(Used In Explosive For Hard Rock Cutting & Blasting
- Electric Bulb (Gls Bulb)
- Electric Energy Meters
- Electric Fan
- Electric Fluorescent Tube
- Electric Gyser
- Electric Mixer
- Electric Motor
- Electric Motor Pumps
- Electric Panel Board (Switch Boards)
- Electric Steam Iron
- Electric Water Heater
- Electrical Accessories (Plugs, Switches, Sockets Etc.)
- Electrical Lamp
- Electrical Panel (Switch Board)
- Electronic Calculator
- Electronic Choke (Ballast)
- Electronic Cut Out For Automobiles
- Electronic Digital Weighing Machine
- Electronic Energy Meter
- Electronic Service Centre
- Electronic Toys
- Emergency Light
- Epabx/Epax System
- Exhaust Fans (Cooler Fan)
- F.H.P. Motors
- Ferrite Magnets
- Fluorescent Tube Starter
- G.L.S. Bulbs/Lamps
- Gas Based Power Project (600 Mv)
- Halogen Lamps
- House Wiring Cables
- Ht & Mv Industrial Cubic Switch Boards
- Hydro Based Power Plant (15mw)
- Immersion Heater
- Information Moving Display (Lead Type)
- Invertors
- Jelly Filled Cables
- Lamp Shades & Chandliers
- Light Emitting Diodes
- M.C.B. (Miniature Circuit Breaker)
- Maintenance Free Re-Chargable Battery
- Micro Oven
- Miniature Transformer
- Multilayer Printed Circuit Board
- Musical Door Bell
- Neon Sign Board Manufacturing
- Optical Fibre Cable
- Optical Pickup Unit
- P.V.C. Stablizers
- P.V.C. Wire & Cables
- Pcb Manufacturing (Flexible)
- Pcb Manufacturing (Multilayer)
- Pcb Manufacturing (Totally Automatic Plant)
- Plastic Coolar Body (Symphony Type)
- Polyurethene Battery Separator
- Portable Television (B & W)
- Portal
- Power Capacitor
- Power Generating Unit From Agricultural Waste Heat Energy
- Power Plant (5 Mw/Hr) By Agro Waste
- Power Plant (Hydro Based) Cap: 10 Mw
- Power Project (100% Foreign Funded)
- Power Supply (Linear Switch Mode)
- Power Transformer
- Printed Cricuit Board
- Pvc Battery Separator
- Pvc Electric Wires & Cables
- Rechargeable Battery - Maintenance Free (Sealed Lead Acid)
- Re-Conditionig Of Fluorescent Tube
- Refrigeration & Mini Refrigeration
- Rewinding Of Burnt Electric Motor
- Rosin Cored Soft Soldering Wire
- Sattelite Receiver
- Soft & Hard Ferrites
- Solar Cooker
- Solar Electrical Cell & Heating Pannel
- Solar Energy Water Heater
- Solar Photo Voltaic System
- Solar Power Plant
- Switch Mode Power Supply
- Tape Recorder's Pinch Roller, Rubber, Drive, Belt Flat
- Telephone (Push Button Type)
- Terminal Connectors
- Transformer/Servomotor/ Relay
- Un-Intrupted Power Supply (Ups)
- Variable Frequency, Variable Voltage A.C. Voltage
- Video Cassette
- Video Compact Disc (V.C.D.)
- Voltage Stablizer (Solid State)
- Voltage Stablizer Using Ic Timer
- Washing Machine
- Washing Machine & Geyser
- Wind Energy Power Project
- Winding Wires Pvc Insulated For Submersible Motors
- Xlpe Cables

Electroplating Industries

- Aluminium Anodizing Plant
- Aluminium Hard-Anodizing Unit
- Chrome Plating
- Electro Polishing Of Steel
- Electroplating Of Gold & Their Chemical Treatment In Golden Colour
- Electroplating Of Plastic
- Electroplating Of Various Metal
- Gold Electroplating On Cheaper Ornaments (Without Using Gold)
- Gold Plated Silver Jewellery
- Gold Plated Silver Jewellery & Cutlery
- Hard Chromium Plating
- Silver & Gold Plating On Pvc And Nylon-6
- Watch Case Buffing

Glass & Cement Industries

- Acrylic Mirror
- Ceramic (Porcelain) Insulator
- Ceramic Hotel Ware Bone China
- Ceramic Thread Guide
- Ceramic Unit
- Glass Ampoules (Distilled Water)
- Glass Bangles & Glass Pressed Wares
- Glass Bottle
- Glass Marble
- Glass Sheet
- Glass Sheet (Automatic Plant)
- Glazed Ceramic Tiles
- Granite Slab & Tiles
- High Alumina Ceramic
- Laminated Safety Glass
- Mirror Colouring (Pink, Black,Golden, Silver)
- Mirrors (Silver, Golden, Pink Black And Yellow Colour)
- Non Glazed Ceramic Tiles
- Optical Glass
- Optical Lenses Manufacture
- Safety Glass
- Watch Glass

Gums & Adhesives

- Acrylic Adhesive
- Adhesive (Fevicol Type)
- Adhesive Based Polyurethanes
- Adhesive Content Pvc Resin & Dop Paste Grade

- Adhesive For All Purpose
- Adhesive For Corrugation (Dry Powder)
- Adhesive For Stickers
- Adhesive From Sodium Silicate
- Adhesive Industries (Laminated Fevicol Sticker And Other Types)
- Adhesive Tape For Hospital Use
- Bopp Pressure Sensitive Self Adhesive Tapes
- Bottle Labeling Gum
- Electrical Insulating Tape Using Bopp Film
- Ester Gum
- Fevicol Type Adhesive
- Glue From Bone Sinews
- Guar Gum
- Guar Gum Powder
- Gum (Liquid) Office Paste
- Gum From Tamarind Seed Powder
- Gums & Adheisve
- Hologram Sticker - 3d
- Hot - Melt Adhesive
- Hot Melt Glue
- Latex Adhesive
- Latex Based Adhesive
- Leather Binder (Resin Based)
- Neoprene Based Adhesive (Rubber Adhesive)
- Office Gum
- Paper Tape
- Plaster Of Paris Bandages & Cotton Adhesive Tape
- Pressure Sensitive Adhesive Tape Binder
- Pvc Electrical Insulating Tape
- Rosin Sizing Agent For Paper Plant
- Rubber Solution
- Starch From Maize
- Synthetic Gum Used In Textile Industry
- Synthetic Rubber Adhesive
- Textile Printig Paste (Gum)

Inks & Stationery Products

- Ball Pen Ink Remover
- Ball Pen Manufacturing
- Ball Point Pen Refills
- Computer Stationery
- Dust Free Chalk Made By Calcium Carbonate
- Exercise Note Book, Register, Pads
- Flexo Graphic Ink
- Flexo Gravure Printing Ink
- Ink For Hot Stamping Foil
- Lead Pencils
- One Time Carbon
- Painting Brush
- Printing Inks
- School Chalk
- Slate Pencils
- Stamp Pad & Stamp Inks
- Staple Pin
- Toner Ink For Xerox M/C
- Wax Crayon

Jute & Jute Based Projects

- Gunny Bags (Jute Bags) Manufacturing
- Gunny Bags From Jute
- Jute Ropes/Sutli
- Jute Shopping Bags
- Jute Tarfelt
- Particle Board From Jute Stick

Leather & Leather Goods

- Leather Garments
- Leather Goods
- Leather Shoes
- Leather Shoes & Chappals
- Leather Shoes (Agra Type)
- Leather Straps For Wrist Watches
- Leather Tanning
- Leather Tanning (Goats &Cows)

Mechanical Engineering Automible Industries

- Activated Alumina
- Activated Alumina Balls
- Agriculture Implements
- Air Cooler
- Air Filter For All Type Of Auto Vehicles
- Air Pressure Gauge (Dial Gauge)
- Aluminium Alloy
- Aluminium Beverages Cans
- Aluminium Blind Rivets & Metal Clips
- Aluminium Bottles Cold Extrusion Of Aluminium
- Aluminium Building Hardware
- Aluminium Caps
- Aluminium Channels, Beading & Pipes
- Aluminium Circle
- Aluminium Collapsible Tubes
- Aluminium Extrusion Plant
- Aluminium Finished Articles (Job Work)
- Aluminium Foil
- Aluminium Gravity Casting
- Aluminium Ingots From Aluminium Scrap
- Aluminium Powder
- Aluminium Pressure Die Casting
- Aluminium Sheet, Circles & Vessels
- Aluminium Utencils
- Aluminium Utensils & Circles
- Aluminium Wire Drawing & Super Enamelling For Winding
- Aluminum Rolling Mill
- Auto Brake Liner
- Auto Head Light
- Auto Leaf Spring
- Auto Wires For 3/2 Wheelers
- Automatic ignition Coil
- Automatic Vending M/C For Hot & Cold Beverages
- Automotive Filters
- Automised Aluminium Powder
- Automobile (Four Wheelers)
- Automobile Battery
- Automobile Brake Shoe
- Automobile Bushes
- Automobile Gaskets
- Automobile Gear
- Automobile Industry (Four Wheelers)
- Automobile Parts (Maruti Vehicles)
- Automobile Piston Rings
- Automobile Products (Processing Metal & Auto Part)
- Automobile Radiators
- Automobile Work Shop/ Garage & Service Station
- Automotive Wiring Harnesses
- Ball Bearing Manufacturing
- Battery For Auto Vehicles
- Battery Plate
- Battery Plate & Assembly
- Bicycle Assembly
- Bicycle Chain
- Bicycle Manufacturing
- Bicycle Rim
- Bidis Manufacturing Unit
- Black And Annealed Wire
- Black Bar To Bright Steel Bar
- Black Pipe Galvanizing Plant
- Body Building (Truck & Bus)
- Brake Liner
- Brass & Aluminium Hinges
- Brass And Copper Tube
- Brass Casting Pollution Control
- Brass Door, Window Fittings
- Brass Novalty
- Brass Pressure Die Casting
- Brass Rolling Sheets
- Bright Bars
- Building Hardware Of Aluminium
- Bus & Truck Body Building
- C.I. Casting Foundry
- C.I. Costing (Foundry) By Induction Furnace
- C.N.G. Cylinders (Storage For C.N.G. Gas)
- C.P. Bathroom Fitting
- Calcined & Activated Alumina
- Carburettor
- Carbon Brushes
- Cargo Containers (For Ship & Train)
- Chains (Bicycle, Scooter, Motorcycle,Moped)
- Clutch Lining For Four Wheeler
- Clutch Plate For Two Wheller
- Clutch, Clutch Plate & Assembly For Four Wheeler
- Cold Rolled Pressed Steel Doors & Windows
- Cold Rolling Of M.S. Strips/Sheet
- Composite Container
- Composite Steel Re-Rolling Mill
- Continuous Electrogalvanising Cold Dip Process Of Steel Strip
- Continuous Copper Rod (Ccr) From Copper Scraps
- Control & Precision Instrumentation
- Cooling Tower
- Copper Foil
- Copper Powder
- Copper Powder & Aluminium Powder
- Copper Rod From Copper Scraps
- Copper Strip Coils From Scraps
- Copper Utensils
- Copper Wire Bars Or Rods From Copper Scraps
- Copper Wire Drawing
- Copper Wire Drawing & Enamelling
- Decoiler And Sheet Shearing Plant
- Diamond & Gem Cutting/ Polishing (All Automatic Machinery)
- Diamond Tools & Wheels
- Die Making For Sheet Metal Working
- Diesel Engine Repairing
- Different Types Of Fire Extinguisher
- Disposable Needles & Syringes

- Bamboo Chips For Paper Mill
- Bamboo Sticks Used For Agarbatti
- Bank (Private Sector)
- Banquet Hall
- Bentonite (Quarrying, Processing & Exporting)
- Bone Crushing Plant
- Buttons From Cattle Houses
- Buttons From Hoves & Horns
- Canvas Shoes
- Car-Leasing & Finance
- Cigarettes Unit
- Cinema Hall
- Coal Washing Unit
- Coir Handicraft
- Cold Storage
- Cold Storage & Ice Plant
- Combine Coke
- Community Hall
- Compozite Carbon Fiber
- Cricket Ball, Bat Manufacturing
- Daily Need Stores
- Departmental Stores
- Diagnostic Centre
- Diamond & Gem Cutting & Processing Unit
- Diamond Cutting & Export
- Dispensary
- Disposable Cigarete Gas Lighter
- Dry Cleaners
- Dry Cleaning And Laundry Unit
- Dry Flowers
- Engineering College
- Expansion Joint Filler
- Eye Hospital
- Fast Food Corner
- Fire Fighting Equipment,Chemicals & Refilling
- Fire Works
- Five Star Hotel (Delux)
- Five Star Hotel Industry
- Flush Door, Chip Board, Hard Board, Insulating Board
- Flush Door, Clip Board & Hardboard
- Games Parlour
- Gas Filling Of L.P.G. Cylinder
- Gems Manufacturing (Original)
- Gold & Silver Jewellery
- Gold Jewellery (100% Eou)
- Handicrafts (Can & Bamboo)
- Hard Board From Saw Dust
- Hawan Samgri
- Health Club & Beauty Parlour
- Health Club Cum Beauty Parlour Cum Hair Saloon
- Heat Chamber Painting
- Holiday Resorts
- Holiday Resorts Cum Ent. Club 4 Star Hotel
- Holiday Village Resort
- Hospital
- Hospital (20 Beds)
- Hospital 300 Beds To 700 Beds Teaching Facility
- Hospital Bed
- Hotel
- Hotel Industries 5 Star, 3 Star Holiday Resorts
- Hotel Unit (Three Star)
- Hotel/Small Motel
- L.P.G. Cylinder Retesting Uint
- L.P.G. Cylinder Testing Centre
- Laminated Partical Board
- Laundry
- Leasing Hire Purchase A/C
- Local Area Bank
- Mfg. Of Coloured Joint Filler Used For Jointing Tiles
- Marketing Arrangement And Distribution Strategy Of Wd-40
- Marketing Of Gram Shilpa
- Match Box Plant (Automatic)
- Medical College
- Medical College Hospital & Research Institute
- Melamine Crockery
- Mineral Fillers For Application Paint, Paper, Rubber, Plastic
- Mineral Wool
- Motel/Small Hotel With Banquet Hall, Restaurant & Catering
- Multistoryed Commercial Complex
- Natural Care Centre
- Nursing Home
- Paeditric Hospital 25 Beds
- Paint Brush
- Particle Board & Block Board With Sanding And Laminating
- Petrol Pump
- Photo Lab. Cum Studio (100% Computerised)
- Plaster Of Paris Bandages
- Plywood
- Plywood & Plyboard
- Plywood (Phenol Bonded)
- Pvc Joint Fillings
- Q.S.S. Colour Lab.
- Quering Of Lime Stone
- Recreation And Health Club
- Residential Appartments
- Restaurant
- Restaurant/Fast Food Parlour
- Rubber Wood Processing Plant
- Saw Mill
- School
- Shellac Manufacturing
- Shoe Uppers
- Slaughter House Beef Processing
- Slimming Centre & Health Club
- Snake Park
- Sport Shoe (Automatic Imported Plant
- Sterilize Bone Meal
- Straw Board
- Stuff Toys
- Sunmica
- Super Market (Commercial Market)
- Synthetic Floating To Fishing Industry
- Synthetic Rubyand Sapphire
- Tennis Ball
- Timber (Wood) Seasoning
- Trading Business (With Packaging Rice, Salt, Pulses, Etc)
- Travelling Agency
- Venetian Blind
- Video Film Studio
- Ware House
- Water Park
- Wind Mill
- Wooden Furniture
- Wonder Fuel (Gel Type)
- Wood Wool Industry
- Wooden Chips For Supplying To Paper Mills
- Wooden Doors Windows Sheets Tv Cabinet
- Wooden Furniture
- Wooden Furniture With Mediocre Automation
- Wooden Furniture With Seasoning Plant
- Wooden Needles For Tooth & Wooden Spoon For Ice Cream
- Wooden Tooth Pick
- Work Shop For Telco Truck

Oils & Fats

- Castor Oil (Batch Process)
- Castor Oil (Extraction & Refining)
- Castor Oil (Refining & Extraction)
- Castor Oil Derivative Oleo Resin
- Coconut Oil From Copra
- Coconut Oil In Containers (Filteration & Airtight Packaging)
- Corn Oil (Maize Oil)
- Cotton Seed Oil
- Cotton Seed Oil (Extraction & Refined)
- Extraction Of Sesame, Rice Bran & Palm Oil
- Extraction Of Oil From Neem Seed
- Extraction Of Oil From Soyabean & Cotton Seed
- Fat Liquor (Sulfated Oil)
- Hydrogenation Of Non-Edible Oil
- Maize Oil
- Margarine/Fat
- Neem Oil From Seeds
- Non-Formal Dye Fixing Oil
- Palm Oil
- Poppy Seed Oil By Expeller Process
- Poppy Seed Oil By Solvent Extraction Process
- Rainbow Colours On Metal
- Refined Oil (Cotton Seed Ground Nut Oil & Sunflower Oil
- Refined, Bleached, Palm Oil From Crude Palm Oil
- Rice Bran Extraction & Refining
- Rice Bran Oil
- Rubber Processing Oil
- Shesham Oil From Shesham Seed
- Shortening & Liquid Palm (Olien)
- Sun Flower Seed Oil
- Turpentine Oil And Rosin

Paints, Pigments, Enamels & Varnishes

- Aluminium Paint
- Anti-Corrosive Thinner & Paint
- Automobile Paints For Car
- Cement Paint
- Chrome Pigments
- Cement Paint
- Clear Transparent Lacquer For Coating On Brass
- Dry Distemper And Cement Paint
- Emulsion Paint (Road Marking & Airodrome Runways -Water Base)
- Insulating Varnish
- Insulating Varnishes & Wire Enamels
- Latex Paints For Roof
- Lead Chrom Pigment From Lead Scrap (97%)
- Lithopone Pigment
- Red Oxide Pigments From Ferrous Sulphate
- N.C. Thinners Used In Auto Parts
- Naphtha Base Thinner

- Offset Printing Press Single Colour
- Offset Printing Press-4 Colour
- Photo Polymer Coating For Plate & Block Making
- Pre-Sensitised (Ps) Plates Of Aluminium For Offset Printing
- Printing On Cartoon
- Screen Printing

Rubber & Plastic Industries

- 100% Polyster Wadding
- Abs Granules
- Acrylic Sheet & Moulded Products
- Acrylic Sheet From Acrylic Waste
- Acrylic Tiles (Extruded)
- Acrylic Yarn
- Air Bubble Packaging
- Armoured Cables
- Auto Tubes
- Automobile Tyre For Bus,Truck,Trolly
- Automobile Tyre Tube & Flaps
- B.O.P.P. Film
- Bakelight Electrical Accesseries
- Bakelite Moulded Products
- Bakelite Powder For Electric Goods & Pressure Cooker
- Bakelite Sheet (Phenolic Sheet)
- Bicycle Tubes
- Bicycle Tyres 4000 Pcs./ 8 Hr.
- Blood Bags
- Blow Moulding (Plastic Containers)
- Bopp Pressure Sensetive Self Adhesive Tape
- Coir Foam (Rubberised Coir)
- Colour Master Batches For Various Plastic
- Conveyor Belting
- Cycle Tyres & Tubes
- Disposable Plastic Cup, Glasses
- Disposable Plastic Syringes
- Epoxy Resin
- Eva (Ethylene Vinyl Acetate Sheet & Sole)
- Expanded Polystyrene
- Expanded Polystyrene Board
- F.R.P. Boat Building
- F.R.P. Product (Fiber Rainforced Plastic Products)
- Fibre Glass
- Fibre Reinforced Plastic Pipes
- Flexible Office Furniture Systems
- Flexible Polyurethane Foam
- Foam & Its Products As Mattresses,Cushion, Pillows
- Frp Auto Scooter Roofs/ Celling
- Frp Sheet & Product
- H.D.P.E. Bags (Stitching)
- H.D.P.E. Film & Sheets
- H.D.P.E. Tarpaulins
- H.D.P.E. Woven Sacks/ Stitching
- Hard Rubber Battery Container
- Hawai Chappal
- Hawai Chappal & Micro Cellular Sheet Manufacturing
- Hdpe Container (1 To 5 Ltr)
- Hdpe Container (All Purpose)
- Hdpe Plastic Tank (Cap.1000 L)
- Hdpe Twine & Rope
- Hdpe/Pp Box Strapings
- Hoses (Air-Based-Welding Hoses & Pesicides Spray Pipe)
- I.V. Cannula
- Injection Moulded Plastic Components
- Injection Moulded Plastic Products
- Intra Venous (I.V.) Sets
- Latex Foam (Rubber) Products
- Latex Rubber Condoms
- Liquid Storage Tank
- Lpg Gas Pipe
- Lpg Rubbr Tube (Pipe) Flexible
- Manufacturing Of Hdpe & Ldpe Pipes & Fittings
- Medical X-Ray Film Slitting And Repacking
- Moulded Luggage
- Moulded Shoe & Hawai Chappal Mfg.
- Multi-Layer 3-Layer Film Printing & Lamination
- Multi-Layer Co-Extrusion, 3-Layer Film With Lamination & Printing
- Neon Sign Board Manufacturing
- Nylon Fish Net
- Nylon Polyester & Polypropylene Rope Making
- Nylone Zip Fasteners
- Optical Fibre
- P V C Bottles
- P.U. Foam (Polyurethane Foams)
- P.V.C. Coating On G.I.Wire
- P.V.C. Conduit Pipe
- P.V.C. Conduit Pipe (Electrical)
- P.V.C. Film
- P.V.C. Granules, Film & Bag (Printed)
- P.V.C. Hand Gloves
- P.V.C. Lining For Metal Crown Caps
- P.V.C. Pipe & Fitting
- P.V.C. Wire & Cables
- P.V.C. Wires And Cables (Flexible)
- Patches Tube Repairing Material
- Pet Bottle
- Pet Bottles From Pre-Form Pet
- Pet Bottles/ Containers
- Pet Pre-Form From Pet Resin
- Plastic Buckets, Bottles & Doli
- Plastic Buttons From Polyester Sheet & Rod
- Plastic Card Mfg. Smart Card, Credit Card, Discount Card
- Plastic Cards (Smart Cards)
- Plastic Cards (Smart Cards) Utilised Credit Cards
- Plastic Collapsible Tube For Tooth Paste & Cream
- Plastic Collopsible Tubes & Printing
- Plastic Corrogated Sheet & Box
- Plastic Fan Guard (Automatic Plant)
- Plastic Felt
- Plastic Films & Sheet With Printing (Flexo & Roto)
- Plastic Granules From Scraps/Waste
- Plastic I. V. Bottles
- Plastic Mats Extruding & Weaving
- Plastic Moulded Furniture
- Plastic Moulded Furniture (Chairs)
- Plastic Moulded Toys
- Plastic Office Products
- Plastic Processing Moulds
- Plastic Sequince
- Plastic Spectacle Frame
- Plastic Sutli
- Plastic Toys
- Plastic Water Storage Tank (H.D.P.E.)(Syntex Type)
- Poly Propylene Measuring Cup
- Polyester Film
- Polyester Polyol Air Foam Mfg.By Using Petroleum Base As Raw Material
- Polyester Resin
- Polyster Film
- Polythene Bags
- Polythene Bags And Automatic Prinitng
- Polythene Pouches For Ghee, Butter, Milk And Oil
- Polythene Printed Bags
- Polythene Printed Bags (Pp & Hm)
- Polyurethane
- Polyurethane Foam & Its Products
- Polyurethane Product (Rigid & Moulded)
- Polyurethane Foam (Flexible)
- Polyurethane Pipe Section,Slab Panels, Rigid Foam, Moulding
- Pvc (Hdpe) Water Storage Tank
- Pvc Bottles For Mineral Water
- Pvc Compound From Pvc Resin
- Pvc Compounding
- Pvc Conduit Pipes
- Pvc Felexible Pipe
- Pvc Footwear
- Pvc From Ethanols
- Pvc Granules & Rigid Pipes
- Pvc Hoses (For Irrigation Purposes)
- Pvc Pipe & Fittings
- Pvc Profiles (Door, Window And Chairs) Decorative Accessories
- Pvc Rexine Cloth
- Pvc Section Hoses
- Pvc Section Pipe
- Pvc Soles
- Pvc Tube
- Rubber (Floor Mat) For Automobile
- Rubber Auto Parts
- Rubber Ball For Childrens
- Rubber Band
- Rubber Band (Disco Type)
- Rubber Baskets
- Rubber Belting (V - Belt)
- Rubber Compound For Automobiles
- Rubber Floor Mat
- Rubber Linning & F.R.P. Linning
- Rubber Powder From Waste Tyres
- Rubber Reclamation Industry
- Rubber Roller & Ebonite Roller
- Rubber Roller For Printing M\C
- Rubber Roller For Rice Mill
- Rubber Rollers
- Rubber Sheet For

HAND BOOK

ON

HERBAL PRODUCTS

(Cosmetics, Toiletries , Medicines & Perfumes)

in 2 Volumes

Vol. II

IMPORTANT STEPS FOR SELECTION OF AN INDUSTRY

- If you are not in a position to decide an appropriate industry within your range of investment then read this book thoroughly. You will find a number of industries of your interest in the book.

- Select few products and keep them in mind for discussion with your friends and family members.

- For the selection you may seek the services of your consultant who can provide you more informations and guidance on the ins and out of all the products which you have selected and help in the final selection of one or two of the products which suits you.

- Although this book provides you basic information, yet before going in for implementation you are advised to assess the latest prices of plant, machinery and raw materials, market position through your own sources.

- For detailed information on manufacturing process, market survey, selection of appropriate plant and machinery, procurement of loan from financial institutions, and other assistance, you must obtain Practical Project Execution Know-How Report which can be availabe from "National Institute of Industrial Research",106 - E, Kamla Nagar, Delhi - 110 007.

HAND BOOK
ON
HERBAL PRODUCTS

(Cosmetics, Toiletries , Medicines & Perfumes)

in 2 Volumes

Vol. II

by

NIIR Board of Technologists

Publicaton Division

नेशनल इंस्टीट्यूट ऑफ इन्डस्ट्रियल रिसर्च

National Institute of Industrial Research

Regd.Office: 106-E, Kamla Nagar, Delhi-110 007(INDIA)

Published by :

National Institute of Industrial Research

Regd. Office: 106-E, Kamla Nagar, P.B. No.2162, Delhi - 110007 (INDIA)
Ph. : 91-11-23843955, 23845654, 23845886, 9811043595
Fax : 91-11-23841561 **E-Mail** : niir @ vsnl.com
Website : www.niir.org

I.S.B.N. : 81-86623-48-5 (Set)

Price Rs. 1500/- (For 2 Volumes)
Us$ 220/-

Printed & Published by **Ajay Kr. Gupta** for "**National Institute of Industrial Research**", Delhi-110007 & Printed at New Gian Offset Printers, Shahzada Bagh, Delhi-35.

Ist(BJJJBAFAA)
IInd(CAAEBCFAA)

CONTENTS

VOL II

10

Ayurveda Siddha Unani Companies and their Products

ADDCCO LIMITED

P.O. Adcconagar, Dist. Hooghly (W. Bengal) Tel - 846298

Product Name : **ASOKE CORDIAL**

Composition : Each 15 ml. contains :

Asoka bark	300 mg.
Berala seth	200 mg.
Simul Flower	200 mg.
Shyamlata	200 mg.
Anantamool	200 mg.
Jaba Flower	200 mg.
Amer ati	200 mg.
Alkushi Big	200 mg.
Posta dhari	200 mg.

Dosage One teaspoon 2-3 times a day.

Product Name : **HAEMOLIN**

Composition : Each 5 ml. contains :

Liquid Ext. 5 g. of Lacca.
500 mg. each of Lodhra, Priyangu,
Rakta chandan, Vasaka.
200 mg. each of Ayapan, Olat kambal

Self Generated Alcohol 10%

Dosage One teaspoon 3-4 times a day.

How Supplied: 10 ml., 30 ml., 60 ml.

Uses : Haemitinic

Product Name : LEUKORA

Composition : Each 10 ml. contains :

Aqueous Extract from 10 mg. each of Bakam, Khadir, Vasaka, Shyamlata, Anantamul, Mango seed, Daruharidra, Chirata, Jira, Bael & Rasanjana, Hirakas.

Dosage 2 teaspoonfuls 2-3 times a day.

How Supplied: 250 ml.

Uses : Leucorrhoea

AIMIL PHARMACEUTICALS (INDIA) LTD.
2994/4, Street No. 17, Ranjit Nagar,
New Delhi - 110 008. Tel - 5701203, 5703041
Fax - (011) 5703064, 5755000

Product Name : AMLYCURE TABLETS

Composition :

Punarnava rakt	50 mg.
Bhringraj	50 mg.
Kasmerd	20 mg.
Bhuimala	20 mg.
Rohitaka	20 mg.
Sarpaunkha mool	20 mg.
Kasni	20 mg.
Chirayata	10 mg.
Katuki	30 mg.
Mandur bhasma	40 mg.
Kakamachi	20 mg.
Limbda chhaal	20 mg.

Dosage : Not Available

How Supplied: 30 tabs., 90 tabs., 1000 tabs.

Product Name : AMLYTONE GRANULES

Composition : Each 10 g. contains :

Shukti bhasma	100 mg.
Loh bhasma	5 mg.

Seb ghansatv	100 mg.
Loh bhasma	5 mg.
Amla	500 mg.
Makhana	500 mg.
Khajoor	500 mg.
Shringataka	100 mg.
Soya conc.	3000 mg.
Dalchini	700 mg.
Jaiphal dist	100 mg.
Elaichi dist	100 mg.

Dosage Not Available

How Supplied: 200 g.

Product Name **: AMRYBION TABLETS**

Composition :

Pushkarmool	40 mg.
Dashmula kwath	20 mg.
Punarnavastaka kwath	20 mg.
Arogyavardhini vati	30 mg.
Chanderprabha vati	15 mg.
Ashwagandha	30 mg.
Shankhapushpi	20 mg.
Shirish	30 mg.
Nagarjunabhi ras	15 mg.
Jaharmohra pisti	10 mg.
Akik pisti	10 mg.
Hradyarnava ras	30 mg.
Arjun chhaal	70 mg.

Dosage Not Available

How Supplied: 30 tabs., 90 tabs.

Product Name **: AMRYCARD CAPSULES**

Composition :

Ghansatva each of :

Tejpatr	100 mg.
Bilvpatr	60 mg.
Vijyasar	40 mg.

Gudmarpatr	20 mg.
Neempatr	20 mg.
Jamunpatr	30 mg.
Giloe	20 mg.
Methi seeds	30 mg.
Trivang bhasma	20 mg.
Sudh shilajeet	20 mg.
Swarn makshik bhasma	20 mg.
Ghansatv of Gularpatr	40 mg.

Product Name : **AMRYGEL TABLETS**

Composition :

Avipatikar churan	100 mg.
Narikel lavan	50 mg.
Satvar Conc.	50 mg.
Amalki rasayan	40 mg.
Madhuyasthi	40 mg.
Sut shekhar ras	20 mg.
Tamra bhasma	15 mg.
Praval pishti	50 mg.
Bhringraj Conc.	15 mg.
Patola Conc.	20 mg.

Product Name : **AMYCLOT TABLETS**

Composition :

Godanti bhasma	30 mg.
Nagkesar	40 mg.
Ashok chhaal	50 mg.
Jeevanti	50 mg.
Praval pishti	10 mg.
Laksha shudha	30 mg.
Gainda pool	20 mg.
Gainda patr	50 mg.
Santra chilka	30 mg.
Kahreva pishti	10 mg.
Sphatika bhasma	20 mg.
Zaharmohra pishti	20 mg.
Dadim chhaal	20 mg.

Mochras	40 mg.
Shukti bhasma	10 mg.
Phool priyangu	40 mg.
Rasaunt	40 mg.

***Product Name* : AMYDIO FORTE SYRUP**

Composition : Each 10 ml. contains :

Extract of Baelgiri	500 mg.
Kutaj	400 mg.
Nagkesar	300 mg.
Indar jav	400 mg.
Sunthi	300 mg.
Saunf	250 mg.
Safed jeera	100 mg.
Ajwain	100 mg.
Katha	100 mg.
Babul gond	50 mg.
Dadim chhaal	100 mg.
Nagar motha	50 mg.
Mochras	40 mg.
Kalimirch	30 mg.
Dhania	30 mg.
Maroorphali	50 mg.
Kala namak	30 mg.

***Product Name* : AMYFLYM TABLETS**

***Composition* :**

Arogya vardhini vati	50 mg.
Purified sulphur	15 mg.
Purified mercury	15 mg.
Nirgundi extract	30 mg.
Loh bhasma	15 mg.
Abhrak bhasma	15 mg.
Triphala	30 mg.
Shilajeet sudh	50 mg.
Guggulu	100 mg.
Chitrakmul	20 mg.
Kutaki extract	60 mg.
Tamra bhasma	20 mg.

***Product Name* : AMYPURE TABLETS**

***Composition* :**

Sudh gandhak	30 mg.
Mahamanjisthadi quath	60 mg.
Yashad bhasma	30 mg.
Ras manikya	40 mg.
Extract of Manjistha	20 mg.
Extract of Aristak	35 mg.
Giloe	35 mg.
Neem chhaal	35 mg.
Chirayata	25 mg.
Daruharidra	15 mg.
Mundi phal	15 mg.
Bakayan	40 mg.

***Product Name* : AMYRON CAPSULES**

***Composition* :**

Loh bhasma	70 mg.
Pravalmool bhasma	30 mg.
Sudh Shilajeet	30 mg.
Shatavar	60 mg.
Varahi kand	60 mg.
Aswagandha	30 mg.
Punarnava mandoor	30 mg.
Ananta mool	40 mg.
Yashad bhasma	10 mg.
Kali Draksh	20 mg.
Soyabeans Conc.	30 mg.
Safed Musli	30 mg.
Praval pishti	10 mg.
Rajmah conc.	20 mg.
Kalachana conc.	20 mg.
Seb ghansatv	15 mg.
Methi	30 mg.
Surajmukhi seeds	20 mg.
Amla	20 mg.
Kesar	2 mg.
Kaunch	30 mg.
Haritaki	20 mg.
Anukurit genhu taila	3 mg.

Product Name : AN-AS-LEU TABLETS

Composition :

Jamun majja ghan satva	25 mg.
Aam majja ghan satva	25 mg.
Rasaunt	15 mg.
Pathani lodhra	35 mg.
Kumari ghan satva	15 mg.
Manjith	15 mg.
Sphatika bhasma	20 mg.
Kumar kas	15 mg.
Praval bhasma	20 mg.
Loh bhasma	25 mg.
Shilajeet shudh	25 mg.
Kuktanadtwak bhasma	40 mg.
Mandur bhasma	40 mg.
Supari chikani	40 mg.
Shatavar	25 mg.

Product Name : ASHREE CAPSULES

Composition :

Kaunch beej	50 mg.
Jaiphal	10 mg.
Javitri	10 mg.
Kesar	0.2 mg.
Shatavar	20 mg.
Safed musli	50 mg.
Gangeran	20 mg.
Lavang	10 mg.
Shilajeet sudh	35 mg.
Dhatura beej	15 mg.
Shalab misri	65 mg.
Sudh vijaya	10 mg.
Ashwagandha	10 mg.
Nagkesar	10 mg.
Pippali	10 mg.
Taj	10 mg.
Gokharu	25 mg.
Makardhwaj	15 mg.
Trivang bhasma	15 mg.
Varahi kand	50 mg.

***Product Name :* ASTHIGON EXPECTORANT SYRUP**

Composition : Each 10 ml. contains Ext. of :

Somalata	200 mg.
Vasaka	200 mg.
Madhuyasthi	200 mg.
Alsi-ke-beej	200 mg.
Jufa	200 mg.
Bhairangi	200 mg.
Akarkara	50 mg.
Naushadar	50 mg.
Yavkshar	30 mg.
Jhatkhatmi	40 mg.
Kaifal	30 mg.
Kakrasingi	100 mg.

***Product Name :* ASHREE FORTE CAPSULES**

Composition :

Makardwaj	20 mg.
Kesar	20 mg.
Jaiphal	20 mg.
Javitri	20 mg.
Shudh shilajeet	20 mg.
Swarn vang	10 mg.
Guduchi extract	20 mg.
Trivang bhasma	10 mg.
Gokhru extract	20 mg.
Kaunch beej	150 mg.
Ashwagandha	30 mg.
Satavar	30 mg.
Safed musli	20 mg.
Shudh bhilwa	30 mg.
Til ghansatv	20 mg.
Varahi kand	20 mg.
Tejpatr	15 mg.
Dalchini	15 mg.
Dhatura beej	10 mg.
Sodhit kuchla	10 mg.
Akarkara	10 mg.

***Product Name* : AYUSH-64 TABLETS**

Composition : Dried aqueous extracts of :

Chirayata	100 mg.
Satona chaal	100 mg.
Kutaki	100 mg.
Karanj beej	200 mg.

***Product Name* : BONIHEAL CAPSULES**

***Composition* :**

Laksha	100 mg.
Asthi shrnkhla	80 mg.
Methi beej	40 mg.
Bidari kand	30 mg.
Praval pishti	50 mg.
Shukti bhasam	20 mg.
Ashwagandha	30 mg.
Sudh shilajeet	50 mg.
Amla	50 mg.
Soyabean conc.	30 mg.
Yashad bhasam	10 mg.
Arjun chaal ghan	20 mg.
Atibala	20 mg.
Nirgundi	20 mg.

***Product Name* : CIDOSEP SYRUP**

Composition : Each 6 ml. contains :

Powder Guggul sudh	80 mg.
Ext. each of Maha rasnadi quath	30 mg.
Manjishtha	15 mg.
Gudichi	14 mg.
Trikatu	13 mg.
Kushka	13 mg.
Amalki	8 mg.
Yashti madhu	6 mg.

***Product Name* : DERMACIN POWDER**

Composition :

Sudh gandhak	14%
Sphatika	10%
Ratanjot	2%
Red chandan	1%

Sangejrahat	2%
Kapoor	0.2%
Tulsi	0.2%
Ajwain	0.2%
Bawachi	2.0%
Gorakhmundi	1%
Nagarmotha	1%
Sudh sohaga	75.4%

***Product Name* : GYCARE TABLETS**

***Composition* :**

Ulat kambal	40 mg.
Hirabol	40 mg.
Manjistha	25 mg.
Kasis sudh	20 mg.
Jeevanti	20 mg.
Ashok ghan	50 mg.
Supari	25 mg.
Elva	50 mg.
Sunthi ghan	50 mg.
Soya	25 mg.
Sohaga	25 mg.
Shilajeet sudh	20 mg.
Rajat parartini vati	30 mg.
Arogyavardhini vati	25 mg.

***Product Name* : FEMEFIT CAPSULES**

Composition :

Mochras	25 mg.
Lodhr pathani	20 mg.
Kutaki	20 mg.
Sudh laksha	20 mg.
Chikni supari	50 mg.
Gokshru	10 mg.
Kutaj chaal	20 mg.
Nyagrodha	20 mg.
Nagkesar	20 mg.
Sheetal chini	10 mg.
Kumari ghrit	50 mg.

Chopchini	30 mg.
Rasonth	10 mg.
Neem chaal	20 mg.
Makoi	20 mg.
Ashok chal ghan	30 mg.
Sunthi	15 mg.
Chauli mool	10 mg.
Bansa	30 mg.
Raal	20 mg.
Anantmool	20 mg.
Mandur bhasam	20 mg.
Praval pishti	10 mg.
Yashad bhasam	5 mg.

AJMERA PHARMACEUTICALS PVT. LTD.

Post Box No. 232, B/9 A, Industrial Estate, Pologround
Indore - 452 003, Tel - 421041, 420227, Fax - (0731) 420227

***Product Name* : ALARGIN FORTE CAPSULE**

Composition :

Ext. Tejpatra	10 mg.
Ext. Saunth	10 mg.
Ext. Chitrakmool	10 mg.
Ext. Bay bidang	10 mg.
Ext. Nagarmotha	10 mg.
Ext. Nishoth	10 mg.
Ext. Neemchhal	10 mg.
Ext. Kut	10 mg.
Ext. Sanay	10 mg.
Ext. Gokharoo	10 mg.
Ext. Neem giloya	10 mg.
Ext. Nagkeshar	10 mg.
Ext. Kutki	10 mg.
Badi Elayachi	20 mg.
Chhoti Elayachi	10 mg.
Dalchini	20 mg.
Haldi	150 mg.
Suhaga	20 mg.
Trifala	10 mg.
Trikatu	10 mg.
Gandhak Rasayan	50 mg.

Dosage 1 to 2 capsule three times a day.

How Supplied: Blister Pack of 6x10 capsules.

Uses : Food allergy, mild urticaria and Dermatographism, Vasomotor rhinities.

Pharmacological Action : Alargin Forte capsule contains natural antihistamines which do not produce drowsiness. Haldi restricts mast cells to release histamines, it is cholaretic and cholagogue, it is very effective against respiratory allergies, useful in mild urticaria and dermatographism Gandhak Rasayan is blood purifier. Badi Elayachi is carminative, stomachic and stimulant, corrects kapha and pitta disorders. Tejpatra works as a germicidal and destroys the pathogenic bacilli. Chitrakmool is nervine, stimulant, diuretic and anthelmintic. Kut is cathartic, stimulant, antiseptic and spasmolytic, it relaxes involuntary muscles and is useful in all types of asthma. Neem chhal promotes the removal of catarrhal matter and phelgm from the bronchial tubes. Kutki is useful in dyspepsia, food allergy and asthma. Restricts mast cells to release histamin. Checks the inflammation of respiratory tract. Provides quick relief from all sorts of discomfort due to allergic attack.

Product Name : **AYOTIC CAPSULE**

Composition :

Godanti Bhasma	50 mg.
Mritunjay Ras	50 mg.
Kajjali	50 mg.
Sutraj Ras	30 mg.
Laxmivilas ras	30 mg.
Laxminarayan ras	30 mg.
Suthshekar ras	30 mg.
Gandhak rasayan	30 mg.
Vishvatapharan ras	30 mg.
Loban	20 mg.
Jaymangal ras	20 mg.
Sanjivani vati	20 mg.
Hartal bhasma	20 mg.
Malla sindur	20 mg.
Samir Pannag ras	20 mg.
Tribhuwan kirti ras	30 mg.

Dosage 1 to 2 capsule two to three times a day.

How Supplied: Blister pack of 6x10 capsules.

Uses : All types of fungal and bacterial infections, Respiratory tract, Skin, soft tissue and Urinary tract infections, Relapsing fever, Conjunctivitis, Primary and secondary syphilis, Severe acne.

Pharmacological Action : Its active ingredients like Loban, Hartal Bhasma, Sutraj ras, Laxmivilas ras, Tribhuvan kirti ras are all effective against Respiratory pathogens, reduce air-ways inflammation, resolve symptoms of cough and fever and restabilise immune defence. Ayotic capsule is effective in common urinary tract infections, its ingredients fight with micro-organisms, flush kidneys, crush calculi and expel them out, rebuild the damaged tissues of the urinary tract. Ayotic capsule is effective against infections of skin and soft tissues. Ingredients like Gandhak rasayn, Loban, Laxmivilas ras are having Anti-allergic, Anti-pyretic, Anti-inflammatory and Fungicidal properties. Ingredients like Godanti Bhasma, Samir pannag ras, Suthshekar ras clean the lungs and detoxify the liver. Ayotic-shows effective bactericidal activity in bronchial secretions thereby resolving symptoms of cough and fever. Kills almost UTI pathogens and maintains prolonged bactericidal levels. Effective against complicated inflammatory dermatitis and eczematous fungal infections.

Product Name : **AYURAL CAPSULE**

Composition :

Kamduddha ras	60 mg.
Sutshekhar ras	50 mg.
Leelavilas ras	50 mg.
Shankh bhasma	50 mg.
Swarnamakshik bhasma	20 mg.
Jeera	60 mg.
Mulethi	20 mg.
Sajjikshar	20 mg.
Avipatikar churna	80 mg.
Yavakshar	20 mg.

Dosage 1 to 2 capsule two times a day.

How Supplied: Blister pack of 6x10 capsules.

Uses : Hyperacidity, Heartburn, Ulcers, Gastritis.

Pharmacological Action : Herbal and other ayurvedic ingredients present in Ayural capsule give quick relief of symptoms such as flatulence, abdominal distention, hyperacidity and heartburn thereby corrects the digestive malfunctioning. Kamduddha ras, Sutshekhar ras, Leelavilas ras are having demulcent, stomachic and antacid properties they help in neutralising the excess acidity to give immediate symptomatic relief. While Jeera, Sajjikshar and Yavakshar improve the digestive function stimulates gastric glands so as to digest food properly. Mulethi, swarnamakshik bhasma and Shankh Bhasma are having anti-inflammatory, antispasmodic, estrogenic and nervine properties they provide relief from heartburn, pain and inflammation due to ulcer. Avipatikar churn and Sajjikshar are fast acting antacids, they also expel out the toxins from gastrointestinal tract. In this way Ayural works on any type of ulcers whether due to hyper acidity or deficiency of the stomach acid.

***Product Name* : GENTLE-S CAPSULE**

Composition :

Ext. Asgandh	50 mg.
Kounch beej	100 mg.
Shatavari	30 mg.
Safed musli	20 mg.
Talamkhana	25 mg.
Vidari kand	25 mg.
Gokharoo bada	25 mg.
Akarkara	10 mg.
Choti Elayachi	10 mg.
Javitri	5 mg.
Lavang	5 mg.
Dalchini	10 mg.
Salam mishri	30 mg.
Keshar	10 mg.
Shudda shilajit	50 mg.
Makardwaj	10 mg.
Loh bhasma	10 mg.
Abhrak bhasma	10 mg.
Swarna bang	10 mg.
Bang bhasma	30 mg.

Dosage 1-2 capsules at night with milk.

How Supplied: Blister Pack of 1x10 capsules.

Uses : Psychic and Functional Impotence. Lack of Sexual Motivation Spermatorrhoea, Nocturnal emissions, Premature ejaculation, Oligospermia Senile debility.

***Pharmacological Action* :** Gentle-S capsule is a well balanced compound of timetested ayurvedic aphrodisiacs, rejuvenator, stimulant, tonic, digestive herbs and minerals for all types of sexual debility in men. Its active ingredients like Kounch Beej, Asgandh, Shatavari and Abhrak bhasma are powerful stimulant and aphrodisiacs. They improve libido and sexual drive, correct nervous debility and psychosomatic disorders and help regain confidence. Shilajeet and Makardhwaj are aphrodisiac and rejuvenators, Loh bhasma increases R.B.C. count. Gokharoo, Choti Elayachi and Dalchini are carminative, diuretic and nerve sedatives Swarna bang and Bang bhasma are general tonics, Javitri and Lavang are antiseptic and stimulants. Gentle-S controls premature ejaculation, develops confidence to perform adequately. Treats nocturnal emission, Controls spermatorrhoea successfully, Corrects psychosomatic disorders, improves general health.

***Product Name* : LEUKODNA CAPSULE**

Composition ;

Ext. of Bavachi beej	50 mg.
Pravad beej	10 mg.
Bay bidang	10 mg.
Belgiri	10 mg.
Trifala	10 mg.
Trikatu	10 mg.
Lal chandan	10 mg.
Jatamansi	10 mg.
Anantmool	10 mg.
Chirayata	10 mg.
Malkangani	10 mg.
Tulsi	10 mg.
Nagarmotha	10 mg.
Arjun chhal	10 mg.
Manjith	10 mg.
Giloy	10 mg.
Bhangra	10 mg.
Haldi	10 mg.
Nishoth	10 mg.
Palash beej	10 mg.
Kut	10 mg.
Indrajaw	10 mg.
Bach	10 mg.
Kutki	10 mg.
Neem chhal	10 mg.

Indrayan mool	10 mg.
Patol patra	10 mg.
Indrayan phal	10 mg.
Bavachi beej	10 mg.
Atis	10 mg.
Makoyä	20 mg.
Kajjali	10 mg.
Loh bhasma	10 mg.
Praval bhasma	10 mg.
Arjun chhal	10 mg.

Dosage 1 to 2 capsule three times a day.

How Supplied: Blister Pack of 6x10 capsules.

Uses : Leucoderma, Psoriasis, Eczema, Skin rashes, Contact dermatitis.

Pharmacological Action : Leukodna capsule is a balanced combination of various herbs and pharmacopoieal medicines. Bavuchi beej is a tonic, stomachic and diuretic, Pavad beej is carminative, anthelmintic, stimulant and antiseptic, it also has a great effect as an alternative in all kinds of skin diseases. Bay bidang is carminative, anthelmintic, and stimulant. Malkangani is alterative, nervine tonic and useful in leprosy. Kutki is used as a bitter tonic, cathartic, stomachic and febrifuge. Neem chhal works as an vermifuge and useful in skin diseases. Loh bhasma increased RBC count. Trifala is a mild laxative and useful in skin diseases. Kajjali is anti bacterial. Praval bhasma is used in calcium deficiency and is also a blood purifier. Leukodna-Accelerates melanim synthesis (MSH activity), Enhances production of vegetable amine substances and thus melanim formation. Corrects 'Pitta' disorder. Regularises digestive system. Eliminates toxins from the intestinal tract, Purifies Blood, Flushes kidneys. Does not produce any side effect.

Product Name : **PREGNITA CAPSULE**

Composition :

Grabha Chintamani Ras	70 mg.
Mandur Makshik Bhasma	70 mg.
Madhu malini	50 mg.
Kamdudha Ras	50 mg.
Garbhapal Ras	70 mg.
Abrak bhasma	20 mg.
Praval pishti	10 mg.
Sitopaladi Churna	30 mg.

Dosage 1 to 2 capsule three times a day.

How Supplied: Blister pack of 6x10 capsules.

Uses : Anaemia in pregnant women, Abnormal vaginal bleeding, Nausea, Vomiting and other complications.

Pharmacological Action : Pregnita capsule is a well balanced formula of various ayurvedic ras and bhasm preparations which are time tested medicines to provide all the nutritive and curative requirements during pregnancy and even after delivery. Garbh chintamani ras and Garphpal ras provides nutrition and protects the foetus. Kamaduddha ras controls heart beat, thereby blood pressure. Abhrak bhasma and Mandur makshik bhasma provide energy and vitality. Praval pishti is natural calcium, which is necessary for lactation and making of bones. This all makes Pregnita capsule an ideal tonic during pregnancy.

Product Name : **RAKTAP CAPSULE**

Composition :

Abhrak bhasma	25 mg.
Loh bhasma	30 mg.
Punarnava Mandur	100 mg.
Swarnamakshik bhasma	15 mg.
Amal ki rasayan	50 mg.
Praval pishti	10 mg.
Kamdhenu ras	50 mg.
Laghumalini basant	50 mg.
Arogyawardhini	75 mg.

Dosage 1 capsule two times a day.

How Supplied: Blister pack 6x10 capsules.

Uses : Hypochronic anaemia, Iron difficiency anaemia, Excessing tiredness & fatigue, breathlessness due to anaemia.

Pharmacological Action : Raktap capsule maintains iron mineral balance in the body, supplies calcium and vitamin C in natural form to fight hypochronic anaemia ingredients like Punarnava mandur, Kamdhenu ras and Swarnamakshik bhasma tonety the liver and maintain digestive fire, restore appetite, improve digestion and assimilation. Praval pishti provides natural calcium. Abhrak bhasma is nervine tonic. Loh bhasma improves RBC count. Amalki rasayan develops body resistance to fight diseases. Arogyawardhini is laxative which detoxifies G.I. tract. Raktap capsule can be prescribed to working women and pregnant ladies to meet their iron, mineral and calcium requirement, it can also be prescribed to women with iron deficiency due to excessive blood loss during menstruation.

***Product Name* : REGULOSE CAPSULE**

Composition :

Ext. Vijasar	10 mg.
Ext. Sheetalchini	10 mg.
Ext. Chopchini	10 mg.
Ext. Amatltas	10 mg.
Ext. Manjith	10 mg.
Ext. Gokharoo (Chota)	20 mg.
Ext. Haldi	20 mg.
Ext. Jamun guthali	20 mg.
Ext. Trifala	20 mg.
Tribang bhasma	20 mg.
Sh. Shilajit	50 mg.
Vrad vangeshwar ras	50 mg.
Prameh gajkesri ras	50 mg.
Shivgutika	50 mg.
Chandraprabhavati	80 mg.

Dosage 1 to 2 capsule two to three times a day.

How Supplied: Blister pack of 6x10 capsules.

***Uses* :** Diabetes Mellitus, Diabetes insipidus.

Pharmacological Action : Regulose capsule is formulated with very effective herbal and other Ayurvedic medicines. Chandraprabhavati a pharmacopoeial preparation is diuretic and blood purifier. Shivgutika is energetic and stomachic. Vrad vangeshwar ras and Tribang bhasma both pharmacopoeial preparations are antidiabetic. Pramesh gajkesri ras is useful in the treatment of excessive urination, U.T. Disorders, Shilajit is anthelmintic, nervine and antidiabetic. Jamun guthli is diuretic and anti-diabetic which checks the pathological convertion of starch into sugar in case of increased production of glucose. Haldi is diuretic, Chopchini is resolvent, stimulant and digestive good for general obesity. Sheetalchini disinfets urine. Vijasar is good for arthritis, diabetes melletus and diabetes insipidus.

Product Name **: R-EXEX CAPSULE**

Composition :

Arogyawardhini	100 mg.
Ext. Dana methi	50 mg.
Ext. Krishna jeera	50 mg.
Shilasindur vati	50 mg.
Laxmivilas ras	50 mg.
Thraiyushnaya loh	50 mg.
Yograj guggal	50 mg.

Dosage 1 to 2 capsule two times a day.

How Supplied: Blister pack of 6x10 capsules.

Uses : Exogenous obesity. Abnormalities in carbohydrate metabolism.

Pharmacological Action : R-exex is a well balanced combination of fat dissolving, digestive, laxative and nervine herbs, its main ingredients like Arogyawardhini controls the function of liver and pancreas and thus checks hyper insulinism, it is also antiperiodic and mild laxative. Methidana is diaphoretic aget it excretes oedema fluid or nitrogenous material retained in body, it also controls the glandular, intestinal, pancreatic secretions. Krishna jeera is useful in treatment of flatulent colic, it also excretes the excessive fluid from the body and thus helps controlling obesity. It is also digestive and diuretic. Yograj guggal is a well balanced mixture of decoction of Triphala and guggalu as a therapeutic agent it maintains cholesterol level and reduces adiposity.

Product Name **: RHEUMALLIN-S CAPSULE**

Composition :

Sh. Kuchala	5 mg.
Malla Sindur	5 mg.
Ext. Indrayan mool	10 mg.
Ext. Negad beej	10 mg.
Ext. neem giloy	10 mg.
Ext. Chop chini	10 mg.
Ext. Indrayan Beej	10 mg.
Ext. Kulinjan	10 mg.
Ext. Asgandha	20 mg.
Ext. Malkangani	20 mg.

Rasaunt	20 mg.
Lahsun	40 mg.
Amavat Prabhadhini Vati	40 mg.
Mahavat Vingasan Ras	40 mg.
Mahayograj Guggal	100 mg.
Yograj Guggal	100 mg.

Dosage 1 to 2 capsule three times a day.

How Supplied: Blister Pack of 6x10 capsules.

Uses : Arthritis, Osteo-Arthritis, Gout, Sciatica, Stiffness in joints, Inflammation, Swelling and Pain, Rheumatoid Arthritis, Flatulence, Lassitude, Sluggish body movements, Digestive disorders.

Pharmacological Action : Its main ingredients Yograj and Mahayograj guggal reduce adiposity, that is the excessive accumulation of fat in the body. It causes an increase of leucocytes in the blood and stimulates phagocytosis. Other ingredient Asgandha works as an anti tumour and sedative agent, helps reducing inflammation and pain. Lahsun is a powerful bactericide and vermifuge that expels intestinal worms, corrects digestive disorders, maintains cholesterol levels thereby provides cytoprotection, it also works as an nervine tonic. Chopchini, Malkangani works as alternative and anti-rheumatism agent. It improves joint function and restores freedom of movement.

Product Name : **SLOGO CAPSULES**

Composition : Each capsule contains :

Jatamansi (Nardostachys jatamansi)	50 mg.
Piplamool (Piper Longum)	30 mg.
Brahmi (Herpestis monniera)	30 mg.
Shankh pushpi (Evoluvulus alsinoides)	30 mg.
Sarpagandhari vati (Pharmacopoeial)	100 mg.
Ichabhedi ras (Pharmacopoeial)	30 mg.
Jaharmohara pishti (Pharmacopoeial)	30 mg.
Amal ki rasayan (Pharmacopoeial)	30 mg.
Praval pishti (Pharmacopoeial)	20 mg.
Sh. Gandhak (Pharmacopoeial)	20 mg.

Dosage 1 capsule three times a day.

How Supplied: Strip of 10 capsules (Blister Pack)

Uses : Moderate to severe essential Hypertension.

Product Name : **AAFRESH CAPSULES**

Composition : Each capsule contains :

Arogyawardhini (Pharmacopoeial)	150 mg.
Ext. Gokharoo (Tribulus terrestris)	60 mg.
Ext. Kukti (Picrorrhiza kurroa)	60 mg.
Ext. Nishoth (ipomoea turpethum)	60 mg.
Ext. Anantmool (hemidesmus indicus)	60 mg.

Dosage 1 to 2 capsules at bed time.

How Supplied: Strip of 10 capsules (Blister pack)

Uses : Chronic constipation, Abdominal gas, Colitis.

Pharmacological Action : AAFRESH is formulated very carefully with timetested mild but effective ayurvedic purgatives and tonics which clean the colon, detoxify the digestive system, nourish the nervous system thereby improve appetite, it solves the problem of weak bowel movements. Arogyawardhini is a pharmacopoeial preparation it is laxative. Gokharoo is cooling, demulcent, diuretic and astringent it releaves nervous tension and headache due to constipation. Kutki is laxative and cathartic. Nishoth is a purgative and tonic which expels out toxins from gastro intestinal tract. Anantmool is alternative and demulcent. AAFRESH can safely be given to treat constipation in obstratic, gynaecological and post partum cases it is safe for pregnant women. AAFRESH does not contain any habit forming ingredient.

Product Name : **U-FIT CAPSULE**

Composition : Each capsule contains :

Shivgutika (Pharmacopoeial)	150 mg.
Asgandha (Withania somnifera)	50 mg.
Shatavari (Asparagus racemosus)	50 mg.
Kaunch Beej (Mucuna pruriens)	50 mg.
Amal ki rasayan (Pharmacopoeial)	50 mg.
Safed musli (Chlorophytum) (Arundinaceum)	30 mg.
Loh bhasma (Pharmacopoeial)	30 mg.
Praval pishti (Pharmacopoeial)	20 mg.
Abhrak bhasma (Pharmacopoeial)	10 mg.
Bang bhasma (Pharmacopoeial)	10 mg.

Dosage 1 to 2 capsules 2-3 times a day.

How Supplied: Blister pack of 10 capsules.

Uses : Debility, Nervous debility, Malnutrition, Anaemia and state of nervous exhastion.

Pharmacological Action : A well balanced combination of timetested Ayurvedic tonics. Aphrodisiacs, Anthelmintics, Blood purifiers, Alternatives, galactagogues and demulcents. Asagandha is an alternative and tonic very useful in nervous and seminal dibility, it is also an aphrodisiac and sedative. Shatavari is tonic, antacid, galactagogue and diuretic it is useful in seminal debility and pulmonary complaints. Safed musli is useful in general debility and in affection of urinogenital system. Kaunch beej is a powerful aphrodisiac, nervine tonic and emmenagogue. Loh bhasma provides adequate iron to the blood cells, useful in anaemia. Abhrak bhasma is vitalizer and rejuvenator maintains youthfulness and strengthens nerves. Shivgutika psychosomatic disorders and weak concentration. Eliminates accumulation of toxins and aggravated humors, Fights deficiencies, Provides vitamin-mineral supplementation in balanced manner, Suitable to both sexes, Provides true fitness.

***Product Name* : HARTONE CAPSULES**

Composition : Each capsule contains :

Arjunchhal (Terminalia arjuna)	100 mg.
Malkangani (Celastrus paniculata)	40 mg.
Jatamansi (Nardostachys jatamansi)	40 mg.
Brahmi (Herpestis monniera)	40 mg.
Shankpushpi (Evolvulus alsinoides)	40 mg.
Prabhakar vati (Pharmacopoeial)	40 mg.
Trinetra ras (Pharmacopoeial)	40 mg.
Kamduddha ras (Pharmacopoeial)	40 mg.
Mukta pishti (Pharmacopoeial)	10 mg.
Praval pishti (Pharmacopoeial)	50 mg.
Kaharava pishti (Pharmacopoeial)	10 mg.

Dosage 1 to 2 capsules three times a day.

How Supplied: Strip of 10 capsules (Blister pack)

Uses : Heart attacks, Stroke, Angina, Arteriosclerosis, Silent Ischaemia, Hypertension.

Pharmacological Action : HARTONE tonifies the heart and the lungs and fights cardiac illness, it maintains cholesterol level, it regulated hypercholesterolemia and hypertrigglycrideaemia by regulating abnormal lipoprotien metabolism it also controls heart beat and palpitation. Its ingredients like Arjun chhal, Brahmi, Kamdhuddha Ras and Prabhakar vati are powerful cardio protectives. Jatamansi is diuretic, nerve sedative, carminative and deobustruent. It fights mental stress, relieves G.I. and urinary tract discomfort. Hartone can be prescribed as a daily health supplement to the patients who are at low energy and cholesterol diet. In ayurvedic terminology it corrects vata, pitta and cough conditions and a real 'tridosh nashak' medicine.

***Product Name* : DAB DAMA CAPSULES**

Composition : Each capsule contains :

Somlata (Ephedra vulgaris)	50 mg.
Haldi (Curcuma longa)	100 mg.
Sh. Suhaga (Pharmacopoeial)	50 mg.
Swaskuthar ras (Pharmacopoeial)	50 mg.
Swasdeman churna (Pharmacopoeial)	100 mg.
Ananbhairav ras (Pharmacopoeial)	50 mg.
Malladi vati (Pharmacopoeial)	50 mg.

Dosage 1 to 2 capsules two/three times a day.

How Supplied: Strip of 100 capsules (Blister pack)

Uses : Bronchitis, Bronchial asthma, Asthmatic bronchitis, Pulmonary emphysema, Other chronic obstructive pulmonary diseases.

Pharmacological Action : DABDAMA capsule is suitable for asthma caused by any of three aggravated humors that is Kapha, Vata, Pitta it has herbal bronchodilators and emetic agents along with tonics to revitalize the lungs. Somlata restores normal breathing and stops paroxysm. Haldi is anti-allergic, antiseptic and stimulant, it also removes the inflammation of epithelial cells, Shudha suhaga is diuretic, astringent and antacid, Swasdaman churn is bronchodilator, it releaves cough of varied etiology, it also removes the lumen blockage, it very useful in case of cardiac asthma, Anand Bhairav ras, Swaskuthar ras and Malladi vati ras are good expectorants and swas-kas har. Dabdama capsule also manages asthma due to psychological or emotional stress as it contains mild but effective nerve sedative and tranquillizers.

***Product Name* : NOBAB CAPSULES**

Composition : Each capsule contains :

Malkangani (Celastrus paniculata)	25 mg.
Kalonji (Nigella sativa)	25 mg.
Kapasjad (Gossypium Herbaceum)	25 mg.

Ulatkambal (abroma augusta)	25 mg.
Gajar beej (Daucus carota)	50 mg.
Muli Beej (Raphanus sativus)	25 mg.
Elwa (Aloe barbadensis)	100 mg.
Sh. Suhaga (Pharmacopoeial)	50 mg.
Trikatu (Pharmacopoeial)	25 mg.

Dosage 1-2 capsules 2-3 times a day.

How Supplied: Strip of 10 capsules (Blister pack)

Uses : Amenorrhoea, Dysmenorrhoea.

Pharmacological Action : NOBAB capsule is a balanced formula of strong emmenagogues, stimulants, anthelmintics, antiseptics and tonics. Malkangani is alternative, stimulant and nervine. Kapasjad, Ulatkambal and Muli beej are emmenagogues. Gajar Beej is antiseptic, blood purifier, aromatic, stimulant and carminative. Trikatu is a pharmacopoeial preparation it is stimulant, useful in dyspepsia, neuralgia and myalgia. Elwa is emmenagogue and anthelmintic. Kalonji is diuretic, stomachic, stimulant, anthelmintic and emmenagogue, it is also useful in the treatment of amenorrhoea and dysmenorrhoea.

Product Name : **JANDUNA CAPSULES**

Composition : Each capsule contains :

Ext. Bhangra (Eclipta alba)	30 mg.
Ext. Punarnava (Boerhaavia diffusa)	20 mg.
Ext. Kalmegh (Andrographis paniculata)	20 mg.
Ext. Chirayata (Swertia chirata)	10 mg.
Ext. Chitrakmool (Plumbago zeylanica)	10 mg.
Ext. Bay Bidang (Embelia ribes)	10 mg.
Ext. Sahajankichhal (moringa Pterygosperma)	10 mg.
Ext. Noshoth (Ipomoea turpethum)	10 mg.
Ext. Neemchhal (Azadirachta indica)	10 mg.
Ext. Gokharoo (Tibulus terrestris)	10 mg.
Ext. Daru Haldi (Berberis aristata)	10 mg.
Ext. Sarfonka (Tephrosia purpurea)	30 mg.
Ext. Dhania (Coriandrum sativum)	20 mg.
Ext. Jatamansi (nardostachys jatamansi)	10 mg.
Saunt (zingiber officinale)	20 mg.
Arogyawardhini (Pharmacopoeial)	100 mg.
Plihanthak loh (Pharmacopoeial)	50 mg.

Tamra bhasma (Pharmacopoeial)	10 mg.
Mandur bhasma (Pharmacopoeial)	50 mg.
Kvath (Pharmacopoeial	10 mg.
Palash beej (Pharmacopoeial)	10 mg.

Dosage 1 to 2 capsules three times a day.

How Supplied: Strip of 10 capsules (Blister pack)

Uses : Jaundice, Hepatitis.

Pharmacological Action : JANDUNA capsule detoxifies liver, purifies blood and regularises the flow of bile. It is a well balanced formula of various ayurvedic herbs and bhasmas. Arogyawardhini is a pharmacopoeial preparation useful in liver disorders and is also a laxative. Plihantak loh is useful in spleen and liver disorders. Tamra bhasma is useful in jaundice and hepatitis, as it controls the production of bile. Mandur bhasma is anthelmintic, blood purifier and tonic, Bhangra and Punarnava are good liver tonics. Punarnava also decreases albuminuria, it is bitter and stomachic. Kalmegh is stomachic tonic, alternative, anthelminitic, antipyretic and cholagogue. Chirayata is a bitter tonic febrigue and astringent. Chitrakmool promotes appetite, it is also digestive and stimulant. Saunth is aromatic, carminative sedative and stimulant. Dhania is aromatic, stimulant carminative and refregreant. Daru haldi is useful in liver enlargement. Gokharoo is a tonic, anthelmintic and inflammatory diuretic and astringent. Nishoth is diuretic, laxative and diaphoretic.

***Product Name :* HERBUSTONE**

Composition : Each 10g. contains :

Ext. Quercus infectoria	0.5 g.
Ext. Saussurea Lappa	0.5 g.
Ext. Acorous calmus	0.5 g.
Ext. Sida spinosa	0.5 g.
Kashishandhy Tail	2 g.
Shriparni Tail	2 g.
Ointment Base	4 g.

Dosage Take a small quantity of Herbustone on to the fingers, gently massage the breasts, one at a time.

How Supplied: Jar of 80 g.

Uses : Nourishes & smoothens wrinkled skin. Stimulates tissues, Provides tonning-Up. Improves voluminous and fullness of bosom due to increased vascularity, Removes dead cells and promotes healthy tissue.

Pharmacological Action : Ext. Quercus Infectoria-Contains tannic acid, an effective astringent, it firms tissues of organs, Ext. Sausseria lappa-its volatitle oil (contains saussurine, tannin etc, which are astringents), provides stiffness to the tissues. Ext. Acorous calmus-Its volatile oil contains X-pinene and camphene which are bitter astringents and cause sweating to the parts applied so that the blood flow in the capillaries increases.

ALARSIN PHARMACEUTICALS
Alarsin House, A/32, Road No. 3, M.I.D.C. Andheri (East),
Mumbai-400 093 ,Tel- 8367804, 8216836

***Product Name :* ALURETIC TABLETS**

Composition : Each tablets contains :

Daruharidra	20 mg.
Punarnava	20 mg.
Haritaki	20 mg.
Guduchi	20 mg.
Suntha	20 mg.
Ikshu mul	20 mg.
Jesthi Madha	20 mg.
Haldi	20 mg.
Anantamul	20 mg.
Saunf	20 mg.
Deodar	20 mg.
Bharangi mul	20 mg.
Gokshura	20 mg.
Kala-kadu	10 mg.
Patola	10 mg.
Nirgundi	10 mg.
Nim pan	10 mg.
Amala	10 mg.
Pashanbhed	10 mg.
Dusparsha	10 mg.
Eranda mul	10 mg.
Vidanga	10 mg.
Apamarga	10 mg.
Shaianjan	10 mg.
Kavach mul	10 mg.
Shankapushpi	10 mg.
Shilajit	30 mg.
Guggul	30 mg.

Dosage 1-2 tablets, 2-3 times a day.

How Supplied: 50 tabs., 75 tabs.

Uses : Increased Blood pressure, Congestive heart failure, Nephritis, Oedema, renal insufficiency.

Product Name : **ARJUN TABLETS**

Composition : Each tablets contains :

Punarnava Co.	37.5 mg.
Apamarg	12 mg.
Anantmul	12 mg.
Katuki Co.	30 mg.
Jatamansi Co.	64.5 mg.
Jyotishmati	48 mg.
Bilva	12 mg.
Arjun	12 mg.
Shilajit	50 mg.
Chandrika	96 mg.
Trifla Co.	36 mg.

Dosage 2-3 tablets, 1-3 times a day.

How Supplied: 50 tabs., 75 tabs.

Uses : Increased Blood pressure.

Product Name : **BANGSHIL TABLETS**

Composition : Each tablets contains :

Chandra prabha Co.	168 mg.
Shilajit	60 mg.
Bang bhasma	80 mg.
Guggul	40 mg.
Kasis	30 mg.
Vanslochan	12 mg.
Svarna makshik bhasma	30 mg.
Sandal Wood Oil	5 mg.

Dosage 2 tablets, 2-4 times a day for 2-3 weeks.

How Supplied: 50 tabs., 100 tabs.

Uses : Burning micturition, Genito urinary tract infections.

***Product Name :* DEKOFCYN TABLETS**

Composition : Each tablets contains :

Shatvari	30 mg.
Piper	30 mg.
Asan	30 mg.
Talispatra	30 mg.
Dagdi pashan Bhed	30 mg.
Galo	30 mg.
Amala	30 mg.
Sudha kachura	30 mg.
Praval Bhasma	30 mg.
Ardushi	15 mg.
Svarnamakshika bhasma	15 mg.
Abhrak bhasma	15 mg.
Ardusi ghan	15 mg.
Suvarna vaṣant malati	1.5 mg.
Haldi	105 mg.

Dosage ½-1 tablets, 3-4 times a day.

How Supplied: 50 tabs., 100 tabs.

Uses : Asthma, Bronchiectasis, Bronchitis, cold, Cough due to varied etiology, Primary complex, Rhinitis, Whooping cough.

***Product Name* : FORTEGE TABLETS**

Composition : Each tablets contains :

Kamboji	56 mg.
Kauncha beej	30 mg.
Sudha kachura	30 mg.
Samudra sosh beej	15 mg.
Vardhara Beej	15 mg.
Asan	15 mg.
Vardhara mool	15 mg.
Laving	7.5 mg.
Piper	7.5 mg.
Vacha	7.5 mg.
Mari	7.5 mg.
Sunth	7.5 mg.
Chini kabab	7.5 mg.

Akalakara	7.5 mg.
Sukhad ver	7.5 mg.
Jaifal	4.5 mg.
javantri	3 mg.
Jeevanti	56.5 mg.

Dosage 1-2 tablets, 2-3 times a day.

How Supplied: 50 tabs., 100 tabs.

Uses : Benign prostatic enlargement, Frigidity (in females), Nocturnal emissions, Prostatism.

***Product Name* : G-32 TABLETS**

Composition : Each tablets contains :

Bakul	80 mg.
Chok	75 mg.
Katha	40 mg.
Lavang	20 mg.
Chikani sopari	20 mg.
Fatakadi	20 mg.
Mayafal	20 mg.
Elaichi	10 mg.
Sonageru	10 mg.
Jiru	10 mg.
Majith	10 mg.
Pashan bhed	10 mg.
Vavding	10 mg.
Pipada Lakh	10 mg.
Samundrafen	10 mg.
Vajradanti	10 mg.
Taj	5 mg.
Mari	5 mg.
Sajikhar	5 mg.
Kulinjan	5 mg.
Piper	5 mg.
Kapur	5 mg.
Kuth	5 mg.

Dosage : 1-2 tablets, to be crushed and massaged over gums, teeth and on the affected parts of the mouth with finger tip and is to be kept for 5 min. and rinsed with fresh water. May be repeated 2-3 times a day.

How Supplied: 50 tabs., 100 tabs.

Uses : Gingivitis, gums, bleeding/swollen/painful/spongy, Leukoplakia, Oran trauma, Pharyngitis. Post oral surgery, Stomatitis, Sub mucous fibrosis, Painful teeth.

Product Name : **SILEDIN TABLETS**

Composition : Each tablets contains :

Brahmi	35 mg.
Shankhpushpi	70 mg.
Jeevanti	17.5 mg.
Chandrika	210 mg.
Kamboji	17.5 mg.
Vacha	18 mg.
Bhirngaraj	52 mg.

Dosage 1-2 tablets, 2-3 times a day.

How Supplied: 50 tabs., 75 tabs.

Uses : Anxiety, Depression, Neurosis, Disturbed sleep, Tension.

Product Name : **MYRON TABLETS**

Composition : Each tablet contains :

Hira Bol	75 mg.
Guggul	30 mg.
Bang bhasma	15 mg.
Kasis	30 mg.
Shilajit	15 mg.
Dhavdi-Flower	15 mg.
Lodhar	15 mg.
Ardusi Leaves	7.5 mg.
Ardsi ghan	7.5 mg.
Raswanti	7.5 mg.
Abhrak bhasma	7.5 mg.

Dosage 2 tablets, 3 times a day.

How Supplied: 50 tabs., 100 tabs.

Uses : Cervical erosions, Girdle pains, Haematinics, Leucorrhoea, Obesity.

***Product Name* : R. COMPOUND TABLETS**

Composition : Each tablets contains :

Suvarnayukta Mahayograj guggul with	
Maharasnadi quath	265 mg.
Haldi	135 mg.

Dosage 2 tablets, 3 times a day.

How Supplied: 50 tabs., 100 tabs.

Uses : Backache, Contusions, Dental pulpitis, Haemarthrosis, Inflammatory conditions, neuromuscular skeletomuscular, Rheumatic diseases, Sprains.

Product Name : **SOOKTYN TABLETS**

Composition : Each tablets contains :

Sookti bhasma	112.5 mg.
Kapur kachli	80 mg.
Jatamansi	40 mg.
Ganthoda	30 mg.
Khurasani ajmo	30 mg.
Kel pan raakh	30 mg.
Vacha	10 mg.
Dhatura Leaves	5 mg.

Dosage : 2 tablets, 3-4 times a day between or after meals.

How Supplied : 50 tabs., 100 tabs.

Uses : Allergy, Loss of Appetite, Dyspepsia (in children), Flatulence (in children), Gastritis, Gripe symptoms (in children), Hard stools (in children).

***Product Name* : DEKOFCYN COUGH SYRUP**

Composition : Each 5 ml. contains :

Aq. Ext. of :	
Talispatra	200 mg.
Kantakari	100 mg.
Satavari	200 mg.
Yastimadhu	100 mg.
Pippali	200 mg.

Tulsi	100 mg.
Ashwagandha	200 mg.
Lavanga	5 mg.
Gurach	200 mg.
Choti elachi	5 mg.
Amla	200 mg.
Gulbanafsa	25 mg.
Kachura	200 mg.
Sunthi	50 mg.
Arusha ghan	100 mg.
Kapur	1 mg.
Haldi	100 mg.
Peperminta ka Phool	1 mg.

Dosage : Adults : 1-2 teaspoonful, 3 times a day.
Children : ½-1 teaspoonful, 3 times a day.

How Supplied: 100 ml.

Uses : Asthma, Bronchiectasis, Bronchitis, Cough due to varied etiology, Laryngitis, Pharyngitis, Sinusitis, Topical eosinophilia, Pulmonary tuberculosis, Upper respiratory tract infections.

AXAR PHARMACEUTICALS
22, Sahjanand Industrial Estate, Muzmuvda, Atladra Road, Vadodara-390 020, Tel - 325711, Fax - (265) 331011

Product Name : **APHORAX CAPSULES**

Composition :

Makardhvaja	15 mg.
Rasa sindhur	15 mg.
Abhraka bhasma	30 mg.
Praval bhasma	30 mg.
Loha bhasma	30 mg.
Bang bhasma	30 mg.
Shudh shilajit	30 mg.
Amruta	30 mg.
Kavacha bija	90 mg.
Yasthimadhu	30 mg.
Shatavari	30 mg.
Ashtavarga	30 mg.
Trifala	60 mg.
Musali sveta	20 mg.

***Product Name :* COLIMAN DROPS**

Composition :

Dalchini	30 mg.
Vacha	80 mg.
Elachi	30 mg.
Pudina	80 mg.
Hingu	40 mg.
Trikatu	80 mg.
Indrajav	80 mg.
Putikaranj	30 mg.
Shatpushpa	40 mg.
Black salt	40 mg.
Yavni	40 mg.
Haritaki	80 mg.
Sindhav salt	40 mg.
Kakmachi	80 mg.
Khaskhas beej	80 mg.

***Product Name :* DY FORTE CAPSULES**

Composition :

Aloes	60 mg.
Abroma augusta	120 mg.
Conesi seeds	120 mg.
Zingiber officinal	75 mg.
Raddish seeds	60 mg.
Carrot seeds	60 mg.

***Product Name :* KOFY SYRUP**

Composition :

Yasthimadhu	15 mg.
Pudina	25 mg.
Salt peppermint	5 mg.
Navsadar	150 mg.
Saubhagya	30 mg.
Yavakshar	15 mg.
Tulsi	20 mg.
Trikatu	20 mg.
Nilgiri	0.02 mg.
Vasa	1 ml.

***Product Name* : MEDIATRIC CAPSULES**

Composition :

Ginseng	150 mg.
Loha bhasma	10 mg.
Shilajit	50 mg.
Ashwagandha	160 mg.
Kaucha	50 mg.
Abhrak bhasma	10 mg.

***Product Name* : SHALTON DROPS**

Composition :

Ashwagandha	120 mg.
Bhringraj	50 mg.
Gakhru	80 mg.
Shatavari	80 mg.
Gulab phool	40 mg.
Jaiphal	30 mg.
Vardharao	80 mg.
Akalkaro	30 mg.
Kaucha beej	80 mg.
Khapat	50 mg.
Chaturjat	30 mg.
Trifala	40 mg.
Trikatu	30 mg.
Ghavandi phool	50 mg.
Rasna	50 mg.
Majith	50 mg.

***Product Name* : VOXAR SYRUP**

Composition :

Sarpankho	50 mg.
Vavding	30 mg.
Galdana	80 mg.
Kadiyatu	10 mg.
Punarnava	80 mg.
Kasni	100 mg.
Kakmachi	100 mg.
Lindipeper	50 mg.
Arujun chaal	100 mg.
Ativish	20 mg.

***Product Name* : SHALTON SYRUP**

***Composition* :** Each 5 ml. contains :

Ashwagandha	120 mg.
Rohitaka	100 mg.
Shatavari	120 mg.
Bhringraj	60 mg.
Astavarg	40 mg.
Gulab phool	50 mg.
Jaiphal	40 mg.
Gakhru	60 mg.
Vardharo	80 mg.
Trifala	40 mg.
Dashmool	40 mg.
Varahikand	40 mg.
Trikatu	30 mg.
Akalkaro	30 mg.
Chaturjat	40 mg.
Lohasav	2 ml.

***Product Name* : VOXAR DROPS**

***Composition* :**

Galo	10 mg.
Ativish	10 mg.
Bhrungraj	40 mg.
Kadiyatu	10 mg.
Lindipeper	40 mg.
Kasni	50 mg.
Ghavandi phool	50 mg.
Dhana	30 mg.
Sarpankho	50 mg.
Kakmachi	50 mg.
Punarnava	40 mg.
Kasundri beej	50 mg.
Gulab phool	50 mg.
Arjun chhal	30 mg.
Chotitakchhal	30 mg.
Khapat	30 mg.
Sunth	30 mg.
Kadachhal	30 mg.
Nasodar	30 mg.
Vavding	30 mg.
Tulsipan	30 mg.

Kalipath	30 mg.
Gokhru	50 mg.
Mendipan	30 mg.

***Product Name* : ZYMAN LIQUID**

***Composition* :**

Draksha	140 mg.
Bhrungraj	140 mg.
Mari	50 mg.
Ashwagandha	160 mg.
Trifala	40 mg.
Sunth	30 mg.
Lindipeper	40 mg.
Lohasav	1.2 ml.
Kumari asav	1.2 ml.

AYULABS PVT. LTD.
Gondal Road, Vavdi, Rajkot-360 004
Tel - 388408, 360628, Fax - (0281) 388461

***Product Name* : AYUPLUS CAPSULES**

***Composition* :**

Extract Ashwagandha, Extract Shemal mushli, Extract Asthavarg, Bang Bhasma, Praval pisti, Makardwaj.

***Product Name* : BACTEFAR CAPSULES**

***Composition* :**

Pulp of Bilwa, Indrajav, Mochras, Kutajaghan, Sweet parpati, Hinga, Extract Isabgul seed, Panchamrut parpati, Ras parpati.

***Product Name* : CHEERUP SYRUP**

***Composition* :**

Ashwagandha, Shatavari, Gokshuru, Vidarikanda, Kaucha, Kulanjan, Triphala, Yashtimadhu, Chaturjat, Jatiphala, Rasna, Shemal mushli, Manjishtha, Suddha shilajit.

Product Name : **DEFET-5 CAPSULES**

Composition :

Tryushanadya loha, Medohar guggul, Muli seed, Extract Triphala, Suddha shilajit, Arogyavardhani ras, Trimurti ras.

Product Name : **FIZZLE CAPSULES**

Composition :

Jethimadh, Somlatachurna, Suddha phatakadi, Suddha tankankhar, Trikatu, Extract Tulsi, Extract Vasaka, Extract Antamul.

Product Name : **LIMIT CAPSULES**

Composition :

Extract Karela, Extract Mamejava, Extract Mudhunasini, Pulp of Jambuseed, Tribang bhasma, Jaiphal, Trikatu, Ashwagandha, Methi, Suddha Shilajit.

Product Name : **NEOGARD DROPS**

Composition :

Trijat, Shatpushpa, Kalmegh, Sauvarchal, Putikaranja, Vaj hinga, Aekhard, Devadali, Bhrami, Dashmool, Saindhav salt, Khurassani ajvanyan, Nimbak salt, Atisisha.

Product Name : **NUTRICH CAPSULES**

Composition :

Bhrungraj Godanti bhasma, Arogyavardhini ras, Dhatriloha, Amlaki, Brahmi, Galo satva, Shemal, Narshinh churna, Abhrak bhasma.

Product Name : **PENWEL CAPSULES**

Composition :

Sallaki ghan, Nirgundi ghan, Maharasnadi ghan, Ashwagandha ghan, Lakshmivilash ras, Mahayogaraj guggul, Samir pannag ras.

Product Name : **PEPCER CAPSULES**

Composition :

Extract Bhrungraj, Extract Patol, Extract Yastimadhu, Extract Shatavari, Extract Amlaki, Extract Haritaki, Extract Ashwagandha, Babbul niryas, Sankha bhasma, Kumdudha ras, Paniyabhaktvati, Sita.

BAN LABS PVT. LTD.

Dr. Vikram Sarabhai Nagar, Gondal Raod (South) Rajkot-360 004
Tel-366411, 366412, 366413, 366414, Fax-(0281) 388477

***Product Name :* CALCUROSIN SYRUP**

Composition :Each 10 ml. Calcurosin Syrup contains:

Nimbak Sat	80 mg.
Navsagar	60 mg.
Saubhagya (Tankan)	60 mg.
Sarjikashar	40 mg.
Sauvarchal (Black Salt)	30 mg.
Moolikshar	20 mg.
Yavakshar	15 mg.
Hingu (Ferula Foetida)	10 mg.
Piperminta Sat	04 mg.

Dosage :Adults:- 2 to 3 Teaspoonfuls three times a day Children:-1 teaspoonful three times a day.

How Supplied : In pack of 100 ml. and 200 ml.

Uses :Disolves and expels calculi, Diuretic Disintegrates calcui into fine particles and expels. Burining micturition Urinary tract. infection

Pharmacological Action :Not be given during pregancy.

***Product Name:* CALCUROSIN CAPSULE**

Composition : Each Calcurosin capsule contain:

Chandra Prabha	140 mg.
Eladi Churma	100 mg.
Trivikram Ras	40 mg.
Saubhagya (Tankan)	40 mg.
Hajrool Yahood Bhasma	80 mg.

Dosage : Adults : 1 to 2 capsules three times a day Children: 1 capsule three times a day: Or as directed by Physician.

How Supplied : Box of 10 blister strips of 10 capsules each

Uses : Dissolves and expels calculi, Diuretic Disintegrates calculi, Diuretic Disintegrates clacui into fine particles and expels. Burning micturition, Urinary tract infection.

Pharmacolgical Action : Not be given during Pregnancy.

Product Name : **COLICARMIN DROPS**

Composition : Each 1 ml. Colicarmin drops contains:

Acorus calamus (vach) Ext.	1 mg.
Hyoscyamus Niger (Khurasani Ajvayan) Ext.	0.75 mg.
Aconitum Heterophyllym (Ativish) Ext.	0.50 mg.
Peucedanum graveolens (Shatpushpa)	4 mg.
Elettaria Cardamomum (Elayachi)	3 mg.
Caesalpinia Crista (Putikarnja)	2 mg.
Black Salt (Sauvarchal)	2 mg.
Ferula Foetida (Hingu)	1 mg.
Sindhav Salt	1 mg.
Nimbak Sat	1 mg.

Dosage :Drops:- To be taken as requred for up to six times a day

Neonatal (3 to 6 months) 2 to 4 drops

Infants :(6 months to 1 year) 3 to 5 drops Children:- 1 to 3 years 4 to 6 drops 5 drops 10 drops or as directed by Physician.

How Supplied : In carton pack of 30 ml.

Uses : Diarrhoea Dysentery, Gripin pain, Digestives, Carminative, Mild Sedatives, Anti spasmodics, Convulsions, Reduces Abdominal disterntion. Other intestinal disorders and discomfort in the stomach

Product Name : **LIVEX TABLET**

Composition : Each Livex Tablet contain:

Terminalia arjuna (Arjuna bark) Ext.	40 mg.
Rhamnus wightii (Rohitak) Ext.	20 mg.
Picrorhiza kurroa (Katuki) Ext.	20 mg.
Boerhaavia diffusa (Punarnava) Ext	15 mg.
Andrographis paniculata (Kalmegh) Ext.	15 mg.
Tephrosia purpurea (Plihari) Ext.	5 mg.
Cichorium intybus (Kasni)	20 mg.
Arogya Vardhini	40 mg.
Mandoor Bhasma	30 mg.
Navayas Loha	15 mg.

Dosage :Adults: -2 to 3 tablets three times a day

Children.:1 tablet three to four times a day Or as directed by Physician.

How Supplied : Box of 10 blister strips of 10 tablets each. and in 1000's pack.

Uses : As a health supplement, Regenerate liver cells, Infective hepatitis, Protect from chemical toxins, Liver protective in chronic alcohol consumers, Pre and post surgical cases.

***Product Name :* LIVEX SYRUP**

Composition : Each 10 ml. Livex Syrup contain :

Andrographis paniculata (Kalmegh) Ext.	20 mg.
Tephrosia purpurea (Plhari) Ext.	10 mg.
Aconitum heterophyllym (Ativish) Ext.	7.5 mg.
Solanum nigrum (Kakmachi) Ext.	5 mg.
Embelia ribes (Vidanga)	50 mg.
Cassia occidentalis (Kasari)	50 mg.
Cichorium intybus (Kasni)	30 mg.
Tamrix gallica (Prans-jhau)	30 mg.
Piper longum (Pippali)	20 mg.

Dosage : Adults:- 1 to 2 teaspoonfuls 3 to 4 times a day. Children:- teaspoonful 3 times a day. Or as directed by Physician.

How Supplied: In pack of 100 ml. and 200 ml.

Uses: As a health supplement, Regenerate liver cells, Infective hepatitis, Protect from chemical toxins, Liver protective in chronic alcohol consumers, pro and post surgical cases

***Product Name :* LIVEX CAPSULE**

Composition : Each Livex Capsule contain :

Boerhaavia diffusa (punarnava) Ext.	80 mg.
Tephrosia purpurea (Plihari) Ext.	40 mg.
Eclipta alba (Bhrungraj) Ext.	40 mg.
Arogya Vardhini	110 mg.
Yakrut plihari loha	50 mg.
Loha Bhasma	80 mg.

Dosage : Adults : 1 capsule three times a day. Or as directed by Physician.

How Supplied: Box of 10 blister of 10 capsules each.

Uses:As a health supplement, Regenerate liver cells, infective hepatitis. Protect from chemical toxins. Liver protective in chronic alcohol consumers. Pre and post surgical cases

***Product Name* : LUCOGYL CAPSULE**

Composition : Each lucogyl capsule contain:

Sarca indica (Ashoka) Ext.	30 mg.
Symlocos recemosa (Lodhra) Ext.	30 mg.
Commiphora myrrha (Hirabol)	40 mg.
Pushyanug Churma	70 mg.
Prodaranatak Loha	60 mg.
Gokshuradi Guggul	30 mg.
Kukkutand watak Bhasma	80 mg.
Loha bhasma	30 mg.
Praval Bhasma	20 mg.
Shilajeet	10 mg.

Dosage : 1 capsules three times a day with milk. Or as directed by Physician.

How Supplied: Box of 10 blister strips of 10 capsules each.

Uses: Back ache and weakness, Non-specific leucorrhoea, Functional uterine bleeding Menstrual irregularities.

***Product Name* : R. PAIRYN TABLET**

Composition : Each tablet contains :

Withania somifera (Ashwagandha)	40 mg.
Mahayograj Guggul	80 mg.
Trayo dashanga Guggul	40 mg.
Maharasnadi Ghan	30 mg.
Shankha Bhasma	30 mg.

Dosage : 2 tablets four times a day. Preferable with milk. Or as directed by Physician.

How Supplied: Box of 10 blister strips of 10 capsules each and in 1000's pack.

Uses: Rheumatic arthritis, Infective polyarthritis, Osteoarthritis, Arthralgia, Lumber spondylosis Gout

Pharmacological Action : It not be used during pregnacy.

***Product Name* : SESA OIL**

Composition : Each bottle of Sesa Oil contains:

Eclipta alba (Keshraj)	3.00%
Trifala	3.00%
Jsminum officinale (Chetika)	2.00%
Citrullus colcynthis (Gavakshi)	1.00%
Indigofera tinctoria (Kalkeshi)	1.00%
Centella asiatica (Saraswati)	1.00%
Abrus precatorius (Krishnala)	0.50%
Berberis aristata (Rasgarbh)	0.50%
Aconsus calamus (Jatila)	0.50%
Lawsomia alba (Henna)	0.50%
Glyeyrrhiza glabra (Mulethi)	0.50%
Pongamia pinnata (Chirbilvak)	0.50%
Azadirachta indica (Paribhadra)	0.50%
Saussurea lappa (Utpal)	0.50%
Nardostachys jatamansi (Tapasvini)	0.50%
Elettaria cardamomum (Sukshma)	0.50%
Ferriper oxidumrubrum (Sinhan)	4.00%
Datura metel (Mahamohi)	2.00%
Dugdha (Milk)	10.00%
Sugandhit dravya	1.50%
Sesamum indicum (Til) Oil	25.00%
Nilibhurngadi Tail	8.00%
Triticum aestivum (Godhuma) Tail	1.00%
Citrus medica (Nimbak) Tail	1.00%
Cocos nucifera (Sadafal)	
Tail Q.S. to	100.00%

Application : Gentle massage on scalp and hair External use only.

How Supplied: In carton pack of 100 ml.

Uses: For nourishment of hair root and scalpImproves blood circulation to hair follicle Stimulates growth of thicker. Healthier and longer hairs checks loss of hair and greying of hair

***Product Name* : VITON "99" SYRUP**

Composition : Each 10 ml. Viton "99" Syrup contains:

Tribulus terrestris (Gokshuru) Ext.	10 mg.
Mucuna pruriens (kavach seed) Ext.	10 mg.

Argyreia speciosa (Bidhara) Ext.	10 mg.
Withania somnifera (Ashwagandha)	60 mg.
Asparagus racemousis (Shatavary)	50 mg.
Pueraria tuberosa (Vidarikanda)	50 mg.
Anacyclus pyrethrum (Akarkara)	20 mg.
Myristica fragrans (Jatifal)	20 mg.
Pluchea lanceolata (Rasna)	20 mg.
Rubia coridfolia (Majishtha)	20 mg.
Chaturjat	20 mg.
Trifala	20 mg.
Trikatu	20 mg.
Shalajeet (Purified)	15 mg.

Dosage : For Adults :- 2 teaspoonfuls 3 times a day. Children :- 1 teaspoonful 3 times a day. Preferably with milk : For 8 to 12 weeks Or as directed by Physician.

How Supplied:In carton pack of 200 ml.

Uses: Post-Natal, Post-Sugery, Malnutrition. Anaemia. Sexual weakness. Feeble circulation, Stimulates appetite, Enchances protein metabolism, Increases weight

BDH INDUSTRIES LTD.
Nair Baug. Akurli Road, kandivli (E), Mumbai - 400101
Tel - 8871370/8870834, Fax - (22) 887085б

Product Name : **FTX TABLETS**

Composition : Each film-coated tablet contains

Commiphora mukul (Guggul)	1 g.
Cyperus rotundus (Musta)	1 g.

Dosage :1 to 2 tablets 3 times a day.

How Supplied: 30 tablets in a glass bottle

Uses : FTX reduces excess fat and thus help an individual to look slim and youthful.

Pharmacological Action : Guggul is an oleoresin secreted by Commiphora mukul. The active constituent of guggul is guggulipid. Guggulipid interferes with cholesterol biosynthesis. Musta is a standardised extract of bulbous roots of Cyperus rotundus. It normalises the equilibrium of free fatty acids & triglycerides. The combination-FTX inhibits the deposition of adipocytes. FTX regulates the imbalance of hormones. FTX is not recommended for children since the relative information and in gastrointestinal disturbances such as diarrhoea and dysentery.

CADILA HEALTHCARE LTD. (Agrovet Division)
201/2/3, 'Saffron', Ambawadi, Ahmedabad - 380006
Tel -6564371-76, 446639, 446649, Fax - (079) 6561659

***Product Name* : FLURRY LIQUID**

Composition :

Ext. of Melia azadirachta (S. Nimba)	17.5%
Ext. of Lawsonia inermis (S.Medika)	17.5%
Ext. of Aloe vera	3%
Ext. of Cocos nucifera	6%

***Product Name* : LIVERUP LIQUID**

Composition :

Phyllanthus niruri	30%
Andrographis paniculata	20%
Acacia catechu	20%
Asparagus recemosus	5%
Tinospora cardifolia	15%

CHARAK PHARMACEUTICALS (INDIA) LTD.
Shed No. 4, G.I.D.C. Industrial Estate
Umbergaon - 396171 (Gujarat), Tel - 4926352

***Product Name* : GULKAND**

Composition : Each 100 g. contains :

Gulkand	99.750 g.
Godanti (Shuddha)	0.200 g.
Praval (pishti)	0.020 g.
Elaichi	0.020 g.
Silver leaves	0.010 g.

Dosage : One tablespoonful every morning and evening.

Uses:Charak gulkand act as cooling agent. Helps relieve burning sensation in the extremities of the eyes. and the whole body in general. Fights overall lethargy alleviates constipation and biliousness acta as blood purifier and a coolant to the brain excellent for bleeding piles.

***Product Name* : Neo Silver Coated**

Composition : Each tablet contains :

Kavach beej shuddha	56.00 mg.
Kuchla Shuddha	20.00 mg.
Hingul shuddha	8.00 mg.
Praval pishti	8.00 mg.
Shilajit shuddha	8.00 mg.
Bang bhasma	2.00 mg.
Loh bhasma	2.00 mg.
Mass extracts derived from	
Shatavari	35.00 mg.
Jethikmadh	8.00 mg.
Bhavana	
Piaz	90.00 mg.
Bhringaraj	16.00 mg.

Dosage : Adults : 2 tablets three times a day for six to eight weeks.
Children : 1 tablet three times a day for four to six weeks.

CONCEPT PHARMACEUTICALS LTD.

167, C.S.T. Road, Santacruz (East), Mumbai - 400098
Tel - 6184378, 6184379, 6184380, Fax - (22) 6114501

***Product Name* : AJAR CAPSULE**

Composition :

Ashwagandha (Withania somnifera)	250 mg.
Arjuna (Teminalia arjuna)	250 mg.
Amalaki (Phyllanthus emblica)	250 mg.
Guduchi (Tinospora cordifolia)	250 mg.
Shatavari (Asparagus racemosus)	500 mg.
Dried powder Shaival- (Spirulina Platensis)	250 mg.

Dosage : 1 capusle once or twice day.

How Supplied: 3x10 capsules

Uses:Ajar capsule in indicated for the stress related conditions that disrupt the physiological neuroendocrino-immuno axis. Ajar is having beneficial effect in patients having high blood pressure. myocardial infarction etc. Ajar is indicated in cholesterlimia. Ajar has antianginal effect. Ajar protects the gastro duodenal mucosa against injurious effects of alcohol, NSAIDS etc.

***Product Name* : Clarex Cream**

Composition :

Yashtimadhu (Glyeyrhiza glabra)	1.60%
Manjishtha (Rubia cordifolia)	1.38%
Arjuna (Terminalia arjuna)	0.36%
Haridra (Curcuma longa)	0.20%
Lodhra (Symplcos recemosus)	0.66%
Powder of Shuddha (Purified zinc)	3.00%
Suitable cream base	q.s.

Application :Apply Clarex on the face after cleaning with mild soap and lukewarm water. It should be applied thickly on the affected area and rubbed gently on the lesion. Thin film of the cream is to be applied on the face for improving complexion

How Supplied: 25 gm collapsible tube in carton.

Uses : It reduces the sebum production Anti inflammatory herbs control the inflammation. Some herbs haiving antibacterial activity thereby quick healing of wounds. No future scar formation.

***Product Name* : KASKOL COUGH SYRUP**

Composition : Each 5 ml. kaskol contains:

Vasa (Adhatoda vasica)	355.4 mg.
Yashitimadhu (Glycyrrhiza glabra)	177.7 mg.
Gojivha (Onosma bractenum)	88.8 mg.
Kantakari (Solanum xanthocarpum)	88.8 mg.
Banafsa (Viola odorata)	44.4 mg.
Pippali (Piper longum)	44.4 mg.
Vacha (Acorus calamus)	44.4 mg.
Shunthi (Zingiber officinale)	44.4 mg.
Bibhitaka (Terminalia belerica)	44.4 mg.
Sariva (Hemidesmus indicus)	22.3 mg.
Madhu (Honey) based syrup	Q.S.

Dosage : Below 2 years up to 2.5 ml. 2 to 3 times day. 2-6 years 2.5 ml-5.0 ml 2 to 3 times day. 6-12 years 5.0 ml - 7.5 ml 2 to 3 times day. Adults 7.5 ml- 10 ml 2 to 3 times day.

How Supplied: 100 ml. bottle

Uses:Upper respiratory tract infections, with cough as predoninant symptom i.e. simple cough remedy in all age group. As an adjunct to broncholdilator therapy in the management of asthma.

CREATION

Mfgrs. & Processor of : Sun Brand Ayurvedic Medicine Narulla CHS Ltd, 1st Floor, Block No. 9, Station Road, Road No. 21, Chembur, Mumbai -400 071, Tel - 5511118, 5552498

Product Name : Isabgol

Composition :

Psyllium Husk	98.03%
Sonamukhi Powder	1.96%

Dosage : 5 to 10 gms of Isabgol can be freely taken accoriding to need with a glass of water. syrup. milk, fruit juice or salted curd or lassi.

How Supplied: 100 g. (3.5 ozs)

Uses: Safe remedy for Constipation, Acidity and Cough.

DABUR INDIA LIMITED

8/3, Asaf Ali Road. New Delhi - 110002,
Tel - 3271001. 3276739

Product Name : **ABLARI SOLUTION**

Composition :Aloes, Postassium Bromide, Hyoscyamus, from Saraca indica, Valeriana Wallichii and Alcohol.

Product Name : **CHYAWANPRASH AVALEHA (SPECIAL)**

Composition : Each 100 g contains :

Dashmool	3.980g
Varahikand	0.796g
Bala	0.398g
Ashwagandha	0.796g
Mudagaparni	0.398g
Shatavari	0.796g
Mashparni	0.398g
Vidarujabd	1.195g
Karkatshringi	0.398g
Amal green	90g
Bhumiamlaki	0.398g
Grit	2.08g

Jivanti	0.398g
Til tail	1.20g
Kushta	0.398g
Sharkara	62.4g
Agarkashta	0.398g
Banslochan	0.8g
Haritaki	0.398g
Abhrak bhasma	0.188g
Guruchi	0.398g
Muktasukti pishti	0.063g
Katchur	0.398g
Akarkara	0.126g
Mustak	0.398g
Pippali	1.12g
Punarnava	0.398g
Negkesar	0.116g
Neelkamal	0.398g
Dalchini	0.116g
Vasak	0.398g
Tejpatra	0.116g
Kakanasa	0.398g
Lavang	0.128g
Yastimadhu	0.398g
Elaichi	0.588g
Chandansaar	0.0092g
Kesar	0.021g
Silver foil	q.s.

Dosage : 5 to 10g or half to one teaspoonful according to age.

How Supplied: 250 g. 500g. 100g.

Uses:Protecting everyday infections, particularly coughs and colds, reducing stress related symptoms and adding to your general well being. It is specially good for growing children.

***Product Name* : DABUR BALM**

Composition :

Menthol	5.20% w/w
Camphor	9% w/w
Methyl salicylate	8.30% w/w
Ajowan Oil	1.25% w/w
Thymol	1.25%

Product Name : DABUR OINTMENT

Composition :

Menthol	3.5 g.
Camphor	5.5 g.
Thymol	0.1 g.
Turpentine oil	1.5 ml.
Eucalyptus oil	1.5 ml.
Nutmeg oil.	0.5 ml.
Paraffin to	100 g.

Product Name **: DABUR-DANT LIQUID**

Compostion :

Phenol	27.9% v/v
Clove oil	18.6% v/v
Camphor	14% w/v
Oil menthol	18.6% v/v
Ajowan Oil	2.3% v/v

Product Name **:DAR-KAN LIQUID**

Composition :

Tincture opium	20% v/v
Tincture aconite	25% v/v
Glycerine	100% v/v
Alcohor	28.6% v/v

Product Name **: NATURE CARE POWDER**

Composition :

Isabgol Husk powder	49%
Amal powder	5%
Sarkara	46%

Dosage : 1 to 3 teaspoon at bedtime for adults and children above 12 years.

How Supplied: 100 g., 200 g., 375 g. 100 g. (Refil)

Uses: Nature care soothes and lubricates the intestinal system. It adds bulk to the final waste product. Regularising motions without cramps or pain.

Product Name : PUDIN HARA CAPSULES

Composition ; Each pearl contains :

Pudin ka satva	180 mg.

Approved colour used.

Dosage : 1-2 Pudin hara pearls as and when required. Swallow them whole with a glass of water.

Product Name : RESTORA LIQUID

Composition : Each 100 ml contains :

Draksha	16.077 g
Elaichi small	0.161 g
Honey	16.077 g
Lavanga	0.161 g
Sugar	16.077 g
Kalamarich	0.161 g
Dhatakipushpa	2.572 g
Tejpatra	0.161 g
Kankol	0.161 g
Nagkesar	0.161 g
Jaiphal	0.161 g
Pippali	0.161 g
Dalchini	0.161 g
Chitrakmool	0.161 g
Chabya	0.161 g
Renuka	0.161 g
Pippalimool	0.161 g
Alcohol content	7-11% v/v

Dosage : Two three tablespoonfull (30-40 ml). twice a day or as required

How Supplied: 50 ml.

Uses: Restora tonic against cough and cold. A stimulant for appetite. An aid to restiful sleep. And a unique source of general well being. Gradually, gently, Restora helps build a natural resistance to most common ailments.

Product Name : RHEUMATIL OIL

Composition :

Mahanarayan Tail	70%
Gandhapuro Tail	10%
Pudina Satva	3%

Neelgiri Tail	2%
Lavanga Tai	2%
Guggulu Sat	2%
Shunti Satva	1%
Oil base	q.s.

Application : Apply oil on affected area. Massage gently till absorbed. For faster results, prior fomentation is recommended. Dip a towel in hot water, squeeze it dry and press against the affected area to open up the pores which will then facilitate better absorpiton.

How Supplied: 60 ml

Uses: Effective for pain associated with rheumatism, arthritis, fibrositis, lumbago, sciatica, cervical and ankylosing spondylitis. stiff necks, frozen shoulders. backaches. muscular sprain and spasms.

Product Name : **RHEUMATIL GEL**

Composition :

Mahanarayan Tail
Gandhapuro Tail
Pudina satva
Neelgiri Tail
Lavanga Tail
Lavanga Tail
Guggulu Satva
Shunti Satva

Product Name : **SARVAGUN LINIMENT**

Composition :

Soft Soap	4.716% w/w
Ammonium Chloride	8.182% w/w
Camphor	5.454% w/w
Turpentine Oil	10.511% w/w
Ammonia soln.	12.273% w/w
Purified water	100% w/w

DECCAN AYURVEDASHRAM PHARMACY LTD

17-1-204-8, Saidabad, Hyderabad - 500059
Tel - 4530414, 4530415, Fax - (040)4532739

***Product Name* : RUMADAP TABLETS, OIL AND GOLD**

Composition : Rumadap Tablets

Mahayograj guggul	200 mg.
Maharasnadi quath	50 mg.
Ashwagandha	40 mg.

Shilajit, Suvarnamakshik Bhasma Manjista, Gambhari, Gokshura, Agnimantha, Patala, Eranda, Aamlavetas, Bala, Parasika

Rumadap with Gold

Mahayograj guggul	200 mg.
Maharasnadi quath	50 mg.
Aswagandha	40 mg.
Shilajit, Suvarnamakshik Bhasma	5 mg.

Manjista. gambhari, Gokshura. Agnimantha, Patala, Eranda, Aamlavetas, Bala, Parasika Rumadap with Gold Rumadap Oil Mahanarayan, gandhapurak, Vatanashak'tailas. Nilgiri tail, Karpoor.

Dosage : Rumadap Tablets-100 and 500 tablets pack. Rumadap with Gold -10 tablets/carton and 100 tablets packing. Rumadap Oil -30 ml., 100 ml., 500 ml. packing

Uses:Osteo-Arthritis, Rheumatoid Arthritis. Spondylitis, Sciatica, frozen shoulder, low backache, myalgias and other sports injuries.

***Product Name* : SHILA FORTE CAPSULES**

Composition : Suvana Bhasma 4 mg, Vanga, Abhraka Bhasma. Ambergis, Makaradwaj. Ashwagandha, Gokshura, Safed musli, Salam Mishri, samal ki musli, Salam punja, Kesar,Jaiphal, Japatri, Akkalakar, Ela, Maricha, Lavang, Karpoor, Ruma Mastagi

Dosage : 1-2 capsules twice a day preferable with milk or directed by the Physician.

How Supplied: In pack of 8 capsules per carton and 30 capsules in container packing.

Uses: Functional impotency, Loss of Libido, Oligo spermia and sexual weakness

***Product Name* : Utrodap Syrup & Tablets**

Composition : Patanga, Ashoka, Lodhra, Ananthamul, Bilva. Khadira, Manjista, Laksha, Shatavari. Ashwagandha, Jatamansi, Bhringaraj. Daruharidra. Triphala, Nagakeshar, punarnava. Gokshura, Palashpushpa, Devadar, Usheera, Padmakasta, Draksha, Chandana, Kharjur, Yastimadhu, Vasa

Dosage : Syrup : 2-3 teaspoonful thrice daily with water or as directed by the Physician. Tablet : 1-2 tablets thrice daily

How Supplied: Syrup : In 200 ml. and 400 ml. packing. Tablet : in 100, and 500 tablets packing.

Uses A powerful and effective Uternine Tonic. Useful in regulating irregular Menstrual cycles. control of non specific leucorrhoea, and other menopausal disorders. A drug of choice in relieving dysmenorrhoes and premenstrual tension (PMT)

DEY'S MEDICAL STORES (MANUFACTURING) LTD.

6-D, Nelly Sen Gupta Sarani. Calcutta - 700 087
Tel - 2499810,2499811, 2499825, 2499827

***Product Name* : Herbodil Liquid**

Composition : Each 5 ml. contains:

Extract of Banaphsa Phool	100 mg.
Tulsi	100 mg.
Hapusha	100 mg.
Sleshmataka	100 mg.
Draksha	25 mg.
Kantakari	100 mg.
Brihati	100 mg.
Pippali	50 mg.
Sunthi	100 mg.
Yastimadhu	200 mg.
Vasaka	200 mg.
Pudina	0.5 mg.
Yamani	0.5 mg.
Shatapushpa	0.5 mg.
Navasadara	100 mg.

Dosage : 1-2 teaspoonful 3-4 times a day.

How Supplied: 110 ml.

Uses:For Choked voice, Cough, Sore throat.

***Product Name* : KEO KARPIN CREAM (Ayurvedic Antiseptic)**

Composition :

Harida	5%
Padmaka	5%
Shimul	5%

Mehndi	2%
In a cream base containing Pusanjan	2%
Chandan Taila	0.2%
Ushira Taila	0.1%
Nimba Taila	0.1%

Product Name : **KEO KARPIN OIL Ayurvedic Massage**

Composition : Each 10 ml. contains :

Daru haridra	50 mg.
Haridra	50 mg.
Manjistha	50 mg.
Arjuna	16 mg.
Karpoor	10 mg.
Lanolin	50 mg.
Neem Oil	0.05 ml.
Sandal Wood Oil	0.03 ml
Arachis Oil	5 ml.
Light Liquid Paraffin	10 ml.
Alcohol	1%
Olive Oil	0.05 ml.

Product Name : **ITONE EYE DROPS**

Composition :

Nimba	5% v/v
Sobhanjana	5% v/v
Bhringaraj	5% v/v
Punarnava	7.5% v/v
Nirgundi	5% v/v
Satapatri	7.5% v/v
Yamani	2% v/v
Haritaki	5% v/v
Vibhitaka	5% v/v
Dhatriphala	5% v/v
Haridra	5% v/v
Karpuram	3% v/v
Pudina	2% v/v
Saindhava Iaban	2% v/v
Mahdu	10% v/v
Ela	5% v/v
Wet chandan	5% v/v
Mukta	1% v/v
Rakta chandan	5% v/v

Hasti sundi	5% v/v
Tulsi patra	5% v/v

Dosage : 1-2 drops, 2-4 times a day.

How Supplied: 10 ml., 15 ml.

Uses: For Belpharitis, Conjunctivitis, Corneal ulcers, Dacryocystitis, Hypermetropix, Keratitis Lenticular opacity.

***Product Name* : LIVINA SYRUP**

Composition : Each 5 ml. contains :

Kakamachi	50 mg.
Indrajava	25 mg.
Sharapunkha	100 mg.
Kalmegh	50 mg.
Guduchi	25 mg.
Haritaki	25 mg.
Kakilakshya	50 mg.
Saptaparna	50 mg.
Daruharidra	100 mg.
Kasni	50 mg.

Dosage : 1-2 teaspoonful, 2 times a day before principal meals.

How Supplied: 100 ml., 220 ml.

Uses: For Fatty liver, Hepatitis, Jaundice, Liver dysfunction, Precirrhotic liver.

DHARMANI DRUGS RESEARCH & TRAINING INSTITUTE,
1133, Sector -IV, Gurgaon -122001
Tel - 329927, 329928

***Product Name* : BRAHMPUSHPI SYRUP (BRAIN TONIC)**

Composition : Each 15 ml. contains:

Evolvulus alsinoides	2 mg.
Hydrocotryle asiatica	0.5 mg.
Nardostachys jatamansi	25 mg.
Salvia egyptiaca	25 mg.
Brunella valgaris	25 mg.
Nepeta ruderalis	25 mg.
Onosma Bracteatum	100 mg.
Sodium Benzoate	12 mg.

Product Name : DIABEC CAPSULES

Composition :

Jawadi Kasturi	25 mg.
Curcuma longa	75 mg.
Phyllanthus embelica	75 mg.
Eugenia jembolana	75 mg.
Jaymnemasylevtris	75 mg.
Exadirecta indica	75 mg.
Aueminium sulphas	100 mg.

Product Name : DIRSTREP CAPSULES

Composition :

Ferula foetida	10 mg.
Piper nigrum	20 mg.
Camphora	10 mg.
Zingiber officinale	10 mg.
Myristica officinale	5 mg.
Carbonate of calcium	300 mg.

Product Name : FANTASY CAPSULES

Composition :

Sawranpatra	0.5 mg.
Jawadikasturi	0.5 mg.
Kesar	0.5 mg.
Jaiphal	10 mg.
Javatri	10 mg.
Akarkara	20 mg.
Bang bhasam	25 mg.
Talmakhana	60 mg.
Musli safed	50 mg.
Salam misri	60 mg.
Shilajeet	40 mg.
Loh bhasma	10 mg.
Ashwagandha	60 mg.
Kaunch beej	60 mg.
Abharak bhasam	5.5 mg.
Sudh kuchla	20 mg.
Satavar	60 mg.

Product Name : FEROPLEX CAPSULES

Composition :

Ferrum	100 mg.
Ferri peroxicum	100 mg.
Ferry sulphas	100 mg.
Purified sugar candy	25 mg.

Product Name : GYNEX CAPSULES

Composition :

Symplocos racemonsa	55 mg.
Guattaria longifolia	55 mg.
Winter cherry	30 mg.
Mesuaferia linn	50 mg.
Gum	30 mg.
Aueminium sulphas	25 mg.
White assenicum sulphidum	25 mg.

Product Name : HERBOGLOBIN SYRUP

Composition : Each 10 ml. contains :

Saffron	0.100 mg.
Ferrum	20 mg.
Sodium Benzoate	50 mg.
Morgorita	20 mg.
Asphaltum panjabinum	0.100 mg.
Citrus aurantium	200 mg.

Product Name : HERBOZYME CAPSULES

Composition :

Sodium Bixarbonate	300 mg.
Ferula feotida	30 mg.
Menthol	3.3 mg.
Beshops weed seed	117 mg.

Product Name : KUFTONE CAPSULES

Composition :

Abis webbiana lindi	150 mg.
Ephedra	15 mg.
Liquorice root	150 mg.
Adhatoda vasica	4.4 mg.
Inula racemosa	150 mg.

EISEN PHARMACEUTICAL CO. PVT. LTD.
34/7, Erandawana, Pune - 411004
Tel - 331174, Fax - (0212) 330024

***Product Name* : ARTICULIN TABLETS**

Composition :

Ashwagandha Powder	450 mg.
Guggul	50 mg.
Jasad bhasma	50 mg.

***Product Name* : ARTICULIN FORTE CAPSULES**

Composition :

Ashwagandha	450 mg.
Guggul shudha	100 mg.
Haldi Powder	50 mg.
Jasad bhasma	50 mg.

***Product Name* : COUGHOREX LIQUID**

Composition : Each 10 ml. contains :

Aqueous ext. of Tulsi	200 mg.
Parijatak	200 mg.
Kantakari	400 mg.
Vasa	400 mg.
Yashtimadh	400 mg.
Dadim twak	100 mg.
Dhatura	100 mg.
Shunti	100 mg.
Mareech	50 mg.
Pippali	50 mg.
Prakshep dravyas : Tankan bhasma	10 mg.
Navsagar	10 mg.
Karpura	5 mg.

***Product Name* : FENUZYME TABLETS**

Composition :

Sunthi	50 mg.
Tankan bhasma	50 mg.
Hingu	50 mg.
Shudha gandhak	50 mg.
Sourvachal	100 mg.
Haritaki	100 mg.

Product Name :NEOSEPTIN TABLETS

Composition :

Twak	12.9 mg.
Ela	25.8 mg.
Pippali	51.6 mg.
Yashtimadhu	103.2 mg.
Sharkara	206.4 mg.

EVEREST HERBAL REMEDIES

184-M/1, Luker Road, Lukerganj, Allahabad - 211001
Tel - 403194,404693, Fax - (0532)404239

Product Name : ASMOCLINE CAPSULES

Composition : Each capsule contains:

Borax (Sohaga)	10 mg.
Adhatoda vasica(Vasaca)	10 mg.
Achyranthes Aspera (Apamarg)	10 mg.
Psoralea Cordifolia (Bavchi	10 mg.
Datura Tatula (Dhatura	10 mg.
Barilla (Sajji Khar)	20 mg.
Piper Nigrum (Kali Mirch)	30 mg.
Ammonil Chloridum (Nausadar)	20 mg.
Trachyspermum Ammi Ajwan	20 mg.
Papaveris Somniferum (Posta Donda)	20 mg.
Potasli Nitras (Kalmi Sora)	20 mg.
Piper longum (Pipal choti)	30 mg.
Calotropis Gigantea (Aak Phool)	20 mg.
Potassium Aluminium (Fitkari)	20 mg.

Processed in : Cow Milk.

Dosage : 1 or 2 capsules each two times a day with warm milk or water, or as advised by the physician.

How Supplied : Available in packs of 25 capsules.

Uses: Bronchial asthma, asthmatic bronchitis, allergic rhinitis, breathlessness, whooping cough, tubercular bronchitis and also prevents the development of cough/phelgum.

Product Name : HERBOLEH TONIC LIQUID

Composition :

Mica bhasma	140 mg.
Feram bhasma	140 mg.
Withania sonifera	3-570 mg.
Zingiber offcinale	1-780 mg.

Asparagus racemosus wild	890 mg.
Pueraria Tuberosa	90 mg.
Piper Longum	90 mg.
Piper Nigrum Linn	90 mg.
Ellecttaria cardamomum	90 mg.
Cinnamomum zeylanicum nees	90 mg.
Caryphollus aromaticus	40 mg.
Myristica fragrans Houtt	40 mg.
Pavonia Odorata	40 mg.
Santalum album Linn	40 mg.
Aegle Marmelos	40 mg.
Bambusa arundinacia	40 mg.
Phyllanthus Emblica	40 mg.
camphora	40 mg.
Plumbago Zeylanica	40 mg.
Root of Piper Longum	40 mg.
Tinospora cordifolia	40 mg.
Boerhaavia Diffusa Linn	40 mg.
Andropogon Muricalus	40 mg.
Styrax Benjoin Drayand	80 mg.
Deshi Ghee	750 mg.
Sugar Base :	Q.S.

Dosage : For adults 10 g. two times a day with milk or water. for children 5 gms two times a day with milk or water.

How Supplied: Avialable in 500 g. containers.

Uses: Dietary deficiencies, malnutrition, post pregnancy care, lactation, retarded growth and underweight.

***Product Name* : LUST-UP CAPSULE**

Composition : Each capsule contains :

Cubeba officinalis (Kankol)	10 mg.
Myristica fragrans (Jaiphal)	10 mg.
Mucuna Pruiens (Kevanch beej)	10 mg.
Sulphuretum hydrargyri	10 mg.
(Hingul Bhasma) Myristica frangrans (Javitri)	10 mg.
Syn. Ptychotis ajowan (Khurasani Ajwan)	10 mg.
Piper longum (Piper)	10 mg.
Mesua ferrea (Naag kesar)	
Crocus sativus (Kesar)	10 mg.
Anacyclus Pyrethum (Akarkara)	10 mg.
Caryophllus Aromaticus (Laung)	10 mg.

Dosage : 2 capsules preferably with milk before 2 hours of sex, is advised for full satisfaction.

How Supplied: Availble in packs of 20 capsules.

Uses: An aphrodisiac sexup is contraindicated in high blood pressure, advanced arterioseterosis, chronic renal diseases and cardiac failure.

Product Name : **MYGRO DROPS**

Composition :

Enhydra flanctuns (Hulhul patti)	0.12%
Nerium odorum (Kaner patti)	0.12%
Abrus precatorius (Gunja safed)	0.12%
Glycyrrhiza glabra(Mulethi)	0.12%
Sapindus trifoliatus (Reetha)	0.24%
Aconitum ferox(Bacch Naag.)	0.06%
Zingiber ofcinale (Adrak)	0.12%
Boerhaavia diffusa (Punarnava)	0.12%
Base q.s. Ad.	100%

Dosage : Mygro drops to be sucked through nose only two drops in each nostril, once a day, or as a advised by the physician. Mygro is for external use only. Not for injection

How Supplied: Available in bottle of 10 ml.

Uses Mygraine, myalgia, hysteria and cerbro, vascular diseases.

Product Name : **STOMYNE CAPSULES**

Composition : Each capsule cotains :

Fossil encrnite bhasma (Sangyahood bhasma)	100 mg.
Potassil carbonas (Yav char)	100 mg.
Raphanus sativus (Muli char)	50 mg.
Dolichos biflorus (Kulthi sat)	50 mg.
Tephrosial purpurea (Safoca char)	50 mg.
Brassica guncea (Raai)	50 mg.
Rehum emodi (Revand Khatai)	50 mg.
Saxifraga liqulata wall (Pakhan bhed)	50 mg.

Processed in : Achyranthes Aspera (Apamarg)

Dosage : 1 capsule each three times a day with water, or as advised by thephysician.

How Supplied **:** Available in packs of 20 capsules.

Uses **:** Stomyne capsule cures urinary tract infections, disintegrates and expels urinary stones, burning micturition, dysuria and nocturia, acute renal colic,kidney dysfunction, acute and chronic nephrotic syndrome, protects the urinary tract from infections by acting on common urinary pathogens, especially E.coli and klebsiella, and prevents recurrence. Stomyne can be safely taken even during pregnancy.

Product Name : **KOSMO PIMPLE CREAM**

Composition :

Hydrargyrum	0.15%
Salphur	0.38%
Bees wax	23.07%
Sesamum Indicum Oleum	76.92%

Plus 0.76 % of each of the following extracts of :

-Ficus religiosa
-Andropogon nuricalus
-Cinnarmomum zeylanicum
-Potassium Alu. Sulphati
-Cinnamomum tamala
-Nelumbium speciosum saffron
-Pterocarpus santalinus
-Shorea robusta resina
-ficus bengalensis
-Blue stone
-Coccus lacca
-Curcuma longa
-Ficus infectoria
-Caesalpinia sappon
-Bole rubra
-Glycyrrhiza glabra
-Mesua orrea
-Butea frondosa
-Santalum album
-Rubia cordifolia
Ficus glomerata
-Real gar
-Yellow arsenic
-Berberis aristata

Dosage : Wash your face with mild soap and warm water, and pat it with a clean towel. Rub 'Kosmo Cream' regularly thrice in the morning, afternoon, and at bed time on the effected parts of the face, till it is well absorbed. You may wipe off the cream from your face with a dry and celan towel after some time.

How Supplied: In 20 g. collapsible tube.

Uses: Kosmo pimples cream is a specific herbal medicine for acne, pimples, blemishes and minor skin ailments. Kosmo cream checks the growth of acne and pimple. It dries and clears away existing pimples. and fights the bacteria which causes pimples. Kosmos cream can be used as an after shave cream to protect the skin from any septic condition. It also has a soothing effect if used regularly. Kosmo cream can be used on dryskin and cracked lips in winter. Kosmo cream gives relief from irritating mosquito bites, bed bugs, and other house-hold insects. Kosmo cream is effective in healing minor cuts, burns, injuries and ringworms, because of its antiseptic effect.

Pharmacological Action : For external use only. Recap tube tightly after use. Avoid constipation. Do not pick or squeeze pimples. Take care to avoid eyes and area around eyes. Store in cool place & keep away from heat and direct sunlight.

Product Name : **KOSMO HAIR VITALIZER**

Composition :

Blue stone (Tutiya)	2%
Abrus precatorius (Ratti bal)	2%
Citrullus colocynthis (Indrayan root)	2%
Solanum searamfamg (Kateri phal)	2%
Caesalpinia bonducella (Karanj phal)	2%
Merium odorum (Kaner root)	2%
Jasminum grandiflorum (Chameli root)	2%
Tinospora cordifolia (Giloi)	2%
Calotropis gigantea (Aak char)	2%
Euphoribia neriifolix (Snuhi char)	2%
Citrus acida (Neebu sat)	5%
Postassil nitras (Kalmi sora)	5%

Dosage : Take two teaspoonfulls of Kosmo and massage gently on the roots ofthe hair and leave it for at least half an hour. Wash your hair, and pat it dry, with a towel. Thereafter you may use any hair oil. It has no side effects. Use regularly for healthy & shining hair.

How Supplied:Available in a 100 ml. attrative flask.

Uses: Kosmo Hair Vitalizer prevents the untimely fall of hair irrespective of any reason. It removes dandruff, and keeps the hair glossy and soft. It also stops further whitening of hair and destroys lice.

Pharmacological Action : For external use only. Take care to avoid eyes. Do not use on raw of blistered areas on the head. Do not drop on the floor and clothes. It is liable to leave stains.

Product Name : **KOSMO BREASTUP OIL**

Composition :

Withania somnifera (Aswagandha)	5%
Punica grantaum (Anar dana)	5%
Punica gran-tum (Anar chilka)	20%
Gmelina arborea (Cambhari chal)	10 %
Sphaeranthus indicus (Gorakh mundi)	10%
Piper longum (Piper Big)	10%
Abutilon indicum (Bala)	5%
Sida cordifolia (Khirethi)	5%
Sassure Lappa (Kut Kaduwa)	5%
Acorus calamus (Bach)	2.5%
Sesamum Indicum Oleum Til oil to make	100%

Dosage : Take 5 ml. (one spoonful)of oil and massage both the breasts gently for at least 10-15 minutes at night daily, before going to bed. then wear a brassiere. After 20-25 days the breasts become tighter and more firmly shaped. then massage after an interval of 2-3 days regularly to maintain the firmness and retain a youthful figure.

How Supplied: Available in 100 ml. attractive flask.

Uses: Sagging and droopy breasts. Breastup Oil helps to tighten the breastmuscles and gives a firm shaps to the body. This gives a more youthful appearance to a ladies figure.

Pharmacological Action : Breastup Oil is free form all side effects. Breastup oil is only for massage.

Product Name : **DAIOCOP CAPSULES**

Composition : Each capsule contains :

Conch bhasma (Sankh bhasma)	50 mg.
Feronia elephantum (Kaitha)	50 mg.
Myristica fragrans (Jaiphal)	50 mg.
Borax (Sohaga)	50 mg.
Holarrhena antidysenterica (Kuda chal)	50 mg.
strychnos nux vomica (Kuchla)	50 mg.
Papaveris sominferum (Posta donda sat)	100 mg.
Symplocos racemosa (Lodha0	50 mg.
Bombax malabaricum (Mochras)	50 mg.

Dosage : Adult : 1 capsule each 4 or 5 times a day with water. till the symptoms are controlled. dosage may be increased in severe conditions. Children: ½ of the above dosage with honey, or as advised by the physician.

How Supplied: Available in packs of 50 capsules.

Uses: Daiocop treats all type of diarrhoea, dysentery (Acute or chronic, bacillary or amoebic), effective in distension and other abdominal disordrs associated with pain and colic, neuro gastritis. Checks fermentation, flatulence, and heaviness in the stomach.

Product Name : **HEPAHERB CAPUSLE**

Composition : Each capsule contains :

Mica bhasma (Abharak bhasma)	10 mg.
Ferum bhasma (Lauh bhasma)	10 mg.
Ras sindoor (Ras sindoor)	10 mg.
Citrus acida (Jambhiri neebu beej)	10 mg.
Aconitum cordatum (Ateesh)	10 mg.
Pterocarpus santalinus (Chandan Lal)	10 mg.
Bergina Ligulata(Pakhan Bhed)	10 mg.
Tinospora cordifolia (Giloi)	20 mg.
Tephrosia Purpurea (Sarfoka Char)	300 mg.
Fumaria parviflora (Pitta Papra)	10 mg.

Dosage :Adult : 1 to 2 capsule two times a day with fruit juice or water. Children : Half or One capsule two times a day with honey, or as advised by the physician.

How Supplied: Available in packs of 50 capsules.

Uses: Hepaherb capsules are advised for protection of the liver against various hepatotoxins, corrects the liver functioning and induces appetitie and growth. Also recommended in gastric upsets, constipation, heartburns, jaundice and diabetes.

Product Name : **DIAMIT CAPSULE**

Composition : Each capsule contains :

Ferum Bhasm	20 mg.
Tinospora cordifolia	20 mg.
Pueraria tuberosa	40 mg.
Phyllanthus emblica ext.	40 mg.
Quercus infectoriaoliv	20 mg.
Elettaria cardmomum	40 mg.

Polypodiaceao	50 mg.
Butea frondosa Ext.	50 mg.
Mesua ferrea	20 mg.
Musa sapientum root	20 mg.
Curculigo orchioides	20 mg.
Asparagus adscedons	20 mg.
Argentum verk	20 mg.
Asphaltum punjabinum	20 mg.
Emblica officinalis	20 mg.
Eguenia jambolana	20 mg.
Euphorobia microphylla H.	20 mg.
Cyperus scariosus	20 mg.
Myristica fragrans	20 mg.
Cannbis sativa linn	6 mg.

Dosage : If blood sugar level is more then 300 mg. then one capsule is to be taken in the morning, affernoon, evening and at night before meals and breakfast, four capsules a day. If blood sugar level is between 300 mg. to 100 mg. then 4 capsules a day, in the above manner are to be taken.

How Supplied:25 capsules.

Uses: Reducing high levels of blood sugar, which finally cures diabetes.

***Product Name* : DENTDROP DROPS**

Composition :

Achyranthes aspera (pamarg)	10%
Embelia ribes (Vaividang)	10%
Piper nigrum (Kail mirch)	2.5%
Bracteated birth cort (Kidamari)	2.5%
Datura stramonium (Dhatura)	105
Jasminum grandiflorum (Chemeli)	10%
Ocimum canmum (Ban tulsi)	5%
Base water	100%

Dosage : 4-5 Drops of Dendrop should be dropped in the car, opposite to the side of the dental pain, twice a day, which should be administered in a lying position.

How Supplied: Available in a 10 ml. Bottle.

Uses In gingivitis, painful gums, carries, and toothaches, etc.

Pharmacological Action : Dentdrop is free from all side effects. Dentdrop is for external use only. Not for injection. Use within 30 days from the date of opening the cap seal.

Product Name **: LEUCOREX CAPSULE**

Composition : Each capsule contains :

Ferfum bhasma (Kant lauh bhasam)	66 mg.
Stannum bhasam (Bang bhasma)	33 mg.
Zincum bhasma (Jasad bhasma)	33 mg.
Vateria Indica (Kaharwa pisti)	33 mg.
Bole Rubra (Geru)	33 mg.
Bombax malabaricum (Mochras)	33 mg.
Shorea Robusta (Safed ral)	33 mg.
Saxifraga ligulata	
Processed by:	
Euphoribia hirta linn (Doob)	
Punica granatum (Anar)	
Emblica officinalis (Amla)	

Dosage : 1 capsule each three times a day with milk, fruit juice or water or as advised by the physician.

Uses: All types of leucorrhoea. Whether irritating, milky mucous slimy smarting thick, watery, yellowish and in menses, any irregularities whether premature, scanty, suppressed, delayed copious, excessive, fiequent, black, clotted, strigy or strong odoured, and for concomitants, like backache, pain, melancholy or depression etc.

Product Name **: HERBOPILES CAPSULE**

Composition : Each capsule contains:

Amorphophallus campanulatus (Suran sat)	122 mg.
Sapindus trifoliatus (Reetha bhasma)	122 mg.
Mimosa catechu (Paparia kattha)	85.4 mg.
Melia azedarach (Bakayan phal)	85.4 mg.
Berberis extractum (Rasaut)	85.4 mg.

Dosage : 1 capsule each taken daily in the morning and night with milk or as advised by the physician.

How Supplied:Available in packs of 25 capusles.

Uses: Herbopiles is effective in haemorrhoids of any kind-whether internal or external, bleeding or nonbleeding, it also helps to reduce agonising pain and inflammation, Its beneficial effect reduces constipation and further gives regular bowels movements.

Uses: Romati Capsule is effective in rheumatic arthritis, rheumatoid arthritis, osteoarthritis, neuralgia, non- articular rheumatism, cervical and lumber spondylosis, gout, frozen shoulder, sciatica,sprains, joints or muscular pains.

GLYCO REMEDIES
C-73, Okhla Industrial Area, Phase-1,
New Delhi -110020, Tel - 6818339,6819834

Product Name **: HERBOCALM CAPSULES**

Composition :

Tagar ghansatav	50 mg.
Vacha ghansatav	30 mg.
Jatamansi ghansatav	50 mg.
Bramhi ghansatav	50 mg.
Pipplamol ghansatav	30 mg.
Arjuna ghansatav	50 mg.
Sarpagandha ghansatav	20 mg.
Shankhpuspi ghansatav	20 mg.
Tulsi ghansatav	20 mg.
Sonpha ghansatav	30 mg.

Product Name **: JAVRIKA CAPSULES**

Composition :

Tribhuvan kirti	50 mg.
Godanti	50 mg.
Trikatu ghansatav	20 mg.
Haritiki ghanstav	20 mg.
Giloy ghansatav	25 mg.
Brahmi ghansatav	20 mg.
Sudarshan churn	50 mg.
Praval	30 mg.
Navjiwan ras	20 mg.
Jeharmohra	20 mg.
Arkshar	20 mg.
Sfatik	30 mg.
Apamargkshar	20 mg.
Chandanadi loha	50 mg.

Product Name **:LAXOCAP CAPSULES**

Composition :

Triphata ghansatav	50 mg.
Nishoth ghansatav	20 mg.
Elwa ghansatav	30 mg.
Indryan mool ghansatav	30 mg.

Jaypital	10 mg.
Kakadana	20 mg.
Sontha ghansatav	20 mg.
Sanaya ghansatav	20 mg.
Sendhawa	20 mg.
Haritki ghansatav	20 mg.

***Product Name* : NO-OBES CAPSULES**

***Composition* :**

Abhya ghansatav	100 mg.
Kalajeeri ghansatav	30 mg.
Punarnnawa ghansatav	30 mg.
Sanay ghansatav	20 mg.
Sonpha	20 mg.
Tankan	20 mg.
Munnaka	20 mg.
Trikatu ghansatav	20 mg.
Trifla	30 mg.
Shudha ghansatav	20 mg.
Yawkshar	20 mg.
Arogya Vardhani	20 mg.
Kaishor guggulu	20 mg.
Navak guggulu	20 mg.
Medohar vidangadiloha	30 mg.

***Product Name* : ROMATI CAPSULES**

***Composition* :**

Mristica fragrans houtt (Jaiphal)	25 mg.
Myristica fragrans (Javitri)	25 mg.
Caryophyllus aromaticus (Laung)	25 mg.
Piper Longum (Piper)	25 mg.
Piper nigrum (Kali mirch)	25 mg.
Zingiber officinal (Sonth)	25 mg.
Anacyclus pyrethum (Akarkara)	25 mg.
Crocus sativus vomica-(Sudha kuchla)	100 mg.
Aconitum ferox (Sudha mitha telia)	20 mg.
Sulphuretum hydrargyri (Singraf)	20 mg.
Cubeba efficinalis (Kankol)	25 mg.
Fam. Leguminosac (Sanai patti)	10 mg.

Terminalia chebula (Pill Harad)syn.	10 mg.
Syn. Turpethum (Nisoth)	10 mg.
Smilax ornata (Uswa)	10 mg.

Processed in : Papaveris somniferum (Posta donda) Citullus colocynthis (Indrayan Phal.)

Dosage : 1 capsule each two times a day , preferably with warm milk to be continued till all traces of pain disappears. Suggested for 4 to 5 months or as advised by the physician.

Product Name : **ULSACAP CAPSULES**

Composition :

Racemos	50 mg.
Glychrrhiza glabra	30 mg.
Ipomoea turpenirum	20 mg.
Hedychiumspicatum	30 mg.
Amalki rasayan	50 mg.
Narikellavan	30 mg.
Sutshekher ras	50 mg.
Kamdudha	30 mg.
Dhatri loh	30 mg.
Avipattikar	50 mg.
Praval	10 mg.
Jahar mohra	10 mg.
Giloy satva	20 mg.
Chotee elaychi	20 mg.
Vavchhar	20 mg.

GROWEL PHARMACEUTICALS
A-31, Talkatora Industrial Estate, Lucknow - 226011
Tle-410308, Fax - (0522) 222051, 210376

Product Name : **CALCUREX CAPSULE**

Composition :Each capsule contains :

Eladi chruma	100 mg.
Chander Prabha	100 mg.
Hajrool Yahud Bhasam	60 mg.
Trivikram Rasa	40 mg.
Kodi Bhasma	20 mg.

Dosage : One capsule for children and two capsules for adults twice a day for one month or till the calculus is flushed out or as directed by the physician.

How Supplied: Pack of 50 capsules

Uses: Helps in disintegration of the renal Calculus. By inducing diuresis-flushes out the calculus particles and crystals. Controls spasm, provides relief from pain. Prevents lithogenesis by restoring crystalloidcolloid balance.

Prevents damage to vital excretory organkidney. Helps in maintaining the normal pH of urine. keeps excretory organs safe from U.T.I.

Product Name : **DERMEX CAPSULE**

Composition : Each capsule contains :

Gandhak Rasayan	100 mg.
Maha Manjishthadi Qvath	100 mg.
Manikya Bhasma	50 mg.
Psoralea Corylifolia 50 mg.	
Praval Panchamrit	50 mg.

Dosage : Depending on the chronicity of case One capsule for children and 1-2 capsules for adults three times a day for one month. After relief also,. the treatment should be continued for some time, may be with reduced doses or as directed by the physician.

How Supplied: Pack of 50 Capsules.

Uses: Eczema (dry & wet) Eczematous and allergic dermatitis Psoriasis White patches due to burn Moles and warts Pimples, Prickly heat and alika skin manifestations Combat the blood diseases and infection of varied unknown etiology. Brings back natural glow & texture of the skin and produces tonic effect.

Product Name : **DISOMA CAPSULE**

Composition : Each capsule contains :

Ptearo Carpus Marsupim	50 mg.
Eugenia Jambolana	50 mg.
Melia Azadirachta	50 mg.
Enicostemma Littorale	50 mg.
Coccinia Indica	25 mg.
Momordica Charantia	25 mg.

Trigonella Foenum-Graecum	25 mg.
Asphaltum Purified	25 mg.
Bang Bhasma	20 mg.
Loha Bhasma	20 mg.
Abhrak Bhasma	20 mg.
Jasat Bhasma	10 mg.
Gold Bhasma	0.5 mg.

Dosage : 1-2 caps three times a day after meals or ad directed by the physician.

How Supplied: Pack of 50 Capsules.

Uses: Disoma capule - A balanced combination of indigenous time proven herbs, specially processed in such a way to bring their potency to maximum. Disoma capsule-Provides safe & comfortable cure even if used for a long period without any side effect. Disoma capsule -Can be introduced very conveniently to the patients on other drugs therapy. gradual withdrawal of drugs is recommended till normal blood sugar level achieved.

Pharmacological action : Disoma capsule Stimulates Betacells of islets of langerhans to secrete more insulin by enabling the pancreas to function at its normal

Product Name **: GASTEX CAPSULE & TABLET**

Composition : Each capsule & tablet contains :

Trifala	5 mg.
Trikatu	5 mg.
Ferula Narthex	20 mg.
Wrightia Tinctoria	20 mg.
Strychnos nux-vomica	20 mg.
Praval Panchamrit	40 mg.
Chitrakadi Churma	50 mg.
Allium sativum	60 mg.

Dosage : Adults- One capsule or one to two tablets after each meal. Children-One capsule after major meal or one tablet after each meal or as directed by the physician.

How Supplied: Pack of 50 Capsules & 100 Tablets.

Uses: Indigestion and Flatulence. Colicky pain and dyspepsias. Gastric distress and abdominal distension. Heartburn and hyperacidity. Neutralise excess acid. Gastric irritation and nausea.

Product Name : **KLOT CPASULE**

Composition : Each Capsule :

Daucus Carota Seed	200 mg.
Clerodendrum Serratum	40 mg.
Ferula Narthex, Trikatu each	40 mg
Aloe Barbadensis	20 mg.
Tankan kshar	20 mg.
Commiphora myrrha	20 mg.
Abroma augusta	20 mg.

Dosage : One to two capsules three times a day foe about 6 days normally, discontinue during menstruation and repeat each cycle till regularised or as directed by physician.

How Supplied: Pack of 20 capsules.

Uses: Assures Menstrual-flow in then ormal natural way.Glandular stimulant and helps to expel undesired substances, from the system. In hypomenorrhoea, oligomenorrhoea. In secondary Amenorrhoea and Priamary Amenorrhoea (Without congential defects). In delayed, difficult and deficient menstruation without apparent cause.

Product Name : **LUCORIN CPASULE**

Composition : Each capsule contains :

Pushyanug Churna	50 mg.
Pradarantak Loha	50 mg.
Saraca Indica	30 mg.
Godanti Bhasma	20 mg.
Gokshuradi Guggul	20 mg.
Loha Bhasma	20 mg.
Asparagus Racemosus	20 mg.
Sysmplocos Racemosa	20 mg.
Kukkutandatwak Bhasma	10 mg.
Praval Bhasma	10 mg.
Commiphora Myrrha	10 mg.
Tribang Bhasma	10 mg.

Dosage : One Capsule thrice a day for seven days followed by one capsule twice a day for 4 to 6 weeks or as directed by the physician.

How Supplied: Pack of 50 Capsules.

Uses: Leucorrhoea of varied etiology. Vicarious vaginal discharges of acute or chronic nature. Checks & Controls obnoxious vaginal discharges Take cares of foul smell from the vaginal discharges. Checks excessive vaginal secretion by reducing permeabillity of vaginal mucosa. Prevents threatened abortions due to Leucorrhoea

Restores vaginal pH. In monalial & protozoal infections. Lucorin capsule is very effective as anadjuvant therepy to antimonalial & antiprotozoal drugs.

Product Name :**LIVOMEX CAPSULE & TABLET**

Composition : Each capsule contains:

Boerhaavia Diffusa	40 mg.
Plumbago Zeylanica	40 mg.
Eclipta Alba	30 mg.
Terminalia Chebula	20 mg.
Holarrhena Antidysenterica	20 mg.
Emblica Officinalis	20 mg.
Asphaltum Purified	20 mg.
Commiphora Mukul	20 mg.
Kajjali	20 mg.
Abhrak Bhasma	10 mg.
Tamra Bhasma	10 mg.
Loha Bhasma	10 mg.

Each tablet contains:

Arogya Vardhani	100 mg.
Mandur Bhasma	40 mg.
Navayas Loha	30 mg.
Eclipta Prostrata	20 mg.
Boerhavvia Diffusa	20 mg.
Andrographis Paniculata	20 mg.

Each 5 ml. syrup contains Extract from:

Boerhaavia diffusa	200 mg.
Eclipta prostrata	100 mg.
Picrorhiza kurroa	100 mg.
Cissampelos pareira	80 mg.
Embelia ribes	80 mg.

Ipomoea turpethum	80 mg.
Plumbago zeylanica	80 mg.
Amoora rohituka	80 mg.
Solanum nigrum	80 mg.
Andrographis paniculata	20 mg.
Piper longum	20 mg.
Tinospora cordifolia	20 mg.
Ocimum sanctum	20 mg.
Berberis aristata	20 mg.
Holarrhena antidysenterica	20 mg.
Flavoured syrup base	q.s.

Dosage :Infants -5-10 drops syrup Children-1teaspoonful (10ml) syrup or 1 tablet Adults-2 teaspoonful (10ml) syrup or 2 tabs. or 1 cap.

How Supplied:Pack of 50 capsules, 100 tablets & syrup 100ml.& 200ml.

Uses A powerful and concentrated formulation of tested & trusted herbs and minerals. Provides faster recovery from malfunction of Liver. Corrects hepatic disorders like hepatitis, Jaundice & Liver Cirrhosis. Corrects anorexia symptoms. Helps in growth failure of organs and the body. Prevents toxaemia in pregnancy. Protects liver from the toxins produced by pathogens.

Product Name : **PILOMA CAPSULE**

Composition : Each capsule contains:

Terminalia Chebula	80 mg.
Curcuma Amada	50 mg.
Emblica Officinalis	50 mg.
Terminalia Belerica	40 mg.
Tinospora Cordifolia	30 mg.

Dosage : Two capsules to be taken early in the morning on an empty stomach about an hour prior to breakfast for 4 to 6 weeks or as directed by the physician. In severe conditions three capsules may be given for 3 to 4 days followed by two capsules for 6 weeks. Avoid foods leading to constipation.

How Supplied: Pack of 50 Capusle

Uses: Provides relief from painful condition Checks bleeding by removing the congestion in the haemorrhoids. Reduces inflamation. Controls & gives relief in ano-rectal pruritus Helps in passing the normal stool due to laxative action. (An important factor to the patients suffering from haemorrhoids) Over and above all advantage provides complete cure from haemorrhoids. Checks the prolapse of the rectum, even of long duration problem.

Product Name : **VIGORIL CAPSULE**

Composition : Each Capsule contains:

Witania Somnifera	100 mg.
Mucuna Pruriens	80 mg.
Anacylus Pyrethrum	30 mg.
Strychnos nux vomica	20 mg.
Asphaltum purificata	20 mg.
Ras Sindur	10 mg.
Suvaran Makshik	5 mg.
Makardhwaj	4 mg.
Jundbedastoor	4 mg.
Crocus Ṡativis	0.1 mg.

Dosage : One to two capsules twice a day with milk for 6 to 8 weeks or as directed by the physician.

How Supplied: Pack of 50 capsules.

Uses: Increases density of semen, ensures satisfactory performance, excites desire, enhances verile power, prolongs retention of semen during sexual congress. Sustains vigour and vitality Improves metabolism and health Non-hormonal therapy free from side effects. Revives depressed Libido. Impotence- functional of idiopathic, premature or delayed ejaculation, sexual- senile-seminal debility, frigidity in the female, involution depression, geriatic tonic in premature senility and at climacteric in both sexes.

Helps in the reconstruction and revitalisation of tissues and cells which have degenerated.

Product Name: **RUMODOL CAPSULE**

Composition : Each capsule contains :

Maha rasnadi Qvath	100 mg.
Maha Yograj Guggul	80 mg.
Triyodasang Guggul	50 mg.
Shankh Bhasma	20 mg.

Strychnos Nux vomica	5 mg.
Suvarn Makshik Bhasma	5 mg.
Ras Sindur	5 mg.

Dosage :Adult-One to two capsule twice a day for 3 to 4 months or as directed by the physician. Children-One capsule once a day or as directed by the physician. Avoid hot condiments and sour fermented articles.

How Supplied:Pack of 50 Capsules.

Uses:Gives satisfactory results by reducing swelling inflammation and stiffness of joints.

Allows the patient to perform his daily routine comfortably and he feels a sense of well being Gives prolonged response when the bonemarrow gets provoked, there occurs breaking pain in fat, bones and joints, arthralgia, ross of flesh and strength, loss of sleep and constant pain.

Can be used for long period as it is safe,nontoxic and does not give any gastrointestinal upsets.In backaches and leg cramps, Ankylosing spondlitis, Frozen shoulder syndrome, sciatica, Fibrositis, Lumbago and all other musculokeletal pains of long duration.

Product Name : **GNOCOL SYRUP**

Composition : Each 5ml. contains:

Hirakasi Shuddha	5 mg.
Saraca Indica	50 mg.
Symplocos racemosa, Inula helenium each	20 mg.
Withania sommifera	20 mg.
Dasmool	40 mg.
Mesuaa Ferrea	10 mg.
Santalum Album	20 mg.
Hemidesmus Indicus	10 mg.
Cedrus libani, Nardostachys Jatamansi each	10 mg.
Cyperus rotundus	20 mg.
Abroma augusta	10 mg.
Flavoured syrup Base	Q.S.

Dosage :Two teapoonful (10ml) three times a day before meals. Treatment should be continued for3-4 cycles or as directed by the physician.

How Supplied:Bottle of 200 ml.

Uses : Delayed puberty Menstrual disorder and uterine dysfunctions. Restores the functions of the ovary and endometrium. Relieves dysmenorrhoea and reduces pelvic congestion. Oligomenorrhoea and dysfunctional uterine bleeding Difficult conception Habitual abortion Helps to minimise the problems of climacteric disturbances at the time of menopause.

Product Name : **LEAF COUGH SYRUP**

Composition: *Each 5 ml. contains:*

Adhatoda vasaka	5 mg.
Glycyrrhiza glabra	5 mg.
Ocimum sanctum	5 mg.
Yavakshar	5 mg.
Piperment sat	5 mg.
Nausadar	100 mg.
Flavoured syrup base	q.s.

Dosage : Infants-5to10 drops Children - One teaspoonful (5ml) Adult-Two teaspoonful (10ml) Three times a day or as directed by the physician.

How Supplied: Bottle of 100 ml

Uses: Natural soothing and anti-tussive Whooping, Allergic,Asthamatic and Spasmodic coughs. Bronchitis, Laryngitis and Pharyngitis Clear chest congestion, sneezing and smokers coughs Expels thick sputum Reduces bronchospasm Suitable in all seasonal Bronchial affections.

Product Name : **TONEX CAPSULE & SYRUP**

Composition : Each capsule contains:

Myristica Fragrans	20 mg.
Cinnamomum zeylanicum	15 mg.
Anacylus pyrethrum	15 mg.
Zingiber officinale	15 mg.
Piper longum	15 mg.
Pistacia lentiscus	10 mg.
Asparagus adscendens	10 mg.

Elettaria cardamonum	10 mg.
Tribulus terrestris	10 mg.
Crocus sativus	4 mg.

Each 5 ml. contains:

Withania somnifera	25 mg.
Asparagus racemosus	20 mg.
Anacyclus pyrethrum	20 mg.
Pueraria Tuberosa	20 mg.
Mucuna pruriens	20 mg.
Rubia cordifolia	15 mg.
Chaturajat	15 mg.
Trikatu	10 mg.
Vanda roxburghii	10 mg.
Trifala	10 mg.
Asparagus adscendens	10 mg.
Santalum album	10 mg.
Flavoured syrup base	q.s.

Dosage : Children - One teaspoonful (5ml) Adults - One capsule or two teaspoonful (10ml) twice a day or as directed by the playsician.

How Supplied: Pack of 50 capsules and Bottle of 200 ml.

Uses: Provides - well balanced natural vitamins, easily absorbed from G.I tract to meet the deficiencies. Helps -: In passing th daily routine life with full of zest, vigour & vitality. Ideal -to people who are unable to take balanced nutrition in day to day life.To pass-long youth life foru oung people. Gives - added advantages to men & women exhausted from work load physical/mental.Tone up- the body of elderly people. Increased-Body resistance to combat with frequent infections of cough, cold etc. For - Speedy recovery during convalescence period.

Product Name : **ZYMEX CAPSULE & SYRUP**

Composition : Each capsule contains:

Ballosperumum Montanum	10 mg.
Piper longum	10 mg.
Carum copticum	10 mg.
Ferula foetida	10 mg.

Stychnos nux-vomica	15 mg.
Kajjali	10 mg.
Plumbago zeylanica	20 mg.
Trikatu	50 mg.
Yavakshar	10 mg.
Conch shell powder	30 mg.
Kaparda bhasma	10 mg.
Punarnava mand	10 mg.
Trifala	20 mg.
Each 5 ml. contains:	
Asparagus racemosus	100 mg.
Withania somnifera	80 mg.
Pueraria tuberosa	50 mg.
Eclipta alba	50 mg.
Trifala	40 mg.
Asparagus adscendens	10 mg.
Plumbago zeylanica	10 mg.
Vitex negundo	10 mg.
Embelia ribes	10 mg.
Myristica fragrans	10 mg.
Cyperus scariosus	10 mg.
Piper longum	10 mg.
Carum coticum	10 mg.
Syzygium aromaticum	5 mg.
Flavoured syrupy base	q.s.

Dosage: Children-One capsule or one teaspoonful (5ml) after major meal. Adult-One capsule or two teaspoonful (10ml) after each meal. If capsule or syrup to be taken before meal to enhance appetite or after meals to help in digestion.

How Supplied: Pack of 50 capsules and bottle of 200 ml.

Uses : Improves and enhances secretion of enzymes at glandular level naturally by stimulating the glands. Restores the natural function of the digestive system organs. increases appetite rapidly and corrects digestion power fully. Checks flatulence and dyspepsia. regulates peristaltic movement and alleviates chronic constipation. Safe and can be used by all including during pregnancy. No toxicity and contraindications.

HALLMARK HEALTHCARE LIMITED

206, Shivai Industrial Estate 89, Andheri-Kurla Road, Sakinaka Mumbai-400072. Tel-8505762, 8503339, 8509232, Fax - (022) 8504363

Product Name : **SATIZYM LIQUID**

Composition : Each 5 ml. contains:

Vidang	40 mg.
Sunth	40 mg.
Mari	30 mg.
Pepper	30 mg.
Kutaj	40 mg.
Kuchala purified	30 mg.
Kutaki	20 mg.
Shonamukhi	80 mg
Papita	50 mg.
Bodiajmod	50 mg.
Chitrak	40 mg.
Amla	100 mg.
Jeshtimadh	100 mg.
Hing	15 mg.
Sajikhar	40 mg.
Sanchal	40 mg.
Jeera	40 mg.
Pudina	100 mg.

Product Name : **VITALYF CAPSULES**

Composition :

Ashwagandha	50 mg.
Shalam	20 mg.
Safed moosali	20 mg.
Kauncha beej	25 mg.
Shatavali	25 mg.
Bala beej	25 mg.
Vidarikand	25 mg.
Jaiphal	15 mg.
Mocharas	25 mg.
Javantri	15 mg.
Kuchala purified	15 mg.
Gokhru	25 mg.
Bhimsheni kapoor	5 mg.
Tribang bhasma	25 mg.
Banga bahsma	20 mg.
Loh bhasma	25 mg.

Praval bhasma	20 mg.
Abharak bhasma	25 mg.
Suvarna makshik bhasma	25 mg.

HAMDARD (WAKF) LABORATORIES

Hamdard Marg Delhi - 110006

Tel - 523337, 523107, 523287, 523497

Product Name : **ZULAMLA HAIR TONIC**

Composition : Each 100 g. contains:

Amla	15 g.
Halela siyah	10 g.
Berg Hina	10 g.
Shikakai	10 g.
Post maulsari	5 g.
Balchhar	5.g.
Gul-e-surkh	3 g.
Sandal safaid	2 g.
Gond keekar	10 g.
Khali sarson	30 g.

Dosage **:**Soak 2½ teaspoonfuls of Zulamla in a cup of water for two hours. Massage on the scalp. Rinse the hair with water after 5 minutes. Use Zulamala atleast thrice a week.

How Supplied: 200 g.

UsesZulamla for men & women, helps to remove dandruff, itching sensations and falling of hair. Keeps the scalp clean and healthy. Nourished the hair follicles to provide natural growth.

Product Name : **JOSHINA**

Composition : Each 10 ml. contains conc. Aq. Extract of:

Gul banafsha (Viola odorata)	1.1 g.
Gaozaban (Onosma bracteatum)	1.5 g.
Khatmi(Althaea officinals)	1.1 g.
Khubbazi (Malva rotundifolia)	1.5 g.
Mulethi(Glycyrrhiz glabra)	1.67 g.
Unnab (Zizyphus vulgaris)	1.1 g.
Sapistan (Cordia latifolia)	3.0 g.
Sugar	1.62 g.

Dosage : 10 ml of joshina mixed with 100 ml warm water, to be taken before breakfast and at bedtime. In case of sore-throat and cough, the dose to be licked. For children, half or less dose may be given according to age.

How Supplied: 100ml.

Uses: Joshima is a readymade, convenient and more effective variation of Joshanda the ago-old, tried and trusted unani remedy for colds, catarrh and sore-throat.

Product Name **:SAFI**

Composition : Each 5 ml. (1 teaspoonful) Contains conc.aq.ext.of:

Senna	201.60 mg
Kalmegh	15.00 mg
Revendchini	162.20 mg
Kassundi	15.00 mg
Turbud	25.00 mg
Mundi	25.00 mg
Nilofar	15.00 mg
Nil kanthi	25.00 mg
Gulab ke phool	25.00 mg
Shahtra	25.00 mg
Sheeshum	15.00 mg
Kachnal	15.00 mg
Sandal surkh	15.00 mg
Neem	15.00 mg
Gilo	15.00 mg
Tulsi	30.00 mg
Harar	15.00 mg
Mazrium	25.00 mg
Narkachoor	15.00 mg
Afsentin	
Chirata	15.00 mg
Roomi	25.00 mg
Turzoon	25.00 mg
Milleh frangi	1.25 g.
Invert sugar	3.40 g.

Dosage : Adult : 10 ml. (2 spoonful) Children ¼ or ½ the normal dosage to be given according to age.

How Supplied: 100 ml

Uses : For skin diseases such as acne vulgaris, boils, skin rashes, blemishes, urticaria etc. Checks nose bleeding, cures constipation, corrects indigestion, improves complexion and helps you stay slim and smart.

Product Name : **SADURI COUGH SYRUP**

Composition : Each 10 ml. contians aq.ext.of:

Vasaka I.P. 66	0.140 g.
Liquorice I.P.66	0.147 g.
Ephedrine Hydrochloride I.P	5.5 mg.
Codeine Phosphate I.P.	7.8 mg.
Menthol I.P.	2.2 mg.
Colour amaranth red	q.s.
Syrup base	q.s.

Dosage : In case above-mentioned troubles, give a 10 ml. (2 teaspoonful) dose of saduri to adults; and a 5 ml. (1teaspoonful) dose to children twice everyday one in the morning and one at night.

Uses : Trusted for years, Saduri provides fast relief form coughs it is effective for curing dry and phlegmetic coughs, accumulated phlegum in lungs bronchitis, children's whooping cough, cold etc.

Product Name : **SUPARI PAK**

Composition : Each 10 g. contains:

Ela laghu	0.91 g.
Anila	0.019 g.
Chandan churan safiad	0.019 g.
Jatamansi	0.019 g.
Bidari kand	0.019 g.
Peepal bari	0.019 g.
Dal chini	0.019 g.
Nag kesar	0.019 g.
Talish patra	0.019 g.
Saunth	0.019 g.
Zeera krishna	0.019 g.
Paraj	0.019 g.
Mirch krishna	0.019 g.
Labang	0.019 g.
Kamal gatta	0.019 g.
Neelotpal pushp	0.019 g.
Gokhru laghu	0.019 g.
Mocharas	0.019 g.
Sikni supan churan	1.0 g.

Sugar	8.0 g.
Majeeth	0.12 g.
Ghee	0.72 g.

Dosage : Take 5 grams morning and evening with milk.

How Supplied: 150 g.

Uses : A well-known medication for female disorders.

Product Name : **JOSHANDA**

Composition : Each packet of 33 g. contains:

Asalussos	3 g.
Berggawzaban	3 g.
Tukhm khubbazi	6 g.
Tukhm Khatmi	6 g.
Sapistan	5 g.
Unnab	6 g.
Gule banafsha	4 g.

Dosage : Mix the entire quantity of joshanda in one and a half cups of water and boil it for twice. Add sugar to taste and drink it lukewarm.

HERBALS (APS) PRIVATE LTD

B.M. Das Road., Patna - 800004 (Bihar), Tel - 650920, 650393

Product Name : **ASHOKA COMPOUND LIQUID**

Composition : Each 29 ml. of fluid contains the extract of:

Saraca Indica (Ashoka)	4.32 g.
Symplocos racemosa (Lodhra)	1.92 g.
Acacia arabica (Babul)	1.92 g.
Terminalia arjuna (Arjun)	1.92 g.
Bombac malabaricum (Shalmali)	1.44 g.
Vitis vinifera (Munakka)	3.25 g.
Woodfordia floribunda (Dhai)	1.45 g.
Viburnum foetidum (Shirporna)	1.25 g.
Nigella sativa (Kalejeera)	2.25 g.
Curculigo orchioides(Musalikand)	1.44 g.
Ferri sulphas (Kasisa)	1.00 g.

Dosage :Adults:2 teaspoonfuls thrice daily with water after meals or as directed by physician.

How Supplied: Bottles of 225 ml. and 450 ml.

Uses Oligomenorrhoea, Dysmenorrhoea, Leucorrhoea, Polymenorrhoea.

Pharmacological Action : The pharmacology of the uterus is complicated Owing to the fact, apart from the nervous influences, the function is controlled and regulated by a complicated arrangement of the different endocrine glands.The cyclic changes in the endometrium and ovaries are regulated by the administration of Asoka compound and it is regarded as tonic to nerovous system also. Asoka compound provides as an astringent and uterine sedative. It is largely used in uterine affections specially in Menorrhagia, Menrorrhagia and post-partum haemorrhage. It acts directly on the muscular fibres of the uterus. It also exhibits stimulating effect on the endometrium and ovarian tissue. This drug arrests uterine haemorrhage and abnormal secretion. Asoka compound also causes relaxation of the uterus indicating the possibility of the drugs being useful in spasmogenic pain associated with uterus, and is of valve in spasmodic and congestive dymenorrhoea associated with other complaints such as pain in the abdomen, vomiting, anaemia, headache and prostration.

Product Name : **CLEMENSTOL LIQUID**

Composition : Each 29 ml. of fluid contains the extract of.

Aloe Indica (Ghrita kumari)	6 g.
Abroma augusta(OlatOkambal)	3 g.
Gossypium Indicum (Kapasmool)	3 g.
Baliospermum axillare(Dantimool)	3 g.
Plumbago zeylanica(Chitamool)	3 g.
Sesamum Indicum (Tila)	3 g.
Raphanus sativus (Mulabeej)	3 g.
Aloes (Musabbar)	3 g.
Bambusa arundinacea (Vansa)	3 g.

Dosage :Amenorrhoea (Primary & Secondary):2 to 3 teaspoonfuls thrice daily after meals.Dysmenorrhoea : 2 to 3 teaspoonfuls thrice daily after meals.

How Supplied: Bottle of 225 ml. and 450 ml.

Uses: Amenorrhoea, Dysmenorrhoea

Pharmacological Action : Clemenstol liquid,a non-hormonal medicament is prepared for oral adminstration from pure fresh vegetable drug which are more powerful in their efficacy in amenorrhoea and Dysmenorrhoea having beneficial effect on endocrine glands relating to sex-organs. The alkalodis and sterols of Clemenstol are assimilated into the blood stream through the vascular capillaries in the villi of intestine and stimulate the Basophil cells of anterior pituitary. The cyclic activity of ovary corresponds with the cyclic changes in the uterus and vagina and this is regulated by the normal secretion of anterior pituitary,gonadotrophic hormones. These hormones, follicular stimulating and luteinizing are responsible for the onset of ovarian activity with liberation of Oesrogen and progesterone. These hormones (Ovarian) bring the growth of the myometrium and endometrium with cyclic changes is menstruation.Thus the drug breaks down hypertophid endometrium causing normal flow of menstrual blood.

Product Name :**HEART SOOTHING LIQUID**

Composition : Each 29 ml. contains the extract of:

Terminalia arjuna (Arjuna)	2.83 g.
Vitis vinifera (Munakka)	0.72 g.
Symplocos racemosa (Lodhra)	0.72 g.
Gmelina arborea (Gambhar)	0.48 g.
Emblica officinalis (Amla)	0.24 g.
Daucus carota (Gajar)	0.24 g.
Asteracantha longifolia (Kokilaaksha)	0.24 g.
Santalum album (Swet chandan)	0.12 g.
Andropogon muricatus (Ushir)	0.05 g.
Sida cordifolia (Berela)	1.15 g.

Dosage : Adults : 2 teaspoonfuls thrice daily after meals. Children : ½ to 1 tespoonful thrice daily after meals or as prescribed by the physician.

How Supplied: Bottle of 112 ml.

UsesPericarditis, Angina, Endocarditis, Mitral Regurgitation.

Pharmacological Action :Sida Cordifolia contains small quantities of alkaloid whose pharmacological action closely resembled that of ephedrine. The stimulant action of this alkaloid on the blood pressure is well known and for this reason it has been used as a cardiac stimulants. The drug produces a well marked beneficial effect when administered to patients in whom the action of heart is weak and compensation is failing. Marked diuresis is produced in those patients in whom the function of kidney is disturbed from in-efficient ciruclation. Terminalia arjuna is a well-known remedy for heart diseases. It has a marked stimulant and tonic action on the heart and is used in all sorts of conditions of cardiac failures and dropsy. The drug is highly recommended in heart diseases complicated with endocarditis, mitral regurgitation.percarditis and angina. It increases the rate and amplitude of contratction of the heart and improves the tone of the cardiac muscle.

Product Name : **HERBOTONE LIQUID**

Composition : Each 29 ml. contains the extract of:

Piper bettle (Pan)	4 g.
Ficus hispida (Kakadumur)	3 g.
Acacia arabica (Babu)	3 g.
Eugenia jambolana (Jamum)	2 g.
Vitis vinifera (Munakka)	2 g.
Areca catechu (Supari)	2 g.
Emblica officinlis (Amla)	2 g.
Carica papaya (Papita)	2 g.

Dosage : Adults : 2 teaspoonfuls thrice daily half an hour before meals. Children : ½ to 1 teaspoonful thrice daily half an hour before meals or as prescribed by the physician.

How Supplied: Bottles of 225 ml.

Uses Dyspepsia, Diarrhoea, Anorexia, Flatulence, Digestive, Disorders, General Debility.

Pharmacological Action :Herbotone liquid is the valuable combination of herbal ingredients which has the extraordinary property of hastening the digestion of protein, fat and carbohydrate diets by proper secretion of enzymes in gastro-intestinal tract. The active principle of carica papaya which resembles pepsin in its physiological properties may be deprived from the extract of the unripe fruit. This substance is called papain and is superior to ordinary animal pepsin in having the peculiar additional advantage of requiring neither the aid of an acid nor an alkali to convert the protein contents of the stomach into peptones. It increases biliary and pancreatic secretion and is beneficial for the treatment of general debility, dyspepsia, flatulence and diarrhoea caused by defective digestion.

Product Name : **LIVOSPIN DROPS**

Composition : Each ml. contains:

Amoora Rohituka (Rohitaka)	8 mg.
Eclipta erecta(Bhringaraj)	8 mg.
Andrographis paniculata (Kalmegh)	15 mg.
Salvia plebeia (Shati)	4 mg.
Hygrophila spinosa	4 mg.
Curcuma longa (Haridra)	15 mg.
Graeceum (Methi)	4 mg.
Berberis aristt (Daruharidra)	4 mg.
Ptychotis ajowan (Jowan)	4 mg.

Dosage : Children : 10 to 30 drops thrice daily after meals.Infants ; 5 to 10 drops thrice daily after meals.

How Supplied: Bottles of 28 ml. 56 ml. and 112 ml.

Uses: Anorexia due to digestive disorders, Fatty or Sluggish liver, pre or Early cirrhotic condition, Nutritional defect of the liver, Hepato-Biliary disorders, Infective and toxic hepatitis with or without jaundice, Habitual constipation.

Pharmacological Action : The liver is by far the largest gland in the body and plays an important part in general metabolism. Any derangement in its function upsets the whole metabolic balance and produces diverse symptoms. Our livospin perfoms the normal metabolism of fat, protein and carbohydrate and accelerates the rate of removal of fat from the liver.Livospin seemed to combine the choleretic and hydrocholagogic action with antiseptic property and thus would be an ideal therapeutic agent in condition ofthe hepato-biliary system and gall bladder due to suspected staphylococcal infection. Our livospin is a powerful hepato-biliary stimulant which markedly increases appetite and improves digestive function, corrects nutritional defect, protects liver against hepatotoxic agent. It increases the functional efficiency of the liver, promotes absorption and improves heaemoglobin, relieves abdominal pain, nausea, vomiting and a regulator of bowel movements. It also controls diarrhoea and dyspepsia associated with gaseous distention of the bowel. The absence of untoward side effects with even prolonged administration makes this drug sage and effective in the management of liver disorders.

Product Name : **LIVOSPIN TABLETS**

Composition : Each tablet contains:

Amoora Rohituka (Rohitaka)	40 mg.
Eclipta erecta (Bhringaraj)	30 mg.
Androgrphis paniculata(Kalmegh)	40 mg.
Salvia plebeia (Shati)	30 mg.
Hygrophila spinosa	40 mg.
Curcuma longa (Haridra)	40 mg.
Graeceum (Methi)	30 mg.
Berberis aristata (Daruharidra)	30 mg.
Ptychotis ajowan(Jowan)	40 mg.
Mandur Bhasma (Oxide of Iron)	30 mg.

Dosage :Adults:2talets thrice daily after meals with water. Children : (From 8 to 12 years) One tablet thrice daily with water after meals or as directed by the pysician.

How Supplied:Container of 100 tablets.

UsesAnorexia due to digestive disorders,Fatty or Sluggish liver, Pre or Early cirrhotic condition,Nutritional defect of the liver,Hepato-Bailiary disorders, Infective and toxic hepatitis with or without jaundice,Habitual constipation.

Pharmacological Action :The liver is by far the largest gland in the body and plays an important part in general metabolism. Any derangement in its function upsets the whole metabolic balance and produced diverse symptoms.Our livospin perfoms the normal metabolism of fat, protein and carbohydrate and accelerates the rate of removal of fat from the liver. Livospin seemed to combine the choleretic and hydrocholagogic action with antiseptic property and thus would be an ideal therapeutic agent in condition of the hepato-biliary system and gall bladder due to suspected staphylococal infection.Our livospin is a powerful hepato-biliary stimulant which markedly increases appetite and improves digestive function, corrects nutritional defect, protects liver against hepatotoxic agent. It increases the functional efficiency of the liver, promotes absorption and improves heaemoglobin, relieves abdominal pain, nausea, vomiting and a regulator of bowel movements. It also controls diarrhoea and dyspepsia associated with gaseous distention of the bowel. The absence of untoward side effects with even prolonged administration makes this drug safe and effective in the management of liver disorders.

Product Name : **NARVINOL CAPSULES**

Composition : Each capsule contains:

Harpestis Monniera (Brahmi)	35 mg.
Canscora decussata (Shankhapushpee)	25 mg.
Rauwolfia serpentina (Sarpagandha)	25 mg.
Acorus calamus (Bach)	20 mg.
Nardostacys jatamansi(Jatamansi)	30 mg.
Alhagi maurorum (Duralava)	30 mg.
Withania somnifera (Ashwagandha)	40 mg.
Asparagus racemosus (Shatavari)	30 mg.
Hemidesmus indicus (Anantamul)	30 mg.
Terminalia anjuna (Arjuna)	35 mg.

Dosage: Adults : 1 Capsule twice or thrice daily after meals or as advised by the physician.

How Supplied:Container of 21 capsules.

Uses: Psychoneurosis, Nervous breakdown, Insomnia, Convulsive affection, Poor memory, Hypochondria, Hypertension, Menopausal syndromes.

Pharmachological Action: Narvinol possesses different alkaloids which has got action on the central nervous system and Cardio-vascular systme. For its well marked hypnotic and sedative properties and Cardio-vascular system. For its well marked hypnotic and sedative properties and also for its blood pressure reducing effect, narvinol has been used extensively in psychiatry for anxious, tense and hyperactive patients associated with hypertension.The main site of action is probably on the hypothalamic level producing an alteration of the sympathetic, parasympathetic balance by suppressing particularly the sympathetic predominance. Narvinol also produces tranquillizing and sedative effect without development of tolerance or addiction. It effectively causes relaxation of the muscles and reduces spontaneous motor activity and aggressiveness.

Product Name : **PARALAPS TABLETS**

Composition : Each tablet contains:

Brihatyogaraj guggul (Guggul & others)	0.165 g.
Ext. of maharasandadi quath	

(Selected drugs)	65 mg.
Glycyrrhiza glabra.(Yastimadhu)	20 mg.
Moringa pterygosperma (Sigru)	10 mg.
Vitex negunda (Nishinda)	10 mg.
Allium sativum (Iasuna)	20 mg.
Asphaltum (Silajit purified)	15 mg.
Gastropoda calcined (Shankha bhasma)	45 mg.

Dosage :Adults : 2 tablets three times daily after meals. Children : (6 to 12 years):1 tablet twice daily after meals or as advised by the physician.

How Supplied: Container of 100 tablets.

Uses Polyarthritis, (Rheumatoid arthritis), Gouty arthritis, Neuralgia, Myalgia, Spondylitis, Aching bones, Sciatica, Periarticular-swelling.

Pharmachological Action :Paralaps tablets consist of cimmiphora mukul which has been found to be a complex mixture of avariety of organic compounds and inorganic ions and number of steroids have been isolated and characterised. The oleoresin portion of the plant posses significant antiinflammatory, antisuppurative and antiarthritic activities. The oleo gum-resin of commiphora mukul lowers serum-cholesterol, serum-lipid phosphorus and effectively lower the serum furbidity.It also protects the patients against cholesterol induced atherosclerosis (at the stage of fatty streek)

Allin, the precursor of anti-bacterial principle of A, Sativum which is used to evaluate the clinical usefulness of the drug in the treatment of rheumatoid arthritis associated with pain and restricted movements in one or major joints. Paralaps also increase the excretion of urate and uric acid in the urine. Also the drug is found to possess an anti-bacterial, analgesic and anti-pyretic activity and its prolonged administration does not produce any toxic effects in the patients.

Product Name : **SOMAPAN SYRUP**

Composition : Each 29 ml. fluid contains the extract of:-

Ephedra vulgaris (Khanda)	6.6 g.
Vitis vinifera (Munakka)	0.6 g.
Saussurea lappa(Kur)	0.4 g.
Adhatoda vasika (Vasak)	0.2 g.

Cordia myxa (Lishora)	0.2 g.
Glyeyrrhiza glabra (Yastimadhu)	0.2 g.
Solanum jacquinii (Kantikari)	0.1 g.
Baliospermum axillare (Dantimool)	0.1 g.

Dosage :Adults : 2-3 teaspoonfuls thrice or four times daily after meals. Children : ½ to 1 teaspoonfuls three or four times daily after meals or as directed by the physician. During attack of Asthma repeat three or four hourly or as directed by the physician.

How Supplied: Bottles of 112 ml.

Uses Bronchial Asthma, Chronic Bronchitis with or without Emphysema, Persistent Hiccough and Cough.

Pharmacological Action : Following up of the anti-spasmodic, bronchodilator and expectorant actions of the drug, it was extensively tried in the treatment of bronchial asthma. It has already been established that the drug thas depressant effect on the vagal tone. The drug has a remarkable effect in controlling attacks of bronchial asthma, especially those of the vagotonic type.At the same time the drug during its excretion into the bronchial mucosa not only relaxes the involuntary muscle fibres ofthe bronchioles but also liquefies the tenacious sputum and produces a well-marked expectorant action. In this way not only is the spasm relaxe but the congestion of the bronchial mucosa is also relieved. The respiratory passages are thus cleared and the attack is subdued. The paroxysms are cut short by the combined action of the alkaloids present in the drug.

Product Name : **SPEMATONE SYRUP LIQUID**

Composition : Each 29 ml. of fluid contains the extract of :

Strychnos nuxvomica (Kuchla)	0.25 g.
Triticum sativum (Wheat)	0.5 g.
Terminalia arjuna(Arjuna)	1.0 g.
Vitis vinifera (Munakka)	2.0 g.
Phaseolous roxburghii (Masha)	0.5 g.
Bombax malabaricum (Shalmali)	0.5 g.
Mucuna pruriens (Banaribeej)	0.5 g.
Withania somnifera(Ashwagandha)	0.5 g.
Anacyclus pyrethrum (Akarkara)	4.0 g.
Asparagus racemosus (Shatavari)	2.0 g.

Dosage :Adults : 2 teaspoonfuls thrice daily after meals or as directed by the physician.

How Supplied:Bottles of 225 ml. and 450 ml.

Uses: Spermatorrhoea, Oligospermia, Seminal-Debility, Loss of libido, Premature ejaculation, Loss of erectile power, In male infertility, fatigubility, male climacteric.

Pharmachological Action :Spematone syrup and forte tablet manily stimulate growth or maintain the primary and secodary sex-characters of the male and sexual drive. Integrity of seminal vesicles, Prostates, epidiymis, testis and cowpers glands are maintained by these drugs. Ths use of Spematone syrup and tablets occasionally overcome the nervous manifestations, some time observed in old people and which are analogous to menopausal syndrome of women. For their protein anabolic effect the drugs are used in both male and female to increase weight in wasting diseases.Both the drugs are rejuvinator and tonic of high potency which induces health vigour also. Thus the drug restores a fertile semen profile, stimulates libido, increases erectile power, improved sexual drive, enhances sexual satisfaction, and protects from fatiguability.

Product Name : **ANGUR SALSA LIQUID**

Composition : Each 29 ml of fluid contains the Extract of:

Vitis vinifera (Munakka)	3 g.
Hemidesmus indicus(Anantamul)	2 g.
Andropogon muricatus (Ushir)	2 g.
Saussurea lappa (Kustha)	1 g.
Sphaeranthus hirtus (Gorakmundi)	1 g.
Fumaria parviflcra(Pittapapra)	1 g.
Acacia catechu (Khadir)	1 g.
Santalum pterocarpus (Rakta chandan)	1 g.
Acacia arabica (Babul)	1 g.

Dosage : Adults : 2 teaspoonfuls thrice daily after meals. Children:- ½to 1 teaspoonful thrice daily after meals or as directed by physician.

How Supplied:Bottles of 225 ml.

Uses : Poor appetite, Mental and Physical stress condition, Fatigue, Wasting diseases, Nutritional defects and anaemia.

Pharmacological Action :Angursalsa is valuable general tonic of high potency for all ages with an improved feeling of physical and mental vigour. The drug raises the serum protein level and increases the body weight and prevents effect of age. The drug is demulcent, cooling, laxative and useful in thirst, heat of the body, cough, hoarseness, consumption and wasting diseases. It augments intake and promotes haemopoesis and is a purifer of blood.

Product Name : **BLOOD VIGOUR LIQUID**

Composition : Each 29 ml. of fluid contains the Extract of:

Hemidesmus indicus (Anantamol)	3.3 g.
Cassia Tora (Chakramarda)	0.6 g.
Melia azedarach (Nimba)	0.6 g.
Psoralea corylifolia (Bakuchi)	0.3 g.
Acacia catechu (Khadir)	1.0 g.
Smilax china (Chobchini)	0.2 g.
Cocculus cordifolius (Gulancha)	0.3 g.

Dosage : Adults: 2-3 teaspoonfuls thrice daily with water after meals.Children : 5 to 30 drops thrice daily with water after meals or as directed by the physician.

How Supplied: Bottles of 225 ml.

UsesItching, Dermatitis, Urticaria, Pemphigus, Scabies, Eczema, Furuculosis, Decolourised skin, Seborrhoeic, Foul sores, Acne vulgaris, Dermatitis.

Pharmacological Action :Blood vigour is deobstruent, resolvent and alexiparmic.It is regarded s purifier of blood and lymph. It has a specific effect on the arterioles of the subcapillary plexuses which are dilated by increased flow of plasma and acts against the skin streptococci. The melanoblasts are stimulated leading to pigment formation of the skin. It exhibits a selective activity against parasitic and fungus infections of the skin. It is also a valuable wound healing agent and soothing preparation for wound, vlcers and dermatoses. It helps to produce a clear granulating wound base necessary for normal repair of tissues and overcome some retarding factors to wound healing.Also, it makes all the cannals, vessels and pores clean and regulated. It has a nutritious and soothing effect upon the circulatory and cutaneous system.

Product Name : **DIARON TABLET**

Composition : Each tablet contains:

Saxifraga ligulata(Pashanbheda)	30 mg.
Crataeva nurvala (Barun)	30 mg.
Cyperus rotundus (Nagarmootha)	30 mg.
Lauha Bhasma (Calcined iron)	20 mg.
Hygrophila spinosa (Gokshura)	30 mg.
Banga bhasma (Calcined tin)	20 mg.
Silajit purified (Asphaltum)	30 mg.
Santalum album (Swet-chandan)	30 mg.

Suvarna makshik bhasma (Iron sulphur compound)	10 mg.
Cubeba officinalis (Kabab chini)	30 mg.
Achyranthes aspera (Apamarga)	30 mg.
Balsamodendron mukul (Guggul)	30 mg.

Dosage : Adults: 2 tablets thrice daily with water after meals. Children (6 to 12 years):-1tablet thrice daily after meals or as directed by the physician.

How Supplied:Container of 100 tablets.

Uses: Genito-urinary affections,Phospaturia, Albuminuria,Haematuria, Urinary, Calculi retention of urine, Strangury, Dysuria, Burning sensation during micturation.

Pharmacological Action :Daron tablet has got a highly, anti inflammatory and antisuppurative properties on acute, sub-acute, and chronic inflamatory condition affecting the glomerulia and tubules of the kidney and other parts of genito-urinary tract also. It is beneficial in phosphaturia, albuminuria and crystalluria, where cast albumin and phosphate diminishes. The drug is effective in removing crystals from ureter and urinary bladder.It also improves the tone of the urinary bladder post operatively.The drug has also exhibited beneficial effect in early obstructive uropathy and neurogenic bladder.It has also been used beneficially to control different symptoms produced by various urinary tract infections. Diaron tablet is effective in the treatment of Nephritis and Nephrosis due to allergic manifestation by the system which become sensitised against the streptococcal toxin. The drug induced diuresis in these diseases. Besides relief in oedema, the patients also show over all improvement.

Product Name : **DYSENTROLIN LIQUID**

Composition : Each 29 ml of fluid contains the Extract of:

Halarrhena anti dysenterica (Kurchi)	2.16 g.
Acacia arabica (Babul)	1.44 g.
Terminalia arjuna(Arjuna)	0.77 g.
Gmelina arborea(Gambhari)	0.45 g.
Eugenia jambolana (Jamun)	0.18 g.
Aegle marmelos (Belgiri)	0.18 g.
Symlocos racemosa(Lodhar)	0.18 g.
Mangifera indica(Amrabeej)	0.18 g.
Emblica officinalis (Amla)	0.54 g.

Pterocarpus santalinus (Rakta chandan)	0.36 g.
Oryza sativa (Lal chawal)	0.18 g.
Cyperus rotundus (Nagar mootha)	1.01 g.

Dosage **:**Adults: 2-3 teaspoonfuls three or four times daily after meals. Children: ½ to 1 teaspoonful three or four time daily after meals or as prescribed by the physician.

How Supplied: 112 ml.

Uses It is valuable remedy in acute and chronic Amobic dysentery with alternate. Diarrhoea and Constipation, Sprue, Colitis, Dyspepsia.

Pharmacological Action : Amoebiasis is a widely prevalant disease particularly in tropical sub-tropical and temperate climates. The protozoa primarily invades the colonic wall, causing ulceration and then may be carried by blood stream to the liver, lungs, brains etc., to form metastatic abscess. Thus the infection may exist mainly in the bowel as intestinal phase or may affect other organs of the body outside the coion and exists as tissus phase.

Our dysentrolin is a well known remedy for the treatment of dysentery both acute and chronic. It acts by virtue of the alkaoid Kurchicine which has a specific lethal action on entamoeba hystolytica. It is effective only on the intestinal phase of the parasites and eradicates vegetative and cystic forms probably by destroying the trophozoites which are the source of the cysts. The drug is valuable in spastic or chronic dysentery with alternate diarrhoea or constipation. It is therefore used in mucous diarrhoea, during convalescence from dysentery and early stage of sprue. The drug also shows marked spasmolytic effect against various spasmogens on gastro intestinal tract.

Product Name : **FEMELIN LIQUID**

Composition : Each 29 ml. of fluid contains the Extract of:

Dashamul (Tenroots)	6.00 g.
Asparagus racemosus (Shatamuli)	2.00 g.
Withania somnifera (Ashwagandha)	2.00 g.
Ipomoea digitat(Bidarikand)	2.00 g.
Tacca aspera (Barahikand)	2.00 g.
Bombax malabaricum (Rakta shalmali)	2.00 g.
Hemidesmus indicus (Anantamul)	2.00 g.
Moschus moschiferus (Kasturi)	0.25.g
Lactus (Milk)	2.00 g.
Berberis aristata (Daruharidra)	6.00 g.

Dosage : Adult:2-3 teapoonfuls thrice daily after meals or as directed by the physician.

How Supplied: Bottles of 225 ml.

Uses Anorexia, malnutrition during pregnancy, Mallactation after delivery, Under developed breasts, Puerperal infection, Disorders associated with pregnancy.

Pharmacological Action : Pregnancy, child birth and lactation are physiological process during which adequate nutrition is essential for the normal development of the foetus as well as the mother. Nutritional life of an infant actually begins in the pregnancy period of the mother and is influenced by the diet of the mother during pregnancy and her status of nutrition to the mother during antenatal and postnatal period and established the nutritional link between the mother and the child. Femelin promotes lactation by stimulating the secretion of prolaction hormone from anterior pituitary. It also increases the weight of mammary glands during pregnancy and exhibits well developed lobuloalveolar tissue with milk secretion. Femelin promotes appetite and digestion improving the general health of the mother.

Product Name : **GREEN PUNARNAWA LIQUID**

Composition : Each 29 ml. of flurid contains the extract of:

Boerhavia diffusa (Punarnawa)	3.6 g.
Hygrophila spinosa (Gokhru)	0.6 g.
Glaega purpurea (Sarapunkha)	0.3 g.
Santalum Album (Swet chandan)	0.6 g.
Curcuma longa (Haridra)	0.3 g.
Cassia lanceolata (Swarna patri)	0.3 g.
Premna integrifolia (Kamika)	0.3 g.
Oxides of iron (Mandur bhasma)	0.62 g.
Moringa oleifera(Sajina)	0.3 g.
Crataeva-religiosa(Barun)	1.9 g.

Dosage : Adults: 2 teaspoonfuls thrice daily after meals. Children : 5 to 30 drops thrice daily after meals, or as advised by the physician.

How Supplied: Bottles of 225 ml. and 450 ml.

Uses Anasarca, Ascites, Elargement and obstruction of liver, Hepatitis, Jaundice, Nephritis, Strangury, renal infection and insufficiency, Affection of joints and the gouty painful condition.

Pharmacological Action : One of the active principle of green punarnawa is punarnavine. There are also large quantities of potassium intake and other potassium salts present in this plant. The diuresis is mainly due to the action of the alkaloids on the glomeruli of the kidneys throughs the heart, increasing the beat and strength and raising the peripheral blood and strength and raising the peripheral blood pressure in consequence. In case of peritoneal and kideny conditions, the drug appears to be very beneficial. The drug is found to be useful in the treatment of nephrotic syndrome. Besides relief in oedema, patients also show overall improvement, such as decrease in albuminuria, rise in serum protein and fall in serum cholesterol level. It induces a very marked and persistent diuresis. The drug exhibits anti-inflammatory activity on oedema and areritis. The alkaloids of the drug significantly inhibit the increase serum aminotransferase activity in arthritic patients. It also increases liver A.T.P. phosphohydrolase activity.

The drug produces anti-infective and anti inflammatory effect in acute inflammatory condition of the urinary passage and deep seated inflammation of liver. It is found to stimulate bile flow by acting as a hydrocholagogue. Absolute values for the entire period of choleresis indicates an increases in total excretion of bile salts, bilirubin and cholesterol. Also by virtue of choleresis property, the drug normalises the jaundice.

Product Name : **GASTODIN TABLETS**

Composition : Each tabelt contains :

Embelia ribes (Biranga)	30 mg.
Zingiber officinale (Sunta)	50 mg.
Cuminum (Safed jeera)	40 mg.
Aegle marnelos (Bel)	65 mg.
Feaula asafoetida purified (Hingu)	20 mg.
Gastropoda calcined (Shankha bhasma)	35 mg.
Triphala (Amla Harra, Bahera)	60 mg.
Ptychotis ajowan (Jowan)	50 mg.

Dosage :Adults : 2 tablets thrice daily after meals. Children : (6 to 12 years) : - 1 tablet thrice daily after meals or as directed by the physician.

How Supplied:Container of 100 tablets.

Uses: Acid dyspepsia, Heart-burn, Nausea epigastric pain, Gastric flatulence, Constipation and digestive disorders.

Pharmacological Action : Gastric secretion is controlled by vagus which contains the secretary fibres, two sets of nerves control the movements of the stomach viz. The vagus or augmentor, stimulation of which causes contraction, and the sympathetic or inhibitor, stimulation of which causes relaxation fo the stomach and of its movement. Hyperchlorhydria is common in patient suffering from gastric syndromes. These are treated by gastric antacid. As a gastric antacid our gastodin tablets are beneficial in gastric syndrome due to hyperchlorhydria with burning sensation in abdominal and cardiac region and epigastric pain are benefitted. It also possess carminative and spasmolytic acitvity on gastro intestinal tract. It regulates secretion of enzymes promoting digestion, corrects constipation and removes flatus from the alimentary tract. It seems to remove the irritating effect of acid, in a better way than alkali. Being a very efficient absorbent, the drug is used for absorption of bacteria and toxins from the intestine thus preventing their absorption.

Product Name **:JWARANTIKA LIQUID**

Composition : Each 29 ml. of fluid contains the extract of:

Cocculus cordifolius (Gulandcha)	2.00 g.
Swertia chirata (Chirata)	2.00 g.
Andrographis paniculata(Kalmegh)	2.00 g.
Alstonia scholaris (Saptaparna)	2.00 g.
Capparis corundas (Karando)	2.00 g.
Crinum asiaticum (Sudarshan)	1.00 g.
Ipomoea turpethum (Trivrit)	2.00 g.
Boerhavia diffusa (Punarnava)	2.00 g.
Nyctanthes Arbortristis (Shefalika)	2.00 g.

Dosage :Adult: 2 teaspoonfuls four times daily after meals or as prescribed by the physician. Children: ½ to 1 teaspoonfuls four times daily after measl or as prescribed by the physician.

How Supplied: 112 ml.

Uses : For the prevention and treatment of malaria with enlarged liver and spleen, Influenza, and other tropical levers.

Pharmacological Action : Jwarnatika has a reputation of being anti perodic and is used for the purpose in chronic malaria fever and other fevers. The action of drug in Malaria is very satisfactory. In cases of malaria, in all of which it causes the temperature to fall steadily to normal in a short-time. No excessive perspiration and over exhaustion of the patient are induced. The drug also seems to produce good effect in cases where the catarrhal condition of the mucous temparature. It is shown that it exercises no synergistic action on quinine. The drug however, is of value as febrifuge.

Product Name : **LECORIN NO.-1 LIQUID**

Composition: Each 29 ml. of fluid contains the extract of:

Prunus puddum (Padmakastha)	1.13 g.
Sida cordifolia (Bala)	1.13 g.
Vitis vinifera (munakka)	0.4 g.
Aegle marmelos (Belgiri)	0.4 g.
Uncaria gambier (Khadir)	0.4 g.
Hemidesmus indicus (Anantamool)	0.2 g.
Hibiscus rosa sinensis (Jabakusum)	0.2 g.
Berberis aristata(Darhaldi)	0.2 g.
Kernel of mangifera indica (Amrasthi)	0.2 g.
Diospyros embryopteris (Gab)	1.00 g.
Crocus sativus (Kesar)	0.2 g.

Dosage **:**Adults: 2 teaspoonfuls three or four times daily after meals or as directed by the physician.

How Supplied: Bottles of 225 ml. and 450 ml.

Uses: Stops non-specific leucorrhoea of actute phase, Checks functional uterine bleeding, corrects antifertility caused by leucorrhoea.

Pharmacological Action: Lecorn 1 restores the normal P.H. of the vaginal canal by virtue of its antibacterial effect and astringent action on the vaginal cannal, cervix, uterus and fallopian tube, reduces the vaginal discharge. It increases appetite and digestive power improving general debility of the patient suffering from non specific leucorrhoea of acute phase. It also improves endocrinal functions.

Product Name : **VASAKSAR LIQUID**

Composition : Each 29 ml of fluid contains the extract of:

Adhatoda vasika (Vasak)	4.00 g.
Vitis vinifera (Munakka)	3.00 g.
Glycyrrhiza glabra (Yastimadhu)	0.60 g.
Asparagus racemosus (Shatavar)	0.60 g.
terminalia arjuna (Arjuna)	0.60 g.
Ocimum sanctum (Tulasi)	0.15 g.
Myrtus caryophyllus (Lavang)	0.15 g.
Piper Longum (Pipul)	0.15 g.
Acorus calamus (Bach)	1.00 g.

Dosage : Adults: 2 teaspoonfuls thrice daily after meals Children : ½ to 1 teaspoonful thrice daily after meals or as directed by the physician.

How Supplied: Bottles of 112 ml.

Uses: Cold, Cough (productive, unproductive, Irritant and allergic), Catarrh, Pharyngitis, Laryngitis, Tracheo bronchitis and Bronchitis.

Pharamcological Action : Vasaka is a stimulant expectorant and bronchial antispasmodic. It is an effective remedy for distressing cough in chronic bronchitis, phthisis and bronchial asthma. It acts by virtue of vasicine which relaxes the bronchial muscles by depressing the vagus endings. It is frequently used in mild pertussis especially when complicates with bronchitis. It is a reliable remedy for cold cough and catarrh.

HIMALYA DRUG CO. (THE)
Makali, Bangalore - 562123
Tel - 8394855, 8396684, 8397823, Fax - (80) 8396057

Product Name : **BONNISAN LIQUID**

Composition : Each 5 ml ocntails:Dill oil 0.0018 ml. plus 0.5 mg. of each of the following significant extracts: Tinospora cordifolia, Piper longum, Cichorium intybus, terminalia chebula, Achillea millefolium Tribulus terrestris, Capparis spinosa, emblica officinalis Cassia occidentalis, Elettaria cardamomum, Tamarix gallica, Boerhaavia diffusa.

Dosage : ¼-3 teaspoonful, 3-4 times a day.

How Supplied: 120 ml.

Uses Digestive complaints (Infants & children)

Product Name : **CYSTONE TABLETS**

Composition :

Extract of Didymocarpus Pedicellata	65 mg.
Saxifraga ligulata	49 mg.
Rubia cordifolia	16 mg.
Cyperus scariosus	16 mg.
Achyranthes aspera	16 mg.
Onosma bracteatum	16 mg.
Vernonia cinerea	16 mg.
Powders of Shilajeet (Purified)	13 mg.
Hajrul yahood bhasma	16 mg.

Dosage : Initially 2 tablets twice daily followed by 1 tablets twice daily or as directed by the physician.

Product Name : **DIAREX TABLETS**

Composition :Activated carbon made from Holarrhena anti-

Dysenterica	0.24 g.
Symplocos racemosa	80 mg.
Helicteres isora	60 mg.
Powder of Pavonia odorata	40 mg.
Punica granatum rind	0.10 g.
Shorea robusta resin	40 mg.
Butea frondosa resin	40 mg.

Dosage : 1-2 tablets, 2-3 times a day

How Supplied: 100 tabs.

Uses Amoebic dysentry

Product Name : **GASEX TABLETS**

Composition :

Aconitum palmatum	65 mg.
Piper nigrum	19 mg.
Cowrie bhasma	32 mg.
Shankh bhasma	32 mg.
Extract Embelia ribes	22 mg.
Triphala	22 mg.
Zingiber officinale	22 mg.

Dosage : 2 tablets twice daily.

How Supplied: 100 tabs.

Uses: For the control of Indigestion, Feeling of fullness, Dyspesia, Nausea, Fiatulence, Hyper acidity.

Product Name : **GERIFORTE TABLETS**

Composition : Each 5 ml. contains:

Chyavan prash conc.	100 mg.
Shilajeet (Purified)	20 mg.
Crocus sativus	7 mg.
Exts. Capparis spinosa	13.8 mg.
Cichorium intybus ext.	13.8 mg
Solanum nigrum ext.	6.4 mg.
Cassia occidentails ext.	3.2 mg.
Terminalia arjuna ext.	6.4 mg.
Achillea millefolium ext.	3.2 mg.
Tamarix gallica ext.	3.2 mg.
Mandur bhasma	5 mg.

Makardhwaj	10 mg.
Asparagus Adscendens	10 mg.
Caesalpinia digyna	10 mg.
Asparagus racemosus	20 mg.
Withania somnifera	30 mg.
Glycyrrhiza glabra	20 mg.
Centella asistica	20 mg.
Terminalia chebula	15 mg.
Mucuna pruriens	10 mg.
Myristica fragrans(mace)	10 mg.
Piper longum	10 mg.
Syzygium aromaticum	5 mg.
Elettaria cardamomum	5 mg.
Carum copticum	5 mg.
Curcuma longa	5 mg.
Ext. Berberis aristata	10 mg.
Ext. Adhatoda vasica	10 mg.
Eclipta alba	10 mg.
Celastrus paniculatus	5 mg.
Argyreia speciosa	10 mg.
Abhrak bhasma	10 mg.
Loh bhasma	5 mg.
Jasa bhasma	10 mg.

Dosage : 2 tablets 2-3 times a day.

How Supplied: 100 tabs.

Uses For anxiety neurosis and Health supplements.

Product Name : **HERBOLAX TABLETS**

Composition :

Extract Ipomoea turpethum	70 mg.
Terminalia chebula	50 mg.
Cichorium intybus	50 mg.
Cassia occidentalis	50 mg.
Solanum nigrum	40 mg.
Glycyrrhiza glabra	40 mg.
Powders of zigniber officinale	45 mg.
Embelia ribes	10 mg.

Dosage : Adults : 2 or 3 tablets ½ an hour before dinner with warm water. The Dosage is best individualized.

How Supplied: 100 tabs.

Uses Corrects chronic constipation gently (Not a pergative)

Product Name : **LIV. 52 SYRUP**

Composition : Each 5 ml. contains:

Extract of Capparis spinosa	34 mg.
Cichorium intybus	34 mg.
Solanum nigrum	16 mg.
Terminalia arjuna	16 mg.
Cassia occidentails	8 mg.
Achillea millefolium	8 mg.
tamarix gallica	8 mg.

Dosage : Children: ½ teaspoonful twice a day Adults: 1 ½ teaspooful twice a day.

How Supplied: 100 ml. 200 ml.

Uses : Protects the liver against various hepatotoxins. Corrects liver dysfunction and damage Promotes appetite of growth.

Product Name : **LIV. 52 TABLETS**

Composition : Each contains powder of:

Capparis spinosa	65 mg.
Cichorium intybus	65 mg.
Solanum nigrum	32 mg.
Terminalia arjuna	32 mg.
Cassia occidentalis	16 mg.
Achillea millefolium	16 mg.
tamarix gallica	16 mg.
Mandur bhasma	33 mg.

Dosage : 2 to 3 tablets three or four times a day. Children: 1 to 2 tablets

How Supplied: 100 tabs.

Uses: Protect the liver against various hepatotoxins corrects liver dysfunctinand damage. Promotes apetite and growth.

Product Name : **LUKOL DS TABLETS**

Composition :

Extract of Woodfordia fruticosa	80 mg.
Astercantha longifolia	80 mg
Asparagus racemosus	80 mg.
Rauwolfia serpentina	40 mg.
Boerhaavia diffusa	20 mg.

Adhatoda vasica	20 mg.
& Powders of: Areca catechu	40 mg.
Myristica fragrans	32 mg.
Elettaria cardamomum	22 mg.
Mesua ferrea	22 mg.
Cuminum cyminum	20 mg.
Santalum album	20 mg.
Shilajeet (Purified)	18 mg.
Praval bhasma	14 mg.
Aegle marmelos	10 mg.
Zingiber officinale	10 mg.
Triphala 10 mg.,Piper nigrum	10 mg.
Balsamodendron mukul	10 mg.
Loh bhasma	10 mg.
trivang	10 mg.
Butea frondosa (Gum)	8 mg.

Dosage : 2 tablets twice daily followed by 1 tablet twice daily or as directed by the physician.

Product Name : **ABANA TABLETS**

Composition : Each contains Ext. of

Terminalia arjuna	30 mg.
Withania somnifera	20 mg.
Tinospora cordifolia	10 mg.
Nepeta hindostana	20 mg.
Emblica officinalis	10 mg.
Terminalia chebula	10 mg.
Dashamoola	20 mg.
Eclipta alba	10 mg.
Glycyrrhiza glabra	10 mg.
Asparagus racemosus	10 mg.
Boerhaavia diffusa	10 mg.
Powders of centella asiatica	10 mg.
Convolvulus pluricaulis	10 mg.
Ocimum sanctum	10 mg.
Nardostachys jatamansi	10 mg.
Cyperus rotundus	5 mg.
Acorus calamus	5 mg.
Embebelia ribes	5 mg.
Piper longum	10 mg.

Carum copticum	10 mg.
Zingiber offcinale	10 mg.
Syzygium aromaticum	5 mg.
Celastrus paniculatus	5 mg.
Santalura album	5 mg.
Elettaria cardamomum	5 mg.
Foeniculum vulgare	5 mg.
Rosa damacena	5 mg.
Cinnamomum cassia	5 mg.
Crocus sativus	2 mg.
Shilajeet (Purified)	20 mg.
Jaharmohra	10 mg
Shankha bhasma	10 mg
Makardhwaj	10 mg.
Abhrak bhasma	5 mg.
Pearl pishti	5 mg.
Agate pishti	5 mg.
Jade pishti	5 mg.
Ruby pishti	5 mg.
Coral pishti	5 mg.

Dosage : 1-2 tablets, 2-3 times a day.

Uses Angina pectoris, Cardiac arrhythmias, Cardiac neurosis, Hyper lipidaemia, Hyper tension. Ischaemic heart disease, Post myocardial infarction, Tachycardias.

Product Name : **DIABECON TABLETS**

Composition :Each contains Ext. each of:

Gymnema sylvestro	30 mg.
Pterocarpus marsupium	20 mg.
Glycyrrhiza glabra	20 mg.
Casearica esculenta	20 mg.
Eugenia jambolana	20 mg.
Asparagus racemosus	20 mg.
Boerhaavia diffusa	20 mg.
Sphaeranthus indicus	10 mg
Tinospora cordifolia	10 mg
Swertia chirata	10 mg
Tribulus terrestris	10 mg
Phyllanthus amarus	10 mg
Gmelina arborea	10 mg.

Gossypium herbaceum	10 mg.
Berberis aristata	5 mg.
Aloe vera	5 mg.
Triphala	3 mg.
Powder each of:	
Balsamodendron mukul (purified)	30 mg.
Shilajeet (Purified)	30 mg.
Vidangadi lauham	27 mg.
Momordica charantia	20 mg.
Piper nigrum	10 mg.
Ocimum sanctum	10 mg.
Abutilon indicum	10 mg.
Curcuma longa	10 mg.
Abhrak bhasma	10 mg.
Praval bhasma	10 mg.
Rumex martimus	5 mg.
Vang bhasma	5 mg.
Akik Pishti	5 mg.
Shingraf	5 mg.
Yashad bhasma	5 mg.
Trikuta	5 mg.

Processed in ficus racemosa, Acacia arabica, Areca catechu, withania somnifera, valeriana wallichi, Oroxylum indicum, Santalum album, zingiber officinale, Eugenia jambolana)

Product Name : **KOFLET SYRUP**

Composition : Each 5 ml. contains:

Meldes pumatum (purified)	1.25 g.
Balsamodendron mukul (Purified)	35 mg.
Extract each of : Vitis vinifera	35 mg.
Ociumum sanctum	25 mg.
Hyssopus officinalis	25 mg.
Tinospora cordifolia	20 mg.
Adhatoda vasica	15 mg.
Myristica fragrans	15 mg.
Glycyrrhiza glabra	15 mg.
Onosma bracteatum	10 mg.
Viola odorata	10 mg.
Triphala	9 mg.
Trikatu	9 mg.
Embelia ribes	8 mg.

Solanum xanthocarpum	8 mg.
Cinnamomum cassia	8 mg.
Navasagara	3 mg.

(Proceed in Onosma bracteatum, Malva sylvestris, Zizyphus sativa, fagonia cretica, ptychotis ajowan)

Dosage **:**Adults: 1-2 teaspoonful, 2-3 times a day. Children: ½-1teaspoonful, 2-3 times a day.

How Supplied: 100 ml.

Uses: For cough.

Product Name **:MENTAT TABLETS**

Composition : Each contains Ext. each of:

Bacopa monnieri	136 mg.
Centella asiatica	70 mg.
Withania somnifera	52 mg.
Evolvulus alsinoides	52 mg.
Nardostachys jatamansi	52 mg.
Valeriana wallichii	50 mg.
Embelia ribes	50 mg.
Prunus amygadalus	50 mg.
Acorus calamus	42 mg.
Tinospora cordifolia	36 mg.
terminalia chebula	36 mg.
Embilica officinalis	36 mg.
Celastrus paniculatus	32 mg.
Powders of:	
Bacopa monnieri	80 mg.
Orchis mascula	18 mg.
Mucuna pruriens	18 mg.
Elettaria pruriens	18 mg.
Terminalia arjuna	18 mg.
Foeniculum vulgare	18 mg.
Ipomoea digitata	18 mg.
Zingiber officinale	14 mg.
Terminalia belerica	14 mg.
Myristica fragrans	14 mg.
Syzygium aromaticum	10 mg.
Mukta pishti	3 mg.

Dosage **:** 2 tablets,2 times a day.

How Supplied: 50 tabs.

Uses: Amnesia, Anti convulsive therapy, Behavioural disorder, enuresis, Hyperkintetic states, Memory disturbances, Psychiatric problems, Speech defects, Stress.

Product Name : **PILEX OINTMENT**

Composition :

Mimosa pudica extract	5%
Vitex negundo extract	3%
Calendula officinalis ext.	2%
Eclipta alba extract	3%
Tankana	1%
Yashad bhasma	1%,2%
Cinnamomum camphora	1.225%
Base q.s. ad.	100%

Dosage: Ointument to be applied locally 1-2 times a day before and after evacuation.

How Supplied: 28 g.

Uses: Anal fissures, Anal fistulae, Harmorrhoids, Proctitis, Thrombophlebitis, varicocele Varicosity, Venous stasis.

Product Name : **RUMALLAYA TABLETS**

Composition :Each contains powders of:

Mahayograj guggual	0.162 g.
Shilajeet (Purified)	16 mg.
Swarna makshik bhasma	5 mg.
Shankh bhasma	65 mg.
Hibiscus abelmoschus	10 mg.
Extracts of Maharasnadi quath	65 mg.
Moringa pterygosperma	16 mg.
Rubia cordi-folia	19 mg.
Tinospora cordifolia	10 mg.
Tribulus terrestris	16 mg.

Dosage : 1-2 tablets, 2-3 times a day.

How Supplied:100 tabs.

Uses: Ankylostomiasis,Akylosing spondylosis arthalgia, Cervical spondylitis, Physicial & mental exhaustion, Fibrositis, Frozen shoulders, Gout, Infective polyarthritis, lumbar spondylosis, Neuralgia, Osteoarthritis.

Product Name : **SEPTILIN TABLETS**

Composition : Each contains powders of:

Balsamodendron mukul	0.162 g.
Shankh bhasma	32 mg.
Extract officinalis emblica	16 mg.
Extract maharasnadi quath	65 mg.
Extract Tinospora cordifolia	49 mg.
Extract Rubia cordifolia	32 mg.
Extract Moringa pterygosperma	16 mg.
Extract Glycyrrhiza glabra	6 mg.

Dosage : 2 tablets, 2-3 times a day.

How Supplied: 100 tabs.

UsesAcne vulgaris, Allergic rhinitis, Aphthous stomatitis, Boils, Carbuncle, common cold, Infractable dermatoses, Eczema fistula, Furuncolosis Health supplement, Infections, mastoiditis, Nasal catarrh, Offerhoea, pyoderma, Recurrent infections, Tonsillitis, Upper respiratory tract infections wounds.

Product Name : **SPEMAN TABLETS**

Composition : Each contains powders each of:

Orchis mascula	130 mg.
Astercantha longifolia	64 mg.
Lactuca scariola	32 mg.
Mucuna pruriens	32 mg.
Suvarnavang	32 mg.
Extracts each of:	
Argyreia speciosa	64 mg.
Tribulus terrestris	64 mg.
Leptadenia reticulata	64 mg.
Parmelia perlata	32 mg.

Dosage : 2 tablets, 2-3 times a day.

How Supplied: 60 tabs.

UsesMale infertility due to oligozoospermia, Prostatic enlargement.

Product Name : **SPEMAN FORTE TABLETS**

Composition : Each contains powders of:

Orchis mascula	39 mg.
Astercantha longifolia	19 mg.
Lactuca scariola	10 mg.
Mucuna pruriens	10 mg.

Mosaic gold	10 mg.
Extracts of:	
Argyreia speciosa	19 mg.
Tribulus terrestris	19 mg.
Leptadenia reticulata	19 mg.
Parmelia perlata	10 mg.

Dosage : 1-2 tablets, 2-3 times a day.

How Supplied: 100 tabs.

Uses: Habitual masturbation, Nocturnal emmisions, Premature ejaculation, Senile sex aberrations, Spermatorrhoea.

Product Name : **STYPLON TABLETS**

Composition : Each contains powders each of:

Chandrakala rasa	0.26 g.
Emblica offcinalis	130 mg.
Praval bhasma	130 mg.
Mesua ferrea	64 mg.
Ruta graveloens	32 mg.
Boerhaavia diffusa salts	12 mg.
Lapis lazuli bhasma	32 mg.
Raphanus sativus salts	12 mg.

(Proceed in Melia azadirachta, Acorus calamus, Spaeranthus indica, Mimosa pudica, Berberis aristat, Alpinia officinarum, Cynodon dactylon, Nalumbium speciosum, Furmaria officinalis, asparagus recemosus.

Dosage : 2-3 tablets, 3 times a day.

How Supplied: 25 tabs

Uses: Bleeding gums, Bleeding piles, Epistaxis,Gastro intestinal bleeding, Haematemesis Hacmaturia intra uterine bleeding, Post operative haemorrhage, Traumatic bleeding.

Product Name : **TENTEX FORTE TABLET**

Composition : Each contains Extracts of :

Hibiscus abelmoschus	10 mg.
Powders of: Withania somnifera	65 mg.
Argyreia speciosa	32 mg.
Mucuna pruriens	32 mg.
Trivang	32 mg.
Shilajeet (Purfied)	32 mg.
Crocus sativus	25 mg.
Strychnos nux vomica (detoxified)	16 mg.

Makardhwaj	16 mg.
Orchis mascula	16 mg.
Anacyclus pyrethrum	16 mg.
Sida cordifolia	16 mg.
Bombax malabaricum	16 mg.
Piper nigrum	5 mg.

Dosage : 2 tablets 2 times a day chewed and with milk or tea.

How Supplied: 10 tabs.

Uses: Cardiac failure, Chronic renal diseases, Arterio sclerosis, Sexual weakness (men).

HIMANI LIMITED

13, B.T. Road, Calcutta-700056 Tel -5530035, 5531509, 5531621
Fax - (133/033) 2480756/5821/2773

Product Name : **BAL GOPAL BABY MASSAGE OIL**

Composition : Each 100 ml. contains:

Aswagandha	0.6 g.
Raktachandana	0.5 g.
Haridra	0.5 g.
Daruharidra	0.4 g.
Anantmool	0.4 g.
Nirgundi	0.4 g.
Shalaparni	0.4 g.
Prishniparni	0.4 g.
Mudgaparni	0.4 g.
Manjistha	0.3 g.
Mashaparni	0.4 g.
Nimba	0.3 g.
Bala	0.3 g.
Atibala	0.1 g.
Sura	0.5 mlts

Product Name : **BABY CARE TONIC**

Composition : Each 5 ml. contains:

Yestimadhu	300 mg.
Guduchi	30 mg.
Ativisa	20 mg.
Vidanga	100 mg.
Haritaki	50 mg.

Product Name : **CHYAWANPRASH PLUS SEMISOLID**

Composition : Each 100 g.contanis:Aqueous extract of : 0.16 each of Agnimantha, Shyonaka, Shalaparni, Haritaki, Vidarikand, Bala,Mudgaparni, Jivanti, Patala, Shati, Bilva, Gambhari, Musta, Punarnava, Prisniparni, Mashaparni, 0.04 g. each of Pippali, goksura, Brihati, Kantakari, Draksa.0.01g. each of Sringi, Bhumyamalaki, Jeevaka, Risabhaka, Riddhi, Ela, Kakoli, Raktachandan, Utpala,Kakanasa, vansalochana, Meda;0.1gm each of Puskara, Aguru; 0.08 g. each of Guduchi,Vasamula;0.35 g. each of Brahmi, Shankhapushpi, Vacha, Jyotimati, Arjun; 0.1 g each of Ghrita, Til tails; Aromatic powders of Pippali 0.55 g., 0.5 gm each of Tvak , Ela,Patra, Nagkeshara; Amlaki pisti 24 g.,

Madhu 0.05 g., Svarna makshik bhasma 0.1 g., 0.1 g. each of Makaradhwaja, Praval bhasmam,Mukta bhasma; Abhrak bhasma 0.02 g., Apple juice Conc 0.05 g., Chhuhara 2 mg., Sura 0.5 ml.

Product Name : **LAL DANT POWDER**

Composition :

Lavanga ka tel	8%
Pudina satva	0.12%
Kapoor	4%
Tomar beej	3%
Babul, Bakul, Vacha, Neem	1% each
Khatika	3%
Tambaku, Pippali, March, Sunthi	6% each
Swarna gairik	0.7% v/w

Product Name : **MEMO PLUS SYRUP**

Composition : Each 5 ml. contains:

Evolvulus alsinoides	400 mg.
Acorus calamus	400 mg.
Glycyrrhiza glabra	400 mg.
Centella asiatica	100 mg.
Withania somnifera	40 mg.
Nardostachys jatamansi	10 mg.
Celastrus paniculatus	10 mg.
Rauwolfia serpentina	10 mg.
Sura	0.025 ml.

Product Name : **SARDIJA INHALER**

Composition :

Pudina satva	30 %
Nilgiri tel	13 %
Gaultheria tel	10 %
Pudina tel	12 %
Karpoor	16 %

Product Name : **SARDIJA COUGH SYRUP**

Composition : Each 5 ml. contains:

Vasa	150 mg.
Tulsi	150 mg.
Pippli	150 mg.
Vacha	150 mg.
Kulinjan	150 mg.
Haridra	70 mg.
Kantakari	70 mg.
Yestimadhu	70 mg.
Kasmard	70 mg.
Somlata	70 mg.
Kayphal	70 mg.
Tejpatra	20 mg.
Lavanga	5 mg
Nvasadar	20 mg.
Pudina	2.5 mg.
Karpoor	0.5 mg.
Madhu	0.0625 g.
Sura	0.025 ml.

Product Name : **SARDIJA VEPORIZING OINTMENT**

Composition : Each 100 g. contains:

Pudina satva	3.3 g.
Karpoor	5.25 g.
Ajowan ka phool	0.1 g.
Lavang ka tel	0.02 ml.
Tarpin tel	5.4 ml.
Adrak tel	0.03 ml.
Nilgiri tel	1.6 ml.
Jatiphala tel	0.06 ml.
Saunf tel	0.07 ml.
Dalchini tel	0.01 ml.

HINDUSTAN ANTIBIOTICS LTD ®Ayurvedic Division
Pimpri, Pune-411 018, Tel - 776511-13, 776521, 772326,
Fax-(0212) 772327

Product Name : **ISOVAC (ISABGOL) POWDER**

Composition: Each 5 g. contains:

Isabgol Psyllium Husk	3.5 g.

Product Name : **RHINAX CAPSULES**

Composition : Herbo mineral formula for Anti-stress, Adoptogenic Rejunuvinative effect.

INDIAN HERBS RESEARCH & SUPPLY CO.(P) LTD.
Post Box No. 5, Sharda Nagar, Saharanpur - 247001
Tel -725044, 725045, 725046, 725429, Fax -(0132) 726288

Veterinary Products:
Product Name : **HIMALAYAN BATISA**

Composition : Each 100. contains:

Katubhadra	0.70
Sahastravedhi	0.070
Mahaushadhu	1.00
Krishna	0.096
Yarnesta	0.50
Ushna	0.048
Katuveera	0.90
Mahishaksh	0.048
Raktapushpak	2.00
Sahastravirya	0.096
Brahamma vriksha	1.00
Utkat	0.096
Lavanajulabi	5.00
Suvarchika	0.048
Aksheev	10.00
Vidiavana	0.048
Manthapak	18.00
Katurohini	0.096
Mangalya	2.00
Dhatukasis	0.096
Amriphal	9.00
Nandini	0.096

Karshaphala	5.00
Kharamanjari	0.077
Yoshitpriya	7.12
Vritakosh	0.096
Kana	0.70
Saubhagya	0.048
Chatra	0.70
Markav	0.500
Dadim	1.50
Maktamal	0.038
Mishreya	1.00
Mridurechni	0.288
Rasayani	1.50
Tikshnagandha	0.048
Yavtikta	1.50
Peeta	0.300
Kanor	0.20
Madhura	0.192
Ramathi	1.00
Gundra	0.192
Tiktak	2.30
Avartini	0.192
Sriphala	2.00
Paravatpadi	0.192
Dipyaka	7.00
Prithupalashika	0.192
Rohini	7.00
Chitra	0.192
Deepani	3.00
Krimighna	0.230
Somraji	1.00
Siddhartha	0.192
Pandurdrum	0.96
Swetpushpa	0.480
Chakri	0.96
Katutikta	0.192
Veervraksha	0.096

Dosage : Cows, Buffaloes, Horses and Mules	40-60 g.
Calves, Foals, Heifers and Pigs	20-30 gms
Sheep and Goats	10-15 g.
Camel and other large animals	80-100 gms

How Supplied: Carton-100 gms, 200 gms, 400 g. Polybag-1kg.

Uses For prevention and treatment of digestive disorders like Anorexia, Dyspepsia, Constipation etc. As an adjuvant therapy along with oral antibiotics, antibacterials, anthelmintica and other chemical drugs. As a digestive tonic to improve digestion Health an productivity.

Product Name : **H.B. STRONG**

Composition : Each 100 g. contains: (in g.)

Katubhadra	1.60 g.
Ashok	0.46 g.
Tiktak	0.90 g.
Bhuteek	0.85 g.
Amrita	0.65 g.
Bhring	0.25 g.
Shatparva	0.25 g.
Vell	0.25 g.
Purah	0.24 g.
Ushan	0.20 g.
Chapla	0.20 g.
Bahupushpi	0.90 g.
Ramsenak	0.70 g.
Hinguniryas	0.90 g.
Bahuparni	0.60 g.
Narsar	0.20 g.
Madhuparni	0.20 g.
Vasuk	0.10 g.

Dosage : Cows, Buffaloes and Horses 10 gms (one sachet) calves, Foals, Heifers and Pigs 5 gms (½ sachet) sheep and Goats:2.5 gms (¼ sachet) Administer orally twice daily for 2-4 days by mixing with feed or jaggery.

How Supplied: Disper carton containing 40x10 gms sachets Sachet 10 g.

UsesAs co-prescription along with any oral or injectable chemical medication, to maintain normal disgestive functions and as a digestive tonic during debility.

Product Name : **RUMBION BOLUS**

Composition : Each 100 g. contains:

Katubhadra	675 mg.
Mangalya	180 mg.
Chakrangi	810 mg.
Kana	135 mg.

Tiktak	540 mg.
Vrishketu	135 mg.
Yavtiktak	360 mg.
Amogha	135 mg.
Dipyaka	360 mg.
Mahishaksh	135 mg.
Jiwanti	270 mg.
Vellaj	112 mg.
Angarak	270 mg.
Upkulya	112 mg.
Mhaushadh	270 mg.

Dosage : Cows, Buffaloes and Horses 2 bolus twice daily sheep and Goats 1 bolus twice daily Rumbion should be adminstered orally with bread(roti) or gur (jaggary) for 2-4 days.

How Supplied: Carton containing 15 strips of 4 boli each strip of 4 boli

UsesSimple indigestion either Acidic or Alkaline, primary or secondary anorexia, ruminal stasis, depraved appetite, after-effects of chemical drugs treatment.

Product Name : **NEBLON**

Composition : Each 100 g. contains :(in g.)

Raktasar	3.5
Sriphala	12.00
Pandurdrum	4.00
Dadim	13.00
Tamrapushpi	7.50
Amritvallari	6.50
Peeta	7.00
Brihatpatra	6.50
Kathini	32.5
Gundra	3.5
Pichcha	1.8
Nagar	0.7
Anjwar	1.5

Dosage :Cows,Buffaloes and Horses 30-50 g. Calves, Sheep, Goats, Folas and Pigs 15-25 gms Dogs and Piglets 2-3 g.

How Supplied: Carton - 100 g., Polybag 1 kg.

Uses: Acute, Subacute or Chronic Diarrhoea and Dysentery of various aetiology; Scours, Non-specific diarrhoea; Symptomatic relief to animals suffering from R.P. and other specific diseases.

Product Name : **TIMPOL**

Composition : Each 100 g.contains :

Ramath	0.75
Dirghjeerak	1.00
Vishva	17.50
Mahaushad	5.00
Raktpushpak	2.00
Dhenuka	1.50
Chatra	1.50
Peeta	6.00
Deepya	6.00
Rohini	2.50
Sriphala	2.50
Chandrika	3.00
Madhura	4.50
Somraji	1.00
lavanjulabi	6.00
Aksheev	20.00
Manthapak	10.00
Tiktak	2.00
Krishna	2.00
Krishn	0.44
Katambhara	0.88
Golomi	1.08
Peetak	0.55
Katuveera	0.44
Markandika	0.44
Ramathi	

Dosage:

Buffaloes and Horses	80 g.
Calves, Foals and Heifers	40 g.
Pig, Sheep and Goats	20-25 g.

How Supplied: Carton - 100 g. Polybag-1kg.

Uses: Gaseous and Frothy Boat\Tympany, Colic, impaction.

Product Name : **LIVOL**

Composition : Each 100 g. contains:(in g.)

Yavtikta	7.00
Raktapushpa	6.00
Dhaval	8.00
Varuni	6.00

Markav	8.00
Ugrangandha	5.00
Rohini	10.00
Manthpak	10.00
Dadimpusphpak	6.00
Gopuadhu	7.00
Vayasi	5.00
Krishna	2.00
Katurohini	1.00
Tamalki	4.00
Vartikta	4.00
Mayurak	5.00
Pichumand	5.00
Kiratikta	1.00

Dosage :

Cows, Buffaloes and Horses	40-60 g.
Calves, foals, Heifers and Adult pigs	15-20 gms
Sheep and Goats	8-12g.

How Supplied:Carton-100 g.,Polybag-1kg.

Uses: Jaundice; Hepatitis; Debility and general weakness; toxaemia;During Convalescece; Fatty liver disease; Leg weakness; For improving feed efficiency, general health and prodction; For better livability; as an adjunct or after antibiotic/anthelmintic/chemical drugs therapy to restore normal detoxification and liver functions.

Product Name :**REPLANTA**

Composition : Each 100 g. contains (in g.)

Krishna	8.5
Ushan	4.0
Espand	5.0
Raktangi	10.0
Payasvini	8.5
Carvi	10.0
Utpal	4.0
Hattavilasini	3.0
Gundra	5.0
Yausahya	8.0
Vanspatri	2.0
Nakuli	5.0
Tundkeshi	10.0

Shakrapushpi	2.0
Paribhadra	6.0
Varuni	1.0
Dhatripatra	4.0
Naktamal	4.0

Dosage :

Cows and Buffaloes	50-60g.
Mares	30-40 g.
Ewes and Does	8-12 g.

How Supplied: Carton -100 g., Polybag-500 g.

Uses: Retained placenta; To promote involution of uterus; For improved breeding efficiency; Supporitve to manual removal;As an ideal uterine cleansing agent and tonic.

Product Name : **GALOG AND GALOG STRONG BOLUS**

Composition :Each 100 g. contains:

Galog Powder:-	
Madhustrava	20.00
Sita	23.00
Sahastravirya	10.00
Misi	6.00
Vajrangi	14.00
Gudhmool	3.00
Madhura	5.00
Sakal	3.00
Gopwadhu	5.00
Yastimadhuk	1.00
Krodkaseruk	1.00
Arista	1.00
Yavnesta	1.00
Madhuparni	1.00
Galog Strong Bolus:-	
Smrita	1.00
Kambojini	1.00
Jiwanti	1.33
Bheeru	0.66
Karvi	0.66

Dosage : Galog Strong Bolus:-

Cows and Buffaloes	3 Boli
Sows	2 Boli
Ewes and Does	1 Bolus

Galog Powder:-

Cows and Buffaloes	50 g.
Ewes and Does	10-15 g.

How Supplied: Galog Strong Bolus:-

Carton Containing 12 strips of 4 boli each.
Galog Powder:
Carton-300 g., Polybag-1kg.

Uses: To enhance the milk production in dairy cattle. To correct failure of regular lactation. Hypogalactia and agalctia. Low level of milk production in apparently healthy animals.

Product Name : **PRJANA HS**

Composition : Each capusle contains:

Mrigakshi	495 mg.
Dharmpattan	55 mg.
Vadehi	55 mg.
Sringaver	55 mg.

Dosage : Cows, Buffaloes, Mares and Heifers 3 capsules. Sows, Ewes and Doses 2 capsules

How Supplied:Carton containing 20 Pouches of 6 capsules each.

Uses : Infertility due to ovarian dysfunction such as anoesturs, silent heat, delayed maturity in heifers etc.

Product Name : **COFECU PLUS**

Composition :

Copper Sulphate	200 mg.
Cobalt Sulphate	40 mg.
Ferrous Sulphate	100 mg.
Manganese Sulphate	400 mg.

Dosage : Cows and Buffaloes 1 Tab daily. Sheep, Goats and pigs ½ Tab daily.

Product Name : **CAFLON**

Composition : Each 100 g. contains (in g.):

Paribhavya	5.00
Mahabharivacha	5.00
Dvijpriya	8.00
Cleetnak	4.17
Nidigdhika	13.00

Vajidanta	25.33
Suvrata	7.00
Eklypto	10.00
Aksha	4.16
Narasar	4.16
Suvarchika	4.16
Swetpushpa	2.05
Dhatripatra	1.94
Golomi	2.00
Bahumanjari	4.00

Dosage : Cows, Buffaloes and Horses 30-40 g. Calves and Heifers 15-20 g. Sheep, Goats,Foals and pigs 6-12 g. Administer orally with gur/treacle or warm water 2-3 times a day.

How Supplied: Carton-100 g. Polybag.-1lg.

Uses Cough, Bronchitis, Coryza and also as supportive therapy in other respiratory disorders.

Product Name :**TEEBURB (Systemic dermatological)**

Composition :Eahc capsule contains:

Parjanya	200 mg.
Nishakhya	200 mg.
Kilim	200 mg.
Saral	100 mg.

Dosage : Cows, Buffaloes and Horses	2 capsules
Dogs, Pigs, Sheeps, Goats and Foals	1 capsules
Camel and other large animals	4 capsules

How Supplied: Vial of 24 capsules

Uses: Ringworm, eczema, Degnalla, Mange, Wounds, Mastitis and other inflammatory conditons.

Product Name : **HIMAX**

Composition : Each 100 g. contains (in g.):

Indradaru	50
Somvalka	24
Absorption Base	q.s.

Dosage : Not Available

How Supplied: Himax Ointment-50 g. tube, 1 kg. Tin.

Himax Lotion-100 ml. bottle.

Himax-D-25 g. tube.

Uses: Sarcoptic Manga, Psoroptic mange, demodectic mange, Chrioptic mange, Surgical wounds, Traumatic wounds, Lacerated wounds, Broken horn, Bite wounds, Sinuses & fistulae, Sores and fissures, Yoke & rope gall Ringwrorm, Dermatomycosis, Eczema, Degnalla, Infected wounds, Septic wounds, Gangrenous wounds, Ulcerated wounds, Foot rot in sheep, Floot lesions in F.M.D, Maggotted wounds, Burn wounds.

INDOEO REMEDIES LTD.

18-A, Mahal Estate, Mahakali Caves Road, Andheri (East),
P.O. Box No. 9467, Mumbai-400093, Tel-8363449, 8363462/64/65
Fax-(22) 8363502

Product Name : **FI-GARD LIQUID**

Composition :Each 5 ml. contains:

Kutaki	100 mg.
Kalmegh	100 mg.
Bhringaraj	500 mg.
Yashtimadhu	500 mg.
Pippali	625 mg.

JAIN AYURVEDIC PHARMACY

15-9-472, Siddiamber Bazar, Hyderabad-500012.(A.P.)
Tel-(040) 4601457, Fax-(040) 4601457

Product Name : **JANODINE**

Composition :Each 10 ml. Contains:

Draksha(Vitis Vinfera)	75 mg.
Khajur(Phoenix sylvestris)	75 mg.
Ashwagandha (Withenia somnifera)	100 mg.
Shatavari (Asperagus racemousus)	100 mg.
Manjistha (Rubia cordifolia)	75 mg.
Bhringraj (Eclipta alba)	100 mg.
Vidarikanḍ (Pueraria tuberosa)	100 mg.
Jeera (Cuminum cyminum)	75 mg.
Ajwain (Carum copticum)	50 mg.
Punarnava (Boerhavia diffuesa)	75 mg.
Sunthi (Zingiberis officianalis)	150 mg.
Marich (Piper nigrum)	150 mg.
Trivruth (Ipomoea turpethum)	150 mg.
Sugar	q.s.

Dosage : Adults : 2-3 teaspoons twice a day before meals or as directed by the physician. Children : ½ teaspoon twice a day or as directed by the Physician.

How Supplied: 200 ml.

Uses: A general health tonic for all ages, seasons, to maintain good health and energy.

JHAWAR CHEMICALS PVT. LTD.
121, Industrial Area, Harda-461331
Tel-(07577)22163, 23366, Fax -(07577) 22722

Product Name : **SISAIROSP**

Composition :

Wrigtia Tinctoria Rox B-R.Br.	1.47 gr.
Azadirchta Indica A.Juss.	0.37 gr.
Hemidesmus Indicus	0.37 gr.
Coconut Oil	71.47 gr.
Hard paraffin	21.05 gr.
Soft paraffin	5.27 gr.

Dosage : To be applied locally

How Supplied: 20 gr. and 100 gr. collapsible tube.

Uses:Indicated in al type of psoriasis.

Pharmachological Action : Wrightia tinctoria possesses antimicrobial properties as well as inhibits the lipoxygenase responsible for the inflammatory/ hyperproliferatre arachidonic acid pathway; sitostarol which resembles vit D 3 Safe, non-toxic, free from side effects/after effects.

Product Name :**DANDRUFF**

Composition :

Wrightia Tinctoria (Roxb) R.Br.	2% w.v.
Hemidesmus Indicus R.Br.	0.5 % w.v.
Azadirachta Indica A. Juss	0.5 % w.v.
Base coconut oil	

Dosage : To be applied locally.

How Supplied: 100 ml.

Uses: Indicated in Dandruff

Pharmachological Action : Anti-inflammatory, anti infective and healing properties. Reduces scaling, Sliminates itching Treats pityrosporum ovale (fungus) infection, Prevents super infecton Safe, non-toxic, free from side effects/after effects.

Product Name : **PYO-CARE**

Composition :

Nagarmotha	4.11 g.
Sonth	2.05 g.
Kalimirch	2.05 g.
Mulethi	2.05 g.
Bhagori katha	2.05 g.
Chhoti harra	2.05 g.
Pudina phool	0.16 g.
Khadiya mitti	85.48 g.
Flavour	

Uses: Indicated in Pyorrhoea

Pharmacolgical Action : Anti-Infective, anti inflammatory, wound healer and local pain killer, relieves tooth ache and prevent caries, reduces acidic pH in the mouth and physically removes debris from teeth and gums. Safe non-toxic, free from side effects/after effects.

JUPITER PHARMACEUTICALS LTD.
25, Dr. Lalit Banerjee Sarani,
(Formerly Eden Hospital Road), Calcutta-700073
Tel-270224, 3510044, 3509026, Fax - (33) 3511076, 260156

Product Name : **CARMINOZYME LIQUID (Carminative Enzyme with Liver Corrective)**

Composition : Each 5 ml. contains:

Carica papaya	50 mg.
Triphala	75 mg.
Agle marmelos	50 mg.
Zingiber offcinale	50 mg.
Andrographics paniculata	50 mg.
Cyperus rotundus	50 mg.
Nux vomica	10 mg.

Oxalis corniculata	50 mg.
Cassia angustifolia	25 mg.
Carum capticum	50 mg.
Hemidesmus indicus	50 mg.
Ferula foetida	5 mg.

Dosage : Not Available

How Supplied:250 ml., 450 ml.

Uses: Carminative, Liver dysfunction

Product Name : **EMCOVINE SYRUP**

Composition :Each 5 ml. contains:

Vitis vinifera	50 mg.
Mucuna pruriens	50 mg.
Withania comnifera	50 mg.
Hemidesumus indicus	50 mg.
Sida cordifolia	50 mg.
Glycyrrhiza glabra	50 mg.
Cassia angustifolia	50 mg.
Curculigo orchioides	50 mg.
Asparagus recemosus	50 mg.
Triphala	60 mg.
Avena sativa	25 mg.
Hydrocotyle asiatics	50 mg.
Ichnocarpus frutescens	50 mg.
Nux vomica	5 mg.
Ipomoea paniculata	50 mg.
Tribulus terrisitis	50 mg.
Coriandrum sativum	50 mg.
Glycerin	105 v/v
Honey	5% v/v
Gaudy Madira 1.5 to Sugar	2% v/v

Dosage : Not Available

How Supplied: 310 ml.

Uses: For Health & Vigour

Product Name : **ENTROCIN DROPS**

Composition : Each 5 ml. contains:

Holarrhena antidysenterica	250 mg.
Vernonia anthelmintica	150 mg.
Embelia indica	250 mg.

Granatum punica	150 mg.
Cyperus rotundus	250 mg.
Arista indica	250 mg.
Aegle marmelos	250 mg.
Podophyllum	66 mg.

Dosage : Not Available

How Supplied: 30 ml.

Uses: For Diarrhoea, Dysentery & Worms

Product Name : **ENTROCIN TABLETS**

Composition:

Holarrhena antidysenterica	30 mg.
Veronianthelmintica	20 mg.
Embelia indica	30 mg.
Granatum punica	20 mg.
Cyperus rotundus	30 mg.
Aegle marmelos	30 mg.
Podophyllum	12 mg.
Arista indica	30 mg.

Uses:

For Diarrhoea,Dysentery & Worms

Product Name : **HEPATEN TABLETS**

Composition :

Solanum nigrum	15 mg.
Eeclipta alba	25 mg.
Aphanamixis polystschya	25 mg.
Andrographis paniculata	25 mg.
Coculus cordifolia	25 mg.
Ptychotis ajowan	50 mg.
Podophyllum	25 mg.
Aloe indica	20 mg.
Luffa bindal	25 mg.
Fumaria perviflora	25 mg.

Uses : For Hepatic Disorders

Product Name : **JRUMAX OIL**

Composition : Each 5 ml. contains:

Calotropis gigantia	50 mg.
Datura alba	50 mg.

Aconitum ferox	25 mg.
Camphora	10 mg.
Saussurea lappa	25 mg.
Cassia fistula	50 mg.
Allium sativum	25 mg.
Sesamum indicum oil	1% v/v
Moringa oleifera oil	0.5 % v/v
Pongamic glabra oil	1% v/v
Anacardium oil	0.5%v/v
jatropha curcas oil	v/v
Brassia campesuri Oil	q.s.

Uses: Rheumatic Massage Oil

Product Name : **JRUMAX TABLETS**

Composition :

Piper longum	25 mg.
Clerodendrum sophonanthus	50 mg.
Solanum xanthocarpum	50 mg.
Saussrea lappa	25 mg.
Moringa akifera	50 mg.
Tribulas terrestris	50 mg.
Withania somnifera	50 mg.
Zingiber officinale	25 mg.
Balsamodendron mukul	50 mg.
Lauha bhasma	25 mg.
Rasa sindur	10 mg.
Abharak bhasma	10 mg.

Uses: For Leuchorroea & Uterine Dysfunctions

Product Name : **JVINE COMPOUND LIQUID**

Composition : Each 5 ml. contains :

Ipomoea digitata	80 mg.
Mucuna pruriens	100 mg.
Vitis vinivera	80 mg.
Avena sativa	80 mg.
Withania somnifera	80 mg.
Phonix dactytifera	80 mg.
Tribulas terrestris	100 mg.

Carica papaya	80 mg.
Berberis asiatica	50 mg.
Musmallo	100 mg.
Sweet Almond	100 mg.
Terminallia arjuna	100 mg.
Indian sarsaparilla	50 mg.
Cardamom	30 mg.

Uses: For Health & Vigour

Product Name : **LIVOSIN LIQUID**

Composition :Each 5 ml. contains:

Andrographis paniculata	50 mg.
Podophyllum emodi	50 mg.
Eclipta alba	50 mg.
Ptychotis ajowan	2.5 gm.
Ferula foetida	2 mg.
Mentha viridis	50 mg.
Zingiber officinale	12.5 mg.
Cassia angustifolia	50 mg.
triphala	60 mg.
Carica papaiya	50 mg.
Hemidesmus indicus	50 mg.
Withania comnifera	50 mg.
Avena sativa	25 mg.
Terminalia arjuna	50 mg.
Embelia indica	25 mg.
Holarrhena antidysenterica	50 mg.
Phyllanthus niruri	50 mg.
Coriandrum sativum	50 mg.
Fumaria parviflora	50 mg.
Tinospora cordifolia	50 mg.
Glycosmis pentaphylla	50 mg.
Glycyrrhiza glabra	25 mg.
Aloe indica	2 mg.

Uses Liver Tonic

Product Name :**LUCOMYN SYRUP**

Composition : Each 5 ml. contains:

Saraca indica	100 mg.
Abroma augusta	100 mg.

Sida cordifolia	50 mg.
Berberis asiatica	50 mg.
Indian sarsaparilla	50 mg.
Mesua roxburgha	50 mg.
Withania somnifera	50 mg.
Avena sativa	50 mg.
Podophyllum emodi	50 mg.
Triphalla	60 mg.
Aloe indica	10 mg.
Cassia angustifolia	10 mg.
Sodhita hirakosh	50 mg.
Terminalia arjuna	50 mg.
Glycerin	10.6 % v/v

Uses: For rhuematism & Arthritis

Product Name : **LUCOMYN TABLETS**

Composition :

Podophyllum emodi	25 mg.
Saraca indica	50 mg.
Abroma augusta	50 mg.
Avena sativa	25 mg.
Withania somnifera	25 mg.
Indian sarsaparilla	25 mg.
Sida cordifolia	25 mg.
Sodhita hirakosh	25 mg.
Cassia angustifolia	5 mg.
Mesua roxburgha	25 mg.
Triphalla	30 mg.
Aloe indica	5 mg.
Berberis asiatica	25 mg.
Terminalia arjuna	25 mg.

Uses: For Leuchorrhoea & Uterine Dysfunctions :

Product Name : **SUGARILL-10 TABLETS**

Composition :

Eugenia jambolana	100 mg.
Abroma augusta	100 mg.
Cephalandra indica	100 mg.
Nux vomica	5 mg.
Emblica officinalis	100 mg.
Pongamia Glabra	25 mg.

Aconitum ferox	5 mg.
Acacia arabica	50 mg.
Abhrak bhasma	25 mg.
Lauha bhasma	25 mg.

Uses : For Diabetes

KAMAL PHARMACY (AYURVEDIC)
1498, Bhagirath Palace, Chandi Chowk, Delhi - 110006
Tel - 2967158, 2969911, Fax - (11) 2969911

Product Name : **BLIDOL TABLETS**

Composition :

Shukti bhasma	60 mg.
Surma bhasma	60 mg.
Aqiq bhasma	30 mg.
Sangira bhasma	52 mg.
Godanti bhasma	45 mg.
Katha	90 mg
Mochras	38 mg.
Parval mul	30 mg.

Product Name : **DESTROL FORTE TABLETS**

Composition :

Mochras	39 mg.
Bale	39 mg.
Podina	49 mg.
Ajowain	29 mg.
Katha	39 mg.
Kurachhal	96 mg.
Inder jau	19 mg.
Sonth	19 mg.
Karpoor	29 mg.
Poast	39 mg.
Kharia	115 mg.
Medicinal opium	9.68 mg.

Product Name : **ENTO-DESTO TABLETS**

Composition :

Bale	49 mg.
Kurachhal	41 mg.
Katha	74 mg.
Saunf	41 mg.
Podina	41 mg.

Kharia	86 mg.
Heeng	8 mg.
Haldi	25 mg.
Mochras	49 mg.
Gond	103 mg.
Poast	82 mg.

***Product Name* : Flurol Tablets**

Godanti bhasma	200 mg.
Tribha\uvan kirti ras	70 mg.
Sphatika shudh	50 mg.
Suhaga shudh	50 mg.
Kutki	10 mg.

***Product Name* : GEXOL TABLETS**

***Composition* :**

Laung	40 mg.
Jaiphal	40 mg.
Chitraka	30 mg.
Nagarmotha	30 mg.
Pipal	30 mg.
Shankh bhasma	60 mg.
Kori bhasma	60 mg.
Shingraf	15 mg.
Podina	40 mg.
Kali mirch	35 mg.
Ajwain	40 mg.

***Product Name* : LAXEEN FORTE TABLETS**

***Composition* :**

Amla	120 mg.
Tankan shudh	10 mg.
Jaiphal	40 mg.
Pipal	10 mg.
Kali mirch	10 mg.
Sonth	20 mg.
Ajwain	20 mg.
Podina	20 mg.

Dosage :

Product Name : **LECORENA PLUS TABLETS**

Composition :

Sanjiarahat bhasma	32 mg.
Loh bhasma	16 mg.
Abhrak bhasma	8 mg.
Kukutanddtwak bhasma	4 mg.
Ashoka	32 mg.
Lodh	32 mg.
Talmakhana	32 mg.
Bij band	64 mg.
katha	40 mg.
Mochras	32 mg.
Shukti pishti	40 mg.
Godanti bhasma	32 mg.
Sphatika shudh	16 mg.

Product Name : **LIV FORTE TABLETS**

Composition :

Chiraita	20 mg.
Kutki	20 mg.
Pipal	10 mg.
Kali mirch	10 mg.
Sonth	10 mg.
Ajwain	10 mg.
Podina	10 mg.
Chitrak	10 mg.
Amla	10 mg.
Bhringraj	20 mg.
Punarnava	60 mg.
Pipla mul	20 mg.
Nishoth	10 mg.
Bhui amla	20 mg.
Shankh bhasma	15 mg.
Mandur bhasma	25 mg.

Product Name : **PILINE TABLETS**

Composition :

Shukti bhasma	28 mg.

Aqiq bhasma	37 mg.
Surma bhasma	66 mg.
Godanti bhasma	47 mg.
Shankh bhasma	19 mg.
Katha	84 mg.
Rasaunt	66 mg.
Mochras	42 mg.
Anjubar	66 mg.
Harrar	47 mg.
Nagkesar	23 mg.

Product Name : **TEXAL TABLETS**

Composition :

Kesar	11 mg.
Makardhawaj	18 mg.
Shilajeet	41 mg.
Rajat bhasma	5 mg.
Vang bhasma	17 mg.
Nag bhasma	9 mg.
Loh bhasma	11 mg.
Praval bhasma	17 mg.
Laung	9 mg.
Jaiphal	9 mg.
Javitri	9 mg.
Salib	23 mg.
Muslisafed	23 mg.
Jarh pan	17 mg.
Asgandh	35 mg.
Nirbsi	5 mg.
Bidhari	23 mg.
Tuj	11 mg.
Shudh vish musthi	17 mg.

KARNATAKA ANTIBIOTICS & PHARMACEUTICALS LIMITED

Dr. Rajkumar Road, 1st Block Rajajinagar Bangalore -560010
Tel-3322123/3322868/3323301, Fax - (080) 8392606

Product Name : **EXOL SYRUP**

Composition : Each 5 ml contains:

Sharupunkha (Tephrosia Purpurea)	50 mg.
Bhringaraja (Eclipta alba)	50 mg.

Bhoomyamalaki (Phyllanthus niruri)	30 mg.
Katuki (Picrorrhiza kurroa)	20 mg.
Rohitaka (Tecommella Undualata)	20 mg.
Punarnava (Boerhaavia diffusa)	20 mg.
Palatable base q.s. to	5 ml

Dosage : 2.5 to 10 ml 3 times a day

How Supplied: 100 ml. Bottle

Uses: Daily health supplement, jaundice, infective hepatitis, cirrhosis of liver, as a hepatoprotective

Product Name :**DYCON TABLETS**

Composition : Each tablet contains:

Punica grantum	75 mg.
Aegle marmelos	20 mg.
Holarrhena antidysenterica	200 mg.
Myristica fragrans	10 mg.
Cuminum cyminum	10 mg.
Zingiber officinale	5 mg.

Dosage : 2 tablets 3 times a day

How Supplied: 30 tablets in container

Uses: Diarrohoea, dysentery and Mixed infections.

Product Name :**ANTAF TABLETS**

Composition :Each tablet contains:

Ystimadhu	150 mg.
Amalaki	150 mg.
Narikela lavana	100 mg.
Shankha basma	100 mg.

Dosage : 30 tablets 3 times a day

How Supplied: 30 tablets in container

Uses Antacid, Antiflualent, Sastric ulcar, Duodenal ulcar, Peptic hyperacidity and Desophagitis

Product Name : **EXOL TABLETS**

Composition : Each tablets contains:

Tephrosia purpurea	100 mg.
Eclipta alba	80 mg.

Phyllanthus niruri	75 mg.
Picrorrhiza kurroa	40 mg.
Tecommella undulata	50 mg.
Boerhaavia diffusa	25 mg.
Azadirachita indica	30 mg.

Dosage : 2 tablets twice a day

How Supplied: 100 tablets twice a day

Uses: Daily health supplement, Jaundice infective hepatitis, Cirrhosis of liver, as a hepatoprotective.

Product Name : **DYCON SYRUP**

Composition : Each 5 ml contains:

Punica granatum	100 mg.
Aegle marmelos	40 mg.
Holarrhena antidysenteri	20 mg.
Myristica fragrans	10 mg.
Cuminum cyminum	10 mg.
Zingiber officinale	5 mg.

Dosage : 2.5 to 5 ml 3 times a day (for paediatric use only)

How Supplied: 60 ml Bottle

Uses Diarrohoea, Dysentery and Mixed infections

Product Name : **VAST SYRUP**

Composition : Each 5 ml. contains:

Tulasi (Ocimum sanctum)	100 mg.
Nvasara	80 mg.
Vasaka	50 mg.
Pushkara moola	50 mg.
Shirisha	50 mg.
Yastimadhu	50 mg.
Bala	20 mg.
Pipali	15 mg.
Srigavera	15 mg.
Palatable base q.s. to	5 ml

Dosage : 2.5 to ml 3 times a day

How Supplied: 100 ml. Bottle

Uses : All types of cough, allergic bronchitis, tracheitis, bronchiolitis

K.S. & SONS (DR.) (Indigenous Pharmaceuticals)
66, Manikkara Street,
Kumbakonam -612001 (T.N), Tel-(0435)21196

Product Name : **ANEMEX TABLETS**

Composition :

Ferrum redactum	70%
Iron	2%
Beleric myrobalans	5.75%
Pepper	5.75%
Indian goose berry	5.75%
Dried ginger	5.75%

Product Name : **ASWAGANDHI LEHEYAM**

Composition :

Withania somnifera	20%
Vitis vinifera	8%
Phoenix dactylifera	8%
Zingiber off+piper Nigrum+ Piper longum	7%
Sandal	1%
Myristica off	1%
Caryophyllum	1%
Amomum Sabulatum	1%
Bark of Caryophyllum	1%
cyprus rotandus	2%
Rhus succedehea	1%
Juglanus regia	1%
Vellamichai	2%
Long Pepper Root of	1%
Chevviyan	1%
Plumbago zeylanica	1%

Product Name : **CANTHALAX TABLETS**

Composition :

Roes buds	65 mg.
Feromia	60 mg.
Marosa	60 mg.

Indian beech	55 mg.
Garlic	55 mg.
Bonduc nut	60 mg.
Dried ginger	60 mg.
Musambar	20 mg.
Hab-ul-salatin	20 mg.
Fruit juice	10 mg.

Product Name : **CHITTUKKURUVI LEHEYAM**

Composition :

Badam	4%
Bistha	4%
Munthri	4%
Acrot	4%
Kasakasa	3%
Sukku	3%
Thippili	3%
Agarakaram	3%
Lavangappathiri	3%
Chittarathai	3%
Jadamanjal	3%
Koraikezangu	3%
Lavangam	2%
Iithikkai	2%
Jathipathiri	2%
Elam	2%
Agil Kattai	2%
Neermulli verai	7%
Poonaikali verai	7%
Badam bisin	3%
Payreetchai	4%
Honey, Ghee, Sugar	q.s.

Product Name : **KARUNAI KEZANGU LEHEYAM**

Composition :

Wild amorphop halus	8%
Phoenix dactyliera	5%
Fig	5%
The Rose flower	5%
Big ink nut	3%
Kadukkai pinchu	3%

Indian goose berry	7%
Fenugreek	5%
Turpeth Root	4%

Product Name : **GINGRAX SEMI SOLID**

Composition :

Three Kadugu	24%
Turmeric	3%
Galangal lesser	3%
Asafoetida	2%
Cloves	3%
Tetran thra roxbergi	3%
Anise seed	3%
Jegititiy	2%
Ink nut	2%
Konnal skin	2%
The Bishops weed	3%

Product Name : **INJI LEHEYAM SEMI SOLID**

Composition :

Inji charu	10%
Cow milk	20%
Mullangi charu	10%
Elumichai charu	10%
Brab sugar	3.5%
Sukku	1.5%
Milagu	1.5%
Thippili	1.5%
Elam	1.5%
Elavangam	1.5%
Cheeragam	1.5%
Vai velangam	1.5%
Thalisapatri	1.5%
Jathikkai	1.5%
Ghee, Honey, Sugar	q.s.

Product Name : **JAMANIRAX SEMI SOLID**

Composition :

Halila	5%
Haleela-e-siyah	5%
Haleela-e-zard	5%
Turbud	10%

Dhanya	10%
Post-e-Bhirah	2%
Post-e-amla	2%
Gul-e-surkh	2%
Thabasheer	2%
Phol-ki-nilufer	2%
Sandal-e-sufeed	1%
Katheera	1%
Safisthan	8%
Gulabi banabsha	5%
Saqmonia	5%

Product Name : **KAYAKALPA LEHEYAM**

Composition :

Thiri kadugu	3%
Kadukkai	3%
Thanikkai	3%
Kazharchikkai	3%
Payetchai	8%
Jathikkai	1%
Jathipathiri	1%
Elam	1%
Karimbu	1%
Amukkra	1%
Bistha	1%
Achroot	3%
Neermulli	2%
Nelappani	2%
Punaikali veethu	2%
Jeeragam	1%
Sombu	1%
Vallarai	3%
Karizalai	3%
Nelli	3%
Ghee, Honey, Sugar	q.s.

Product Name : **MANORA TONIC LIQUID**

Composition :

Jequitity	0.5 g.
Dried ginger	0.5 g.
Stone flower	0.5 g.
Nut gras	0.5 g.

Anise seed	0.5 g.
Cumin seeds	0.5 g.
Indian gooseberry	0.5 g.
Cardamom	0.5 g.
Valerian root	0.5 g.
Tail pepper	0.5 g.
Grapes	0.5 g.
Pinju kadukkai	0.5 g.
Chebulic-myrobalans	0.5 g.
Big-ink nut	0.5 g.
Beleric myrobalans	0.5 g.
Coriander seeds	0.5 g.
Feromia	1 g.
Persian rose	1 g.
Ferrum readactum	1 g.
Iron	1 g.
Ghee	17 g.
Syrup	41 g.
Honey in base	41 g.

KUMAR AYURVEDIC (PHARMACY) TRADING CO.
Gulab Devi Hospital Road, Jalandhar-14408
Tel-(0181) 254195, 253700, 252437, 252383

Product Name : **NAVRATNA FORTE CAPSULES**

Composition :

Makardhwaj	5 mg.
Saffron	5 mg.
Jund	5 mg.
Ras Sindur	5 mg.
Gokhru	20 mg.
Shattavar	20 mg.
Tal Makhanan	20 mg.
Bang Bhasma	20 mg.
Abhrak Bhasma	20 mg.
Loh Bhasma	20 mg.
Long	20 mg.
Jaiphal	20 mg.
Tinduk	30 mg.
Konch Beej	30 mg.
Jawitri	30 mg.

Beej Band	30 mg.
Ashawagandha	30 mg.
Swarna makshik Bhasma	30 mg.
Shilajeet	40 mg.

Dosage : Two capsules a day with milk or as directed by the Physician.

How Supplied: 25 capsules.

Uses: Navratna Forte helps an aged person to feel young by regaining his strength & vitality. It is especially effective in general debility.

Product Name : **SEXSONA FORTE CAPSULE.**

Composition :

Makardhwaj	10 mg.
Saffron	8 mg.
Jund	7 mg.
Ras Sindur	10 mg.
Shudh Kuchla	60 mg.
Bang Bhasma	25 mg.
Abhrak Bhasma	25 mg.
Loh Bhasma	25 mg.
Long	20 mg.
Jaiphal	50 mg.
Konch Beej	50 mg.
Jawitri	30 mg.
Beej Band	50 mg.
Ashwagandha	30 mg.

& bhavan Panra, Dhatura
Ashawagandha & Shilajeet.

Dosage :Two capsules a day with milk & continue treatment for 3 months

How Supplied: 25 capsules

Uses: Sexsona Forte provides youthful vigour & vitality for men & women. Improves body resistance in old age & during winters.

Product Name : **KATCHOPHOS SYRUP**

Composition : Each 5 ml contains liquid ext. of:

Shankh Pushpi	500 mg.
Brahmi	125 mg.
Sarpgandha	125 mg.

Ashawagandha	125 mg.
Distilled extracts of:	
Ajwain	125 mg.
Pudina	125 mg.
Zeera	125 mg.
Sugar, preservatives Colour & flavour	q.s.

Dosage : Adults : One tablespoonful twice a day before meals. Children : One teaspoonful twice a day before melas.

How Supplied: In packs 100 ml. 200 ml, 450 ml & 4500 ml.

Uses: It ensures normal growth and development during infancy and childhood, Malnutrition caused by inadequate diet, anorexia and other causes. It is a supplement of vitamins in specific fevers and infections, prior to operation and during convalesence, Effective in nervous breakdown, loss of vigour & vitality, loss of appetite, general weakness. It acts as a brain tonic.

Product Name : **LIVOREX-K TABLET**

Composition : Each coated tablet contains:

chitrakmool	17 mg.
Kashni	47 mg.
Mako	8 mg.
Arijan	32 mg.
Kutki	20 mg.
Punarnva	20 mg.
Kalmegh	10 mg.
Bansa	10 mg.
Haritaki	10 mg.
Bhringraj	30 mg.
Kachur	10 mg.
Vavding	20 mg.
Mandur Bhasma	30 mg.

Dosage :1 to 2 tablets twice daily with milk or water.

How Supplied: In packs of 100 tablets & 1000 tablets.

Uses: Livorex-K tablet is a compound of thirteen famous herbal and mineral drugs which have been used since several years for the treatment of liver disorders, loss of appetite, growth failure, constipation etc. Punarnva is a powerful diuretic, antiinflammatory laxative & antispamoidc. It is useful in depression. Kashni is haematinic and is usedful in enlargement of liver and spleen. Effective in indigestion, anorexia, flatulence, toxic hepatitis & jaundice.

Product Name : **KATCOZYME TABLET**

Composition :

Sanjivani Vatti	60 mg.
Agni Tundi Vatti	40 mg.
Shankh Vatti	40 mg.
Pipla Mool	30 mg.
Hing	20 mg.
Trikuta	50 mg.
Sajjiskharr	20 mg.
Sounth	20 mg.
Inderjav	20 mg.
Naushadar	20 mg.
Shodh Kuchla	20 mg.
Lahsum	20 mg.

Dosage : 1 to 2 tablets 3 or 4 times daily after meal.

How Supplied: 10x10tabs. 50x10 tabs. (Blister)

Uses: Effective in flatulene,dyspepsia, abdominal distention, hyperacidity & other digestive disorders. It improves appetite & digestion.

Product Name : **RAKSHOD SYRUP**

Composition : Each 5 ml contains liquid ext. of:

Mundi	250 mg.
Sarna Patter	125 mg.
Vavding	62 mg.
Nagar Motha	125 mg.
Daru Haridra	125 mg.
Kalmegh	125 mg.
Guruchi	125 mg.
Neem	125 mg.
Trifla	125 mg.
Trikuta	125 mg.
Red Candan	125 mg.
Pit Papra	125 mg.
Chiraita	125 mg.
Sugar, premitted	
Preservatives & flavour	q.s.

Dosage : Children : ½ to 1 teaspoonful 3 or 4 times a day Adult : 2 to 3 teaspoonful 3 or 4 times a day.

How Supplied: In packs of 100 ml & 200 ml.

Uses: Rakshod is made from thirteen herbs. Rakshod acts internally as a powerful antiseptic, anti-bacterial, astringent, laxative & stimulant to purify the blood. Regular use of Rakshod can cure even chronic skin disorders. Rakshod is an effective blood purifier and a remedy for skin diseases e.g. pimples, summer boils, pruritis, urticaria and nose bleeding, corrects digestion, improves complexion.

Product Name :**ASHOKA CORDIAL SYRUP**

Composition : Each 5 ml contains:

Ashoka	375 mg.
Lodhra Pathani	250 mg.
Jeera	62.5 mg.
Nagarmotha	62.5 mg.
Moch Ras	62.5 mg.
Nagkesar	62.5 mg.
Ulat Kambal	125 mg.
Daru Haridra	125 mg.
Babul Chaal	125 mg.
Sugar,	
Preservative & flavour	q.s.

Dosage **:**1 to 2 teaspoonfuls thrice a day with water.

How Supplied: In packs of 100 ml. 200 ml & 450 ml.

Uses: Ashok Cordial reduces permeability of the vaginal mucosa and diminishes vascularity and congestion in the pelvic region. Restores the pH of vaginal mucosa and provides a bacteriostatic action. This makes it useful in leucorrhoea, general run down condition and backache caused by over-flowing whites.

Product Name : **NARI JIWAN FORTE SYRUP**

Composition : Each 5 ml contains liquid ext. of:

Ashoka	500 mg.
Dashmool	100 mg.
Lodhra	500 mg.
Arjana	250 mg.
Ashawagandha	250 mg.
Bidari Kand	100 mg.
Supari	100 mg.

Mochras	100 mg.
Chitrak	100 mg.
Bansa	100 mg.
Red Chandan	100 mg.
Nagarmotha	100 mg.
Kamal Keshar	100 mg.
Shatavar	100 mg.
Jata Manshi	100 mg.
Belgiri	100 mg.
Manjishtha	100 mg.
Sugar,	
Preservative & flavour	q.s.

Dosage :1 to 3 teaspoonfuls 3 times a day or as directed by the physician.

Uses: Nari Jiwan Forte cures female ailments, such as burning of feet & hands, backache, headche etc. Restores health, beauty & is useful in fuctional gynecological disorders. Nari Jiwan Forte is a useful effective, non-toxic oral treatment of indigenous origin for leucorrhoea, vicarious discharges during pregnancy or confinement, menstrual disorders, tox of pregnancy and prevention of miscarriage. Tone up uterus. Develops bustline.

Product Name : **SOMKALP MADHU SYRUP**

Composition : Each 5 ml contains liquid ext of:

Mulathi	125 mg.
Karka Singhi	125 mg.
Kantkari	125 mg.
Pushkarmool	125 mg.
Bharangi	125 mg.
Tulsi	60 mg.
Unab	60 mg.
Lasorian	250 mg.
Vibihitak	250 mg.
Bansa	250 mg.
Somlata	250 mg.
Neelgiri Tail	0.006 ml
Sat Pudina	0.006 ml
Suhaga	10 mg.
Sugar, Preservative & flavour	q.s.

Dosage : 1 to 2 teaspoonfuls 3 to 4 times daily with water or as directed by the physician.

How Supplied: In packs of 60 ml, 100 ml, 450 or 4500 ml.

Uses: The combination of Som Kalp Madhu is very useful in chronic cough and cold. Bharangi, mulathi, and somlata have been successfully used as expectorants while sat pudina is helpful in giving soothing, effect. It is very safe for all ages. Bronchial asthma, status asthmaticus, emphysema, spastic bronchitis and in bronchospam of various etiologies.

Product Name : **KUMAR COUGH EXPECTORANT**

Composition : Each 10 ml syrup contains liquid ext. of:

Bansa	0.5 g.
Bahera	0.25 g.
Somlata	0.25 g.
Lasurian	0.25 g.
Saunf	0.125 g.
Mulathi	0.125 g.
Kakrasinghi	0.125 g.
Jar Paan	0.125 g.
Kuthmithi	0.125 g.
Joofa	0.125 g.
Kantkari	0.125 g.
Kapoor	0.005 g.
Sat Pudina	0.005 g.
Sat Loban	0.0375 g.
Shoudit suhaga	0.0375 g.
Oil Sat Podina	0.0125 ml
Oil Neel Giri	0.0125 ml
Sugar colour, preservative & flavour	q.s.

Dosage : One to Two teaspoonfuls three times a day for adults. Half to one teaspoonfuls three times a day or as directed by the Physician.

How Supplied: In packs of 100 ml, 450 & 4500 ml.

Uses: It is a cough syrup providing the most potent antitussive, decongestant and bronocodilator drugs in an optimally balanced combination. Somlata-one of them most potent antitussive agents-acts on the cough centre and relieves the irritating cough very effectively. Joofa checks the allergic component of cough. It also acts as a decongestant and decreases nasal stuffiness and helps breathing by causing dialation of air passages, reduction in viscosityy of bronchial secretions ensuring their easy expulsion. Bharangi soothens the irritated and inflammed mucosa due to its local anaesthetic effect. It is effective in all types of cough (Productive and dry) & cold, fever, bronchitis, asthma & smokers cough. In cough due to tuberculosis as adjunct therapy.

***Product Name:* LIVOREX-K SYRUP**

***Composition*:** Each 5 ml contains liquid Ext. c.;

Kantkari	125 mg.
Kashni	125 mg.
Arijan	125 mg.
Punarnva	125 mg.
Bhring raj	125 mg.
Trifla	125 mg.
Kutki	125 mg.
Revandchini	125 mg.
Bansa	125 mg.
Sonth	125 mg.
Kalmegh	125 mg.
Naushadar	25 mg.
Sugar, Preservatives & flavour	q.s.

Dosage*:* 1 to 3 teasponful 2 times daily or as directed by the Physician.

How Supplied: In packs of 100 ml, 200 ml, 450 ml & 4500 ml

***Uses*:** LIVOREX-K is useful in the treatment of various liver disorders. It corrects sluggish and enlarged liver, induces a healthy appetite with improved assimilation. It also prevents the damage of liver due to chronic alcohlism. It is absolutely harmless even on prolonged treatment. It is effective in indigestion, anorexia, flatulence, constipation, toxic-hepatitis, jaundice & hyperacidity.

***Product Name:* KATOZYME SYRUP**

***Composition*:** Each 10 ml contains liquid ext. of

Adrak ka ras	200 mg
Ajmod	50 mg.
Lemon juice	100 mg.

Nagar motha	50 mg.
Trikuta	150 mg.
Vavding	50 mg.
Jeera	100 mg.
Naushadar	50 mg.
Pudina	100 mg.
Saunf	25 mg.
Haritaki	100 mg.
Saindhava	25 mg.
Anardana	50 mg.
Pipla mool	25 mg.
Phool gulab	25 mg.
Kapoor	5 mg.
Sugar, permitted preservatives & Flavour	q.s.

Dosage: Before meals to stimulate appetite and after meals to aid digestion. Children: 1/2 to 1 teaspoonful with equal quanity of water. Adults: 1 to 2 teaspoonful with equal quanity of water.

How Supplied: In packs of 100 ml, 200 ml, 450 ml & 4500 ml

Uses: KATACOZYME is a reputed drug for its unique and quick action in digestive disorders. It assures prompt relief from flatulence, dyspepsias, trapped wind and abdominal distension. It also relieves common symptoms of hyperacidity like heart burns and fullness etc. It stimulates appĕtite and improves digestion.

Product Name: **KUMAR BAL JANAM GHUTTI SYRUP**

Composition: Each 10 ml contains:

Sarna patri	150 mg
Vatch	100 mg.
Harar	300 mg.
Bansa	100 mg.
Mulathi	150 mg.
Lhisaurhy	100 mg.
Amaltas	200 mg.
Soya	100 mg.
Saunf	100 mg.
Sobagia	150 mg.
Vavding	100 mg.
Niri kishar	100 mg.
Sugar, preservative & Flavour	q.s.

Dosage:

1 month to 3 months	10 drops
4 months to 6 monhs	15 drops
7 months to 1 year	20 drops
1 year to 2 years	1/2 teaspoonful
2 years to 3 years	1 teaspoonful

One dose of Kumar bal janam ghutti mixed with two teaspoonfuls of warm water should be given in the morning and evening. If no relief is obtained givea double dose similarly, three times a day.

How Supplied: In packs of 30 ml, 60 ml & 100 ml.

Uses: Kumar bal janam ghutti is extremely useful in the disorders of new borns and children. For years it has been successfully used in digestive disorders, symptoms due to teething, weaning flatulence, acidity, vomiting of clotted milk, and gripes. It is also indicated in common cold & couth and in infantile diarrhoea, stomatitis, thrush and constipation.

Product Name: **KASALEEN COUGH TABLET**

Composition: Each tablet contains liquid ext. of

Mulathi	100 mg.
Sat Pudina	3 mg.
Bansa	100 g.
Nilgiri oil	3 mg.
Sugar	q.s.

Dosage: Keep one tablet in the mouth & let it dissolve.

How Supplied: In packs of 100 tablets

Uses: Cough tablets Kasleen soothes the throat and respiratory passages, reduces bronchial mucosal irritability. Effective in all types of productive and non productive cough of varied actiology.

Product Name: **KUMAR BAL AMRIT SYRUP**

Composition: Each 5 ml. contains distillates of

Soya	50 mg.
Ajwain	50 mg.
Podina	50 mg.
Saunf	50 mg.
Jeera	50 mg.

Bari Illaichi	25 mg.
Gulab phool	50 mg.
Sugar, permitted colour, Preservative & flavour	q.s.

Dosage: One to two teaspoonful thrice a day.

How Supplied: In packs of 100 ml.

Uses: Bal Amrit is a balanced clinically proven digestive tonic for infants and children which improves appetite promotes weight gain, healthy growth and keeps babies free from digestive upsets, gas, teething defects, colics, gripes, cough, diarrhoea and constipation. When children are weeping for unknown reasons give Bal Amrit and within a few minutes the children become quiet, calm and sleepy.

***Product Name* : KAYRON SYRUP**

Composition: Each 10 ml contains liquid ext. of

Punarnva	200 mg
Sonth	100 mg.
Ashwagandha	100 mg.
Nagar motha	100 mg.
Unab	100 mg.
Anant mool	25 mg.
Amla	100 mg.
Bidari kand	100 mg.
Haritki	100 mg.
Majitha	100 mg.
Shataur	100 mg.
Sugar, preservative colour & flavour	q.s.

Dosage: 1 teaspoonful thrice a day for children upto 3 years of age. 2 teaspoonfuls thrice a day for adults or as directed by the physician.

How Supplied: In packs of 100 ml, 200 ml, 450 ml.

Uses: Nutritional anaemia, loss of weight & growth, dyspepsia, neurasthenia.

***Product Name*: DIADYN TABLET**

Composition: Each tablet of 500 mg contains:

Mochras	36 mg.
Kutajghan	30.34 mg.
Bilkath	43 mg.
Hing	8 mg.

Saunf	43 mg.
Goond kikar	85 mg.
Podina	43 mg.
Haldi	35 mg.
Katha	43 mg.
Kharia	124 mg.
Opium	9.66 mg.

Dosage: Adults : 2 tablets twice a day or as directed by the physician

Uses: Highly valuable in treating profuse diarrhoea (with mucous and blood) summer diarrhoea, epidemic diarrhoea, infantile diarrhoea, and senile diarrhoea, acute or chronic bacillary dysentery or amoebic dysentery.

Product Name: **HEPATONE DROPS**

Composition:

Bhring raj	300 mg.
Harar	300 mg.
Guruchi	300 mg.
Tulsi	200 mg.
Rose phool	300 mg.
Revanchini	100 mg.
Saunf	300 mg.
Soya	100 mg.
Kachur	300 mg.
Nishoth	100 mg.
Kalmegh	300 mg.
Ajwain	100 mg.
Punarnava	300 mg.
Shunthi	100 mg.
Vaviding	300 mg.
Tankan	100 mg.
Adusa	300 mg.
Arvind	200 mg.
Sugar, Preservative & Flavour	q.s.

Dosage: Infant: 3 to 5 drops with milk thrice a day; Children: 8 to 12 drops thrice a day.

How Supplied: In packs of 30 ml.

Uses: Hepatone is a unique preparation formulated after wide experience and has proved that it protects hepatic paranchyme, accelerates metabolic activity, regenerates liver cells, increases growth, corrects liver disorder. Useful in pre & early cirrhotic lever & jaundice Hepatone (Drops) is prophylactic against drugs and chemicals which are hepatotoxic. It reduces the side effects of over use of the antibiotics. Useful in anorexia, growth failure, sluggish liver dysfunction due to various causes.

***Product Name:* AMRIT PAIN BALM**

***Composition*:** Each 12 gm contains:

Sat pudina	2%
Neel giri oil	5%
Sat ajwain	2%
Dalchini oil	%
Oil gultheria	5%
Tarpeen oil	5%
Kapoor	3%
Petroleum jelly	q.s.

Dosage: *For cold:* Rub in Amrit pain balm on chest, back, throat and inside nostrils. *In severe colds:* A teanspoonful of Amrit pain balm should be melted in boiling water and its vapours inhaled.

***How Supplied*:** In packs of 12 g.

***Uses*:** For aches & pains: Like headache, lumbago, backache, stiffneck, muscular ain, insectbite, swelling, tooth ache & rheumatic paint etc.

LIBRA DRUGS (INDIA)

145/146/92-B, Mangalwar Peth, Pune-411 011
Tel : 637668, 335134 Fax: (0212) 627668

***Product Name:* CARMIL LIQUID**

***Composition*:** Each 5 ml contains:

Extract of Gnger	0.0012 g
Extract of Embelia ribes	0.0012 g.
Extract of Hingastak	0.012 g.
Drakshasav	3.75 ml.

***Product Name:* LIBRA'SADULSA COMPOUND LIQUID**

***Composition*:** Each 5 ml contains:

Extract Adhatoda vasica	2.5 ml.

Extract Terminalia chebul	0.15 ml.
Extract Terminalla balerica	0.15 ml.
Extract Dashmul	0.30 ml.

Product Name: **LIPOCHEN SYRUP**

Composition: Each 10 ml contains:

Aqueous Extracts of

Vitex agnus castue	50 mg.
Holarrhena antidsentrica	50 mg.
Tephrosia purpurea	100 mg.
Terminalia arjuna	100 mg.
Tinospora cardifolia	100 mg.
Boerhavia diffusa	100 mg.
Tribulus terrestris	100 mg.
Caparris spinosa	100 mg.
Solanum nigrum	100 mg.
Piper longum	100 mg.
Acorus calamus	100 mg.
Ipoeca turpenthum	100 mg.
Terminalia chebula	100 mg.
Ammora rohitaka	200 mg.
Eclipta prostata	200 mg.
Plumbago zeylanica	200 mg.
Picrozhia kurooa	200 mg.
Embelia ribes	200 mg.

Product Name: **UTROSAN LIQUID**

Composition: Each 10 ml. contains:

Saraca indica	200 mg.
Symplocos racemosa	200 mg.
Asparagus racemosus	200 mg.
Impomoea digitata	200 mg.
Terminalia arjuna	200 mg.
Rubia cordifolia	200 mg.
Berberis aristata	200 mg.
Piper longum radix	150 mg.
Acorus calamus	150 mg.
Hemidesmuns indicus	150 mg.
Bambusa orundinaoea	150 mg.

Tribulus terrestris	100 mg.
Boerhaavia diffusa	100 mg.
Pterocarpus santalimus	100 mg.
Dashmoolas	500 mg.

LUCENT PHARMACEUTICALS (INDIA) PVT. LTD.
310, Murli Bhawan, Ashok Marg, Hazratganj, Lucknow-226 001
Tel : 275003, Fax: (0522) 300483

***Product Name:* LUCENLIV CAPSULE**

***Composition*:** Each capsule contains:

Katuka	30 mg.
Bhringraj	40 mg.
Kasani	40 mg.
Madarmool	20 mg.
Shatpushpa	20 mg.
Musthak	30 mg.
Kakmachi	40 mg.
Kalmegh	40 mg.
Apamarg	30 mg.
Harithaki	40 mg.
Sharpunkha	40 mg.
Rohithak	40 mg.
Parpat	40 mg.
Punarnava	40 mg.
Madhur bhasma	10 mg.

Dosage: 1 to 2 capsules twice or thrice daily or as directed by the physician.

***How Supplied*:** 10 capsules in a blister and 100 capsule packs.

***Uses*:** Indicated in enlarged liver, inflammation of the liver, discomfort of the liver after hepatitis, jaundice and constipation, clayey stools, congestion of the liver and also prevents dropsy.

***Product Name*: LUCENT BEAU CAPSULE**

***Composition*:** Each capsule contains:

Sariva	40 mg.
Manjistha	40 mg.
Mundi	40 mg.
Kusht	35 mg.

Aargwadh	40 mg.
Amrita	40 mg.
Kalmegh	40 mg.
Katuka	30 mg.
Khadir Twak	40 mg.
Nimb Twak	35 mg.
Kiraththirkth	30 mg.
Harithki	40 mg.
Apamarg	40 mg.
Rasanjan	10 mg.

Dosage: 1 to 2 capsules twice or thrice daily or as directed by the physician.

How Supplied: 10 capsules in a blister pack.

Uses: Purifies blood, removes acne, pimples dark rings around eyes, improves brightness of skin, removes skin rashes.

Product Name: **NERVOMINE CAPSULE**

Composition: Each capsule contains:

Aakar karbh	80 mg.
Kapikachhu	80 mg.
Puthramjeev	80 mg.
Kumkum	10 mg.
Jathiphal	20 mg.
Shilajith	50 mg.
Kasturi	05 mg.
Bang bhasm	50 mg.
Ras Sindoor	25 mg.
Yasad bhasm	50 mg.
Swarn maakshik Bhasm	50 mg.

Dosage: One capsule twice a day or as directed by the physcian

How Supplied: Blister packings of 10 capsules each.

Uses: Indicated in general nervous condition, melancholia, tendency to weep, nervousness, during menopause, drowsiness and headache, jerking and twitching in all parts, premature ejaculation.

Product Name: **NURSING MOTHER HERBAL BODY MASSAGE OIL**

Composition: Each 10 ml. contains:

Bala	400 mg.
Athibala	400 mg.
Mustak	400 mg.
Ashwagandha	240 mg.
Nirgundi	400 mg.
Rasna	400 mg.
Shatavari	240 mg.
Tulsi	400 mg.
Shankhpushpi	400 mg.
Thil thail	10 ml.

Dosage: For external use only

How Supplied: Supplied in 100 ml and 200 ml unbreakable and elegant bottles.

Uses: Strengthens muscles and nerves during post-natal period and prevents bulging of stomach.

Product Name: **HERBAL BABY MASSAGE OIL**

Composition: Each 10 ml. contains:

Ashwagandha	200 mg.
Shakpushipi	200 mg.
Rasna	200 mg.
Vidari	200 mg.
Varahi	500 mg.
Kamal	080 mg.
Rakthchandan	120 mg.
Kunth	200 mg.
Sugandhbala	200 mg.
Rasone	200 mg.
Van pandu	200 mg.
Harida	120 mg.
Mash	200 mg.
Misthak	200 mg.
Yashtimandhu	080 mg.
Deodaru	080 mg.
Laksha	200 mg.
Rattanjoth	200 mg.
Thil thail	10 ml.
Karpur	01 mg.

Dosage: For external use only.

How Supplied: Supplied in 100 and 200 ml bottles.

Uses: Indicated in rickets, dry skin, also strengthens muscles and nerves.

Product Name: **CONSTOCIN (Powder/Churan)**

Composition: Each 100g contains:

Amalaki	5 g.
Harithki	20 g
Ishdugol	10 g.
Yavani	5 g.
Shunthi	10 g.
Shatpushpa	10 g.
Swarnapathri	20 g.
Saidhav	20 g.
Sauvarchal	10 g.

Dosage: Recommended dose of constocin 3 to 6 g. once or twice daily or as recommended by the physician.

How Supplied: Not available

Uses: Indicated in nervous gastric complaints, chronic constipation with heaviness, constant urge to pass stool without success, acidity

Product Name: **LUCENT HERBAL HAIR OIL**

Composition: Each 10 ml. contains:

Thagar	166 mg.
Darusitha	066 mg.
Ushir	166 mg.
Yashtimadhu	166 mg.
Amaalki	166 mg.
Shatavari	166 mg.
Shunti	100 mg.
Chandan sweth	033 mg.
Harithaki	166 mg.
Karpur kachari	066 mg.
Jatamansi	166 mg.

Erandmul	166 mg.
Vibhathik	166 mg.
Kankol	066 mg.
Musthak	166 mg.
Lodhra	166 mg.
Madyantik	166 mg.
Manjishta	166 mg.
Shikakai	066 mg.
Raktachandan	133 mg.
Priyangu	066 mg.
Kethak	033 mg.
Bhringraj	166 mg.
Tharuni	166 mg.
Rattamjoth	166 mg.
Thil thail	10 ml.
Lavang thail	0010 g.
Peppermint	01 g.

Dosage: For external use only

***How Supplied*:** Lucent herbal hair oil is supplied in 100 and 200 ml unbrekable bottles.

***Uses*:** Maintains natural colour of hair, maintains health and natural thickness, prevents dandruff, provides nutrines and strength.

***Product Name:* FEMIGLOW Syrup**

Composition: Each 10 ml. contains:

Ashok	222 mg.
Lodhra	222 mg.
Arjun	139 mg.
Ashwagandha	083 mg.
Shatavari	139 mg.
Yavani	139 mg.
Amaalki	222 mg.
Ulatkambal	222 mg.
Dhataki	139 mg.
Shunthi	139 mg.
Gokshuri	139 mg.
Mishreya	056 mg.
Harithki	139 mg.

Chini	400 mg.
Abrak bhasm	004 mg.
Loh bhasm	0008 mg.
Sodium benzoate	008 mg.

Dosage: Adults: 10 to 15 ml twice or thrice daily or as directed by the physician.

How Supplied: Supplied in 200 ml and 450 ml bottles.

Uses: Indicated in uterine debility, vaginal itching, leucorrhoea, menorrhoea, dismenorrhoea, anaemia, insomania, sexual weakness, loss of appetite, atony, yellowish and white skin.

***Product Name:* GASORUP Syrup**

Composition: Each 10 ml. contains:

Kutaj	169 mg.
Bilb	169 mg.
Dhathaki	101 mg.
Avarthini	169 mg.
Marich	034 mg.
Bidang	169 mg.
Harithai	169 mg.
Shunthi	101 mg.
Shatpushpa	169 mg.
Yavani	169 mg.
Putheena	160 mg.
Chitrak	101 mg.
Zeerak	034 mg.
Trivath	169 mg.
Shukthi bhasm	008 mg.
Kapard bhasm	008 mg.
Hing	0041 mg.
Chini	3.99 mg.
Sodium benzoate	008 mg.
Erithrocin colour	0004 mg.

Dosage: *Adult:* 10 to 20 two to four times daily. *Children:* 5 ml to 10 ml two to four times daily or as directed by the physician.

How Supplied: Gasorup syrup is supplied in 200 ml bottles.

Uses: Indicated in acidity, constipation, gastro enteritis, belching.

Product Name: **LUCENT HERBAL HAIR WASH (Powder-Dry Shampoo)**

Composition: Each 10g. contains:

Bhandir	15 g.
Bhringraj	15 g.
Aamalaki	15 g.
Thriphala	15 g.
Shikakai	25 g.
Arishtak	15 g.

Dosage: For external use only

How Supplied: Supplied in 100g. packings.

Uses: Prevents dandruff, premature greying and for long and silky hair.

LUPIN LABORATORIES LTD.
159, C.S.T. Road, Kalina, Santa Cruz (East), Mumbai-400 098
Tel: 6102722, 6113391 Fax: (22) 6114008

Product Name: **ONE-BE Capsules**

Composition: Extract equ. to Shatavari	950 mg.
Ashwagandha	550 mg.
Vidarikand	550 mg.
Kaunch beej	275 mg.
Varahikand	275 mg.
Vriddhdaru	275 mg.
Suddha shilajit	275 mg.
Pippali	235 mg.

LYKA LABS. LIMITED
77, Nehru Road, Vile Parle (East), Mumbai-400 099
Tel: 6105900-01-02, 6105999-6003 Fax: (22) 6105281/6111024

Product Name: **DANCLIN LOTION**

Composition:

Kushtha	5%
Mehndi	2%
Nagkesara	2%
Haridra	2%
Brahmi	2%
Amla	2%
Vaj	2%
Rasanjan	0.2%

Chaulmugra	2%
Neem	2%
Karanj	2%
Badam	5%
Proc. Jasat bhasma	8%

MEDILA PHARMACEUTICALS
24 Sneh Nagar Indore-452 001, Tel: 461616, 46600

Product Name: **CHOKKA HERBAL Capsules**

Composition:

Sudh shilajeet	60 mg.
Keshar	5 mg.
Akalkara	20 mg.
Jayaphal	30 g.
Jawitri	30 mg.
Lavang	20 mg.
Swarna makshik bhasma	30 mg.
Bang bhasma	20 mg.
Loh bhasma	10 mg.
Konch beej	30 mg.
Gokhru	25 mg.
Moosli	40 mg.
Satavar	30 mg.
Talmakhana	25 mg.
Pipli	15 mg.
Kapoor	5 mg.
Satvas: Amla	15 mg.
Ashwagandha	40 mg.
Bahera	15 mg.
Yastimadhu	20 mg.
Harad	15 mg.
Bhavna: Paan	

Product Name: **ENERGIC PHOS Capsules**

Composition:

Shudh shilajeet	50 mg.
Ashwagandha	75 mg.
Amla, Sheetal chini each	25 mg.
Haldi, Gokhru chota each	20 mg.
Safed chandan burada	15 mg.

Dalchini, Dautimoolm Swarna Makshik Bhasma, Bhanshlochan, nagarmotha, Tejpat, Chilka Daro-Haldi, Choti elayachi, Dhania, Sonth, Safed moosli, Bari elayachi, each 10 g Burada devdaro, Baobidang, Chav,, Atish mitha, Kala namak, Giloi, Sambhar namak, Gajpippal, Lodhra pthani, Sajjkhar, Sendha namak, Kali Mirch each 5 mg.

***Product Name:* FEMI PHOS Capsules**

***Composition*:**

Lodhra pathani	60 mg.
Ashok chal	50 mg.

Alum Chikni supari, Lajwanti, Dhakgondh, Geru, Mochras, Talmakhana, Trifla, Gokru chota each 30 g, Majophal, Kuk-Kutavagta bhasma, Tribang bhasma, Lal chandan, Gondh each 20 mg Loh bhasma, Mulehthi each 10 mg.

***Product Name:* SONA HERBAL Hair Oil**

***Composition*:**

Ext. of Brahami	10%
Amla	8%
Sugandhbala	2%
Bhangra	10%
Jatamansi	2%
Gulab patri	2%
Nimb patra	1%
Mehandi patra	2%
Babchi	1%
Majeeth	2%
Nagarmotha	2%
Talish patra	2%
Ratanjot	1%
Anantamool	2%
Charila	2%
Chandan	1%
Agar	2%
Chameli tel	2%
Sariso tel	5%
Jatoon tel	1%
Til tel	q.s.

Prduct Name: **VIGOPHOS Capsules**

Composition:

Shudh shilajeet	60 mg.
Moosli	50 mg.
Ashwagandha	40 mg.
Satavar, Konch beej each	30 mg.

Swarna makshik bhasm, Jawitri, Talmkhana, Gokhru, each 25 mg. Bang bhasma, Akalkara, Jayaphal, Lavang, Melethi satva each 20 . Pipli, Harad satva, Ala satva, Bahera satva each 15 mg. Abhrak bhasma, Loh bhasma each 10 mg. Keshar, Bhimsaini kapoor each 5 mg.

Product Name: **VITAZIL Capsules**

Composition:

Ashwagandha 60 mg. Shudh shilajeet, Moosli,Sheetal chini, Lodhra pathani each 40 mg. Shatavar,Talmakhana, Amla, Gokhru each 30 mg. Bang Bhasma,Kuk-Kutangvtak bhasma, Alum bhasma, Kontha beej each 15 mg. Choti Pippal, Badi elaychi each 15 mg. Geru, Bahera,Harad each 10 mg.

MEDIAWAYS PHARMACEUTICALS
Sirsaganj-205 151, Firozabad, U.P.
Tel: (05675 22035, 22225 Fax: (0562) 381637

Product Name: **GROTHAN syrup**

Composition:

Foebiculum vulgare	50g.
Viola odorata	50 g.
Terminalia arjuna	20 g.
Terminalia chebula	50 g.
Terminalia belerica	50 g.
Embica officinalis	50 g.
Cinchorium intybus	50 g.
Piper longum	10 g.
Tinospora cordifolia	50 g.
Cyperus rotundus	50 g.
Aconitum hetrophyllum	50 g.

Product Name: MEDIBURN Ointment

Composition:

Linum usitiassimum	150 mg.
Shorea robusta	150 mg.
Trachyspermum ammi	100 mg.
Camphora officinarum	100 mg.
Sikth oil	50 g.

Product Name: MEDIDIX Ointnment

Composition:

Aloe barbadensis	100 mg.
Borex	100 mg.
Curcua aromatica	100 mg.
Sikth oil	75 g

Product Name: MEDIFER Syrup

Composition:

Emblica officinalis	50 g
Terminalia chebula	50 g.
Withania somnifera	50 g.
Terminalia arjuna	50 g.
Tinospora cordifolia	50 g.
Sida cordifolia	50 g.
Abutilan indicura	50 g.
Vitis vinifer	30 g.
Leptadenia retivulta	50 g.
Phascolus trilobus	50 g.
Termamnus labiali	59 g.
Purearia tuerosa	50 g.
Dioscorea bulinogra	50 g.
Camella asiatics	50 g.
Piper longum	20 g.

Product Name: MEDIKOF Syrup

Composition:

Ephedra giradiana	50 g.
Pistasis integerrima	50 g.
Piper longum	20 g.

Adhaoda vasica	50 g.
Ocimum sanctum	50 g.
Glycyrrhiza glabra	50 g.
Terminalia belerica	50 g.
Solanum surathense	50 g.
Zingiber Officinlale	30 g.
PIper nigrum	10 g.
Cordia mysa	50 g.
Viola ororat	50 g.
Onosoma bractaetum	50 g.
Cassia occidentialis	50 g.

Product Name: **MEDILIME tablets**

***Composition*:**

Opercullina turpethum	45 mg.
Trachyspermum ammi	45 mg.
Emblica offininalis	45 mg.
Terminalla chebusa	45 mg.
Zingiber officinale	40 mg.
Foeniculum vulta	45 mg.
Glychrrhiz glabr	45 mg.
Mentha spicata	45 mg.
Trichosanthes dioica	45 mg.
Tinosporac cordifolia	45 mg.
Adhatoda vasicsa	45 mg.

Product Name: **MEDILIV Syrup**

***Composition*:**

Cinchoium intybus	50 g.
Solanum nigrum	50 g.
Terminalia arjuna	50 g.
Tinospor cordifolia	50 g.
Fumaria vasillantil	50 g.
Emblica officinalis	50 g.
Boerhavia diffusa	50 g.
Nyctanthes arbortristis	50 g.
Eclipta alba	50 g.
Achryanthes aspera	50 g.
Andrographis paniculata	50 g.
Tephrosia purpurea	50 g.
Picrohiza kurroa	30 g.

***Product Name:* METORRHOEA Tablets**

***Composition*:**

Aegle marmelos	50 mg.
Embelia ribes	40 mg.
Beberis aristata	50 mg.
Heticteres isora	50 mg.
Foeniculum vulgare	50 mg.
Trachyspermum ammi	30 mg.
Oroxylum indicum	50 mg.
Woodfordia fructicosa	50 mg.
Plumbago zelyanica	20 mg.
Cyperus rotundus	50 mg.

MOUNT METTUR PHARMACEUTICAS LTD.
63/1, 2nd Main Road, Gandhi Nagar, Adhyar, P.B. No. 2069
Chennai-600 020, Tel: 4915388, 49013588, 4911404

***Product Name*: ENE-LIV Tablets**

***Composition*:**

Picrorrhiza kurroa	25 mg.
Tinospora cordifolia	25 mg.
Andrographis paniculata	25 mg.
Solanum nigrum	25 mg.
Galega furpurea	25 mg.
Beriberis aristata	25 mg.
Phyllanthus camurs	25 mg.
Aloe litoralis	25 mg.
Rincinus communis	25 mg.

***Product Name*: FLAMET Capsules**

***Composition*:**

Maha yograj guggal	50 mg.
Berberis aristata	25 mg.
Withania somnifera	25 mg.
Trikatu	50 mg.
Tribulus terrestris	25 mg.
Tinospora cordifola	25 mg.
Rinifinus communis	25 mg.
Tribala	50 mg.

***Product Name*: GYLOMIN Capsules**

***Composition*:**

Saraca indica	75 mg.
Berberis aristata	75 mg.
Symplocos racemosa	50 mg.
Ocimum sanctum seeds	10 mg.
Tribulus terrestris	25 mg.
Acacia catechu	25 mg.
Bombax malabaricum	25 mg.
Kasisa (Ferrous Sulphate)	50 mg.
Adhatoda vasika	50 mg.

***Product Name*: PIL-REL Capsules**

***Composition*:**

Plumbago zeylanica	50 mg.
Holarrhena antidysentrica	50 mg.
Cissampelos pereira	25 mg.
Picorrhiza kurroa	50 mg.
Abutilon indicum	100 mg.
Terminalia chebula	50 mg.
Berberis arisata	50 mg.

MYNCIL PHARMACEUTICALS
S, 17/331-P, Vijay Nagar,Maldahiya,
P.O. Box No. 2084, Varanasi-221 002,
Tel : 344577, Fax: (542) 342944

***Product Name*: DYSBEL Granules**

***Composition*:** Each 10 ml. contains:

Beal guddi	300 mg.
Kurchi	300 mg.
Sauf	100 mg.
Haratki	100 mg.
Isabgol	750 mg.
Indrajav	300 mg.
Nagarmotha	50 mg.
Sontha	100 mg.
Dhania	25 mg.
Ayapan	50 mg.

Ajwain	100 mg.
Dhai ka phool	50 mg.
Methi	100 mg.
Mehandiseed	25 mg.
Kapoor	3 mg.
Pipermint	3 mg.
Mochras	10 mg.
Pudina	50 mg.

Product Name: **GASTRIP Syrup**

Composition: Each 10 ml contains:

Giloi	50 mg.
Atish	100 mg.
Revand chini	25 mg.
Saunf	100 mg.
Siyah Jira	100 mg.
Triphala	100 mg.
Chitmul	50 mg.
Hing	2.5 mg.
Ajwain	100 mg.
Dalchini	10 mg.
Pipal	50 mg.
Pipla mool	50 mg.
Chitrak	100 mg.
Kali mirich	50 mg.
Bach	100 mg.
Nagarmotha	100 mg.
Laung	5 mg.
Dried milk of papita	60 mg.
Beal guddi	100 mg.
Daruhalid	100 mg.
Rohitak	50 mg.
Methi	100 mg.
Radhuni seed	50 mg.
Sontha	100 mg.
Chabya	50 mg.
Haldi	50 mg.
Tejpat	10 mg.
Elachi	5 mg
Nagkeshar	10 mg
Jayaphal	10 mg
Draksha	50 mg.
Jamun ka sirka	0.5 ml.

Product Name: **GYNEMYN Liquid**

Composition: Each 5 ml. contains:

Ashok bark	400 mg.
Lodh	400 mg.
Dhai ka phool	200 mg.
Patang	25 mg.
Beal guddi	25 mg.
Anantmool	50 mg.
Shyam lata	50 mg.
Daruhaldi	100 mg.
Mango seed	50 mg.
Bala	50 mg.
Jeevanti	50 mg.
Satavar	50 mg.
Semar ka phool	50 mg.
Nagar moth	50 mg.
Rasaut	25 mg.
Tagar	100 mg.
Khair wood	25 mg.
Chandan wood	10 mg.
Aswagandha	50 mg.

Product Name: **HEPTAMYN Drops**

Composition: Each ml. contains:

Kasani	20 mg.
Makoi	8 mg.
Kasaudi	6 mg.
Pittapapra	40 mg.
Sanai patti	8 mg.
Arjuna bark	20 mg.
Gadah purna	40 mg.
Ajawain	40 mg.
Methi	40 mg.
Daru haldi	50 mg.
Satauna	20 mg.
Sontha	20 mg.
Guruch	40 mg.
Sarpunkha	20 mg.
Choti piper	12 mg.
Kusum phool	20 mg.
Bhangra	20 mg.
Radhuni seed	12 mg.

Triphala	60 mg.
Rohera bark	20 mg.
Jhau	20 mg.
Atish	10 mg.
Kalmegh	20 mg.
Ghrit kumari	100 mg.

***Product Name:* HEPTAMYN syrup**

***Composition*:** Each 10 ml. contains:

Kasani	100 mg.
Makoi	30 mg.
Kasaudi	20 mg.
Pitpapra	200 mg.
Senai patti	50 mg.
Arjuna bark	100 mg.
Gadahpurna	100 mg.
Ajwain	100 mg.
Methi	100 mg.
Daruhaldi	200 mg.
Satauna	100 mg.
Guruch	100 mg.
Sontha	100 mg.
Sarpunkha	100 mg.
Chotipiper	50 mg.
Kusum phool	100 mg.
Bhangra	100 mg.
Radhuni seed	50 mg.
Amla	100 mg.
Harra	100 mg.
Bahera	100 mg.
Rohera bark	100 mg.
Jhau	100 mg.
Ghrita kumari	500 mg.
Kalmegh	100 mg.
Jamun ka sirka	0.5 mg.

***Product Name*: MINNITONE liquid** (Baby Tonic)

Compositio: Each ml. contains:

Ajwain	10 mg.
Kasni	20 mg.
Makoi	20 mg.
Amla	10 mg.

Harra	10 mg.
Bahera	10 mg.
Punarnavae	20 mg.
Ghrit kumari	40 mg.
Pipal mool	10 mg.
Bach	10 mg.
Pipal	10 mg.
Chitrak mool	20 mg.
Kali mirch	10 mg.
Sauf	20 mg.
Nagarmotha	20 mg.
Aswagandha	20 mg.
Satawar	20 mg.
Bidarikand	20 mg.
Bala	20 mg.
Baibidong	50 mg.
Atish	10 mg.

Product Name: **MYNCIL ASHOKA Compound Liquid**

Composition: Each 10 ml contains:

Ashoka bark	800 mg.
Lodh	500 mg.
Dhai ka phool	500 mg.
Dharuhaldi	100 mg.
Tagar wood	50 mg.
Mango seed	50 mg.
Khair wood	50 mg.
Nagarmotha	50 mg.
Ashwagandha	50 mg.
Bala	50 mg.
Ananthmool	50 mG.

Product Name: **OCTIN EXPECTORANT Liquid**

Composition: Each 10 ml. contains:

Banafasa	200 mg.
Kantikari	800 mg.
Adusa leaves	1000 mg.
Choti piper	40 mg.
Kakrasingi	50 mg.
Bari kateri	50 mg.

Javasa	100 mg.
Mulethi	100 mg.
Guruch	200 mg.
Kulanajan	50 mg.
Lishora	200 mg.
Ghorbach	50 mg.
Bahera	100 mg.
Gajpipar	50 mg.
Ajwain	100 mg.
Bhagra	100 mg.
Na kesdar	50 mg.
Jatamasi	25 mg.
Talish patra	50 mg.
Adrakh	400 mg.
Tulshi leaves	250 mg.
Nausadar	300 mg.
Pipermint	2.5 mg.

***Product Name:* VINOMYN Liquid (General Tonic)**

Composition: Each 10 ml. contains:

Satavar	100 mg.
Gokhuru	50 mg.
Safed musali	50 mg.
Kali musali	50 mg.
Bidari kand	150 mg.
Aswagandha	200 mg.
Kala munnakka	100 mg.
Dashmul	100 mg.
Kevanch seed	50 mg.
Baryara	100 mg.
Atish	50 mg.
Gambhari	50 mg.
Sugandha bala	50 mg.
Jatamasi	50 mg.
Bhumi avala	50 mg.
Kamal gatta	100 mg.
Maulsari chal	25 mg.
Babul gum	100 mg.
Brahmi	100 mg.
Bhringraj	100 mg.

Nag keshar	5 mg.
Kabab chini	10 mg.
Akarkara	10 mg.
Guruch	10 mg.

NATCO PHARMA LTD.

Natco House, Road No. 2 Banjara Hills, Hyderabad-500 003
Tel: 247532 (14 lines) Fax: (040) 248 243

Product Name: **CLENZ Syrup**

Composition:

Azadirachta indica extract	1% w/w
Pongamia glabra extract	2% w/w
Glycyrriza glabra extract	0.5% w/w/
Santlum album	0.5% w/w
Circuma longa	1% w/w

Product Name: **REVIVIN TABLETS**

Composition:

Ashwagandha extract	50 mg.
Satavari extract	30 mg.
Yastimadhu extract	30 mg.
Kaunch beej extract	15 mg.
Vidari kanda extract	10 mg.
Drakshadi churnam	35 mg.
Yasheda bhasma	5 mg.
Bala beej	1.5 mg.
Akarakara	30 mg.
Jati phal	10 mg.

NATURO HERBAL REMEDIES

3/33, Iyer Line, Swarnapuri, Salem-4 Tel (0427) 446674

Product Name: **DEFLAMM Capsule**

Composition:

Extracts	
Cardiospermum Helicacabum	5 mg.
Daemia extensa	5 mg.
Delonix alata	5 mg.

Powders	
Anethum sowa	50 mg.
Embellia ribes	25 mg.
Gingiber officinalel	50 mg.
Sodium Chloride	25 mg.
Alpinia galanga	50 mg.
Cidrus deodara	50 mg.
Tinospora stem	50 mg.
Balasaodendan mukul	90 mg.
Titration	
Maha Rasnadi kashayam	5 mg.
Valuluvai kashayam	5 mg.
Dasamula kashayam	5 mg.

Dosage: 1-2 caps thrice daily

How Supplied: Pack of 100 caps.

Uses: Inflammatory conditions of joints. Low back Pain, rheumatoid arthritis, Osteo Arthritis, Sciatic, Lumbago, Muscular pain & stiffness

Pharmacological Action: Deflamm has an effective combination of drugs to neutralise the "Amam" held in the joints which according to Indian Medicine is the basic cause for Arthralgia. Deflamm successfully resolves pain, stiffness & Inflammation. Deflamm helps prevent sclerotic changes in the joints. Deflamm strengthens synovial membrane & Cartilagenous tissues of the joint. Deflamm IS FREE FROM ANY SIDE EFFECTS-even on prolonged use.

Product Name: **ETIOMENT LEPAM**

Composition: Each 30 g. Contains:

Vitex Nigundu	2.5 g.
Dolonix alata	2.5 g
Cardiospermum	2.5 g
Daemia extena	2.5 g
Tinospora cordyfolia	2 g.
Pavonia Zeylanica	2 g.
Withania somnifera	2 g.
Alpinia galanga	2 g.
Balasamondram mukul	5 g.

Camphorum	0.05 g.
Eucalyptus oil	0.05 g.
Pudina ka Phool	0.05 g.
Sesame Oil	22.85 g.
Bess wax	Q.S.

Dosage: Gentle massage on the affected part twice or thrice after a wash with warm water.

How Supplied: Pack aof 20 gms & 40 gms.

Uses: Rheumatoid arthritis, Osteo arthritis, Low back pain, sciatica, Muscular sprains, Joint stiffness etc.

Pharmacological Action: Etioment is a time tested unique combination of Herbs to relax the muscles and relieve pain. Etioment improves blood circulation in the affected part. It retards regenerative process in the joints. Etioment combats effectively spasm and stiffness of muscles. Etioment is safe even on long term use.

Product Name: **SUPER MEMO Capsule**

Composition:

Extracts	
Bacopa monneri	100 mg.
Hydrocotyle Asiatica	100 mg.
Powders	
Evolvulus alsinoids	50 mg.
Achorus calamus	20 mg.
Clitoria ternatea	20 mg.
Nar jatamansi	20 mg.
Valerina vallichi	20 mg.

Dosage: Adults 1-2 caps, bds, Children 1 cap oid

How Supplied: 100 caps pack

Use: Memory disturbances, Lack of attention, Depressive state, stress syndrome etc.

Pharmacological Action: Super memo improves mental alertness Super memo relieves Anxiety, Depression & psychosis, Super memo alleviates stress syndrome, Mental fatigue, and sleep disturbances.

***Product Name:* NEO PUSHTI granules**

Composition:

Withania somnifera (boiled in milk)	50 mg.
Asparagus racemosus	30 mg.
Cucurligo root	30 mg.
Ipomea digitata	20 mg.
Orchis mascula	20 mg.
Astracantha longifolia	10 mg.

Dosage: Mix one teapsoon full with a cup of hot milk.

How Supplied: 100 grams per pack

Uses:

Pharmacological Action

1. Enhances the child's Immunity
2. Promotes Healthy growth in children
3. Meets the energy requirements of working people
4. Supplements vital Nutrients for the aged

***Product Name:* PRANA Pills**

Composition:

Tylopora Asthmatica	39 mg.
Tinospora cordyfolia	39 mg.
Ocimum sanctum	40 mg.
Adathoda Vasica	41 mg.
Sol. Trilobatu	65 mg.
Sol. Xanthocarpum	65 mg.
Dasamula kashayam	10 mg.
Calyx of Pravala	10 mg.

Dosage: 5-10 grams twice or thrice daily

How Supplied: 100 pills per pack

Uses: Bronchial Asthma, Chronic bronchitis, Allergic bronchitis etc.

Pharmacological Action: Exhibits Broncho-dilatory action; has anti-spasmodic activity. Depresses the vagal endings and provides control over cough reflex; Corrects the imbalance of vatha & kapha by improving the state of Pitta, to restore normalcy in respiration; In long term use it enhances patient's immunity, thus reduces his hypersensitivity to allergens.

***Product Name*: COSY COUGH Syrup**

***Composition*:** Each 5 ml. contains:

Ocimum sanctum	0.65 ml.
Adathoda vasaca	0.65 ml.
Sol. Xanthocarpum	0.65 ml.
Sol. Trilobatum	0.65 ml.
Mukia scarvarilla	0.20 ml.
Eclipta alba	0.50 ml.
Tylophora asthamatics	0.50 ml.
Piper betel	0.50 ml.
Decoction	
Glycerrhyza glabra	0.20 ml.
Sassures lappa	0.20 ml.
Alpinia galanga	0.30 ml.
Sugar base	q.s

Dosage: 5-10 ml. (2 teaspoons) twice or thri\ce daily

***How Supplied*:** 60 ml, 100 ml. bottles

***Uses*:** Dry cough, Productive cough, cough associated with common cold, Bronchitis and other infections of the respiratory tract.

Pharmaclogial Action: Cosy is a successful combination of drugs formulated to pacify the increased Vatha in the throat and remove the dryness and give a SOOTHING EFFECT.

Cosy also acts by liquifying the hardened kapha and gives an ANTITUSSIVE/EXPECTORANT ACTION.

Cosy is a non habit forming, non sedative, and non constipating cough formula. Cosy gives an excellent Bronchodilator effect for a prolonged time.

***Product Name:* DIGEST Lozenges**

***Composition*:**

Kaqvikkal churnam	100 mg.
Ashta churnam	100 mg.
Madhuyashti churnam	50 mg.
Pirandai churnm	50 mg.
Lavanbhaskara churnam	50 mg.
Panchalavana baspam	30 mg.
Sana bapsam	20 mg.

Dosage: 1-2 chewable lozenges twice or thrice daily

How Supplied: Pack of 100 lozenges

Uses: Acidity, Gastritis Loss of appetite, Indigestion, Flatulence etc.

Pharmacological Action: Has an antacid, Anti-flatulant and antispasmodic action. Checks Hyer acidity, Relieves spasm, Pain & Anxiety. Protects th Mucosa from ulceration. Can be given as an adjuvant to other antiinflammatory & anelgesic drugs.

***Product Name*: SUGNIL Capsule**

***Composition*:**

Extract	
Euginia jambolana	20 mg.
Aristolochia Bracteatea	20 mg.
Gymnema sylvestris	40 mg.
Cassia auriculata	40 mg.
Memordica charantia	20 mg.
Powders	
Murraya koenigli	60 mg.
Curcua longa	60 mg.
Cosinium fenestratum	60 mg.
Andrograpis paniculata	60 mg.
3 myrobalans	60 mg.
Seendil sarkarai	50 mg.
Calyx of asphalt	20 mg.

Dosage: 1-2 capsules twice daily

How Supplied: 100 caps/apck

Uses: Mild to moderate NIDDM. Can be given along with other medicines in uncontrolled diabetes.

Pharmacological Action: Sugnil is an efficient combination of Herbo-Mineral hypoglycemics used since ages Sugnil gives excellent results in reducing blood glucose level in moderate cases of Non-Insulin dependent diabetes Mellitus which fact has been clinically recorded. Sugnil gives significant remedy in controlling general weakness, constipation, palpitation, anorexia, Insomania etc.

***Product Name:* NEO FERTILIS-M Capsule**

Composition:

Asphaltum (Pure)	100 mg.

Withania somnifera	100 mg.
Micuna pruriens	100 mg.
Asparagus racemosus	30 mg.
Ipomea digitata	30 mg.
Moringa oleflora	30 mg.
Myristica officinalis	20 mg.
Orchis mascula	20 mg.
Milk of ficus glomerulata	20 mg.

Dosage: 1-2 capsules twice daily

How Supplied: 100 capsules per pack

Uses: Management of Male functional Infertility, Oligospermia, Spermatorrhoea etc.

Pharmacological Action: Promotes youthful vigour & vitality improves motility of sperms. Increases the quantity & quality of semen Assures sustained adequacy in performance.

Product Name: **SLIMSURE Capsule**

Composition:

Pariera brava	180 mg.
Balasamondron mukul	150 mg.
Terminalia chebula	50 mg.
Embilica officinalis	50 mg.
Terminalia Bellarica	50 mg.
Embellia ribes	10 mg.
Sida cordyfolia	10 mg.
Zingiber officinalis	1 mg.

Dosage: 2-4 capsules twice daily

How Supplied: 100 capsules per poack

Uses: Reduces blood cholesterol level. Reduces excessive fat from the body.

SAGAR PARMACEUTICALS
"Varada", 375, 1st "B" Main, 1st Phase, Girinagar, Bangalore-560 085
Tel: 6721031 Fax: (080) 6720139

Product Name: **ANULOMA Tablet**

Composition: Each tablet contains:

Ajamoda (Ptychotis ajowan seeds)	8 mg.

Jeeraka (Cuminum cyminum seeds)	8 mg.
Balharda (Black erminalia chebula Fruit)	8 mg.
Yashtimadhu (Glycyrrhiza glabra root)	8 mg.
Ginger (Zingiber officinale rizome)	8 mg.
Saindhav salt (Natural potassium nitricum)	10 mg.
Senna (Cassia lanaceolata leaf)	550 mg.

Dosage: 1 to 3 tablets at bed time

How Supplied: Aluminium strips of 12×10×10' s cntainers of 3×500's.

Uses: Pils old age, after operation, pregnancy, psychiatry, hear diseases.

***Product Name:* ANULOMA tablet**

Composition: Each 1.5 g powder contains:

Ajamoda (Ptychotis ajowan seeds)	80 mg.
Jeeraka (Cuminum cyminum seeds)	80 mg.
Balharda (Black terminalia chebula Fruit)	80 mg.
Yashtimadhu (Glycyrrhiza glabra root)	80 mg.
Ginger (Zingiber officinale rhizome)	80 mg.
Saindhav salt (Natural potassium nitricum)	100 mg.
Senna (Cassia lanceolata leaf)	1 mg.

Dosage: 1/2 to 1 teaspons at bed ime (0.75 gm to 1.5 gm)

How Supplied: Containers of 12×50 gm, Cartons of 1×1 kg.

Uses: Piles, old age, after operation, pregnancy, psychiatry, heart diseases.

***Product Name:* ARTHNEX Tablet**

Composition: Each tablet contatins:

Raasna (Pluches lanceolata root)	60 mg.
Guduchi (Tinospora cordifolia stem)	60 mg.
Erandamoola ext. eq. (Ricinus communis root)	60 mg.
Deodar ext. eq. (Cedrus deodara stem)	50 mg.
Ginger (zingiber officinale rhizome)	60 mg.
Balamoola ext. eq. (Sida cordifolia stem)	60 mg.
Guggul ext. rq. (Commipora mukul gum)	60 mg.
Processed in ajamoda (Ptychotis ajowan seeds)	

Dosage: 2 tablet 3 times a day for 4 to 6 weeks or more. after the symptoms subside taper off the dose to 1 tablet t.i.d. upto 6 months or till adequate improvement is noticed.

How Supplied: Containers of 12 × 100's, Containers of 6 × 500's

Uses: Articular inflammatory diseases, articular degenerative diseases, non-articular rheumatism, musculo-skeletal inflammatory conditions.

Product Name: DECAZYME tablet

Composition: Each tablet contains:

Pippali (Piper longum berry)	1.5 mg.
Ginger (Zingiber officinate rhizoe)	15 mg.
Maricha (Piper nigrum seedP	16 mg.
Cardamom (Elettaria cardamomum fruit)	15 mg.
Chitrak (Plumbago zeylanica root)	20 mg.
Jeeraka (Cuminum cyminum seed)	20 mg.
Amalakee (Emblica officinalis dried fruit)	25 mg.
Vacha (Acorus calamus root)	50 mg.
Garlic ext. eq. (Allium sativum bulb)	50 mg.
Kapardik bhasma (Conc. sheel calcinate)	15 mg.
Sugar	100 mg.

Dosage: 2 tablets 3 times a day for about 6 weeks. 1 tablet 3 times a day as a supportive treatment.

How Supplied: Containers of 12×100's, Containers of 6×500's

Uses: Indigestion, Flatulence, Hyperacidity,Anorexia, Loss of absorption of food and drugs.

Product Name: GORANCHI Tablet

Composition: Each tablet contains:

Madhunashinee (Gymnema sylvestre) Leaf ext. eq.	50 mg.
Madhunashinee root ext. eq.	50 mg.
(Gymnema sylvestre)	50 mg.
Jambuphala ext. eq.	

(Eugenia jambolana seed)	120 mg.
Amakalee	
(Emblica officinalis dried fruit)	60 mg.
Haridra (Curcuma longa dried rhizome)	60 mg.
Saptarangi ext. eq.	
(Caseriana esculenta root)	20 mg.
Mamejav et. eq.	
(Enicostemma littorale herb)	20 mg.
Shilajit ext. eq. (Asphaltum)	30 mg.

Dosage: 2 tablets 3 times a day for 6 months or till adequate stability of urine sugar and blood sugar is achieved. Later mainteance dse 1 tablet 3 times a day.

How Supplied: Containers of 12×100's; Containers of 6×500's

Uses: Diabetes mellitus, polyurea

Product Name: **GYNOVEDAN Capsule**

Composition: Each capsule contains:

Swarna makshik bhasma	40 mg.
Vanga bhasma	10 mg.
Karpoora (Camphor I.P.)	250 mg.
Ashok ext. eq. (Saraca indica stem)	50 mg.

Dosage: 1 capsule two times a day during three consecutive menstrual cycles only. Start soon after the menstrual flow begins and continue for 3 days. Repeat during the next two subsequent periods. In obstinate cases a second course of further 9 days may be necessary. A ripe banana or chikku fruit has to be taken with each dose of Gyynovedan capsule to counter the smell of camphor.

How Supplied: Blisters of 12×10×10's; Containers of 12×100's

Uses: Menstrual pain, premenstrual tension, no repetitions of episodes, useful in secondary infertility in females due to dysmenorrhoea.

Product Name: **NASOLLERIN Capsule**

Composition: Each capsule contains:

Kachora (Curcuma zedora root)	85 mg.
Ginger (Zingiber officinale rhizome)	60 mg.
Haridra (Curcuma longa rhizome)	70 mg.

Maricha (Piper nigrum died fruit)	50 mg.
Khurasani ajamoda	
(Hyociamus niger seed)	50 mg.
Bhumyanalaki ext. eq.	
(Phyllanthus niruri herb)	70 mg.
Tulsi ext. eq. (Ocimum sanctum leaf)	50 mg.
Pippalee (Piper longum berry)	10 mg.
Talispatra (Abis webbiana leaf)	25 mg.
Jatipatra (Myristica fragrance seed testa)	05 mg.
Karpoora (Camphor IP)	05 mg.

Dosage: Not available

How Supplied: Blisters of 12×10×10's; Containers of 3×500's

Uses: Nasal and respiratory congestion, common cold sneezing, sinusitis, vasomotor and allergic rhinitis; fever and flu as a supportive drug.

***Product Name:* OLEUM ARTHNEX**

Composition: Each 5 ml oil contains:

Katuveera ext. eq.	
(Capasicum annum fruit)	1 mg.
Nirgundi ext. eq.	
(Vitex nigundo leaf)	1.75 g
Eucalyptus oil	
(Oil of eucalyptus globulus)	0.5 ml.
Camphor I.P.	0.05 mg.
Rasna ext eq.	
(pluchea lanceolata root)	200 mg.
Base	q.s.

Dosage: Apply on the affected part and massage if necessary as directed by the physician.

How Supplied: Shipper of 10030 ml bottoles.

Uses: For external application in muscioskeletal pains, strainsand headache.

***Product Name:* REJUVITE capsule**

Composition: Each capsule contains:

Kapikachchu	
(mucuna prurience seed)	200 mg.
Ashwagandha (Withania somnifera root)	100 mg.

Kokilakhsa exf. eq.	
(stracantha longiflolia seed)	100 mg.
Guduchi ext. eq.	
(Tinospoa cordfolia stem)	50 mg.
Gokshura ext. eq.	
(Tribulus terresris fruit)	50 mg.
Shikhi ex. eq.	
(Blepharis edulis seed)	50 mg.
Lvan (Syzygium aomaticum	
Flower bud)	10 mg.
Shilajit ext. eq.	
(Natural asphaltum)	10 mg.
Jatiphala	
(Myristica fragrance kernel-Nutmeg)	05 mg.
Kehsar (crcus sativus stemen)	01 mg.

Dosage:One to two capsules per day followed by milk.

How Supplied: Blister of 5×1×10's

Uses: Functional impotence, depressed libido, sexual neurasthenia, premature ejaculation, unsatisfactory erection, unsatisfactory sexual perofmance, rigidity in women, ooligosphermia

***Product Name*: SAGARLIC PEARL**

Composition: Each pearl contains:

Rasona (Allium sativum bulbsP	200 mg.
Tila taila base	
(Oil of sesamum indicum seed)	250 mg.

Dosage: 1 to 2 pearls 3 times a day.

How Supplied: Containers of 12 × 50's

Uses: Sagarlic pearl can be employed individually or as an adjuvant in several clinical conditions with good bnenefit. Sagarlic pearl is of immense use as a carminative, gastric stimulant to aid digestion and absorption of food and as a long term treatment in diseases of respiratory tract. Sugarlic pearl is useful in treatment of malginant tumours, fractured bones, diabetes mellitus, typhoid, fis and vata vyadhis.

***Product Name:* SANGWAYU Capsule**

Composition:

Ashwagandha ext. eq.	250 mg.
(Withania somnifera root)	
Vidarikand	
(Pueraria tuberorsa tuber)	250 mg.

Amalakee (Emblica officinalis dried fruit)	250 mg.
Shatavaree (Asparagus racemosus root)	250 mg.
Loha bhasma (Ayurvedic iron)	25 mg.
Jasada bhasma (Ayurvedic zinc)	25 mg.

Dosage: 1 capsule 2 times a day. Children: 1 capsule 2 times a day.

How Supplied: Containers of 12×50's

Uses: Sangwyu capsule is indicated in all conditions where administration of multivitamin, B-complex, zinc and haematinics are needed. Such conditions include convalescence, chronic alcoholism, old age,prolonged antibiotic therapy, debilitating diseases, surgery, anaemia, pediatrics and gynaecology. Sangwayu is a valuable adjuvant in diabetes mellitus, tuberculosis and chronic diseases. Sangwayu relieves vague aches and pain. Sangwayu therefore is an all purpose tonic for men women and children.

***Product Name:* TANTU PASHAN tablet**

Composition: Each tablet contains:

Maricha (PIper nigrum berry)	180 mg.
Chavya (Piper chabab stem)	80 mg.
Tantu pashan bhasma	140 mg.

Dosage: *Massive Dose with pathya (Diet):* 4 tablets morning and 4 tablets evening for 3 days. 3 tablets morning and 3 tablets evening for 7 days to 10 days.

Maintenance dose without pathya: 1 tablets morning and 1 tablets evening for 30 days.

How Supplied: Containers of 12 × 100's

Uses: Grandmal, petitmal, focal epilepsy, myoclonic jerks

***Product Name*: TEJODERM Capsule**

Composition: Each capsule contains:

Haridra (Curcuma longa rhizome)	40 mg.
Daruharida (Berberis aristata bark)	40 mg.
Hareetakee (Terminalia chebula dried fruit)	40 mg.
Vibheetaka (TErminalia belerica dried fruit)	40 mg.
Amalakee (Emblica officinalis dried fruit)	40 mg.
Vidanga (Embella ribes berry)	40 mg.
Vakuchi (psoralia corylifolia seed)	20 mg.

Guggul (Basaodendron mukul gum)	60 mg.
Vasaka ext. eq.(Adhatoda vasica leaf)	40 mg.
Nimbatwak ext. eq. (melia azedarach stem)	100 mg.
Khadira bark (Acacia catechu bark concentrate	10 mg.
Patolapatra ext. eq. (Trichosanthes Cucumeena plant)	20 mg.
Manjishta xt. eq (ubia cordifolia root)	20 mg.
Chopchini ext. eq. (Smilax china tuber)	20 mg.

Dosage: 1 capsule 3 to 4 times a day for a week in acute conditions and minimum 6 weeks or more in chronic conditions.

Children: 1-2 capsules

How Supplied: Containers f 12 × 100's Containers of 3 × 500's

Uses: Acute and chronic eczema,itching, excessive sweating, acne vulgris, pigmentary disorders of skin, allergic dermatitis, bacterial, fungal, viral infections of skin, initial stages of psoriasis.

Product Name: **TONSARI capsule & TONSARI THROAT PAINT capsule**

Composition: Each capsule contains:

Daruharidra (Berberis aristata stem)	110 mg.
Indrajav (Holorrhina antidysentrica seed)	110 mg.
Karanja twak (pongamia glabra bark)	110 mg.
Nimba twak (Melia azedarach bark)	110 mg.
Hareetakee (TErminalia chebula fruit)	110 mg.
Pippale, (Piper longum berry)	110 mg.
Nimba taila (Oil of melia azedarach fruit)	300 mg.

Dosage: a) Tonsari capsule: 2 capsules 3 times a day for 6 weeks; Children above 5 years 1 capsule 2 to 3 times a day. b) Tonsari throat paint capsule: 1-2 capsules 3 times a day. The capsule is cut open and the contents squeezed onto the throat internally or on the wounds and injury externally or used as a gum massage oil. Tonsari throat paint capsule not designed to be awallowed whole. However the contents are safe to be sallowed.

How Supplied: Tonsari capsule 7 tonsari throat pain capsule in contaienrs of 12×50's.

Users: 1. Acute and chronic bacterial and viral infection of lymph glands, tonsils, uvula, pharynx, throat pain, travelles throat pain, opainful swallowing, sensation of foreign body, enlarged and tender lymph glands at the angle of mandibles; in short for all diseases of throat; 2. After removal of tonsils if pain persists; 3. Acne vulgaris, pimples; 4. As a supportive therapy in bronchial asthma and ski diseases; 5. Ear discharge.

***Product Name:* VIKAS Syrup**

Composition: Each 10 ml. contains:

Vibheetaka (Terminalia belerica fruit)	200 mg.
Bharangamoola (Clerodendron serratum root)	100 mg.
Kantakari (Solanum xanthocarpum fruit)	100 mg.
Kushta (Saussurea lappa stem)	100 mg.
Vasaka ext. eq. (Adhatoda vasica leaf)	100 mg.
Tulsi ext. eq. (ocimum sanctum leaf)	100 mg.
Yashtimdhu (Glycyrrhiza glabra root)	100 mg.
Pippalee (Piper longum berry)	100 mg.
Raasna (Pluchea lanceolata root)	100 mg.
Ginger (Zingiber officinale rhizome)	20 mg.
Maricha (Piper nigrum seed)	10 mg.
Nawasagar (Ammonium chloride)	125 mg.
Menthol	0.001 mg.
Neelgiri taila (Oil eucalyptus)	0.005 mg.

Dosage: *Adults:* 2 teaspoonful 4 times a day. *Infants:* 1/4 teaspoonful 2 to 3 times a day. *Children:* 1 teaspoonful 3 times a day.

How Supplied: Shipper of 60 ×100 ml bottles; Jery cans of 1×45 litres.

Uses: Catarrhal affections of the respiratory tract (cough dry or wet) laryngitis,Pharyngitis, smokers cough, naso-respiratory allergy, irritating couth of tuberculosis and all couths of unknown aetiology.

SANDHU BROTHERS PRIVATE LIMITED
Chembur, Mumbai-400 071
Tel: 5563554, 5564402

***Product Name:* ASHOKA Compound**

Composition:

Saraca indica (Ashoka chal)	125 mg.
Berberis aristata (Daruhaldi)	125 mg.
Woodfordia fucticosa (Dhai)	125 mg.
Symplocsa racemosa (Lodhra)	25 mg.
Ficus glomerata (Umber chal)	25 mg.
Adhatoda vasica (Adhulsa)	12.5 mg.
Cedrus deodara (Deodar)	12.5 mg.
Fagonia cretica (Dhamasa)	12.5 mg.
Tecoma undulatci (Rohitak chal)	12.0 mg.
Rasanjan (Rasanjan)	10.0 mg.
Rubia corditolla (Manjith)	6.25 mg.
Vetivera zizaniodes (Khus)	6.25 mg.
Santalum album (Safed chandan)	6.25 mg.
Cyperus rotundus (Musta)	6.25 mg.
Cuminum cyminum (Kalajeera)	6.25 mg.
Tribulus terrestris (Gokharu)	6.25 mg.
Ocimum sanctum (Tulsi)	3.125 mg.
Nelumbo nucifera (neel kamal)	3.750 mg.

Dosage: 4 teaspoonfuls twice a day with equal quantity of war water or as advised by the Physician. In the treatment of menorrhagia, start on the th day of the monthly period and continue till bleeding stops. Shake the bottle well before use.

How Supplied: 250 ml., 450 ml.

Uses: Ashoka compound has thus become an excellent formulation of the above mentioned various potent drugs and during the last many decades has been clinically found to be very useful in the treatment of feminine disorders like Leucorrhoea, Menorrhagia etc.

Pharmacological Action: It is a powerful astringent and a uterine sedative and acts directly on the mascular fibres of the uterus. It also exerts a stimulaing effect on the endometrium and the ovarian tissue. It also stimulates the uterine tissue making the contractions more frequent, and prolonged and without producing tonic contractions as in the case of ergot or pituitary extracts. Besides Ashoka, the other drugs like lodhra, patranga and Dhayati also, are noted for their use in the treatment of Menorrhagia (excessive bleeding during menstruation) and Metrorrhagia (excessive uterine bleeding at any or age. Ashoka compound is absolutely non-toxic.

***Product Name*: BERB ENTERONE COMPOUND**

Composition

Berberis aristara (Daruhaldi)	875 mg.
Holarrhena antidysentrica (Kudachal)	1000 mg.
Punica gratum rind querdus (Anar chal)	125 mg.
Querus infecoria (Majuphal)	125 mg.
Myristica fragrans (Jatiphal)	100 mg.
Eugenia caryophyllus (Laug)	50 mg.

Dosage: 2 tables 3 to 4 times a day or as directed by the Physician. In case of acute dysentery with plenty of mucus and blood or in chronic dysentery, it may be employed along with bilvavaleha for very satisfactory results.

How Supplied: 50 and 1000 tablets in a plastic container.

Uses: The powerful astrigents employed immediately bring down the frequency of stool, while the antibacterial and antiamoebic principle deal simultaneously with the causative agent. The carminatives intensity the agni, thereby causing a Pachan of Aam while at the same time giving the patient a relief from abdominal colics. Berb-Enterone compound there may be confidently relied, on as a comprehensive complete and effective therapy for dysentery and diarrhoea.

Pharmacological Action: Berberis aristata (Daruhaldi), the chief ingredient in this composition has always been known to Ayurved for its extremely useful action in diarrhoea and dysentery. The antibacterial effect of Berberine compares very favourably with that of Chloramphenicol and Teracyline. In fact in many clinical studies Berberine was seen to have a distinct superiority over Chlormphenicol (Lahri S.C. & Dutta N.K.J.L.M.A. Vol 48, No. 1 Jan 67 PH. 111) Berberine has also been shown to have an excellent antibacterial effect against dysentery bacilli and also against cocci (Such as streptococci and staphylococci) Further Berberine was seen to have no action on the para-sympathetic nerve fibers supplying the gastro intestinal tract. Berberine has another advantage over the antibiotics in that it neither interferes with the normal intestinal flora, nor gives any unpleasant (Adverse) side effects or toxic reactions that are so common with antibiotic therapy. Kurchi is another ancient drug employed by the traditional Ayurvedic in combating Dysentery and which has been fully accepted by the Modern Medicine for treatment of amoebic dysentery.

Kurhicine the active principle of Kurchi, has been shown to arrest amoebic growth in dilutions of 1 in 10 i.e. 10,00,00,000 (Brown 1924). The total alkaloids of Kurchi as well as the decoction of the bark have been seen to be very effective when given by mouth in acute as well as chronic amoebic dysentery and particularly so in the chronic and longstanding cases. The drug is very well tolerated and no unpleasant or toxic effects have been noted.

***Product Name*:** **BERB-ENTERONE PAEDIATRIC SUSPENSION**

Composition: Each 5 ml. contains:

Berberis aristata (Daruhaldi)	625 mg.
Holarrhena antidysentric (Kuda chal)	625 mg.
Aconitum heterophyllum (Atis)	333 mg.
Cyperus rotundus (Musta)	333 mg.
Funica gratum rind (Anarchal)	333 mg.
Quercus infectoria (Majuphal)	333 mg.
Zingiber officinale (Saunth)	167 mg.
Embelia ribes (Vayvidang)	125 mg.
Myristica fragrans (Jatiphal)	63 mg.

Dosage: Children between 1-2 years 1 ml. Children between 2-4 years 2 ml.

Children 4 years 5 to 8 ml. as per age, three or four times a day as per physicians advice.,

How Supplied: 50 ml bottles.

Uses: Berb-Enterone Paediateric syrup has been extensively tried clinically against diarrhoea, dysentery and similar other intestinal disorders of infants and children and has been proved to be very efficacious.

Pharmacological Action: Berb-Enterone Paediatric suspension is an extension of the formula for Berb-enterone compound to suit the special requirement of paediatric therapy of diarrhoea and dysentery. With this view in mind drugs like Ativish, Nagarmotha, Vavuding has been added to earlier formula while the proportion of the other have been suitably revised. Of the above, drugs like ativish, Nargarmotha are known to be stomachic and Aam Nashak, while Vading is noted to be excellent kriminashak (Anthelminthic). The syrupy form and pleasant palatability of this suspension make it easily acceptable to the children.

***Product Name*:** **PANCHASAV DIGESTIVE POWER TONIC**

Composition: Each 15 ml. contains.

Vitis vinifera (Kali draksha)	543 mg.
Piper longum (Pippali)	222 mg.
Piper longum root (Pippali mul)	222 mg.
Piper retrofractum (Chabh)	222 mg.
Plumbago zeylonica (Cheeta)	222 mg.
Glycyrrhiza glabra (Mulhati)	93 mg.
woodfordja fructicosa (Dhaiphool)	150 mg.

Dosage: 2 teasponds twice a day after meals.

How Supplied: Available in 450 ml. Pack.

Uses: Panchasav improves digestion, stimulates appetite, as well as secretion of digestive enzymes. Panchasav, therefore, is useful in alleviating digestive discomforts such as indigestion, loss of appetite flatulence constipation and other functional disorders.

Pharmacological Action: Panchasva is free from any harmful effect, even in log term use.

***Product Name*:** **EPHENIN TABLET**

Composition

Ephendra vulgaris (Somalata)	1080 mg.
Solanum xanthocarpum (Choti kateri)	90 mg.
Pistacia integerrima (Kakarsingi)	60 mg.
Alpinia gaianga (Kulinijan)	60 mg.
Shwas kuthar rasa	60 mg.
Praval bhasma (Agniputi)	60 mg.
Adhatoda vasica (Adusa)	34 mg.
Dhatura metel leves extract (Dhatura)	34 mg.
Ammoumum choride (Nausadar)	15 mg.

Dosage: 1 tablet 3 to 4 times a day with honey or warm water or as directed by the physician.

How Supplied: 50 tablets, 100 tablets in plastic containers.

Uses: Absolutely safe and nontoxic within prescribed limits.

Pharmacological Action: Shwas Kuthar Ras is a Rasayana prepared in strict conformity with the Shastric process described in the standard Ayurvedic Text "Ras Chandanshu" Ras Chandanshu" described this drug as Shwas Haraka, Kapha nashaka, Agnit Deepaka and Jwar Nashaka. Ayurvedic clinicians always rely on this Rasayan for controlling asthmatic parxoysms and also in the treatment of other inflammatory aumaments of the respiratory tract. Somavalli)Ephedra vulgaris a drug very well known for its action on Ashtma. The active principle of Somavalli is ephedrine. The phamacological action of ephedrine is very similar to that of adrenaline though ephedrine is much less toxic and a lot safer than adernaline. The formulation of Ephenin (Improved Formula) makes use of the whole drug Somavalli (Ephendra vulgaris) rather than the isolatd active principle. The whole drug clinically has the same efficacy (if not better) as active principle, and yet the former is much safer than the latter. Somavalli stimulates the respiratory centre and relives the feeling of tightness in the chest by dilating the bronchial tubes. This also helps in expectoration Somavalli is also a heart stimulant and restores sufficiency in an insufficient heart. Another excellent bronchodilatory drug is Koshtha (Alpinia galanga). Its pronounced the treatment of Ashtma, difficulty in breathing, dry cough etc. Navsagar is a mild expectorant which acts fast due to its rapid absorption in the alimentery tract. It increases the secretion of the bronchial mucus and gives relief in dry coughs. Choti kateri is an ingredient of ten famous Dashmools and is noted for its tonic, alterative and expectoratnt action. Karkatak shringi is particularly useful in dry cough and inflammatory condition of the respiratory tract. Praval bhasma is known for its alterative soothing and tonic properties. It also helps the other ingredients for a better and synergistic action. Ephenin (Improved Farmula) thus becomes a valuable tool in the hands of the physician in the treatment of Asthma & other similar respiratory troubles.

Product Name: **HAEMIL FORTE TABLET**

Composition

Punamava mandur	116 mg.
Loha bhasma	58 mg.
Praval bhasma agniputi	116mg.
Tamra bhasma	29 mg.
Abhrak bhasma 100 puti	14.5 mg.
Shuddha para	20 mg.
Shuddha gandhak	87 mg.
Zingiber officinale (Saunth)	12.57 mg.

Piper nigrum (kali mirch)(	12.50 mg.
Terminalia chebula (Harad)	12.50 mg.
Terminalia belerica 9Baheda0	12.50 mg.
Emblica officinalis (Amalak9)	12.50 mg.
Cyprus rotundus (Musta)	12.50 mg.
Embelia ribes (Vayvidang)	12.50 mg.
Plumbago zeylanica (Cheeta0	12.50 mg.
Strychnos nuxvomica (Kuchala shuddha0	12.50 mg.
Gomutra	0.773 ml.

Dosage: One tablet twice a day after meals preferably with milk or fruit or as per Physician's adive.

How Supplied: 25,50,100 tablets in plastic container.

Uses: Haemol Forte is useful in: Indadequte intake of iron, Inadequate absorption of ingested iron, Defective functioning of the organs taking part in the complex process of blood formation i.e. damaged liver, spleen, bone marrow etc. in conditions like Bright's disease and uremia, there is a severe anaemia due to the effect of the disease upon blood formation, Nutritional defects like nonavailability of certain vitamins like folic acid and vit. B12, Deficiency of anti anaemic factor (haematinic principle) in the Liver.

Pharmacological Action: The formulation of Haemol Forte has been done with a view to meeting the requirements of most of the above conditions. Punarnava Mandur is recognised as an excellent liver stimulant. The importance of liver in the process of blood formation cannot simply be over emphasised. Liver stores within itself the haematinic principle, so vital for correct R.B.C. formation. Liver also produces heparin and vitamin K which are necessary for healthy blood conditions. Purnava Mandur reactivates a sluggish liver by toning and stimulating it. It has always been a drug of choice in the treatment of anaemia, Jaundice, spleen disorders. etc. Punarnava Mandur as well as Loha Bhasma are iron supplying drugs. The iron in these drugs, due to the special Ayurvedic treatments involved in the preparation of these drugs, becomes extremely finely divided. In conjuction with the many vegetable and animal origin durgs employed, this iron becomes readily assimilable. Besides it does not give any tendency towards constipation.

***Product Name*: HEMOCLEEN**

Composition: Each 10 ml. contains.

Acacia catechu (Khadircha)	188 mg.

Hmidesumus indicus (Anantmul)	88 mg.
Smilax china (Chabh)	63 mg.
Swertia chirayita (Chirayata)	88 mg.
Andrographis paniculata (Kalmegh)	88 mg.
Adhatoda vasica (Adulsa)	125 mg.
Picrorhiza kurroa (Katuki)	100 mg.
Valeriana wallichi (Tagar)	63 mg.
Pterocarpus santalinus (Lal chandan)	100 mg.
Azadirachta indica (Kadava neem)	250 mg.
Rubia cordifolia (Manjith)	250 mg.
Tinospora cordifalia (Giloya)	100 mg.
Pongamia pinnata (Karan)	75 mg.
Operculina turpethum (Nishoth)	38 mh.
Pterocarpus marsupium (Vijaysar)	38 mg.
Beeberis aristtata (Daruhaldi)	38 mg.
Fumaria valliantil (Pitapapada)	38 mh.
Embelia ribes (Vayvidang)	38 mg.
Curcuma long (Haldi)	38 mg.
Psoralia corylifolia (Bavachi beej)	38 mg.
Terminalia chebula (Choti harad)	125 mg.

Dosage: 2 teaspoonful (approx 10 ml.) twice a day with equal quantity of lukewarm water or as advised by the physician. Shake the bottle well before use.

How Supplied: 20 ml., 450 ml.

Uses:

1. All types of Rakta Pitta Vikar, Rakta shuddhi.
2. Ailments arising out of impure blood like skin inflammating, rash, eruptions, burning or itching of the skin, Erysipelas etc.
3. In the treatment of skin diseases like dermatits, wet or dry eczemas, scabies, ringworm etc. If during the treatment with Hemocleen, Elegance oil is used for massaging the affected parts externally, better and quicker results are obtained. Clinical trials have proven that a regular treatment with Hemocleen and a little Bawachi churna (to be taken internally) can be efficacious in the treatment of Leucoderma.
4. Hemocleen is an excellent preparation for prevention and cure of Acne Pimples.

Pharmacological Action: Hemocleen has been formulated to take care of this very function. Drugs like Khadir, Anatmul, chopchini, Manjistha are very effective blood purifiers. Bitter tonics like Chirayata, Katuki, Amrita are excellent liver stimulants. They improve the general tone of the digestive system Neem bark is well known for its beneficial effects on skin diseases. Haridra is not only a good anti-Inflammatory agent but it also cures skin diseases and gives the skin its natural health and glow.Vasaka is alternative, cooling and a blood purifying agent. A balanced and judicious combination of all these potent drugs has made Hemocleen an exceedingly effective blood purifier. It stimulates digestion, improves appetite, cleans the bowels, cleans the blood of its irritant toxins and makes the blood healthy and pure.

Product Name: **PREG-UTERO**

Composition: Each 5 ml. contains:

Uraria picta (Pithvan)	171.875 mg.
Sida cordifolia (Bala)	189 mg.
Adhatoda vasica (Adulsa)	92 mg.
Centella asiatica 9Brahmi)	45 mg.
Withania somnifera (Asagandh)	45 mg.
Woodforida fructicosa (Dhaiphool)	17 mg.
Glycyrrhiza glabra (Mulhati)	15 g.
Kelakand	15 mg.
Asparagus racemosus (Shatavar)	15 mg.
Emblica officinalis (Amalaki)	9.5. mg.
Tinospora cordifolia (Giloya)	9.5 mg.
Fumaria vaillanti (Pitpapada)	8 mg.
Prunus cersoides Padmakath)	8 mg.
Acacia catechu (Khadirchal)	8 mg.
Tribulus terrestis (Gokharu)	8 mg.
Terminalia belerica (Baheda)	8 mg.
Ficus glomerata (Umberchal)	17 mg.
Acacia arabica (Babulchal)	8 mg.
Vetivera zizanioidis (Khus)	8 mg.
Cuminum cyminum (Jeera)	8 mg.
Mentha spicata (Pudina)	8 mg.
Picorrhiza kurroa (Katuki)	8 mg.
Embelia ribes (Vayvidang)	4 mg.
Santalum album (Safed chandan)	4 mg.

Dosage: 2 to 4 teaspoonfuls twice a day with equal quantity of warm water or as directed by the physician.

How Supplied: 200 ml. and 450 ml. bottles.

Uses: Checks tendency for miscarriage or abortion, Purifies blood. Stimulates the development of the mammary glands and ensurses a normal lactation after delivery. It therefore affords an excellent clinical protection both for the mother as well as for the foetus.

Pharmacological Action: Preg-Utero, which is judicious combination of the choicest of the herbs from the Ayurvedic pharmacopoeia, which have been reputed to be efficacious in protecting from such complaints affords the clinician a valuable tool in the treatment of these complaints. Besides the above, Preg-Utero is an excellent uterine tonic during the pregnancy condition & is also beneficial to the growth of the foetus. Brahmi is a nervine tonic, most useful in disorders of the nervous and circulatory system. Ashwagandah (Askand) is a sedative and a nervine and muscular tonic. It is a sovereign Ayurvedic medicine for general debility conditions and particularly for maintaining the muscular and body energy when the body is subjected to vigorous stresses as in pregnacy. Shatavari is a nutritive tonic, galactogogue, said to tone up the hormonal control of the genital apparatus of women. It is refrigerant and antispasmodic as well. Lodhra is a uterine tonic, prevents miscarriage and Toxaemia durig pregnancy. Madhuyasthi (Jaishthmadha)is a laxative, expectorant emollient tonic and useful in genito urinary disoder. The many other herbs that have been employed are selected for their digestive carminative and tonic action. Preg-Utro therefore is particularly efficacious in preventing common complaints during pregnancy, like morning sickness, diddiness, lack of appetite and enthusiasm, cramps and swelling in the legs. Anaemia and general debility during pregnancy, girdle pains, weak digestion and constipation etc. Tones up uterine muscles, nourishes the foetus and ensures its healthy development. Preg-Utero is non-toxic.

***Product Name:* VIMFIX TABLET**

Composition

Mucuna pruiens (Kawach beej)	145
Asteracantha longifolia (Talimkhana)	75 mg.
Blepharia edulis (Utangan beej)	100 mg.
Strychnos nuxomica (Shudha kuchala)	5 mg.
Datura terrestirs (Shudha kala ddhotra)	5 mg.
Tribulus terrestris (Gokharoo)	100 mg.

Pueraria tuberosa (Buikohala)	150 mg.
Asparagus adscendens (Safed Musali)	100 mg.
Asparagus racemosus (Shatavari)	100 mg.
Withania somnifera (Ashwagandha)	150 mg.
Nakeshar	2 mg.
Crocus sativus (Keshar)	3 mg.
Myristica fragans (Jaipal)	20 mg.
Cinnamomum camphora (Kapur)	5 mg.
Rasa sindur	30 mg.
Shudhha shilajeet	20 mg.

Dosage: 1 tables twice a day with milk.

How Supplied: 25,50,100 and 1000 tablets in plastic container.

Uses:

1. As a sexual tonic for the treatment of sexual debility, weak libido and a weak physical response to sexual stimulli, spermatorrhoea. nocturnal emissions, decrease retentive power and sexual stamina etc.
2. As a general tonic in geriatric therapy in senile conditions or premature senility, disturbances of climaceteric in men, depressive and asthenic condition etc.
3. An excellent nervine and glandular tonic to correct sexual exhaustion due to nocturnal emissions, spermatorrhoea, masturbation or excessive sexual indulgence.
4. It can also be taken by normal males for added Vim, Vigour and Vitality and for that extra pep and zest which all men so much want to have.

Pharmacological Action: Abhrak Bhasma (Sahastraputi) is considered to be a sovereign Ayurvedic tonic for nerves, muscles and liver. It's tonic action probably lies in its capacity to stimulate the intracellular metabolism. It is always indicated in the treatment of sexual neurasthenia and spermatorrhoea. Shilajeet is a reputed urinogenial tonic and is considered to be a specific against spermatorrhoea. Vang bhasma is a potent sedative aphrodisiac, which tones up the sexual organs, there by increasing the sexual libido as well. Vang bhasma is also considered to be a specific against spermatorrhoea and nocturnal emmissions, it is a good general tonic also. Ras sindoor decreases the oxidation and wear and tear of tissues, increases the R.B.C. count of blood and also improves digestion and assimilation of food. It is a good nervine, cardiac and liver stimulant too. The aphrodisiac, properties of all the remaining vegetable drugs like Kavacha beeja, Talimkhana, Utangana beeja, Bhui kohala, Gokharu, Shatavari, Ashwagandha are realy to well known to be mentioned here. Absolutely harmless and non-toxic within prescribed limits. It is also non-habit forming.

***Product Name:* VASA SYRUP**

Composition

Adhatoda vasica (Adulsa)	400 mg.
Piper longum (Pippal)	75 mg.
Glycerrhiza glabra (Mulhati)	50 mg.
Ocium snactum (Tulsi)	50 mg.
Zingiber officinale (Saunth)	50 mg.
Terminalia belerica (Baheda)	34 mg.
Borax (Suhaga)	25 mg.
Cinnamomum cassia (Dalchini)	7 mg.
Eugenia caryophyllus (Laung)	5 mg.

Dosage: For children ½ to 1 teaspoonful and for adults 2 to 4 teaspoonful 3 to 4 times a day or as advised by the Physician.

How Supplied: 100 ml, 200 ml glass bottles.

Uses: Due to the synergistic action of all the above ingredients Sandhu Vasa Syrup can be employed with great advantage...

1. In the treatment of wet as well as dry cough.
2. To bring relief from hoarseness of throat irritation that accompanies dry cough.
3. To liquify the thick sputum and ensure easy breathing.
4. To control the severe paraxysms of Bronchitis.

Pharmacological Action: The Ayurvedic clinical approach is therefore not as much towards the mitigation of the manifested symptoms as towards the removal of the root cause of these and thereby the restoration of the Tridosha Balance. Sandu Vasa Syrup has been specially formulated with this view in mind. And the direct clinical experience with this product, over the last many years has indeed justified and indicated this approach. Vasa has been considered even by the modern medicine as an excellent antispasmodic expectorant, thanks, to its persistent bronchodilatory and sputum, liquifying action. It is therefore of great use in the treatment of Bronchitis, where it liquifieds thick, sticky and tenacious sputum, thus aiding in its easy expectoration. Vasaka also controls the cough reflex by depressing the vagal endlings, giving the patient an immediate relief from the presistent and troublesome praroxysms. The various aromatics employed intensify the Agni and in conjuction with Glycyrrhiza (Jeshthamadha) with its pleasantly demulcent action, go to soothe the inflammed and irritated air passage thus affording a functional relief to the patient. Arjuna is considered by Ayurved to be Tridosha Nashaka and cardiac tonic.

Product Name: **BILVA VALEHA**

Composition: Each teaspoonfull contains:

Aegle marmelos (Beelphal)	3.33 mg.
Avaleha (Sugar Based) q.s.	15 g.

Dosage: 1teaspoonful there to four times a day or as directed by the physian.

How Supplied: 200 gms, 400 g.

Uses: It is therefore particularly indicated in case when there is a copious discharge of blood and mucus. Sandhu Bilvavaleha has been also found to be useful in pre-sprue conditions or early cases of spure. Due to its delightful palatablity, sandhu Bilvavaleha is accepted even by children, with relish.

Pharmacological Action: Baelphal (Bilva fruit, Baelfructus, Aegele Marmelos fruit), thanks to its astringent, stomachiec kashayaa and grhi qualities had always been considered by the ancient Ayurvedic clinicians as a very valuable tool in their combat against diarrhoea and dysentary especially the chronic type. Sandu bilvavaleha, in such cases can be a very useful adjunct. Due to its astringent action, it discourages any further tendency to watery stools, while at the same time, due to its demulcent nature it aids in relieving any constipation thus allowing the ulcerated surface to heal firmly.

Product Name: **OSTEON-D**

Composition: Each tablet contains:

Laghu Maini vasant	40 mg.
Swarna makshika bhasma	40 mg.
Praval bhasma (Chandraputi)	40 mg.
Shouktika bhasma	40 mg.

Guduchi satva	40 mg.
Dashamool choorna	240 mg.
Shankha bhasma	40 mg.

Dosage: Below 4 yrs. 1 tablet per day. Between 4-8 years 1 tablet twice a day. Above 8 years 1 tablet thrice a day or as directed by the physician.

How Supplied: 50 and 1000 tablets in plastic container.

Uses: Osteon-D a general tonic for all children. It improves appetite and digestion, intensifies metabolism and thus ensures a correct growth and development of children. Due to its content of assimilable calcium drawn from natural sources osteon-D is useful in cases of calcium deficiency. It provides assimilable iron and hence is useful in anaemia low vitality and general weakness in children. Osteon-D also increases resistance to infection. Osteon-D has been found to be very effective in conditions like Bal Shosha. Osteon-D has also been seen to show astonishingly good results in cases of low vitality and lack of energy and stamina in children owing to excessive body heat conditions.

Pharmacological Action: Laghu malini vasant along with praval chadraputi and gulvel satva is a combination recognised to be a souvereign tonic for children. Ayurvedic clinicians particularly favour to combination particularly for its very gentle and yet equally efficacious action. This combination is also known to counteract the ill effects of excessive body heat in chidren, caused by environmenta as well as clinical factors. Praval bhasma ikn conjunction with shankha bhasma and shauktik bhasma supplies calcium in an extremely finely divided colloidal form and hence is easily assimilable. These bhasma also supply minute quantities of other trace minerals which are necessary for a proper cellular metabolism, growth and general development. Suvarna makshika bhasma affords a clinically effective source of iron and being mild in action is very well tolerated by the delicate constitutions of children. Dasha moolas are a group of ten famous and really invaluable herbs which as a group are considered to be extremely effective, rejuvenative and stimulant tonic. Ayurveda considers this combination as Tridosh Nashaka, and particularly good for lungs and nerves. It is gentle in action and hence can safely be employed for small children.

Product Name: **SYRUP JAUNDEX**

Composition: Each 5 ml. contains:

Ricinus communis (Erand patra)	625 mg.
Phyllanthus urinaria (Bhuiamalaki)	188 mg

Terminalia chebula (Choti harad)	188 mg.
Tinsoporat cordifolia (Giloya)	175 mg.
Picrorrhiza kurroa (Katuki)	125 mg.
Swertia chiraita (Chirayta)	125 mg.
Rhamnus wightti (Lal roheda)	125 mg.
Berberis aristata (Daruhaldi)	125 mg.
Yavskhsar (Javkhar)	33 mg.g
Calatropis procera leaves (Aak patra)	25 mg.
Ammonium chloride (Nausadar)	6 mg.

Dosage: One teaspoonful (approx 5 ml.) thrie a day with equal quantity of lukewarm water or as directed by the physician.

How Supplied: 100 ml. and 200 ml. bottles.

Uses: Syrup jaundex is a liver tonic par excellence for the treatment of jaudice, Hepatitis, Sluggishness of liver and all cases of hepatic dysfunctioning.

Pharmacological Action: Syru jaundex with its very potent liver stimulant and cholagogue herbal principlefs, offers a comprehensive and total therapy for jaundice. It immediately stimulates and tones up the bile circulation and relieves and hepatic or bile duct congestion. The normal flow of the bile thus restored, digestion automatically improves. Appetite is restored, the tongue clears and digestion distrubances subside. The stools return to their normal colour and consistency. The urine also returns to its normal colour. The yellow discolouration of the skin and eyes gradually disapppers. Syrup jaundex also tones up the normal liver metabolism, with liver again functioning smoothly, the patient soon experiences a general feeling of well being. Syrup jaundex is absolutely safe and nontoxic and does not give any harmful side effects even after a protracted period of treatment.

***Product Name*:** **VANARI KALPA**

Composition: Each teaspoonful contains:

Kavach Beej (Mucuna pruriens)	1.560 g.

Dosage: 1 to 2 teaspoonful twice a day with milk.

How Supplied: 100 gms, 200 gms, 400 gms Granules in plastic.

Uses: Extremely potent spermatogenetic and aphrodisiac tonic to correct various conditions of sexual exhaustion. Its regular use corrects the defects and insufficiences of the semen and makes it healthy and pure. It has been experienced that a regular use of Vanari Churna results in the increase of sperm-count in the semen. This kalpa therefore, will be very useful for the treatment of male sterility due to ineffective semen or to the too low sperm count. It can be used as a general tonic geriatricx therapy in senile conditions, climacteric insufficiences of males etc.

Pharmacological Action: The spermatogenetic, seman purifying and aphrodisiac properties of Vanari (Kavach beeja) have been known to the ayurvedic clinicians for a long time. It is with a view to remove this and similar other traditional drawbacks and to present the product in a more convenient and freely acceptable from, that we have developed the present kalpa.

Product Name: **WHOOPING COUGH MIXTURE**

Composition: Each teaspoonful contains:

Vitis vinifera (Draksha)	400 mg.
Ficus carica (Angeer)	385 mg.
Glycerrhiza glabra (Mulhati)	275 mg.
Solanum xanthcorpum (Choti kateri)	13 mg.
Aconitum heterophyllum (Atis)	11 mg.
Pistacia intergerrima (Kakarshingi)	11 mg.
Borax (Suhaga)	13 mg.
Mimusops elengi (Bakool sal)	38 mg.
MImosa pudica (Lajaloo)	38 mg.
Aplinia galanga (Kulingan)	11 mg.
Adhatoda visica (Adulsa)	57 mg.
Embelia ribes (Vayvidang)	11 mg.

Dosage: 20 drops for infans, ½ to 1 teaspoonful for children (as per age), 2 teaspoonful for adult, thrice a day.

How Supplied: 100 ml, 200 ml glass bottles.

Uses: Whooping cough is a distressing infectious disease, very common in the young but by no means uncommon with adults. The initial dry troublesome cough (with sometimes a cold in the head) soon develops into the characterisitic 'whoop's accompanied by the characteristic whooping sound. These paroxysms may follow one another rapidly and at the end the exhaused child may expectorate a little very sticky sputum and may even vomit. As secondary effects of this disease the child may get thoroughly emaciated, may loose all its natural resistance to diseases and may become a victim to infections like broncho-peumonia. Heart and lung infections may also follow.

Pharmacological Action: Drugs like Adulsa, choti kateri known to be very effective expectorants. Adulsa particularly acts on the sticky and tenacious phlegm, thus liquifying it and helping int its easy expectoration. Koshtha Kolinjan has a marked bronchodilatory and antispasmodic action. Drugs like anjeer, Draksha and Liquorice are well known demulcents and helps to give the patient relief throat irritation, which indirectly causes the frequency of the parozysm bouts to diminish. Draksha and Anjeer are also mild though effective laxatives and in conjuction with the many other constituents employed, go to build up the patient's stamina against the infection, thus aiding in his speedy recovery. Whooping cough Mixture is absolutely non-toxic.

Product Name: **SHATAVARI KALPA**

Composition

Asparagus racemosus (Shatavari)	2 g.
Glycerrhiza glabra (Mulhalti)	0.4 g.

Dosage: Not available.

How Supplied: 200 gm, 400 gm, 1 kg in attractive plastic container.

Uses: Shatavark kalpa because of its demulcent property is uses as adjuvant therepy in gastritis, ulcer, hyper acidity. It is considered to be a tonic for women, as Shatavari exerts beneficial effects on genito urinary tract and is useful as tonic.

Pharmacological Action: Shatavari Kalpa has three distinctive actions which help mothers during lactation. Lactopoesis, Lactogenesis, Lactokinesis. The above action of Shatavari Kalpa makes it a durg of choice for increasing lactation after the delivery.

Product Nake: TEJRAS

Composition: Each 5 ml. represent extract of:

Convolvulus pluricalus (Shankhapushpi)	125 mg.
Centella asiatica (Brahmi)	125 mg.
Eclipta alba (Bhringaraj)	160 mg.
Cynodon dactylon (durva)	100 mg.

Asparagus racemosus (Shatavari)	75 mg.
Withania somnifera (Asgandha)	60 mg.
Nardostachvs jatamansi (Jatamansi)	60 mg.
Acorus calmus (Bacha)	20 mg.
Zingiber officinale (Saunth)	50 mg.
Vetiveria zizanioodis (Khus)	20 mg.
Celastrus paniculatus (Malkangani)	20 mg.
Iron suppliment (Hirakas) (Shudha)	50 mg.
Calcium suppliment (Praval pisti)	40 mg.

Dosage: Children between 4 to 8 years 1 teaspoonful twice a day. Children between 8 years & Adult 2 teaspoonful twice a ay. Higher dosage may be recommended in acute and chronic conditions.

How Supplied: 200 ml, and 450 ml. Bottles.

Uses: Tejras formula has been developed so as to help the individual to restore mental peace. Tejras: Improves mental alertness Enhances concentration and attention: Removes mental fatigue. Increase memory span Suppliments iron and calcium to restore good health. Tejras helps the individual to combat stress effectively.

Shree Baidyanath Ayurved Bhawan Ltd.
Gwalior Road, Jhansi-284004
Tel.: 440665, 440934, 441076, 441478

Product Name: **SURAKTA**

Composition: Each 5 ml. contains ext. of:

Indian sarsaparilla (Anantool)	750 mg.
Saraca indica bark (Ashoka)	250 mg.
Senna (Senna)	100 mg.
Indian rhubarb (Revand chini)	70 mg.
Indian jalap (Nishodh)	70 mg.
Myrabolan (Herre)	100 mg.
Cassia fistula (Amaltas)	100 mg.
Andrographis (Kalmegh)	30 mg.
Paniculata Swertia (Chirata)	30 mg.
Chirata tinospora (Geloy)	30 mg.
Cardifolia Indian lilac (Neem)	30 mg.
American sarasaparilla (Ushva)	30 mg.
Smilaz china (chopchini)	30 mg.

Spheranthus indicus (Garakh mundi)	30 mg.
Indian madder (Mazeeth)	30 mg.
Berberis aristata (Rasant)	30 mg.
Neel kanthi (Neel kanthi)	30 mg.
Cassia occidentalis (Kasaundi)	30 mg.
Acacia catechu (Khadirsaar)	30 mg.
Bauhinia tomentosa (Kachnaar)	30 mg.
Turmeric (Haldi)	30 mg.
Pterocarpus (Rakta chandan) Santalinus	30 mg.

Dosage: Two or three teaspoonfuls twice a day.

How Supplied: 200 ml.

Uses: A herbal blood purifier that works towards a healthy, glowing skin by attacking the root cause of pimples, acne and other skin problems. If has a pleasant tase. A salt-restricted or saltfree diet is advised for better results.

***Product Name:* KABJA HAR GRANULES**

Composition:

Sanaay	50% w/w
Choti harre roasted	5% w/w
Nishoth	10% w/w
Kala namak	15% w/w
Sendha namak	5% w/w
Viavidang	5% w/w
Ajwayan	10% w/w

Dosage: 2 teaspoonful with water at bed time.

How Supplied: 100 g.

Uses: Laxative.

***Product Name*: Shankh Pushpi**

Composition: Each 15 ml contains:

Shankha puspi	2 gm.
Bramhhi	0.5 gm.
Jatamanbi	25 mg.
Tukhme Balunga	25 ng.

Ustekhudus	25 mg.
Badranj Boya	25 mg.
Gavjaba	100 mg.
Sat Loban	12 mg.

Colour: Apple green conc.

Unjha Ayurveda Pharmancy

H.O. Unjha, 384170 (N. Gujrat)

F/75 Riico Ambaji Ind. Area, Abu Road (Raj.)

Dosage: 20 to 30 ml. twice a day with water or as directed by the physician.

How Supplied: 200 ml.

Uses:

1. Impromotes concentration.
2. Improves grasping power.
3. Increases capacity to recall quickly.
4. Keeps you alert and sharp.

Skap Pharmaceutucals (P) Ltd.

E-3, UPSIDC Industrial Area

Hardwar-249401 (U.P.)

Tel. : (0133) 424762

Fax: (0133) 425262

Product Name: **APPELIV TABLET**

Composition

Each tablet contains:

Telphrosia purpuria (Sarphunka)	30 mg.
Cichorium intybus (Kasni)	30 mg.
Eclipta alba (Bringraj)	16 mg.
Picrorhiza kurroa (Kutki)	12 mg.
Phyllanthus urinaria (Bhumyamla)	12 mg.
Tinospora cordifolia (Giloy)	12 mg.
Terminalia chebula (Haritki)	12 mg.
Fumaria oficinalis (Parptak)	12 mg.

Andrographis paniculata (Kalmegh)	16 mg.
Mandoor bhasma (Mandoor bhasma)	15 mg.
Acacia arabica	Q.T.

Dosage: Adult—2 tablets thice daily. Children—1 tablet thrice daily.

How Supplied: 100 tabs. packed in glass bottles.

Uses: Appeliv herbal aid to liver ailments, Protects liver from Hepatodic drugs, Alcohol infections & toxins, Stimulate appetite, digestion, Promote Hepatocellur regeneration, Bile secretion, Elimanate jaundice and associated symptoms, Recommended as a daily health supplement also.

Product Name: **APPELIV SYRUP**

Composition: Each 5 ml. syurp contains:

Tephrosia purpuria (Sarphunka)	10 mg.
Cichorium intybus (Kasni)	10 mg.
Eclipta alba (Bringraj)	10 mg.
Picrorhiza kurroa (Kutki)	8 mg.
Phyllanthus urinaria (Bhumyamla)	8 mg.
Tinospora cordifolia (Giloy)	10 mg.
Terminalia chebula (Haritki)	10 mg.
Fumaria oficinalis (Pitpappda)	10 mg.
Andrographis paniculata (Kalmegh)	10 mg.
Cane sugar	14 mg.

Dosage: Adult—2 teaspoon thrice daily. Children—1 teaspoon thrice daily.

How supplied: 100 ml, 210 ml., packed in glass bottles.

Uses: Appeliv herbal aid to liver ailments, protects liver from Hepatoxic Drugs, alcohol infections & toxins, Stimulate appetite, digestion, Promote Hepatocellur regeneration bile secretion, Eliminate jaundice and Associated symptoms, Recommended as a daily health supplement also.

Product Name: **LAXOL TABLET**

Composition: Each 250 mg. contains:

Gercinia morella (Kakuth)	15 mg.
Aloe vera (Grith kumari)	15 mg.
Terminalia chebula (aritki)	10 mg.
Terminalia belerica (Vibhitki)	10 mg.

Emblica officinale (Amalki)	10 mg.
Cassia fl Et angustxfolia (Sanayki)	15 mg.
Hyoscyamus raticulatus (Parsik yavani)	15 mg.
Ipomea Hederacea (krishna beej)	15 mg.
Foemoeulu vulgare (Mishraya)	20 mg.
Picrorhiza hurroa (Kutki)	15 mg.
Calotropis procera (Arak pusp)	15 mg.
Glycyrrhiza glabra (yastimadhu)	15 mg.
Zizyphus nummularia (Karkantu)	20 mg.
Jujulia fruit (Kubal)	15 mg.
Opercitina turphethum (Trivart)	20 mg.
Indian plum (Badar)	15 mg.
Shudh tankan (R.T.)	10 mg.

Dosage: 2 tablets twice a day or as directed by physician.

How Supplied: 100 tablets in glass bottles.

Uses: Mild Laxative.

Product Name: **MENSULE**

Composition: Each capsule contains:

Aloevera (Alva)	40 mg.
Zingiber officinale (Sounth)	50 mg.
Abroma agusta (Ulat)	80 mg.
Derrhean antisenterica (Indra jao)	80 mg.
Raphanus sativus (Mulee)	40 mg.
Daucus carota (Gajar)	40 mg.
Ricinus communis (Arandi)	400 mg.

Dosage: 1 capsule B.D. for 2 days in the morning on an empty stomach with milk.

How Supplied: 4 capsules packed in glass bottles.

Uses: A perfect non-hormonal Mensuration Regulator.

Product Name: **Nitya Churn**

Composition: Each 100 g. contains:

Cassia angustifolia (Sanayki)	10 g.
Terminalia chebula (Haritki)	5 g.
Operculina turpenthum (Nishoth)	6.35 g.
Glycyrrhiza glabra (Madhu yasti)	5 g.

Embelia officinalis (Amalki)	6.25 g.
Zingiber officinale (Sunthi)	6.25 g.
Rosa gaptifolia (Savati)	6.25 g.
Emblica ribes (Bybidang)	6.25 g.
Piper nigrum (Krishna marich)	1.25 g.
Amomum subulatum (Ela vahrat)	1.25 g.
Piper longum (Pippli)	1.25 g.
Syzygium aromaticum (Lawang)	1.25 g.
Foeniculum vulgare (Misraya)	6.25 g.
Ipomea hederaceal (krisna beej)	6.25 g.
Trigonella foenum graecum (Mayika)	1.25 g.
Punica granatum (Darim beej)	6.25 g.
Plumbago zeylanica (Chitrak)	2.5 g.
Sodium bicarbonate (Sajjishar)	2.5 g.
Black salt (Krisna lawan)	6.25 g.
Cane sugar (Misri)	12.5 g.

Dosage: 5 to 10 g. Twice a day with water.

How Supplied: 100 g. in plastic boxes.

Uses: Useful in acidity, Indigestion, Constipation & General gastric troubles recommended as natural health suppliement.

***Product Name:* NATUROVAC**

Composition: Each 100 mg. contains:

Plantago ovata (Isapgol husk)	2 g.
Cassia angu (Sonamukhi)	0.35 g.
Terminalia chebula (Harad)	0.50 g.
Cassia fistula (Amaltas)	0.50 g.
Liquorice (Mulhethi)	0.25 g.
Aegle marmelos (Bael)	0.40 g.
Rosac centifolia (Gulab dal)	0.25 g.
Foeniculam vulgre (Sounf)	0.25 g.
Sugar (Sharkara)	0.42 g.
Fennel oil (Saunt taila)	0.05 g.
Sodium benzoate (Sodiumbenzoate)	0.03 g.

Dosage: 1-2 heapfuls with plain or warm water at bed time.

How Supplied: 100 g. in plastic boxes.

Uses: Habitual constipation and irregular bowel habits constipation associated with prolonged illness.

***Product Name*: Studd Capsule**

Composition: Each 500 mg. contains:

Withania somnifera (Ashwagandha)	50 mg.
Asparagus adcendens (Safadmusli)	50 mg.
Mucuna prurita (Kounch beej)	50 mg.
Orchis latifolia (Salam panja0	20 mg.
Argyria speciosa (Samundra sosh)	20 mg.
Astercantha longifolia (Tal makhana)	20 mg.
Anacyclus pyrethrum (Akarkara)	20 mg.
Strychnos num-vomica (Shudh kuchla)	20 mg.
Asparagus racemosus (Satawari)	20 mg.
Argyria speciosa (Vidhra mool)	20 mg.
Sida cordifolia (Bala)	20 mg.
Acacia arabica (Babool phali)	20 mg.
Myristica fragrans (Japhal)	15 mg.
Myristica fragrans (Javitri)	15 mg.
Cinnamomum zeylanicum (Dal chini)	20 mg.
Ocimum sanctum (Tulsi beej)	20 mg.
Crocus sativus (Kesar)	5 mg.
Vivery divethalin (Jundhadastar)	5 mg.
Shudh silajit (Shudh shilajit)	50 mg.
Tribang bhasma (Tribang bhasma)	10 mg.
Abhrak bhasm (Abhrak bhasma)	10 mg.
Makardwaj (Makardwaj)	20 mg.

Bhawna Dravya
Bombax ceiba Shalmati
Pueraria tuberoea Vidarikand
Pedalium murex Gokshru
Piper betal Pan
Asparagus adcedens Musli

Dosage: 1 to 2 capsule in a day or as directed by physician.

How Supplied: 30 capsules glass bottle.

Uses: Useful for general debility.

***Product Name:* SHISHU PRABHA**

Composition: Each 5 ml. contains:

Piper longum (Pippli)	20 mg.
Foencuium vulgare (Mishraya)	10 mg.
Terminalia chebula (Haritkilaghu)	15 mg.

Vitis vinifera 9Munnaka)	20 mg.
Mentha spicata (Podina)	10 mg.
Rosa centifolia (Gulab)	20 mg.
Casia fistula (Amaltas)	15mg.
Pistacia integerrima (Kakrasringi)	10 mg.
Glycyrhiza glabra (Yastimadhu)	25mg.
Zizyphus vulgare (Unnav)	10 mg.
Anethem sowa (Shatpuspa)	10 mg.
Viola odorata (Gulbanapsha)	10 mg.
Iris ensata (Buch)	20 mg.
Aconitum hetrophylum (Atish karvi)	20 mg.
Nelumbo nucifera (Kamak pusp)	10 mg.
Cyprus rotundus (Mustak)	10 mg.
Trachyspermum ammi (Yavani)	10 mg.
Honey (Honey)	1.5 g.
Cane sugar (Sugar)	2 g.

Dosage: 2 teaspoonful two or three times a day.

How Supplied: 100 ml. packed in glass bottles.

Uses: Improves appetite, promotes weight gain, healthly growth in new borns and infants & helps babies from digestive troubles, gas, collic, gripes, diarrhoea & constipation.

***Product Name:* VENTI SYRUP**

Composition: Each 1000 ml. syrup contains:

Viola odorata (Banpsa)	45 g.
Ocimum sanctum (Tulsi)	13.5 g.
Junieperus communis (Hapusa)	50 g.
Vitis vinifera (Draksa)	20 g.
Solanu zanthozylum (Kantkailaghu)	75 g.
Solanum indicum (Vhratki)	75 g.
Piper longum (Pippli)	50 g.
Zingiber officinale (Sunthi)	50 g.
Glycyrrhiza glabra (Yastimadhu)	200 g.
Adhatoda vasica (Vasaka)	200 g.
Mentha spicata (Poudina)	.5 g.
Trachyspermum ammi (Yawani)	.5 g.
Anethum sowa (Satpuspa)	.5 g.
Sudha amonium chloride (Shud narshar)	15 g.
Myrica esculentabuch (Kayphal)	15 g.

Pistica integerrima (Kakra sringi)	15 g.
Cane sugar (Sugar)	150 g.
Shudh sphatika	20 g.

Dosage: 2 teaspoonsful two or three times a day.

How Supplied: 120 ml., 210 ml. in glass bottle.

Uses: A soothing expectorant for productive unproductive, dry & spasmodic cough, smokers cough, throat irritation.

Product Name: **VORMIN CAPSULE**

Composition: Each 500 mg. capsule contains:

Embilica Ribes (Vidang)	20 mg.
Azadirachta indica (Nimbhtwak)	20 mg.
Pongamia pinnata (Karanj beej)	20 mg.
Butea monsoperma (Palash)	20 mg.
Moringa oelifera (Sringu)	20 mg.
Holarrhena antidysenterica (Kutaj)	20 mg.
Premna mucronata (Agnimanth)	20 mg.
Carum xoxburghianum (Ajmodh)	20 mg.
Trachyspermum ammi (Yavani)	20 mg.
Cyperus rotundus (Mustak)	20 mg.
Aegal Marmelos (Vilbhphal)	20 mg.
Berberis aristata (Darvi)	20 mg.
Ferula foetida (Shudh hingu)	10 mg.
Operculina turpethum (Nishodh)	10 mg.
Terminalia belerica (Vibhitki)	20 mg.
Terminalia chebula (Haritki)	30 mg.
Holarrhena antidysenterica (Indryav)	20 mg.
Citrus aurantium (Nagrang)	20mg.
Mallotus philippinensis (Shudh kampilak)	20 mg.

Dosage: 2 capsules thrice a day for seven days or as directed by Physician.

How Supplied: Packed 100 capsule in glass bottles.

Uses: Antiameobic, antiworms.

Product Name: **Chyawan Praksh**

Composition: Each 10 g. contains:"

Emblica officinalis gaertn (Amalaki)	4.750 g.

Sugar (Sarkara)	5.700 g.
Ghee (Ghrit)	570 mg.
Sesamum indicum linn (Til tail)	570 mg.
Honey (Madhu)	570 mg.
Tugakshiri (Tugakshiri)	152 mg.
Piper longum linn (Pippali)	190 mg.
Cinnamomum zeylanicum blume (Tvak)	95 mg.
Elettaria cardamomum maton (Ela)	95 mg.
Cinnamomum tamala nees & Eberm (Patra)	95 mg.
Mesua ferea linn (Nagkesar)	95 mg.
Aegle marmelos corr. (Bilva)	95 mg.
premna integrifolia roxb. (Agnimanth)	95 mg.
Oroxylum indicum vent (Syonak)	95 mg.
Stereospermum suaveolens D.C. (Patali)	95 mg.
Gmelina arborea linn (Gambhari)	95 mg.
Desmodium gangeticum D.C. (Shalparni)	95 mg.
Uraria picta desb. (Prishnipani)	95 mg.
Solanum indicum linn (Gokshura)	95 mg.
Solanum xanthocarpum schard & Wendl (Kantkari)	95 mg.
Tribulus terestris linn (Gokshura)	95 mg.
Phaseolus trilobus ait (Mudgaparni)	95 mg.
Teramnus labialis spreng 9Mashparni)	95 mg.
Sida cordifolia linn (Bala)	95 mg.
Piper longum linn (Pippali)	95 mg.
Pistacia integerrima stew.ex Brandis (Shringi)	95 mg.
Phyllandthus niruni linn (Tamalaki)	95 mg.
Vitis vinifera linn (Draksha)	95 mg.
Inula racemosa hook. F. (Pushkara)	95 mg.
Aquilaria agallocha roxb. (Agru)	95 mg.
Termanalia chebula retz. (Haritaki)	95mg.
Tinospora cordifolia willd. miers. (Guduchi)	95 mg.
Habenaria intermedia d.don (Ridhi)	95 mg.
Microstylis mucifera ridlay (Jeevak)	95 mg.
Microstylis wallichii lindl. (Rishabhak)	95 mg.
Polygonatum cirrhifolium royle (Meda0	95mg.
Lilium polyphyllum d.don. (Kakoli)	95 mg.
Leptadenia reticulata W.& A. (jeevanti)	95 mg.
Hedychium spicatum ham ex smith (Shati)	95 mg.
Cyperus rotundus linn (Musta)	95 mg.
Boerhaavia diffusa linn (Punarnava)	95mg.
Flettaria cardamomum maton (Ela)	95 mg.

Santalum album linn (Chandan)	95 mg.
Nelumbo nucifera gaertn (Utpala)	95 mg.
Pueraria tuberosa D.C. (Vidari)	95 mg.
Adhatoda vasica nees (Vasa)	95 mg.
Pentatropis microphylla W.&A. (Kaknashika)	95 mg.

Dosage: 2 teaspoonful twice a day with milk (According to age).

How Supplied: ½ kg, 1 kg. In plastic Boxes.

Uses: Perfectly balanced health tonic of Ayurveda. An ideal tonic for body and mind suited for entire family. Fortified with natural vitamin-C and calcium.

Spectromed Pharmaceutical Manufacturers
M-36/1, 7th Cross Street, Besant Nagar
Chennai-600090
Tel.: 4914775, 4919943
Fax: (44) 4915382

***Product Name:* SPEC**

Composition: Each SPEC capsule contains:

Dasamoola kwatha extract	300 mg.
Ashtavarga kwatha extract	200 mg.
Withania somnifera (Ashwagandha)	300 mg.
Tinospora cordifolia (Guduchi)	200 mg.
Tinospora cordifolia (Guduchi)	200 mg.
Centella asiatica (Mundooka parni)	200 mg.
Tribala	50 mg.
Trikatu	50 mg.
Teminalia arjuna (Arjuna)	100 mg.
Spirulina fusiformis	200 mg.

Dosage: 1-3 capsules daily in run-down conditions followed by 1-2 capsules as maintenance for general well-being or as directed by the Physician.

How Supplied: Blister of 10 capsules in a carton.

Uses: In fatigue conditions, adjuvant supplement during tuberculosis, along with chemotherapy drugs in the treatment of cancer, during convalescence, after surgery, during pregnancy, after delivery, during lactation, during and after menopause, in wight loss, in dementia memory loss, senile debilities. To improve retention and recall of memories in school going children. To relieve stress and strain in active executives, housewives and as a general body toner for all age group.

Product Name: REMIND

Composition: Each Remind capsule contains:

Acorus calamus (Vacha)	50 mg.
Celastrus paniculata (Jyothismati)	100 mg.
Bacopa monnieri (Brahmi)	300 mg.
centella asiatica (Mundooka parni)	300 mg.
Spirulina fusiformis	200 mg.
Evolvulus alsinoides (Vishnu Kranti)	100 mg.

Dosage: 1-2 capsules daily initially, followed by 1 capsule daily as maintenance dose for 45 days or as directed by the Physician.

How Supplied: Blister of 10 capsules in a carton.

Product Name: RHEUMINAX

Composition: Each capsule contains:

Dasamoola kwatha extract	200 mg.
Ashtavarga kwatha extract	100 mg.
Mahayogaraja guggulu	100 mg.
Chandra prabhavati	100 mg.
Sida retusa (Bala)	100 mg.
Withania somnifera (Ashwagandha)	100 mg.
Alpinia galanga (Rasna)	100 mg.
Tinospora cordifolia (Guduchi)	100 mg.

Dosage: 1-2 capsules daily followed by one capsule as maintenance dose for 45 days or as directed by the Physician.

How Supplied: Blister of 10 capsules in a carton.

Uses: Inflammatory conditions of musculoskeletal systems, rheumatoid arthritis, osteoarthritis, sciatica, lumbago, soft tissue inflammations, dental pain, dysmenorrhoea, sports injuries, sprains and back ache.

Pharmacological Action: Mild gastric irritation in rare cases. The drug should be given in reduced dose (in divided doses) after food.

Product Name: TYLOSOL

Composition: Each capsule contains:

Tylophora asthmatica (Pitamart)	150 mg.
Solanum xanthocarpum (Kantakari)	150 mg.

Adhatoda vasica (Vasa)	100 mg.
Ephedra vulgaris (Somavalli)	100 mg.
Inula racemosa (Pushkaramool)	25 mg.
Albizzia lebbek (Shirish)	50 mg.
Glycyrrhiza glabra (Yashtimadhu)	25 mg.
Piper longum (Pippali)	10 mg.
Curcuma longa (Haridra)	25mg.

Dosage: 1-2 capsules 6 hourly in acute phase of asthma and 1-2 capsules daily in chronic asthma and 1-2 capsules as maintenance dose for 45 days or as directed by the Physician.

How Supplied: Blister of 10 capsules in a carton.

Uses: Bronchial asthma, bronchitis, bronchiospasm, bronchiectasis, allergic asthma, smokers cough and other allergic respiratory syndromes.

Pharmacological Action: Nausea, vomiting and gastric irritation in rare cases.

***Product Name*: U-NITE**

Composition: Each Unite capsule contains:

Asparagus racemosus (Satavari)	400 mg.
Tribulus terrestris (Gokshura)	300 mg.
Mucuna pruriens (kapikatchu)	200 mg.
Sida retusa (Bala)	100 mg.
Asteracantha longifolia (Kokilaksha)	100 mg.
Withania somnifera (Ashwagandha)	600 mg.
Curculigo orchiodes (Kalamusli)	200 mg.
Puereria tuberosa (Vitarikhand)	100 mg.
Myristica fragrans (Jathi Phala)	50 mg.
Shilajit	100 mg.

Dosage: 1-2 capsules at bed time with milk for a minimum period of 45 days followed by 1 capsule daily as maintenance dose or as directed by the Physician.

How Supplied: Blister of 10 capsules in a catron.

Uses: In neurogenic, vasculogenic and psychogenic impotency, in both male and female. Loss of libido in men and anorgasima in women. In deficiency of penile erection, premature ejaculation and impotency due to varied etiologies, in decreased libido due to beta blocker therapy, diabetes.

***Product Name*: Hem Stop**

Composition: Each hemstop capsule contains:

Rubia cordifolia (Manjistha)	200 mg.
Cyperus rotundues (Mustha)	100 mg.
Adhatoda vasica (Vasa)	100 mg.
Symplocus racemosa (Lodhra)	100 mg.
Saraca indica (Ashoka)	100 mg.
mimosa pudica (Lajjalu)	50 mg.
Laceifer lacca (Laksha)	50 mg.
Cedrus deodara (Devadaru)	100 mg.
Aegle marmelos (Bilwa)	100 mg.
Andrographis paniculata (Karatatiktaka)	100 mg.

Dosage: 1-2 capsules 2-3 timesa day for 4-5 days or till the bleeding subsides or as directed by the Physician.

How Supplied: Blister of 10 capsules in a catron.

Uses: In bleeding of gums, bleeding due to active peptic ulceration, post surgical bleeding, excessive bleeding due to traumatic conditions, menstrual excess bleeding and leucorrhoea.

Pharmacological Action: Abdominal distress like nausea and vomiting has been reported in 1% patient. The dosage and frequency of administration should be reduced in these cases.

Sri Surya Ayurveda Nilayam Pithapuram 553450
E.G. Dt. (A.P.)
Tel. : (08869) 51260

***Product Name*: Varnika Capsules**

Composition: Each capsule contains:

Abhraka Bhasmam	30 mg.
Machikka powder	30 mg.
Loha kalpa	30 mg.
Tintrinee beeja bhasmam	30 mg.
Bala leap powder	70 mg.
Black turpeth powder	30 mg.
Sukti bhasmam	30 mg.
Triphala decoction	q.s.
Ex. CP.	250 mg.

Dosage: Adult: 1 capsule 3 or 4 times a day. Child: ½ capsule 3 or 4 times a day.

How Supplied: 30 capsules.

Uses: Piples, Bleeding piles, Pain and buring sensation of anal region, Prolapse rectum, Continued use will shrivel up pile-mass.

***Product Name*: SWARNI CAPSULES**

Composition: Each capsules contains:

Swarni sindooram	30 mg.
Khurasani omam	40 mg.
Kantakari samoola choornam	40 mg.
Vartaki samoola chooram	40 mg.
Haritaki choornam	350 mg.
Decoction of vasaka	
Kustha; Taleesapatri	q.s.

Dosage: Adult: 1 caps. 3 to 4 times a day. Child: 1 caps. twice a day.

How Supplied: 30 caps.

Uses: Bronchial Asthma, Bronchitis, Eosinophilia, Whooping cough, Dry spasmodic cough, Recurrent sneezing, Recurrent allergic rhinitis and nasal block.

***Produce Name*: PRADARI TABLES**

Composition: Each tablets contains:

Sankha bhasmam	35 mg.
Jasada bhasmam	35 mg.
Swarnavangam	35 mg.
Kaseesam	35 mg.
Tankanam	35 mg.
Baboola twak choornam	70 mg.
Nyagrodha twak choornam	70 mg.
Ex. CP	185 mg.

Dosage: 1 tab. 3 times a day.

How Supplied: 10 tabs.

Uses: Cures leucorrhoae in women (white discharge), Palvic inflammatory disease, Cervicitis, urinary tract infection.

***Product Name*: SWETANI CAPSULES**

Composition: Each capsules contains:

Mayura sindooram	30 mg.
Lohakalkpa	30 mg.
kaseesam	30 mg.
Kaphari	30 mg.
Tamra bhasmam	10 mg.
Psoralea seed powder	100 mg.
Decoction of bhringaraj and Guduchi together	100 mg.
Thrikatukam	70 mg.

Dosage: Adult: 1 cap. 3 or 4 times a day.

Child: 1 cap. 2 times a day.

How Supplied: Not Available.

Uses: Cures vitiligo (leucoderma).

***Product Name*: CANTER CAPSULES**

Composition: Each capsules contains:

Shatguna sindooram	30 mg.
Abharaka bhasmam	30 mg.
Pravala bhasmam	30 mg.
Calx of hen's egg shells	30 mg.
Dried ginger powder	130 mg.
Aswagandhi choornam	150 mg.
Triphala choornam	100 mg.
Decotion of Yastimadhu	q.s.

Dosage: 1 cap. 3 to 4 times a day.

How Supplied: 30 capsules.

Uses: Rejuvinator, Vajeekarna durg, Increases libido, Sex. Stgamina and body vigour, Prevents premature ejaculation, Keeps the body strong, Verile and active, Increases sperm count, Good drug or oligo spermea, Improves blood and nerve functions, Imparts good sleep, Cures weakness, Vague fears and paopitations, To keep one self strong Healthy and sexually vigourous a course of canter can be taken for 2 months once in every year.

***Product Name*: MAHATI PILLS**

Composition: Each pill contains:

Aconite powder	50 mg.
Rasna powder	50 mg.
Black pepper powder	50 mg.
Bhallataki oil	50 mg.
Parpatee rasam	50 mg.
Tamra bhasmam	10 mg.
Mahishkshi guggul	130 mg.
Decoction of sigrubark and guduchi	q.s.
Lusunam (Garlick)	130 mg.

Dosage: Adult: 1 pill 3 times a day. Child: ½ pill 3 times a day.

How Supplied: 30 pills.

Uses: Vata diseases, Joint diseases, Osteo-arthritis, Cervical or lumbar spondylosis, rhumatiood arthritis, Neuromuscular pains, Frozen shoulder sydrome. Heel pain, Sciatica, Non-specific joint pains, Infected arthritis, Chronic (functional) lumbago.

***Product Name*: CHARMI CAPSULES**

Composition: Each capsules contains:

Vyavdhi Harana rasam	40 mg.
Gandhaka choornam	100 mg.
Pravala bhasmam	75 mg.
Nimbapatra choormam	135 mg.
Yevani	100 mg.
Kiratatikta	50 mg.

Dosage: Adult: 1 cap. 3 to 4 times a day. Child: ½ cap. 3 to 4 times a day. Or ½ cap. Twice a day.

How Supplied: 30 capsules.

Uses: Psoriasis, Puritic skin lesions, blood impurities, Urticaria, Eczema, Fissaries heads & feet.

***Product Name*: VIGARIN CAPSULE**

Composition: Each capsule contains:

Bala neelam, musta, Paraseeka yavani, Ajamedam, Krishna jeerkam, Methi, Satavari, Vacha equal parts.

Dosage: Adult: 2 capsules two times a day. Child: 1 capsules two or three times a day.

How Supplied: 30 capsules.

Uses: Improves general health, Improves appetite, digestion and liver functions, Improves memory and brain functions, strengthens and hardens the body, increases mental strength, Imparts good sleep, Keeps the body active, Removes vague fears, recurrent headaches.

***Product Name*: SOOLARI PILLS**

Composition: Each pill contains:

Kuberakshi	30 mg.
Hing	30 mg.
Lasun	30 mg.
Nagaram	30 mg.
Vampuvvu (Thymol)	30 mg.
Parasaeeka yavavi	30 mg.
Karpooram	30 mg.
Musambaram	30 mg.
Ardrakaswarasm juia	q.s.

Dosage: 1 pill 3 or 4 times a day before food.

How Supplied: 30 pills.

Uses: Colic abdomen, Recurent abdominal pain, Indigestion, Distension of abdomen, Peptic ulcers.

***Product Name*: SORIN TABLETS**

Composition: Each tab. contains:

Purified Hingulam	60 mg.
Purified thalakam	10 mg.
Fried tankamam	20 mg.
Purified soweeram	1 mg.
Sankha bhasmam	30 mg.
Mareecha choornam	30 mg.
Guduchi decoction	q.s.
Ex. Cp.	394 mg.

Dosage: Adult: 1 tablet 3 or 4 times a day. Child: ½ tablet 3 or 4 times a day.

Uses: Cures psoriasis, fungal infections of skin, Pruritic skin lesions, Eczema, Hypopigmented skin areas, Ashtadasa kushta rogam.

Swastik Formulations Pvt. Ltd.
C.K. 36/1-A, Banasphatak
P.B. NO. 1022, Varanasi-221 001
Tel.: 352258, 352754, 352460
Fax : (542) 323877

***Product Name*:** **ASHOKA COMPOUND LIQUID**

Composition: Each 5 ml. contains:

Aqueous Extract of each of contains

Ashoka bark	0.5 ml.
Lodh	0.50 ml.
Arjun bark	0.60 ml.
Mulethi	0.25 ml.
Jatamanshi	0.25 ml.
Daruharidra	0.25 ml.

Dosage: Not Available.

How Supplied: 450 ml.

Uses: Restorative Herbo-mineral compound for females—Specially useful in menstrual disorders and in leucorrhoea.

***Product Name*:** **GRO LIQUID**

Composition: Each 5 ml. contains:

Kalmegh	62.5 mg.
Kulekhera	40 mg.
Brahmi	25 mg.
Pitpapra	50 mg.
Bhringraj	100 mg.
Pipli	30 mg.
Kashniphol	30 mg.
Sunthi	30 mg.
Makoi	20 mg.
Punarnava	100 mg.

Dosage: Not Available.

How Supplied: 100 ml.

Uses: Hepatoprotective and in convalescence, Improves auto-immune system.

***Product Name*: Gynesol Capsules**

Composition: Dry Extract of followings:

Ashoka	1 g.
Sugandhabala	500 mg.
Mulethi	500 mg.
Satavar	200 mg.
Ọlatkambal	200 mg.
Lodh	500 mg.
Loh bhasma	15 mg.

Dosage: Not Available.

How Supplied: 60 capsules.

Uses: In menstrual disorders, excessive vaginal discharges, secondary sterility, restores normal pH of vagina, checks emotional and anxiety states during menopause.

***Product Name*: GYNESOL LIQUID**

Composition: Each 5 ml. contains:

Ashok Bark	0.20 ml.
Lodh	0.20 ml.
Jatamanshi	0.25 ml.
Mulethi	0.20 ml.
Ashwagandha	0.15 ml.
Dhatki	0.10 ml.
Jeevanti	0.10 ml.
Ulat kambal	0.10 ml.
Satavari	0.10 ml.
Hara kashish	100 mg.
Nausadar	50 mg.
Neebu ka satva	75 mg.

Dosage: Not Available.

How Supplied: 240 ml.

Uses: In menstrual disorders, excessive vaginal discharges, secondary sterility, restores normal pH of vagina, checks emotional and anxiety states during menopause.

***Product Name*: PREPETONE LIQUID**

Composition: Each 5 ml. contains:

Patola	450 mg.
Amla	450 mg.
Hareda	450 mg.
Kutki	450 mg.
Bhringraj	450 mg.
Chirayata	450 mg.
Sunthi	450 mg.
Pittpapda	450 mg.
Baheda	450 mg.

Dosage: Not Available.

How Supplied: 240 ml.

Uses: "Bitter" tonic. Pure herbal decoctions of all bitters. In Jaundice, Drug induced hepatomegaly and alcoholism.

Synthochem
7--B, Shahajahanpur Road
Bareilly-243 005
Tel.: 476388
Fax: (0581) 471901

***Product Name*: COS COUGH SYRUP**

Composition: Each 5 ml. contains:

Extract each of Tej Pat	2 g.
Bahera chhal	2 g.
Talsih patra	0.5 g.
Kantkari	1 g.
Kulinjan	0.5 g.
Sonth	0.25 g.
Khurasani ajwain	0.5 g.
Dhatoora seeds	200 mg.
Mentha oil	q.s.

Dosage: 5-10 ml. T.D.S.

***Product Name*: DIGEST SYRUP**

Composition: Each 10 ml. contains:

Papain	250 mg.

Chitrak	500 mg.
Tirkatu	50 mg.
Sugar	9 g.
Sodium Benzoate	5 mg.

***Product Name*: GYNEC-20 SYRUP**

Composition: Aq. Extract each of:

Ashoka	20%
Lodh	10%
Shatavari	12.5%
Asgandh	12.5%
Khadi	10%
Supari	10%
Vellerian	25%
Sugar as Syrup base	4.5%

***Product Name*: GRYPEX SYRUP**

Composition: Aq. Extract each of:

Ashwagandha	25%
Musli	25%
Shatavari	25%
Haritaki	10%
Lime water	20%
Aq. Ptychotis	5%
Sugar 4.5%	

***Product Name*: Livosyn Tablets**

Composition

Chitrak	30 mg.
Sarjikshar	30 mg.
Amla	25 mg.
Kali kutki	30 mg.
Chuna	20 mg.
Papra khar	160 mg.
haritaki	25 mg.
Shunthi	30 mg.
Kalmegh	10 mg.
Mandoor bhasma	10 mg.

Dosage: 1-2 tablets thrice daily.

How Supplied: 100 tablets.

Uses: All types of liver disorders such as hepatomegaly Sirrhosis of liver due to chronic alcoholism, viral hepatitis, Jaundice, dypepsia, growth retardation in children due to calcium defficiency/liver disfunction.

***Product Name*: LUCOSYNTH-O CAPSULES**

Composition

Extract Acacia	10.5%
Alum detoxicated	10%
Quercus intectoria	30%
Extrate Ashoka	15%
Lodh	15%
Loh bhasma	5%
Tamra bhasma	4%
Tagar	10.5%

***Product Name*: LIVOSYN SYRUP**

Composition: Each 5 ml. contains:

Chitraks	30 mg.
Sarjikakshar	30 mg.
Amla	20 mg.
Kali kutki	30 mg.
Chuna	20 mg.
Parakhar	260 mg.
Haritaki	25 mg.
Shunthi	30 mg.
Kali mirch	30 mg.
Mandur bhasma	10 mg.
Kalmegh	10 mg.
Sugar	4.5 g.

Dosage: 5-10 ml. three time a day.

Uses: All types of liver disorders such as hepatomegaly cirrhosis of liver due to chronic alcoholism, viral hepatitis, Jaundice, dyspepsia, growth retardation in children due to calcium deficiency/liver disfunction.

***Product Name*: LIVOSYN DROPS**

Composition: Each 5 ml. contains:

Chitrak	20 mg.

Kali marich	15 mg.
Amla	20 mg.
Kalmi shora	5 mg.
Papadakhar	175 mg.
Kali kutaki	15 mg.
Haritaki	15 mg.
Sugar as syrup base	q.s.

Dosage: 10 to 30 drops T.D.S.

How Supplied: 100 ml.

Uses: All types of liver disorders such as hepatomegaly cirrhosis of liver due to chronic alcoholism, viral hepatitis, Jaundice, dyspepsia, growth retardation in children due to calcium difficiency/liver disfunction.

***Product Name*: SUPERTINE SYRUP**

Composition

Moosli safed	10%
Moosli kali	10%
Asgandh	10%
Chitraka	1%
Mandukparni	10%
Brahami	5%
Sonth	5%
Pippli	5%
Shatawari	18%
Guduchi	7%
Bharanjraj	12%
Kasis	1%
Sodium Benzoate	2%

***Product Name*: VEDNIL CAPSULES**

Composition

Shudh kuchla	50 mg.
Shudh guggul	30 mg.
Chitrak mool churan	50 mg.
Sonth churan	50 mg.
Haridra churan	50 mg.

***Product Name*: Vitrisan Syrup**

Composition: Each 10 ml. contains:

Sodium chloride	350 mg.
Potassium cirate	250 mg.
Sucrose	2.5 g.
Orange	0.02 ml.

***Product Name*: WHOOPEX CAPSULES**

Composition

P. vasicum	90%
Dudhi bhasma	10%

Themis Chemicals Ltd.
(Phyto Medica Division)
11/12, Udyog Nagar Industrial Estate
S.V. Road, Goregaon (W)
Mumbai-460062
Tel.: 8757836, 8755676, 8756949
Fax: 8746621, 8743643

***Product Name*: CUROPILE OINTMENT**

Composition: Extracts derved from:

Acorus calamus	100 mg.
Plumbago zeylanica	50 mg.
Azadirachta indica	30 mg.
Achyranthes aspera	30 mg.
Mimosa pudica	100 mg.
Symplocos recemosa	30 mg.

***Product Name*: Curopile Tablets**

Composition

Extracts derived from

Acorus calamus	100 mg.
Amorphophallus campanulatus	100 mg.
Semecarpus anacrdium	100 mg.
Mesua ferrea	100 mg.
Terminalia chebula	50 mg.
Plumbago zeylanica	50 mg.
Terminalia belerica	50 mg.
Piper longum roots	100 mg.
Sesamum indicum	50 mg.

***Product Name*: Daash Capsules**

Composition

Extracts derived from	
Withania somnifera	1000 mg.
Bacopa moniera	500 mg.
Mucuna pruriens	500 mg.
Ocimum sanctum	500 mg.
Shuddha shilajit	250 mg.
Chyuvanprash	500 mg.

***Product Name*: Digiped Syrup**

Composition: Each 5 ml. contains:

Dil oil	0.0018 ml.
Fennel oil	0.0125 ml.
Extract derived from	
Tinospora cordifolia	250 mg.
Pyllanthus emblica	150 mg.
Acontium heterophyllum buds	25 mg.
Carum roxburghianum	50 mg.
Piper longum roots	50 mg.
Zingiber officinale	100 mg.
Cuminum cyminum	100 mg.
Embelia ribes	50 mg.
Alpinia galanga	50 mg.

***Product Name*: Globinol Syrup**

Composition: Each 30 g. contains:

Withania somnifera	150 mg.
Ipomoea digitata	500 mg.
Asparagus racemosus	500 mg.
Glycyrrhiza glabra	200 mg.
Tribulus terrestris	250 mg.
Zingbier officinale	50 mg.
Plumbago zeylanica roots	10 mg.
Piper longum roots 50 mg.	
Convulvulus pluricaulis	50 mg.
Narodostachys jatamansi	2.5 mg.
Bacopa moniera	50 mg.
Godanti bhasma	150 mg.
Elettaria cardamomum (Elaichi)	10 mg.

Myristica fragrans (Jaiphal)	5 mg.
Crocus sativus (Kesar)	1 mg.

***Product Name*: Herbokof Syrup**

Composition: Each 10 ml. contains:

Extracts derived from	
Ocimum sanctum	100 mg.
Adhatoda vasica	250 mg.
Glycyrrhiza glabra	50 mg.
Solanum xanthocarpum	200 mg.
Berberis aristata	50 mg.
Piper nigrum	50 mg.
Pepermint oil	0.002 ml.

***Product Name*: LIVOCURE LIQUID**

Composition: Each 5 ml. contains:

Extracts derived from	
Andrographis paniculata	125 mg.
Picrorrhiza kurroa	125 mg.
Phyllanthus niruri/amarus	150 mg.
Boerhaavia diffusa	125 mg.
Eclipta alba	250 mg.
Tinospora cordifolia	125 mg.
Glycyrrhiza glabra (Film coated)	250 mg.

***Product Name*: OSTEOGARD CREAM**

Composition

Extracts derived from	
Commiphora mukul	5% w/w
Boswellia serrata	5% w/w
Ricinus communis oil	20% v/w
Vitex Negundo	5% w/w
Citrullus colocynthis	0.33% w/w
Gaultheria fragrantissima	10% v/w

***Product Name*: OSTEOGARD TABLETS**

Composition

Extracts dervied from

Commiphora mukul	200 mg.
Boswellia serrata	200 mg.
Ricinus communis roots	100 mg.
Pluchea lanceolata	100 mg.
glycyrrhiza glabra	100 mg.
Picrorrhiza kurroa	50 mg.
Zingiber officinale	50 mg.

Trio Pharma
Ayurvedic Division
3008, G.I.D.C. Phase IV, Vatva
Ahmedabad-382445
Tel : 5830178, 5831069

***Product Name*: ARGONE CAPSULE**

Composition

Abha Guggul	125 mg.
Lakshadi Guggul	125 mg.
Pushpadhanvaras	10 mg.
Mahdumalini vasant	100 mg.
Kidore Guggul	50 mg.
Kukkutandatwak Bhasma	50 mg.
Praval bhasma	40 mg.
Excipients	Q.S.

Dosage: 1 to 2 capsules a day after meals, oras directed by the Physician. Can also be given 2 to 3 does if required, initially.

How Supplied: A box containing 10 blister packs each of 10 capsules.

Uses: The above wholesome compound renders excellent treatment in acute and chronic stages in planned management of rheumatic, arthritic and collagen complaints, such as osteoarthritis, neuralgia, Sciatica, ankylo-Spondilitis, fibrositis, back-ache, gout, joint and muscular aints. Guggul therapy, pain absorber with high degree of safety, accelerates healing process in bone fracture, and specially useful in osteomalacia, osteoporosis, rickets, and to enrich bonemarrow, as a Calcium reinforcement. Long-acting with no side effects.

Pharmacological Action: Abha guggul: Helps healing of bones and improves the integrity of the joints. Guggul is prominent, has anti-inflammatory and analgesic action. Lakshadi guggul: Helps the reunion of fractured bones, reduces pain and inflammation, and strengthens the bones system. Pushpadhanvaras: is useful in calcium deficiency particularly in menopausal syndrome which results in Osteoporosis. Due to osteoporosis a little limping is seent in a walking, and a little lump is noticed. All these symptoms are corrected. Mahdumalini vasant: Very useful in rickets, and treating weak bones. Corrects calcium deficiency improves overall bodily functions. Kishore guggul:L The drug of choice as an analgesic and anti-inflammatory. Useful to treat Rheumatism, Arthritis and Govt. Kukkutandatwak bhasma: A Natural calcium reinforcement. One of the best general tonics for both the sexes. Corrects calcium deficiency, improves muscle tone, increases debility and appetite. Praval Bhasma: Natural calcium. Useful in rickets and other calcium deficiencies. In bone T.B. along with kukkutandatwak bhasma, is very beneficial given for longer period.

***Product Name*: COLIMIN DROPS**

Composition: Each ml. contains:

Black salt (Sauvarchal)	2 mg.
hingu (Ferula foetida)	1 mg.
Saindhav salt	1 mg.
Nmbak sat	1 mg.
Aconitum heterophyllum ext. (ativisha ext.)	0.5 mg.
Hyoscyamus niger ext. (Khurasani ajawayan Ext.)	0.75 mg.
Ellataria cardamomum (Elayachi)	3 mg.
Peucedanum graveolens (Shatpushpa)	4 mg.
Acerus calamus Ext. (vach ext.)	1 mg.
Caesalpinia crista (puti karania)	2 mg.
Flavoured syrup base	Q.S.

Dosage: 4 to 10 drops five to six times a day or as directed by the Physician. In severe conditions, dosage can be increased and no adverse effects found.

How Supplied: IN 30 ml. Glass Bottle.

Uses: Colic Pains, abdominal distension and discomfort, green diarrhoea, indigestion, griping pain, checks vomiting.

Pharmacological Action: Black salt: stomachic, digestive, purgative, demulcent, carminative. Useful in dyspepsia, colic in abdominal tract. Hingu: carminative. Expells worms. Useful in colic, dyspepsia gastric affections. Relieves abdominal distension. Saindhav salt: carminavtive, tonic stomachic, Useful in enlargement of liver and spleen, Anti-flatulent and anti-spasmodic and digestant. Nimbak sat: aromatic, carminative, stomachic, checks chloresis and thirst and abdominal distension. Source of VIT-C. Helps general health and promotes resistence. Ativisha

Ext.: anti-spasmodic. Anti-diarrhoeal, stomachic. Tonic and gives astringent action. Khurasani ajawayan Ett.: Digestive, astringent aniemetic, laxative, carminativ, anti-spasmodic and relieves diarrhoea. Elayachi: Aromatic, stimulant, carminative, stomachic, diuretic, has mild purgative action. Shatpushpa: Carminative, stomachic, aromatic, dill water prepared from the fruit is stimulant, diuretic. Relieves flttulence, hiccup, colics, abdominal pain, griping, diarrhoea and dysentery situations. Vacha Ext: useful in dyspepsia, flatulence, loss of appetite, atonic diarrhoea, choleric diarrhoea, nervine sedative, carminative, anti--septic. Puti karanja: Bitter tonic, anti-spasmodic, febrifuge and anthelminitic.

***Product Name*: EMPROMIN CAPSULE**

Composition: Each capsule contains:

Ashwagandha Ext.	110 mg.
Ashtavarga	20 mg.
Amala Ext.	15 mg.
Bhrungraj Ext.	25 mg.
Brahmi Ext.	15 mg.
Bala beej	20 mg.
Dashmul	10 mg.
Kavach seed	20 mg.
Manjishtha Ext.	20 mg.
Makardhwaja	30 mg.
Punarnava Ext.	20 mg.
Rasna	20 mg.
Shatavary	50 mg.
Trifala	40 mg.
Trikatu	25 mg.
Vidarikanda	40 mg.
Yashtimadhu Ext.	20 mg.
Excipients	Q.S.

Dosage: Grown up Children: 1 capsule three times a day with milk.

Adults: 2 capsules three times a day with milk after meals, or as directed by the physician.

***Product Name*: EMPROMIN SYUP**

Composition: Each 10 ml. contains:

Ashwagandha	100 mg.
Akakara	20 mg.
Ashtavarga	20 mg.

Amla	15 mg.
Bhrungraj Ext.	25 mg.
Brahmi	15 mg.
Bala	25mg.
Chaturajat	20 mg.
Vidarikanda	40 mg.
Gokshuru Ext.	10 mg.
Jatifal	10 mg.
Kavach seed	25 mg.
Manjishtha	20 mg.
Punarnava	20 mg.
Rasna	20 mg.
Shatavary	50 mg.
Trifala	40 mg.
Trikatu	25 mg.
Utangan	25 mg.
Dashmul	10 mg.
Yashtimadhu	20 mg.
Flavoured syrup base	Q.S.

Dosage: Infants: 3 drops 3 to 4 times a day with milk. (nursing mothers must take to benefit their infants).

Children: 1 teaspoonful 2 times a day with milk, fruit juice or diet. Adults: 2 teaspoonfuls 2 to 3 times a day with milk, or, after diet.

How Supplied: In glass bottle of 200 ml. sweet and delicious syrupy base.

Uses: An enriched combination of Herbo-Mineral compounds from natural sources, to fulfil the demand of an ideal tonic, towards Holistic treatment. For young and old. Either Sex. Stunted growth, malabsorption syndrome, & Wasting diseases, Stabilising long-lasting constructive process. Cross section of a tonic: Brings in perfect cohesion in digestive, nervous, circulatory and respiratory systems of the body. Infuses dynamism, energy, vigour and vitality afresh. Empromin builds up resistance power and strengthens Inner Strength to combat disease, and toxic effects arising from overdrugging and anti-biotic treatment. Useful in Anaemia, Calcium, Iron-protein and Vitamin deficiencies at all stages. Strengthens assimilation and absorption & Evacuation. Highly beneficial to run-down patients with a low key. Patients who are subjected to low B.P. with swoons and giddiness and faints. Makes mind alert and body active. Good appetiser. Delicious. Treatment commences right form the Taste on the tongue. Glandular stimulant. Empromin styup: that everyone needs today.

***Product Name*: GALACTIM CAPSULE**

Composition: Each capsule contains:

Shatavary	100 mg.
Jivanti	100 mg.
Ashwagandha	50 mg.
Praval bhasma	50 mg.
Kukkutandatwak bhasma	50 mg.
Mandur bhasma	50 mg.
Excipients	Q.S.

Dosage: 2 capsules t.i.d. with milk, or as advised by the Physician (Right from 5th Month of pregnancy).

How Supplied: A box containing 10 blister packs each of 10 capsules.

Uses: General weakness during pregnancy and after delivery. Galactagogue of choice. Promotes involution of Uterus. Tones up abdominal muscles. Assures galactogenesis and ensures better lactation. Reinforces Natural Iron and Calcium essential during nursing period, and post operative conditions. helps to contract and strengthen uterine muscles after delivery by exerting astringent action on elasticity of tissues of muscles towards a feeling of virginity. Improves nutritional status. Guards mother and child from infection. Helps mother to maintain normal shape and figure. Restores tension of nerves and muscles system of mammary gland (Breasts) on prolonged use.

Pharmacological Action: Shatavari: Has good quantity of lactose. Increases milk secretion by mammary gandular functions. Nutritive Appetiser and Restorative. Has antioxytoxic activity and tones uterine muscles, & Helps maintain rigidity. Jivanti; Milk supplement, stimulant, tonic. Ashwagandha: Rejuvenative. Infuses fresh vigour and vitality in the worn-out system. Stimulates various metabolic activities. Promotes synthesis of carbohydrates and proteins. Secures status of health. Tones up neuro-muscular activity. Mild nervine sedative. Induces natural sleep. Praval bhasma: A natural calcium reinforcement, towards stronger bones, strength and stability to the skeleton of mother and child. Kukkutandartwak bhasma: Natural source of calcium and phosphorous. Stimulates calcium metabolism and ensures proper absorption. Corrects digestion and malnutrition in anaemic condition. Mandur bhasma: Rich source of Natural iron. Easily assimiable. Tolerated & absorbed. Improves concentration of haemoglobin and RBC count. Essential in post natal cases with no side effects. Irons-out iron deficiency.

***Product Name*: LIVGARD CAPSULE**

Composition: Each capsule contains:

Punarnava Ext.	80 mg.
Arogya vardhini	110 mg.
Loha bhasma	80 mg.
Yakrut plihari loha	50 mg.
Plihari Ext.	40 mg.
Bhringaraj Ext.	40 mg.
Excipients	Q.S.

Dosage: 1 capsule 3 times a day for adults, or, as per the advice of the Physician.

How Supplied: A box containing 10 blister packs each of 10 capsules.

Uses: In hepatitis, Jaundice, sluggish liver, anorexia as a digestant & Tonic, Detoxifier and safety measure to be given with any antibiotic therapy.

Pharmacological Action: Punarnava Etx.: Natural diuretic, Anti-inflammatory. Decreases albuminurea. Rises serum protein while lowers serum cholesterol, is note-worthy. Arogya vardhini: A vertuous compound. Tonic, Appetiser, Enhances bile secretion. Useful in enlargement of liver. A scientific prepartion of Mercury, Sulphur, Loha-abhrakTamra Bhasmas, Triphala, Shilajita, Guggul, Chitrak and Katuki-Compound. Loha bhasma: Blood enricher, stimulates vital organs, and glandular system in the body. In debilitating conditions is a standby. Increases RBC count and haemoglobin. In Iron-deficiency and dysfunctions of liver. Yukrut plihari loha: A special compound evolved to maintain and put liver & spleen in order. Bile secretion is regularised, Antiseptic. Useful in infective hepatitis, and to reduce billirubin content of blood and urine. Plihari ext.: treats enlargement of liver, and obstructive jaundice. Exerts mild laxative action. Bhringaraj Etx.: Effective in derangement of liver and Gall bladder, and puts in order. Exerts rapid action in Jaundice.

***Product Name*: LIVGARD DROPS & SYRUP**

Composition: Drops each ml. & Syrup each 10 ml. contains:

Drops

Ativisha Ext.	1 mg.
Kalmegh Ext.	2 mg.
Plihari Ext.	1.5 mg.

Kakmachi Ext.	0.75 mg.
Kutaj Ext.	2 mg.
Pippali	2 mg.
Kasari	3 mg.
Kasni	3 mg.
Pransjhau	3 mg.
Vidanga	3 mg.
Gokshuru	2 mg.
Flavoured syrup base	Q.S.
Syrup	
Ativisha Ext.	7.5 mg.
Kalmegh Ext.	20 mg.
Plihari Ext.	10 mg.
Kakmachi Ext.	5 mg.
Kutaj Ext.	—
Pippali	20 mg.
Kasari	40 mg.
Kasni	30 mg.
Pransjhau	30 mg.
Vidanga	50 mg.
Gokshuru	—
Flavoured syrup base	Q.S.

Dosage: Neonates: 4 to 6 drops t.i.d. Infants: 5 to 10 drops t.i.d. Children: 10 to 20 drops t.i.d. Adults: 1 to 2 teaspoonfuls 3 times a day or as directeed by the Physician.

How Supplied: Drops in glass bottle of 30 ml. Syrup in glass bottle of 100 ml. & 190 ml.

Uses: Stimulates liver functions, induces bile formation, improves digestion, enhances assimilation, improves appetite, promotes metabolic activities, prevents hepatic damage and disorders. When the Liver is sluggish and spleen functions are not upto the meark. Cirrhosis of liver, jaundice and infantile liver disorders. As a dependable anabolic agent during convalescence period, and to combat toxic effects of Antibiotics and over-drugging.

Pharmacological Action: Ativisha Ext. Valuable in debility, tonic in postinfantile jaundice and illness and fevers. Useful in enlargement of liver. Also an anthelmintic. Kamlegh ext.-Prominent ingredient. stomachic, cholagogue, febrifuge, alterative, anthelmintic, antipyretic, and is useful in sluggish liver. Plihari ext.-durg of choice in liver enlargement, obstructive jaundice. Mild laxative. Kakmachi Ext.-Reduces oedema. Diuretic and laxative. Useful in liver enlargement. Pipplali-

regulates liver and spleen functions. Kasari-Cooling, laxative, diuretic, reduces oedema, useful in intestinal obstruction. Kasni-Stimulates bile secretion. Tones up liver functions. Checks jaundice, and spleen enlargement. Pranjhau-useful in bile disorders. Diuretic and astringent. Vidanga-Helps normal abdominal functions. Diuretic, laxative and anthelmintic. Gokshuru-Tones up kidney functions. Diuretic.

***Product Name*: Mobic Capsule**

Composition: Each capsule contains:

Ras parpati	15 mg.
Panchamrit parpati	20 mg.
Swet parpati	20 mg.
Bilwa pulp	100 mg.
Maradashingi	10 mg.
Kutaj Ext.	50 mg.
Mochras	20 mg.
Indrajva	100 mg.
Hingu	15 mg.
Excipients	Q.S.

Dosage: 2 capsules 3 times a day for 7 to 10 days or as directed by the Physician.

How Supplied: A box of 10 blister packs each of 10 capsules.

Uses: Mobic capsule is effective in both-cyst and motile form of amoeba and quickly eradicates amoeba from lumen and tissues. Mobic has a multipronged action and hence provides a high cure rate. Mobic controls frequency of stools very fast alongwith its concomitant symptoms like abdominal pain and associated flatulence. Mobic is free from gastric upset, metalic taste like synthetic drugs metronidazole and tinidazole. Moreover Mobic has demulcent and binding action on stools. Mobic is effective in diarrhoea, dysentery, amoebiasis, trichomona, giardia and amoeba, amoebic colitis and nonspecific diarrhoea. It resolves the infammation of mucus membrance, improves digestion and checks abdominal discomfort. It is effective vet a safe drug.

Pharmacological Action: Daru haridr ext.-is a very powerful astringent and checks diarrhoea very fast. It is stomachic, tonic antiperiodic, diaphoretic, antipyretic and alterative. Ras parapati: Is is useful in amoebic as well as ulcerative colitis. Rasparpati enhances the actions of panchamrit parpati. Panchamrit parpati: It is useful in chronic dysentery, diarrhoea, nausea and vomiting. Swet parpati: It is useful in chronic diarrhoea and has astringent action. Bilwa pulp: The durg is useful in diarrhoea and dysentery. The drug absorbs toxins and irritating substances released by bacteria. Kutaj Ext.: It is antiamoebic and antibacterial and hence checks amoebic and bacillary diarrhoea and dysentry. Indrajav: the drug is useful in amoebic dysentery and amoebic diarrhoea. It has direct action on entamoeba histolytica, trichomona and because of the systemic action, the drug is useful even in cyst form of amoeba as well as the amoeba hidden in the lumen of the intestine.

***Product Name*: Multibex Drops**

Composition: Each 5 ml. contains:

Bhringraj Ext.	20 mg.
Amruta Ext.	20 mg.
Pippali Ext.	15 mg.
Punarnava Ext.	20 mg.
Sunth Ext.	15 mg.
Vidang Ext.	25 mg.
Tulsi Ext.	20 mg.
Gokhru Ext.	20 mg.
Suva Ext.	15 mg.
Ashwagandha Ext.	20 mg.
Dashmul	12.5 mg.
Flavoured syrupy base Q.S.	

Dosage: Infants: 10 to 15 drops 2 to 3 times a day. Children: 15 to 30 drops 2 to 3 times a day preferably with milk, or fruit juice, or as directed by the Physician.

How Supplied: Pilfer-proof glass bottle of 30 ml.

Uses: A multi complex tonic for infants and children. in retarded growth, loss of appetite, indigestion, abdominal distension, colic & griping pain, constipation, diarrhoea, impaired liver and renal functions and carbohydrate indigestion, also as an adjuvent.

Pharmacological Action: Bhringraj etc.: Useful in derangement of liver & gall bladder. Regulates their functions, enhances secretion of bile, present in blood and thus exerts to clear jaundice. Amruta ext.: Also known as giloy. Stomachic. Bitter tonic, alterative & hepatic tonic. Increases appetite and digestion. Best known to be tonic of choice for entire body. Brain sharpener. Pippali ext.: stimulates spleen and liver functions. Helps secretion to bile. Punarnava ext.: carminative and digestive action. Corrects assimilation of food and digestion. Antiflatulent.

Vidang ext.: maintains normal functions of abdomen. Diuretic, laxative and anthelmintic. Tulsi ext.: The durg is anti-tussive, expectorant, and anti-bacterial. Promotes digestion, appetite, as cholagogue diuretic. Pulmonary antiseptic. Suva Ext.: Carminative, stomachic, stimulant. Given in hiccup, indigestion, flatulence, colic & griping. Appetiser. Gokhru ext.: diuretic. Tones up functions of kidneys. A tonic ashwagandha Ext.: Nervine tonic and alternative. Mild sedative. Controls hyperactivity. Growth is faster and gives strength to body and mind. Dashmul: Virtuous combination of "TEN ROOTS" of important medicinal values. Useful in asthma, cold, cough, headache, insomnia, inflammation, fevers, abdominal distension, and works as a coordinator of all systems in the body.

***Product Name:* NEEMI CAPSULE**

Composition: Each capsule contains:

Sarsaparilla (Hemidismus indicus)	150 mg.
Hemkshiri (Argemone mexicana)	100 mg.
Neem Ext. (Melia azardichata)	125mg.
Excipients	Q.S.

Dosage: 1 to 2 capsules 2 to 3 times a day along with Neemi cream; or as directed by the physician.

How Supplied: A box containing 10 blister packs each of 10 capsules.

Uses: For better, faster and definite action, it is suggested to use Neemi capsule internally and Neemi cream extremely in chronic skin diseases, localised bacterial and fungal infections, acne, pimples, boils, carbuncles, skin ulcers, bed sores, ulcers and wounds, cracked nipples, chilblains and as a blood purifier. Neemi capsule and Neemi cream improves the complexion and because of the rubefacient action, brings a glow on the face.

Pharmacological Action: Sarsaparilla: The drug is useful for skin ulcers as it clears the same and because of the antibacterial and antifungal action it cures the ulcers, it helps in healing ulcers and wounds. Hemkshiri: The drug heals blisters, excoriation and indolent ulcers. It is used in herpetic conditions and other skin diseases. Neem ext.: The drug is insecticide and antiseptic. The drug is cathartic, bitter and anthelmintic. It has a diuretic action and is astringent and stomachic.

Product Name: NEEMI CREAM

Composition

Neem Ext.	10%
Sarasparilla	2%
Hemkshiri	2%
Haldi Ext.	2%
Cream Base Q.S. to make	100%

Dosage: To apply the cream, clean the affected part properly with luke-warm water, dry it with a dry cotton cloth; apply Neemi Cream so that deeper penetration of the drug takes place, for better and faster action. Apply two to three times a day; or as per the direction of the physician.

How Supplied: Collapsible tube of 15 g.

Uses: The Neemi cream is the Neem cream marketed for the first time to treat acne, pimples, boils, carbuncles, bacterial or fungal infections like, eczema, ringworms, itching, skin infections.

Pharmacological Action: Neem Ext.: The drug when applied locally has stimulating effects, insecticide and antiseptic and used as a dressing for foul ulcers as liniment to rheumatic affections and to the head in headache. Sarasparilla: For ulcers and swellings it cleanses and cures. It helps in healing ulcers and wounds. Hemkshiri: Relieves, blisters, heals excoriation and indolent ulcers, herpetic conditions and other skin diseases. The drug checks itching and pruritus and checks and blisters. Haldi Ext.: It is applied to recent wounds, bruises, leechbites. In smallpox and chicken pox a coating the ointment is applied to facillitate the process of scabbing.

Product Name: NUFLAM CAPSULE

Composition: Each capsule contains:

Maharasanadi quath	100 mg.
Pathiadi Quath	100 mg.
Shulgajkesri Ras	75 mg.
Shulvarjini Ras	75 mg.
Shringa bhasma	75 mg.
Abharak bhasma	15 mg.
Ras sindur	15 mg.
Bang bhasma	15 mg.
Shankh bhasma	15 mg.
Godanti bhasma	15 mg.
Excipients	Q.S.

Dosage: 2 to 3 capsules a day with water, or as directed by the Physician.

How Supplied: A box containing 10 blister packs each of 10 capsules.

Uses: Inflammation, stiff joints, abdominal pain, gall bladder pain, headache, chest pain due to colds and congestion an dphelegm, low back pain, lumbago, sciatica, mirgraine, fever, dry cough, neuralgia etc. Nuflam is a deep acting analesic, antipyretic, anti inflammatory and anti spasmodic and answer to the thousand pricks of pain.

Pharmacological Action: Maharasanadi quath: The drug of choice in acute cases of rheumatism. Safest remedy in all pains acute or stubborn. Pathiadi quath: Digestive. Antispasmodic. Effective in headache, migraine, antipyretic. Can be prescribed safely during pregnancy in lieu of quinine.

Shulgajkesri ras: Anti-spasmodic. Useful in abdominal colic. Shulvarjini ras:
Antispasmodic. Effective in abodiminal colic and renal colic. Shringa bhasma : useful also in asthma cough bronchial affections, influenza, pyonhoea, rickets, Powerful anti-spasmodic and anti-pyretic effects. Even in T.B., Plurecy, controls fever, cough, and strengthens lungs and bronchii. Checks excessive secretion. Clears phlegm, and phlegmatic conditions, from the system. Abhrak bhasma: anti-inflammatory, anti-spasmodic. Strengthens nerves and treats neuralgia and chronic cough. Ras sindur: Reliable drug in painful conditions, and spasmodic affections. A cardiotonic, also useful in abdominal & renal colic and postntal pains. Bang bhasma: Weakness in urinogenital system, relaxes spasm, calms diwn pain in prostate and remvoes inflammation. Shankh bhasma: in abdominal colic, and diarrhoea due to bad digestion and gases. Godanti bhasma: antipyretic, analgesic, relieves dry cough, low fever, headache, high fever, low back ache, in females due to menstrual problems. Has good effect in burning sensation of the body, excessive thirst, aches, high BP, insomnia, stress.

***Product Name*: OBELIN CAPSULE**

Composition: Each capsule contains:

Guggul (Purifie)	200 mg.
Triphala	60 mg.
Chitrak	30 mg.
Vavding	30 mg.
Sindhav	30 mg.
Loha bhasma	40 mg.

Trikatu	30 mg.
Nagarmoth	30 mg.
Salt	30 mg.
Kadu	20 mg.
Excipients	Q.S.

Dosage: 1 to 2 capsules, 2 or 3 times a day, or as directed by the Physician.

How Supplied: A box containing 10 blister packs each of 10 capsules.

Uses: Obesity, abnormal deposition of fats, corrects assimilation and elimination process, treats "Vaat prakriti", increases energy output, and burns fat deposition. Assures normal activity, normal life and normal fat deposition. Useful in Obesity due to heredity, long sickness, menstrual irregularities like amenorrhoea, and in endothermic constitutions gives Exothermic effect.

Pharmacological Action: Guggul: Its anti-obesity action due to thyroid stimulating activity of its keto-steroids had disinfectant and blood purifying properties. Triphala: Is an age old remedy for G.I. system, with its unique astringent action on intestine; constricts the veilli tissues causing reduced absorption of fat. Chitrak: an appetiser and gastric stimulant. Alterative, given in flatulence and rheumatism. Vavding: Anthelmintic, removes obstruction by worms. Carminative, laxative, stimulant, useful in flatulence and dyspepsia. Loha bhasma: haematinic, nutritive, tonic invigorates vital orgns, corrects debility, caused by dietic restrictions. Stimulates metabolic activities and relieves lassitude. Nagarmoth: Liver-corrective, bowel-regular, relieves heat and thirst, and has fast dissolving properties.

***Product Name*: PLUM SYRUP**

Composition: Each 5 ml. contains:

Til oil	0.0018 ml.
And 5 ml. of extract obtained	
From 6 mg. combined powders of:	
Tribulus terrestris	8.33%
Capparis spinosa	8.33%
Phyllanthus emblica	8.33%
Cassia occidentalis	8.33%
Elettaria cardamomum	8.33%
Tamarix gallica	8.33%
Boerhaavia diffusa	8.33%

Tinospora cordifolia	8.33%
Piper longum	8.33%
Cichorium intybus	8.33%
Terminalia chebula	8.33%
Achillea millefolium	8.33%
Flavoured syrup base	Q.S.

Dosage: Neonates: 4 to 10 drops, 3 to 4 times a day. Infants: 1 to 2 teaspoonfuls, 3 to 4 times a day. Children: 2 to 3 teaspoonfuls, 3 to 4 times a day. Or as directed by the Physician.

How Supplied: In glass bottle of 120 ml.

Uses: All the above ingredients are primarily digestives, carminateves, Astringents, Mild sedatives, Aromatics, Soothing in action, Antiflatulants, Nutrients, alternatives, Mild laxatives, Diuretics, antiperiodics, and help to remove gases, spasms, useful in oedema, liver disorders, loose diarrhoea, and allied giestive ailments, common to the infants and children, at the growing stage. Safe and do not have addiction or side effects, and free from alcohol, and Narcotics.

***Product Name*: Regulet Capsule**

Composition: Each capsule contains:

Gajar seed (Daucus carota)	300 mg.
Ruphanus sativas	50 mg.
Aloes indica	20 mg.
Carica papaya	30 mg.
Hingu (Ferula foetida)	30 mg.
Suddha saubhagya	25 mg.
Trikatu	25 mg.
Excipients	Q.S.

Dosage: 2 capsules 3 times a day, for 2 or 3 days, to be followed with 2 capsules twice a day, for 3 days, or as directed by the Physician.

How Supplied: A box containing one blister pack of 10 capsules.

Uses: Amenorrhoea, oligomenorrhoea, dysmenorrhoea, and menorrhagia.

Pharmacological Action: Gajar seed: Helpful in abortion. Clinical trials showed 7 days course. Possesses antioestrogenic and antiprogesteronic activity. Clears the uterus and regulates the menstrual cycle. It is contra-indicated during pregnancy. Ruphanus sativas: diuretic, laxative, lithontriptic, having emmenagogua properties. Regulates menstrual cycle. Aloes indica: Diuretic, mild laxative, and an emmenagogue. Tones liver functions and regulates menstrual cycle. Carica papaya: Powerful emmenagogue, Helps also as a digestant specially of proteins. Hingu: Exerts emmenagogue action. Anti spasmodic, mild diuretic and laxative, and digestant. Suddha saubhagya: Is known for its diuretic action. Anthelmintic and emmenagogue. Trikatu: Improves digestion. Liver stimultant. This drug should be avoided during pregnancy.

***Product Name*: Trim up Capsule**

Composition: Each capsule contains:

Ashoka	130 mg.
Dashmul	40 mg.
Lodhra	40 mg.
Ashwagandha	30 mg.
Shatavary	30 mg.
Hirakasis	10 mg.
Nagpushpa	20 mg.
Bala	20 mg.
Guduchi	20 mg.
Bhrungraj Ext.	20 mg.
Excipients	Q.S.

Dosage: One capsule two to three times a day or as directed by the Physician.

How Supplied: A box containing 10 Blister packs each of 10 capsules.

Uses: A safe non hormonal remedy to correct all the gynaecologic disorders. The drug enhances the internal secretion of hormones and normalises the body function.

***Product Name*: TRIM UP SYRUP**

Composition: Each 5 ml. contains:

0.5 ml. of extract obtained from combined powders of	800 mg.
Ashoka	46%
Nagrmoth	2%
Dashmul	10%
Sunth	2%

Lodhra	7%
Manjishtha	2%
Ashwagandha	4%
Lavang	1%
shatavary	4%
Nagkeshar	1%
Hirakasis	1%
Nishoth	1%
Jatamansi	2%
Pippali	1%
Amala	2%
Twak	1%
Baheda	2%
Daru harida	1%
Bhrungraj	2%
Chiraita	0.4%
Harde	2%
Guduchi	0.4%
Chandan	2%
Rasna	0.4%
Jeera	2%
Vacha	0.4%
Vidanga	0.4%
Flavoured syrup base	Q.S.

Dosage: One to two teaspoonfuls two to three times a day or as directed by the physician.

How Supplied: A glass bottle of 200 ml.

Uses: Trim up syrup offers lasting comfort and checks of dysmenorrhoea. Trim up syrup is indicated in premenstrual tension, dysmenorrhoea, irregular menstrual cycle, oligomenorrhoea, menorrhagia, pelvic inflammation, habitual abortions, general debility, leucorrhoea.

***Product Name*: TULCOF CAPSULE**

Composition: Each capsule contains:

Tulsi Ext. (Ocimum sanctum)	50 mg.
Yashtimadhu Ext. (Glycyrrhiza glabra ext.)	50 mg.
Vasaka (Adhatoda vasika ext.)	50 mg.
Sudarshan ghan	35 mg.
Sitopaladi churna	60 mg.
Sunth (Zingiber officinale)	25 mg.

Khurasani ajawayan(Hyoscyamus niger)	20 mg.
Pippali (Pipper longum)	50 mg.
Rasna (Vanda roxburghii)	10 mg.
Excipients	Q.S.

Dosage: Children: One capsule 2 to 3 times a day. Adults: Two capsules 2 to 3 times a day or as per the direction of the Physician.

How Supplied: A box containing 10 blister packs each of 10 capsules.

Uses: Tulcof prevents the frequent asthmatic attacks because of the anti-spasmodic effect and allows better breathing. Tulcof reduces inflammation, soothes sore throat, provides round the clock anti-cough effect to patients. The drug is safe for hypertensive, cardiac, diabetic patients and even for children.

***Product Name*: TULCOF SYRUP**

Composition: Each 10 ml. fluid contains:

Glycyrrhiza glabra ext. (Yashtimadhu)	20 mg.
ocimum sanstum ext. (Tulsi)	10 mg.
Adhatoda vasika ext. (Vasaka)	10 mg.
Oil of eucalyptus globulus (Nilgiri Oil)	0.007 ml.
Piperminta sat (Menthol)	5 mg.
Navsagar	200 mg.
Flavoured syrup base	Q.S.

Dosage: Infants & Children: ½ to 1 teasponful of Tulcof, 3 to 4 times a day. Adults: 1 to 2 teaspoonfuls 3 to 4 times a day, or as directed by the Physician.

How Supplied: In pilfer-proof glass bottle of 100 ml.

Uses: Cough, cold, congestion, acute and chronic bronchitis, allergic coughs, laryngitis, pharyngitis, and as a chief adjuvant in dealing with pulmonary affections. Reduces mucosal inflammation, relieves chest congestion, pyrexia, and body aches. Checks out excessive mucous secretion, as a digestive, decongestant & Diuretic.

Pharmacological Action: Glycyrrhiza glabra ext.: Demulcent, soothing, anti-inflammatory, soothes irritated throat and hoarsensess of voice, anti spasmodic and expectorant and helps to expel sputum. Ocimum sanctum ext.: The drug of repute, for bronchial affections. Tulsi is useful in acute and chronic coughs, and catarrhal conditions. Adhatoda visika ext.: Well establised expectorant, antiasthmatic, antispasmodic, and very useful in chest affections and bronchitis. Oil of eucalyptus globulus: Reduces glandular swellings, soothens sore throat, congestion, inflammation in throat, chest and pulmonary region. Piperminta sat: soothes irritated throat and bronchial muscosa. navsagar: A known diuretic, having anti-cough and mucolytic properties.

***Product Name*: Zymoliv Syrup**

Composition: Each 10 ml. contains:

Kulanjan	100 mg.
Ashwagandha	100 mg.
Bhringraj	100 mg.
Nagar	100 mg.
Chitraka	100 mg.
Ajmoda	100 mg.
Mandukparni	100 mg.
Pippali	60 mg.
Anartwak	60 mg.
Elaychi	60 mg.
Twakpatram	60 mg.
Nagpushpa	60 mg.
Flavoured syrupy base	Q.S.

Dosage: Children: ½ to 1 teaspoonful twice a day after meals. Adults: 1 to 2 teaspoonfuls twice or thrice a day, as convenient, or as directed by the physician.

How Supplied: Pilfer-proof glass bottle of 170 ml.

Uses: Zymoliv syrup is a wholesome digestive tonic. Useful in anorexia, indigestion, food allergy, G.I. spasma, bloating, flatulence, heartburn, hyper-acidity, irregular bowel movements, abdominal distension and carbohydrate indigestion.

Pharmacological Action: Kulanjan: Stimulant, aromatic, bitter and possesses carminative activity. Useful in dyspepsia. Ashwagandha: An ideal neuro-dynamic, which helps digestion, converting food into energy, as it is a tonic and alterative. Bhringraj: treats dearrangement of liver and gall bladder. Chitrak: Increases digestive power and promotes appetite. Nagar: Carminative, stimulatant gastro-intestinal tract towards proper functions. Ajmodea: Bitter & pungent. Stimulant. Tones the G.I. system. Mandukarni: appetite stimules, tonic, digestive, nervine tonic, and has tranquillizing action. Pippali: Stimulant, carminative, laxative, alterative. Anartwak: Bitter, tonic, antibilious, stomachic and astringent. Useful in billious dyspepsia, and functional inactivity of liver. Twakpatram: Carminative, anti-spasmodic, aromatic. It is a vascular and nervine stimulant. Nagpushpa: Mild laxative, removes inflammation in the intestines, improves peristaltic movement.

T.T.K. Pharma Ltd.
(Indian Medicine Division)
91, Santhome High Road
Chennai--600028
Tel.: 4937458, 4938057, 4938205

***Product Name*: COFREM LIQUID**

Composition: Each 5 ml. contains:

Adhatoda vasica	100 mg.
Ocimum sanctum	100 mg.
Berberis aristata	2 mg.
Curcuma longa	35 mg.
Glycyrrhiza glabra	35 mg.
Terminalia belerica	50 mg.

***Product Name*: ELCARIM DROPS**

Composition

Total water soluble extracts derived from

Phyllanthus emblica	90 mg.
Zingiber officinale	4 mg.
Embelia ribes	8 mg.
Acorus calamus	3 mg.
Terminalia chebula	4 mg.

***Product Name*: ELCARIM ELIXIR**

Composition: Each 5 ml. contains:

Total water soluble extracts derived from

Phyllathus emblica	160 mg.
Zingiber officinale	75 mg.
Embelia ribes	15 mg.
Acorus calamus	5 mg.
Terminalia chebula	80 mg.

***Product Name*: LACTARE CAPSULES**

Composition

Asparagus racemosus	200 mg.
Withania somnifera	100 mg.
Glycyrrhiza glabra	50 mg.
Trigonella foenumgraceum	50 mg.
Allium sativum	20 mg.

***Product Name*: MUSTONG TABLETS**

Composition

Mucuna pruriens	155 mg.
Withania somnifera	100 mg.
Glycyrrhiza glabra	25 mg.
Myristica fragrans	15 mg.
Tribulus terrestris	25 mg.
Tinospora cordifolia	30 mg.

Tulison Pharma
118-H, East Moti Bagh, Sarai Rohilla
Delhi-110007
Tel.: 3545190, 7773086

***Product Name*: KAS MADHU**

Composition: Each 5 ml. teaspoon contains:

Yashti Madhu	50 mg.
Gul banafsha	50 mg.
Kaiphal	50 mg.
Nagar motha	50 mg.
Vasaka	50 mg.
Jupha	50 mg.
Karka singi	50 mg.
Pan-ke-patte	50 mg.
Unnab	50 mg.
Pipal	25 mg.
Sat loban	25 mg.
Karpoor	2.25 mg.
Sat podina	2.25 mg.
Sugar	q.s.

Dosage: Adult: 2 teaspoonful every after 4 hrs a day with equal warm water. Children: ½-1 teaspoonful thrice a day with equal warm water. Infants: ¼ teaspoonful thrice a day with equal warm water.

Product Name: SWARNA VATI

Composition

Makardhuwaj	25 mg.
Karpoor	10 mg.
Shatawari churna	125 mg.
Maju churna	50 mg.
Garuchi satwa	20 mg.
Shilajit purified	25 mg.
Kapilu purified	25 mg.

Dosage: 2 tablets twice a day with warm milk.

Product Name: Bal Rashak Sudha

Composition

Vanshpatri	50 g.
Nagar motha	50 g.
Vai varing	50 g.
Soya	50 g.
Sauhf	50 g.
Phool gulab	50 g.
Chhoti ilaichi	25 mg.
Kheel suhaga pudina	25 mg.
Kesar	0.5 mg.

Dosage: Infants from one month to 3 montsh ¼ to ½ teaspoon ful, From 3 months to 2 years or above 1 to 2 spoon ful twice or thrice a day.

Product Name: PATHANI GHUTTI

Composition

Phool gulab	50 gms.
Saunf	50 gms.
Nagar motha	50 gms.
Amaltas-ka-guda	50 gms.
Vai varing	50 gms.
Sanai	50 gms.
Chhoti harar	50 gms.
Bari harar	50 gms.
Maror phali	25 mg.
modkii	25 mg.
Kakra Singhi	25 mg.

Ajwain	20 mg.
Kala namak	10 mg.
Kheel suhaga	10 mg.

Dosage: Babies: From 1month to 3 months ¼ to ½ teaspoon. From 3 months to 2 years 1 to 2 spoon with warm water twice or thrice a day.

***Product Name*: KAMINI SUDHA**

Composition

Ashoka	10%
Dhai-ke-Phool	2%
Dashmool	2%
Maju	0.2%
Majistha Iodhra	0.2%
Nagkesar	0.2%
Kala jeera	0.2%
Chhoti ilaichi	0.2%
Sonth	0.2%
Shiv lingi	0.2%
Amla	0.2%
Chandan safed	0.2%
Shatawar	0.2%
Sugar	q.s.

Dosage: Two teaspoon full with equal water morning & evening after meals.

***Product Name*: KESH JEEVAN TEL**

Composition

Bhangra	10%
Amla	10%
Brahmi	10%
Chhilka bari ilaichi	2%
Talis patra	2%
Jatamasi	2%
Nagar motha	2%
Khas	2%
Tagar	2%
Kapoor kachri	2%
Burada safed sandal	1%
Kapoor 1%	
Mehendi ki patte	1%
Til tel	50%
Tel Paniri	1%

Product Name: TULISON COMPOUND SYRUP

Composition

Beej band	125 mg.
Moosli safed	125 mg.
Arjun	125 mg.
Shatavar	75 mg.
Behman safed	75 mg.
Salem Misri	175 mg.
Sheetal chini	175 mg.
Gokhru	92 mg.
Ilaichi chhoti	120 mg.
Shankh pushpi	100 mg.
Dalchini	82 mg.
Chandan safed	25 mg.
Brahmi konch-ke-beej	150 mg.
Ashwagandha	95 mg.
Pipla mool	95 mg.
Tal makhana	100 mg.
Kesar	30 mg.
Sugar	q.s.

Product Name: RAKTABH

Composition

Chirata	130 mg.
Gul banafsha	130 mg.
Usba	130 mg.
Sanai	110 mg.
Nilofer	110 mg.
Sandal surkh	90 mg.
Gilo	84 mg.
Mundi	144 mg.
Tulsi	80 mg.
Manjeesth	70 mg.
Saunf	70 mg.
Unnab	95 mg.
Hasura	112 mg.
Sugar	q.s.

Dosage: 1 or 2 teaspoonful twice or thrice a day with equal water.

Product Name: FLU TAB

Composition

Tribhuvan kirti rasa	50 mg.
Lakshmi vilas (Nardiya)	50 mg.
Shring bhasma	50 gm.
Garuchi satva	50 gm.
Harital bhasma (Godanti)	50 gm.
Sudarshan churna (Prepared in the decoction)	50 gm.

Dosage: Two tabs twice or thrice a day with warm water.

Universal Medicanments Pvt. Ltd.
P.O. Box No. 308, 545, Shantinagar
Nagpur440 002
Tel. : 768512, 764597, 762589, 765128
Fax: 0712) 763212

Product Name: KARNIM CAPSULES

Composition

Momordica charantia (Karela)	150 mg.
Azadirachata indica (Neem)	75 mg.
Ociumum sanctum (Tulsi)	75 mg.
Picrorhiza Kurroa (Kutki)	35 mg.
Zingiber officinale (Sounth)	30 mg.
Pure commpiphora mukul (Shudha Guggul)	35 mg.

Dosage: One capsule two times a day for freshly diagnosed non-complicated diabetes. One capsule three times a day for the cases of other oral hypoglycemic failure & insulin resistance.

How Supplied: Pack of 100 capsules.

Uses: Karnim is indicated for patients with maturity onset diabetes mellitus. It is especially useful in cases of insulin resistance & oral antidiabetic failure. It can be used singly or in combination with other oral antidiabetic drugs for smoother control of diabetes. Karnim is also useful for obese diabetic in whom sulfonyl ureas are contraindicated.

Pharmacological Action: Karnim acts on different sites in different ways to effectively control factors and pathways leading to diabetes mellitus.

1. Karela-Normilizes the deficiency of insulin.

2. Neem & Sounth-Stimulated beta cells of pancreas to secrete insulin.
3. Tulsi-Reduces peripheral resistance to insulin.
4. South & Guggul-Prevents narrowing of vessels by lowering systemic levels of cholesterol and free fatty acids.
5. Guggul & Neem-Normalizes the body immune system. Karnim has no toxic effects.

***Product Name*: VALILIV TABLETS**

Composition

Kabar (Capparis spinosa)	65 mg.
Kasni (Cichorium intybus)	65 mg.
Makoy (Solanum nigrum)	32 mg.
Kasondi (Cassia occdentails)	16 mg.
Arjun chhal (Terminalia arjuna)	32 mg.
Gandhana (Achillea millifolium)	16 mg.
Tamarix gallica	16 mg.
Mandur bhasma	33 mg.

Dosage: Adults: 2-3 tablets thrice daily. Children: 1-2 tablets thirce daily.

How Supplied: 100 x 1000 tablets.

Uses: infectious/Viral Hepatitis, Post hepatitis, syndrome, Obstructive jaundice, Cirrhosis, Aalcoholic & drug induced/liver damage, and other disturbances of liver cell functions.

Pharmacological Action: Valiv is a combination of heptoprotective and tonic substances. They are known to enhance regeneration of liver cells promoting early recovery. These protect the liver cells from damaging agents like alcohol, drug & chemicals and revert the damage already occurred and stimulate hepatic function. Some of these substances, are known to be cholegogues, improving bile secretion & consequently relieving intrahepatic obstruction lessening the severity of jaundice.

***Product Name*: U-GYANESTONE SYRUP**

Composition: Each 5 ml. contains:

Ashok Chhal	200 mg.
Ashwagandha	50 mg.
Rakt chandan	15 mg.

Munnakka	50 mg.
Lodhra	20 mg.
Shatawari	40 mg.
Musli	20 mg.
Harde	20 mg.
Bheda	20 mg.
Amla	20 mg.
Nishottar	10 mg.
Anantmool	10 mg.
Pippali	10 mg.
Aam ki guthali	10 mg.
Bad chhal	10 mg.
Mochras	10 mg.
Sunthi	20 mg.
Nilkamal	20 mg.
Milethi	20 mg.
Haldi	20 mg.
Chitrakmool	20 mg.
Jeera safed	10 mg.
Rasna	5 mg.
Daruhaldi	50 mg.
Vasaka	5 mg.
Netrabala	5 mg.
Gambhari	5 mg.
Padmakh	5 mg.
Pathamool	5 mg.
Chirayata	5 mg.
Vavding	5 mg.
Khairchhal	5 mg.
Vach	5 mg.
Jamunbeej	40 mg.
Vidari kend	30 mg.
Kababchini	10 mg.
Ushir	10 mg.
Dalcchini	10 mg.
Nagkesar	10 mg.
Safed chandan	20 mg.
Kamal	20 mg.
Nagarmotha	20 mg.
Kali mirch	20 mg.
Lavang	5 mg.
Jatamansi	5 mg.
Shudh Harakasis	10 mg.
Syrup Base	Q.S.

Dosage: Therapeutic use: 2 Teaspoonful t.i.d. in all cases.

Prophylactic use: 1 teaspoonful t.i.d.

Uses: Therapeutic: For secondary Amenorrhoea, Dysmenrrhoea, metrorrhagia, menorrhagia, Non specific and puerperal leukorrhoea & Anovulation, Post I.U.C.D., Bleeding. Prophylactic: Adjuvant to psychotropic medication, stress induced disorders like irritability, fatigue, hypertension, G.I.T. disturbances etc.

Pharmacological Action: Its gynaec, endocrinological related corrective actions may possibly be through Adaptogenic, Anitstress, Immunostimulant and Hepatoprotective properties of the ingredients of U-Gyanestone. These activities are further supported by Antiinflammatory, Antispasmodic, Hemostatic and hematinic properties for quick relief. Moreover U-Gyanestone has carminative property to relieve the associated symptoms. U-Gyanestone has no adverse effects.

***Product Name*: UNICOUGH SYRUP**

Composition: Each 5 ml. Syrup contains:

Khair chhal (Acacia catechu wild)	150 mg.
Vach (Acorus calamus linn.)	15 mg.
Elaichi (Elettaria cardamomum maton)	15 mg.
Dalchini (Cinnamomum zeylenicum)	5 mg.
Nagkeshar (mesua ferrea)	15 mg.
Sonth (Zingiber officinale)	25 mg.
Pippli (Piper longum)	20 mg.
Kabab chini (Piper cubeba)	10 mg.
Talisapatra (Abies weebbiana)	60 mg.
Vasaka patra (Adhatoda vasica)	150 mg.
Mulethi (Glycyrrhiza glabra)	100 mg.
Somlata (Ephedra geradianan wall)	100 mg.
Dhatura panchag (Dhatura metel)	2.5 mg.
Tulsi (Ociumum sanctum)	60 mg.
Ajwan sat (Thymo)	1 mg.
Pudina sat (Menthol)	1 mg.
Syrup base q.s.	
Colur Caramel	

Dosage: Adults: 1-2 teaspoonful 2-3 times daily. Children: ½ to 1 teaspoonful 2-3 times daily.

How Supplied: Bottle of 100 ml.

Uses: Bronchitis, Asthma

***Product Name*: MORALAC CAPSULES**

Composition

Allium sativum (Lasun)	50 mg.
Puraeria tuberosa (Vidharikand)	250 mg.
Trigonella foemumgraecum (Methi)	100 mg.
Withania somnifera (Ashwagandha)	100 mg.
Euphoribia hirta (Dhudi)	50 mg.
Leptadinia reticulata (Jivanti)	150 mg.
Spirulina	100 mg.

Dosage: Two capsules 3 times a day or as directed by the physician.

How Supplied: 1 bottle of 100 capsules.

Uses: In all cases of diminished milk secretion & ejection due to nutritional/psychological and/or emotional factors.

Pharmacological Action: Action of morolac is overcoming the oligogalactia is multifold. Ingredients of Morolac have prolactin increasing effects, oxytocin, tranquilizers nutritional, appetite stimulating actions. No toxic effects have been reported.

Vasu Pharmaceuticals Pvt. ltd.
967/4, GIDC Makarpura
Vadodara-390010
Tel.: 644459, 645772
Fax: (0265) 644171

***Product Name*: ALERTI CAPSULE**

Composition: Each 300 mg. capsule contains:

Celastrus paniculata (Jyotishmati Oil)	75%
Cow Ghee	21%
Shuddha Amalsari Gandhak	4%

Made siddhi with Acorus calamus,
Convolculus pluricauis (Shankh Puship)
Nardostachys Jatamanshi, Eclipta alba (Bringraj)

Dosage: Children—one capsule/day, with milk. Adults—one to two capsuels/day with milk or as directed by the physician.

How Supplied: Blister Pack of 10 x 10 capsules.

Uses: Stress and strain, anxiety, tension, insomnia, brain fag, loss of memory, improvement of learning process.

***Product Name*: BONTON CAPSULES**

Composition: Each 500 mg capsule contains:

Abha guggal	125 mg.
laxadhi guggal	125 mg.
Madhu Malini Vasant	100 mg.
Kishor guggal	50 mg.
Kakudantwak bahsma	50 mg.
praval bahsma	50 mg.
Pushpa Dhanva Ras	10 mg.

Dosage: One to two capsules/day with milk or as directed by the physician.

How Supplied: Blister Pack of 10 x 10 capsules.

Economy Pack of 250 capsules.

Uses: Fracture Healing, osteoporosis, osteomalacia, Girdle Pain, Inflammation of joints.

Product Name: CASPA DROPS

Composition

Peucedanum graveolens (Suva, Dill)	100 mg.
Embelia ribes (Vidanga)	30 mg.
Trijat (Twak, Tamalpatra, Elayachi)	30 mg.
Apium graveolens (Ajmoda)	30 mg.
Sanchal (Blacksalt)	20 mg.
Ferula assafoetida (Hingu)	15 mg.
Sindhalun (Rock salt)	15 mg.
Citrus acida (Lemon)	10 mg.
Flavoured Syrup base	Q.S.

Dosage: Infants below six months: 5 to 10 drops, 15 minutes before feed, 3 to 4 times a day. Six months to twenty four months: 10 to 20 drops, 15 minutes before feed, 3 to 4 times a day.

How Supplied: A glass bottle of 30 ml. with dropper.

Uses: Colicky pain, Flatulence, Abdominal distention, G.I. Spasm.

***Product Name*: DAZZLE CAPSULE**

Composition: Each 350 mg. capsule contains:

Boswellia serrata (Sallaki) Ext.	200 mg.

Vitex negundo (Nirgundi) Ext.	100 mg.
Withania somnifera (Ashvagandha) Ext.	25 mg.
Maharasnadi Ghan	25 mg.

Dosage: One Capsule 2-3 days or as directed by the Physician.

How Supplied: Blister Pack of 10 x 10 capsules Economy pack of 250 capsules.

Uses: Rheumatoid arthritis, Spondylitis, Gouty Arthritis Sprains.

***Product Name*:** **MERYTON SYRUP**

Composition: Each 10 ml. contains:

Saraca indica (Ashoka)	400 mg.
Symplocos racemosa (Lodhra)	400 mg.
Withania somnifera (Ashvagandha)	150 mg.
Asparagus racemosus (Shatavari)	100 mg.
Glycyrrhiza glabra (Yashtimadhu)	100 mg.
Sida cordifolia (Bala)	50 mg.
Tinospora cordifolia (Guduchi)	50 mg.
Mesua ferrea (Nagpushpa)	50 mg.
Hemidesmus indicus (Sariva)	50 mg.
Berberis aristata (Daruharidra)	50 mg.
Dashmool	50 mg.
Valeriana wallichi (Tagar)	50 mg.
Nardostachys Jatamansi (Tatamansi)	50 mg.
Leptadenia reticulata (Jivanti)	50 mg.
Flavoured syrup base	Q.S.

Dosage: Two to three teaspoonfuls three times a day after meals with milk or as directed by physician.

How Supplied: Pilfer proof glass bottle of 190 ml.

Uses: Menstrual disorder, menorrhagia,Leucorrhoea, Amenorhoea, Metrorhagia, General debility, Oligomenorrhoea, Low back pain.

***Product Name*:** **PLUGIT CAPSULE**

Composition: Each 500 mg capsule contains:

Maharasanadi Quath	100 mg.
Pathyadi Quath	100 mg.

Shulgaikeshri Ras	75 mg.
Shulvarjini Ras	75 mg.
Shrung Bhasma	75 mg.
Abharak Bhasma	15 mg.
Ras sindur	15 mg.
Bang Bhasma	15 mg.
Shankh Bhasma	15 mg.
Godanti Bhasma	15 mg.

Dosage: Two to three capsules a day or as directed by the physician.

How Supplied: Available in blister Pack of 10 x 10 capsules Economy pack of 250's capsules.

Uses: Influenza, Headache, Neuralgia, Low back pain, Sciatica, Myalgbia, Lumbago, Inflammation, Dysmenorrhoea, Abdominal colic, Toothache, Pyrexia.

***Product Name*: SPARK CAPSULE**

Composition: Each 500 mg. capsule contains:

Makardhwaj	15 mg.
Ras sindur	15 mg.
Abhrak Bhasma	30 mg.
Praval Bhasma	30 mg.
Loha Bhasma	30 mg.
Bang Bhasma	30 mg.
Shilajita	30 mg.
Amrutasatva	30 mg.
Withania somnifera (Ashwagandha) Ext.	20 mg.
Mucuna pruriens (Kavcha) ext.	30 mg.
Asparagus racemosus (Satavari) ext.	20 mg.
Glycerrhiza glabra (Yashtimadhu) ext.	30 mg.
Ashtavarga	60 mg.
Trifla	60 mg.
Asparagus adscendens (Musli)	Q.S.

Dosage: Two or three capsules a day with milk or as directed by the physician.

How Supplied: Blister Pack of 10 x 10 capsules. Economy pack of 250 capsules.

Uses: Oligospermia, premature aging, Loss of libido, General debility, premature ejeculation.

Product Name: WRANGER SYRUP

Composition: Each 10 ml. contains:

Asparagus racemosus (shatavari) Ext.	50 mg.
Eclipta alba (Bhrungraj) Ext.	25 mg.
Mucuma Pruriens (Kavcha Beej) Ext.	25 mg.
Withania somnifera (Ashwagandha) Ext.	200 mg.
Tinospora cordifolia (Rasayani)	100 mg.
Tribulus terrestris (Gokshurak)	100 mg.
Dioscorea bulbifera (Varahikand)	75 mg.
Ipomoea digitata (Vidarikand)	50 mg.
Hygrophila spinosa (Talamkhana)	25 mg.
Sida cordifolia (Beej Band)	25 mg.
Belphari sedulispers (Utongan)	25 mg.
Alpinia galanga (Kulanjan)	25 mg.
Trikatu	25 mg.
Bombax malabaricum (semal Musali)	20 mg.
Myristica fragrans (Jatifal)	10 mg.
Chaturjat	10 mg.
Hibiscus abelomsshus (Kasturidana)	10 mg.
Flavoured syrup Base	Q.S.

Dosage: 2-3 teaspoonfuls per day with milk or as directed by physician.

How Supplied: Plifer proof glass bottle of 200 ml.

Uses: General debility, Muscular weakness, loss of memory, Anaemia, Loss of body weight.

Product Name: ZEAL SYRUP

Composition: Each 10 ml. contains:

Ocimum santum (Tulsi)	200 mg.
Adhatoda vasika (Vasaka)	200 mg.
Glycyrrhize glabra (Yashtimadhu)	200 mg.
Ephedra vulgaris (Somvally)	100 mg.
Solanum xanthocarpum (Kantkari)	100 mg.
Rhus Kakrasingi (Karkatashrungi)	100 mg.
Inula racemosa (Pushker mool)	100 mg.
Trikatu	50 mg.
Hyoscymus raticulatus	10 mg.
Sat Piparmint	6 mg.

Nilgiri Oil	0.006 mg.
Navsagar	200 mg.
Flavoured Syrup base	Q.S.

Dosage: 1 to 2 teaspoonful 3 times a day. Children: 1 teaspoonful (5ml) 3 times a day. Infants: 5 to 10 drops three times a day or as directed by the physician.

How Supplied: Plifer proof glass bottle of 100 ml.

Uses: Productive cough, Non productive cough, Asthmatic cough, Spasmodic cough, Bronchitis, Respiratory infection.

***Product Name*: TRICHUP OIL**

Composition

Sesamum indicum (Til) Oil	80%
Cocos nucifera (Tranaraj) Oil	20%
Made siddhi with:	
Eclipta alba (Bhrunguraj)	1%
Emblica officinalis (Vrushya)	1%
Indigofera tinctora (Nilpushpa)	1%
Centella asiaticas (Mandokparni)	1%
Cyperus rotundus (Nagarmotha)	1%
Jasminum officinale (Jatichetika)	1%
Abrus precatorius (Gunja)	1%
Glycyrrhiza glabra (Yashtimadhu)	0.5%
Crateeva murvala (Varunbark)	0.5%
Pongamina pinnata (Karanj beej)	0.5%
solanum indicum (Bruhati Laxmana)	0.5%
Citrulus colocuthis (Indravaruni)	0.5%
Dhatura	2.5%

Dosage: Wash the hair thoroughly, dry it and apply the oil and massage gently for a minute or two so as to reach the skin deeply. Same may be repeated during night hours, for better and faster effects. Simultaneously, Trichup capsules may be taken two to three capsules a day with cold milk after meals for three to four months.

How Supplied: Pilfer proof glass bottle of 120 ml.

Uses: Falling and premature greying of hair, Dandruff, Alopecia, Mild infections of the scalp.

***Product Name*: BLUMIN SYRUP**

Composition: Each 10 ml. contains:

Sida cordifolia (Bala)	140 mg.
Argyria speciosa (Vruddhadruka)	140 mg.
Foeniculum vulgaris (Mishreya)	100 mg.
Holarrhena antidysentrica (Indrajav)	100 mg.
Acorus cocculus cordifolius (Guduchi)	100 mg.
Calamus (Vacha)	80 mg.
Trikatu	80 mg.
Zizyphus valgaris (Saubir)	80 mg.
Apium graveolens (Aimoda)	80 mg.
Ashtavarga	80 mg.
Gardenia lucida (janntuka)	80 mg.
Hydrocotyle asiatica (Mandookparni)	80 mg.
Convolvulus mycrophyllus (Shankhpushpi)	60 mg.
Terminalia chebula (Haritaki)	50 mg.
Rhus suecedanea (Karkatshrungi)	40 mg.
Aconitum hetrophylum (Ativisha)	20 mg.
Myristica flower (Jatipatri)	20 mg.
Phyllanthus emblica (Vrushya)	20 mg.
Elettaria cordamomum (Elayachi)	20 mg.
Flavoured syrup base	Q.S.

Dosage: Infant–½Teaspoonful 2-3 times a day. Children–1-2 Teaspoonfuls 3 times a day or as directed by physician.

How Supplied: Pilfer proof glass bottle or 100 ml.

Uses: Abdominal pain, Indigestion, Retarded mental & physical growth, Debility of poliomyletis.

***Product Name*: CUTIS CAPSULE**

Composition: Each 500 mg. capsule contains:

Gandhak rasayan	100 mg.
Azadirachta indica (Neem) Ext.	70 mg.
Rubia cordifolia (Manjista) Ext.	70 mg.
Mimosa Pudica (Lajalu) Ext.	70 mg.
Cassia tora (Chakramarda seeds) Ext.	50 mg.
Psoralea corylifolia (Bawachi seeds) Ext.	50 mg.
Argemone mexican (Darudi panchang) Ext.	50 mg.
Berberis aristata (Rasanjan)	40 mg.

Dosage: 1 capsule two to three times a day preferably with milk after meals or as directly by the physician.

How Supplied: Available in blister pack of 10 x 10 capsules. Economy pack of 250 capsules.

Uses: Atopic and sebhorric skin disorder, Allergic dermatitis, Boils, Caruncles, Eczema, Icthyosis, Psoriasis, Pruritus, Urticaria, Pyoderma.

***Product Name*:** **DIGIT CAPSULE**

Composition: Each 300 mg. capsule contains:

Celastrus paniculata (Jyotishmati) Oil	90.0%
Alium satium (Garlic) Oil	00.20%
Ricinus communis (Castor) Oil	09.80%

Made siddhi with: Terminalia arjuna (Arjuna), Rauwolfia serpentina (Sarpagandha)

Dosage: Two or three capsules a day with milk or after meals or as directed by the physician.

How Supplied: Available in blister pack of 10 x 10 capsules.

Uses: Anxiety, Hypertension, Cholesterolemia, Arrhythmia, Cardiac disorder, Angina.

***Product Name*:** **MERYTON CAPSULE**

Composition: Each 500 mg. capsule contains:

Saraca india (Ashoka Ext.)	150 mg.
Symplocos racemosa (Lodhra Ext.)	150 mg.
Withania somnifera (Ashvagandha) Ext.	100 mg.
sparagus racemosus (Shatavari) Ext.	50 mg.
Tinospora cordifolia (Guduchi Ext.)	25 mg.
leptadenia reticulata (jivanti Ext.)	25 mg.

Dosage: One or two capsules per day or as directed by the physician.

How Supplied: Blister pack of 10 x 10 capsule.

Economy pack of 250 capsules.

Uses: Menstrual disordeer, Pelvic inflammation. Metrorrhagia, menorrhagia, Dysmenorhaea, General debility, Low back pain.

***Product Name*: PEP-UP SYRUP**

Composition: Each 10 ml. contains:

Alpinia galanga (Kulinjan)	100 mg.
Withania somnifera (Ashwagandha)	100 mg.
Eclipta alba (Bhrungraj)	100 mg.
Zingiber officinale (Nagar)	100 mg.
Plumbago zeylanica (Chitraka)	100 mg.
Apium graveolens (Ajmoda)	100 mg.
Hydrocotyle asiatica (Mandookaparni)	100 mg.
Piper longum (Pipli)	60 mg.
Punica granatum (Anartwak)	60 mg.
Elettaria cardamomum (Elayachi)	60 mg.
Cinnamomum zeylanicum (Tvakpatram)	60 mg.
Mesua ferrea (Nagpushpa)	60 mg.
Flavoured syrup	Q.S.

Dosage: Two teaspoonsfuls three times a day or as directed by the physician.

How Supplied: Pitfer proof glass bottle of 200 ml.

Uses: Indigestion, Dyspepsia, Flatulence, Abdominal distention, Indigestion of protein and fat, Anorexia and digestive disturbances.

***Product Name*: STEP CAPSULE**

Composition: Each 450 mg. capsule conrtains:

Vranpahari Ras	105 mg.
Gandhak Rasayan	80 mg.
Arogyavardhini	50 mg.
Chopchini	50 mg.
Godanti Bhasma	50 mg.
Suvarna Makshik Bhasma	50 mg.
Sat loban	20 mg.
Kamdudha Ras	15 mg.
Kasish Bhasma	15 mg.
Shrung Bhasma	15 mg.

Dosage: One or two capsule, two to three times a day with milk, or as directed by the physician.

How Supplied: Available in blister pack of 10 x 10 capsules. Economy pack of 250 capsules.

Uses: Acute and chronic bronchitis, Upper respiratory tract infections like tonsilitis, Pharyngitis, Pneumococcal infections, Sinusitis, Urinary tract infections, nephritis, Urethritis, Oophritis, Gastro-Intestinal tract infection, Otitis media, Sexually transmitted diseases.

***Product Name*: STEP SYRUP**

Composition: Each 10 ml. contains:

Maharasnadi quath	200 mg.
Argemone mexicana (Hemkshiri)	160 mg.
Smilaxchina (Dvipantarvacha)	160 mg.
Commiphora mukul (Guggul)	100 mg.
Sphearanthus indicus (Shravani)	80 mg.
Tinospora cordifolia (Guduchi)	70 mg.
Hermidesmus indicus (Sariva)	70 mg.
Saussurea lappa (Kushtham)	70 mg.
Glycyrrhiza glabra (Yashtimadhu)	30 mg.
Emblica officinalis (Vrushya)	50 mg.
Trikatu	50 mg.
Flavoured syrup base	Q.S.

Dosage: One teaspoonful three times a day or as directed by the physician.

How Supplied: Available in pilfer proof glass bottle of 100 ml.

Uses: Pneumonia, Other U.R.T.I., R.T.I., G.I.T.I., skin and soft tissue infections.

***Product Name*: TRICHUP CAPSULE**

Composition: Each 500 mg. capsule contains:

Eclipta alba (Bhrunguraj) Ghan	210 mg.
Hydrocotyle asiatica (Mandook parni) Ghan	100 mg.
Arogya vardhini	50 mg.
Saptamrut loha	50 mg.
Narshinh churna	40 mg.
Embliya officinalis (Vrushya) Ext.	25 mg.
Abhrak bhasma	25 mg.

Dosage: One capsule two to three times a day with cold milk or as directed by physician.

How Supplied: Available in blister pack of 10 x 10 capsules. Economy pack of 250 capsules.

Uses: Dandruff, Falling of hair, Premature greying, Alopecia.

***Product Name*:** **VASULIV CAPSULES**

Composition: Each 500 mg. capsule contains:

Phyllanthus urianaria (bhumiamia) conc.	120 mg.
Tephrosia purpurea (Sarpankha) conc.	100 mg.
Boerhavia diffusa (Punarnava) conc.	100 mg.
Eclipta alba (Bhrungraj) conc.	90 mg.
Andrographis paniculata (Kalmegh) Concentrate	30 mg.
Cichorium itybus (kashi) conc.	30 mg.
Picrorrhiza kurrooa (Katuki) conc.	30 mg.

Dosage: 1 to 2 capsule, thrice daily, preferably before meals or as directed by the physician.

How Supplied: Plifer proof glass bottle of 100 ml.

Uses: General liver dysfunction, Loss of appetite, hepatomengaly, Jaundice, Acute & Chronic viral hepatitis, Liver dysfunction because of alcohol consumption, Pre-cirrhotic conditions of liver.

Venkarteswara Ayurveda Nilayam Private Limited
Chintaluru-533 232 (Andhra Pradesh)
Tel.: (08855) 48429, 48592
Fax: (08855) 48429

***Product Name*:** **SIDHAMAKARADHWAJA PILLS**

Composition: Swarnabhasma (Calcined gold) 1 part, Sudha Parada 6 parts, Sudha Gandhaka 12 parts, cooked and collected in calcinated stage. Then Sidhamakaradhwaja, Jatiphal, Ela each one part, Pachakurpura half part collected and blended with the decoction of Sandalwood and made into pills.

Dosage: One pill twice daily for adults. To be chewed and swallowed, preferably with milk. One pill per day for 13 to 25 yrs. age group people.

How Supplied: 25 pills (Sealed tin pack)

Uses: Helps to enrich memory, potency, complexion. Imparts vigour to total body.

***Product Name*: POORNACHANDRODAYA PILLS**

Composition

Swanabhasma (calcined gold) 1 part, Sudha parada 3 parts, Sudha gandhaka 6 parts cooked and collected in calcinated stage. Then purnachandrodaya Abhrakabhasma, Vangabhasma each one part, Vidari, Pachakarpura, Bamboo camphor, Salamisri each half part collected in a vessel and blended. After blending the medicine will be made into pills.

Dosage: One pill twice a day, to be chewed and swallowed only. One pill in a day for 10 to 15 yrs. One pill twice in a day from 15 yrs. onwards.

How Supplied: 25 pills (sealed tin pack).

Uses: Helps to cure spermatorrhea, Nervousness and weakness.

***Product Name*: NO. 4 VASANTAKUSUMAKARA PILLS**

Composition

Swarnabhasma ¼ part, Mouktikabhasma (Pearls), Pravalabhasma (Corals), rajatabhasma (Silver), Abhrakabhasma (Sataputa) etc., one part each. The prepared vasantakusumakara, Sudha shilajit, Abhrakabhasma one part each, well and made into pills.

Dosage: One pill after breakfast and one pill after dinner with water.

How Supplied: 25 pills (sealed tin pack).

Uses: a wonderful remedy in weakness due to diabetes. Enriches memory, works well on Debility and general weakness. Helps to act well on urinary disturbances.

***Product Name*: PANCHABANARASA PILLS**

Composition

Swarnabhasma ½ part, Pravalabhasma (Corals), Mouktikabhasma (Pearls), Rajatabhasma (Silver), Sudha shilajit, Jayphal, Ikshugandha etc.,One part each collected, blended and made into pills.

Dosage: One pill twice a day to be chewed and swallowed. For better results take milk (or) any fruit juice (or) any vegetable soup after swallowing the pill.

How Supplied: 25 pills (sealed tin pack)

Uses: An aphrodisiac. Works well on impotency. Helps to enrich semen count. Improves Vim Vigour and Vitality.

***Product Name*:** **BRUHADWAQTACHINTAMANI PILLS**

Composition

Rasa Sindura, Rajata (Silver) bhasma, Mouktikabhasma (pearsl), Abhrakabhasma (Satapura), Pravalabhasma (Corals) each one part and Swarnabhasma (calcined gold) half part. Rasna powder, Guggul Mahisakshi ¼th part collected, blended with the decoction of Rasna and made into pills.

Dosage: One pill twice in a day with water.

How Supplied: 25 pills (sealed tin pack).

Uses: A good remedy in arthritis & Rheumatism. Controls nervous disorders.

***Product Name*:** **KC 2 PILLS (MAMACHUDAMANIRASA PILLS)**

Composition

Swarnabhasma ½ part, Rajata (Silver) bhasma, three parts, Mouktikabhasma one part, Jatiphal, tejpatra, Ela ¼th part each. These ingredients are collected, blended and made into pills.

Dosage: One pil twice in a day. For better result milk is advisable to consume along with.

How Supplied: 25 pills (sealed tin pack).

Uses: Removes sexual debility and thus helps to control impotency. An aphorodisiac.

***Product Name*:** **CHYAVANAPRASALEHYA (A CONFECTION)**

Composition

Fresh amla, aswagandha, Dasmula, Chaturjath, Karkatakasrinigi,

Vidari, Jivanti, Vasaka, Satavari and other valuable 19 herbs, Sarakara, Madhu, Tilataila and ghruta.

Dosage: One spoonful (10 gms.) twice in a day. Preferably with milk.

How Supplied: 300 g. bottle.

Uses: Relieves stress and strain. Prevents debility and vitalises the entire system. A well acclaimed product for respiratory disorders.

***Product Name*: ASWAGANDHADILEHYA (A CONFECTION)**

Composition

Aswagandha	10 gms.
Swetapunanava	900 mg.
Trikatuka	1.365 g.

Jatiphal, Chavika, Ela, Vidanga, Kushta, Lavang, Vamslochan, Sariba, Rasna, Musli, Jiraka, Krishnajiraka, Satavari, Yavanika, Pippalimula, Kanne komali, Hribera 7.735 g.

Sarakara	40 g.
Madhu	25 g.
Chruta	15 g.

Dosage: One spoon ful (10 gms) twice in a day. Preferably with milk.

How Supplied: 300 gms. bottle.

Uses: Acts as anti-stress and anti-anxiety Neurosis. Restores vigour and energy.

***Product Name*: RATNAPURUSHALEHYA (A CONFECTION)**

Composition

Ratnapurusha	10 g.

Aswaganda, Vidari, Ela, Satavari, Sariba, Tejpatra, Usira, Kannekomali, bhusarkara, Musli, Jeeraka, Ikshuraka, Rupamastaki, Sounphu, Salamistri, Sabja, Badamnut, Jatipatri, Gokshura, Musta, Beejabandhu, Akshotnut, Swarnapati Gulabi, Sudhamuli and Trikatuka 10 g.

Sarkara	40 g.
Madhu	25 g.
Ghruta	15 g.

Dosage: One spoon ful (10 gms.) twice in a day.

How Supplied: 300 gms bottle.

Uses: For Vim, Vogour and Vitality. Energing tonic. Imparts strength to body.

***Product Name*:** **MADEEPHALA RASAYANA**

Composition

Dhania 1 part, Jeera 1 part, Ardraka 3 parts, Sarakara 22 parts, Saindhavalavana 0.16 parts. These ingredients are collectec and items no 1,2,3 are soaked well and juice was collected proportionately. Then sugar and saindhavalavana are added, stirred well, and fire was given. Then paka is prepared.

Dosage: One spoon ful twice in a day.

How Supplied: 200 ml. bottle.

Uses: Useful in distaste. Cures nausea. A well recommended medicine for women in pragnency.

Vijay Pharmaceutical Works
Kalpana Building, Old Subzi Mandi
Sirsa-125 055
Tel,L 20458, 31669, 27458
Fax: (1666) 20458

***Product Name*:** **Blood-up-Capsules**

Composition

Tapyadi lauh	80 mg.
Navayas lauh	80 mg.
Arogya vardhini	80 mg.
Punarnavadi mandoor	80 mg.
Dhatri lauh	80 mg.

Dosage:

How Supplied: 10 caps.

Uses: Anaemia, Iron deficiency, Convalescence, General debility, Loss of Appetite, Exhaustion, Neurasthenia.

Product Name: DASTROL PLUS TABLETS

Composition

Bael	60 mg.
Saunf	30 mg.
Nagar Motha	50 mg.
Hing	5 mg.
Haldi	45 mg.
Kharia	90 mg.
Kura Chhal	40 mg.
Nag Kesar	10 mg.
Sudh Kuchla	10 mg.
Opium Seed	50 mg.
Lodhra	40 mg.
Ral	20 mg.

Dosage: Not Available.

How Supplied: 500 tabs.

Uses: Entero-colities, Summer Diarrhoea, Acute and chronic, Amoebic & Bacillary dysentry, other Abdominal Disorders.

Product Name: KCR GOLD CAPSULES

Composition

Kaam churamani ras	200 mg.
Ashwagandha	100 mg.
Safed musli	100 mg.
Pure gold	100 mg.

Dosage: Not available.

How Supplied: 10 capsules.

Uses: Tonic for sexual Debility in Male & Female. Premature ejaculation, Concentrates Semen, Debility, Vaginismus, Frigdity, Dry Vagina & Lack of Emotion.

Product Name: KUFGYL SYRUP

Composition: Each 10 ml. contains:

Somlata	250 mg.
Mulethi	200 mg.

Sobhanjan	100 mg.
Tulsi	100 mg.
Vasa	30 mg.
Kanthkari	30 mg.
Sat pipermint	5 mg.
Loban	5 m.g
Gandhpatri tail	5 mg.

Dosage: Not available.

How Supplied: 110 ml.

Uses: Acute & Chronic Bronchities, Laryngitis, Pharyingitis, Asthamatic Cough. Tonsillitis, Spasmodic & Whooping Cough, Expectorant.

***Product Name*: LEUCOFLY SYRUP**

Composition: Each 10 ml. contains:

Ashoka	2000 mg.
Lodhra	200 mg.
Satavar	200 mg.
Lal chandan	25 mg.
Ulat kambal	200 mg.
Elaichi	10 mg.
Brahmi	200 mg.
Manjith	50 mg.
Vidharikand	100 mg.
Daru haldi	100 mg.
Dashmool	200 mg.

Uses: Leucorrhoea, Rundown conditions, irregular menstruation, Back-ache due to over flowing of whites & a general female tonic.

***Product Name*: VIJLIV CAPSULE**

Composition

Kutki	50 mg.
Mandoor Bhasam	50 mg.
Sankh Bhasam	30 mg.
Jawakhar	30 mg.
Parwal Bhasam	40 mg.
lauh Bhasam	50 mg.

Dosage: Not available.

How Supplied: 10 capsules, 30 capsules.

Uses: Anorexia, Hepatic dysfunctions, Growth failure, Hepatitis & Adjunct to hepatotoxic drugs.

***Product Name*:** **VEEJOTONE SYRUP**

Composition: Each 10 ml. contains:

Ashwagandha	150 mg.
Sankh Pushpi	100 mg.
Brahmi	100 mg.
Sheelajit	150 mg.
Long	3 mg.
Jaiphal	3 mg.
Dal chini	3 mg.
Kesar	2 mg.

Dosage: Not available.

How Supplied: 200 ml.

Uses: Anaemia, Loss of Weight, Nervous Debility, Run down conditions, Restorative & Invigorative Tonic for all ages.

Yamuna Pharmacy
Jagadhri Road
Yamuna Nagar-135001
Tel.: 23501
Fax: (01732) 50750

***Product Name*:** **GYNAFLIX SYRUP**

Composition: Each 100 ml. Contains:

Ashok–Goolar 4.167 g Each
Rasaunt-Pipaltwak-tatjata-Patang-Shwet jeerak-Krishan Jeerak-Jatamansi-Nagarmotha Nilmakal-Devdaru-Hartiri-Vibhitak-Asmraguthli-Adusa-Chandan-Gudhal-Ashvagandha--Shatavari-Jiyapota-Nagkesar-Samudra sock-Lodhra 416.7 mg. Each, Laakhpipal 2.816 g. In syrup base.

Dosage: 10-15 ml. Three or four times a day from 15 days to 90 days depending upon severity of the case.

How Supplied: 200 ml. 450 ml.

Uses: * Menorhagia * Metrorrhagia * Polymenorrhoea * Post IUCD bleeding * Idiopathic bleeding from uterus * Uterus prolapsus * Displacement of uterus & Leucorrhoea * Endometritis accompanied with severe bleeding * General weakness of women patients * Menopausal syndrome.

***Product Name*: M.M. FORTE CAPSULE**

Composition

Makardhwaj	05 mg.
Al-ahmer	25 mg.
Lauha bhasma	30 mg.
Shudh kupilu	30 mg.
Lavang	30 mg.
Jaiphal	30 mg.
Jaivitri	30 mg.
Kulinjan	30 mg.
Khrurasani ajwain	30 mg.
Harnal	35 mg.
Majuphal	35 mg.
Samudra sokh	35 mg.
Daalchini	45 mg.
Aqarqara	50 mg.
Kaunchbeej	60 mg.

Dosage: 1 capsule twice a day for 3 to 4 days, Subsequently 1 capsule a day, with milk or its various forms. For Fatigue, Syndrome: One capsule a day.

How Supplied: 10 capsule sealed packs.

Uses: *Functional or Psychogenic Impotence *Sexual, senile or seminal weakness *Lack of sexual interest in women.

***Product Name*: ANTHECID SYRUP**

Composition: Each 5 ml. contains aqueous ext.

Palashpapda	200 mg v/v
Vidang	200 mg v/v

Dicamali	200 mg v/v
Dadimmooltwaq	200 mg v/v
Kalijiri'	200 mg v/v
Sennaleaf	200 mg v/v
Mustak	150 mg v/v
Ounderkani	150 mg v/v
Kirmani ajowain	150 mg v/v
Triphala	150 mg v/v
Nimbatwaq	150 mg v/v
Kampillak	100 mg v/v
Sahijan	100 mg v/v
Poogam	100 mg v/v
Devadaru	100 mg v/v
Ajowain	50 mg v/v
Indrayav	50 mg v/v

in sugar base.

Dosage: Infants: ½ teaspoon TDS for 7 days. Children: 1 teaspoon twice or thrice a day for 7 days. Adults: 2 teaspoon TDS for 7 days.

How Supplied: 100 ml.

Uses: Roundworm, Threadworm, Whipworm, Tapeworm, Strongloides & ill effectrs caused by helminthiasis viz. Fever, Flatulence, diarrhoea, Urticaria, Asthma, Bronchitis, Convulsion etc.

***Product Name*: COFEX EXPECTORANT**

Composition: Each 10 ml. contains ext.

Vasaka	600 mg v/v
Kantakari	600 mg v/v
Madhu yashti	300 v/v
Lisodha	30 mg v/v
Somlata	150 mg v/v
Khatmi	150 mg v/v
Tulsi	150 mg v/v
Navsadar	200 mg v/v
Tankan	20 mg v/v
Satva pudina	0.006 mg.

in sugar base.

Dosage: 1-2 teaspoonsful with warm water.

How Supplied: 50 ml., 100 ml., 450 ml.

Uses: Cough, Cold, Asthma, Spasmodic productive cough with tenacious sputum.

***Product Name*:** **EPIDERMOIL OIL**

Composition

Chakramarda	277 mg.
Nimbachhal	277 mg.
Chiraita	277 mg.
Haldi	277 mg.
Drauhaldi	277 mg.
Raktachandan	277 mg.
Vaasa	277 mg.
Harar	277 mg.
Baheda	277 mg.
Aamla	277 mg.
Chameli patra	277 mg.

In fused aqueous extract form oil.

Dosage: Used extremally only. Quantity sufficient to apply to affected part and massaged.

How Supplied: 50 ml.

Uses: Pruritus vulvo–et.-ani, Contact dermatits, Exfoliative dermatitis, Radiation dermatitis, eczematous lesions, Napkin rashes, dandruff.

***Product Name*:** **HEMCYTONE SYRUP**

Composition: Each 10 ml. contains aqueous extract derived from:

Arjuna	200 mg v/v
Ashwagandha	200 mg v/v
Mishreyak	200 mg v/v
Nibushwaras	200 mg v/v
Lauha bhasma	200 mg v/v

In syrup base

Dosage: ½ to 2 teaspoons twice a day with water after principal meals.

How Supplied: 100 ml., 200 ml.

Uses: Iron deficiency anaemia, Psychosomatic weaknesses, Palptitation of heart in anaemia, Habit of eating non-foods.

Product Name: HEMOCLIN SYRUP

Composition: Each 5 ml. contains ext.derived:

Unnao	94.33 mg v/v
Parpat	94.33 mg v/v
Sharpunkha	94.33 mg v/v
Mundi	94.33 mg v/v
Khairchhal	94.33 mg v/v
Harar	94.33 mg v/v
Raktachandan	94.33 mg v/v
Mehandi	94.33 mg v/v
ndrayav	94.33 mg v/v
Nimb	94.33 mg v/v
Daruharidra	94.33 mg v/v
Sanaya	94.33 mg v/v
Haridra	94.33 mg v/v
Brahmdandi	94.33 mg v/v
Chiraita	94.33 mg v/v
Gulab	94.33 mg v/v

in syrup base.

Dosage: 2 teaspoonful twice or thrice a day with simple water, milk or fruit juice.

How Supplied: 200 ml.

Uses: Skin diseases associated with liver troubles viz: Acne, Pimples, Napkin rashes, Herpes zoster Leucocytosis, Hepatitis, hepatotoxicity, toxaemia, skin infections, Prurigo (itching) in jaundice.

Product Name: LIVOL SYRUP

Composition: Each 5 ml. contains ext. from:

Rohish	34.7 mg v/v
Apamarg	34.7 mg v/v
Saunfmool	34.7 mg v/v
Kasanimool	34.7 mg v/v
Mulethi	34.7 mg v/v
Punernavamool	34.7 mg v/v
Karfas	34.7 mg v/v
Sanaya	43.05 mg v/v
Amlica	86.8 mg v/v
Anjir	76.8 mg v/v

Each in syrup base.

Dosage: Infant: ¼ to ½ teaspoonful. Children: 1 teaspoonful. Adults: 2 to 3 teaspoonful two to four times a day for 30 days.

How Supplied: 100 ml., 200 ml., 450 ml.

Uses: Anorexia, Malnutrition, Growth failure, Liver dysfunction, Liver inflammation, Jaundice, Alcoholism, Fatty infiltration of liver.

***Product Name*: MENSULIX SYRUP**

Composition: Each 10 ml. contains ext. derived from:

Mishreyak	90 mg. v/v
Hapusha	90 mg. v/v
Harmal	90 mg. v/v
Kalajaji	90 mg. v/v
Jatamansi	90 mg. v/v
Moolibeej	90 mg. v/v
Ergot	90 mg. v/v
Manjishta	180 mg v/v
Kapasmoltwaq	180 mg v/v
Gajarbeej	180 mg v/v
Ulatkambal	180 mg v/v
Sitab	180 mg v/v

Each in sweet syrup base.

Dosage: 15-20 ml. BD/TDS with hot water for 15-20 days from 14th day of last cycle.

How Supplied: 200 ml.

Uses: Amenorrhoea, Premenstrual tension, Dysmenorrhoea, Congestive painful menstruation, Oligomenorrhoea, Delayed menarche.

Zandu Pharmaceutical Works Ltd.
70, Gokhale Road South (Dadar)
Post Box No. 9144
Mumbai-400 025
Tel.: 4307021, 4304518, 4304517
Fax: (22) 4375491

***Product Name*: ABHAYASAN TABLETS**

Composition

Asafoetida	10 mg.

Cummin seeds	10 mg.
Dill	10 mg.
Nutgrass	10 mg.
Ptychotis	10 mg.
Turpenthum	20 mg.
Coriander	30 mg.
Fennel	30 mg.
Triphala	30 mg.
Myrobalan	40 mg.
Senna leaf	40 mg.
Trikatu	60 mg.
Chaturjat	80 mg.

***Product Name*: ALPITONE LIQUID**

Composition: Each 5 ml. contains:

Ashwangandha	200 mg.
Bala	200 mg.
Shatavari	100 mg.
Draksha-Black resin	50 mg.
Chitrak	50 mg.
Gokharu	50 mg.
Rasna	50 mg.
Amruta	25 mg.
Sunthi	25 mg.
Alcohol	11% v/v

***Product Name*: BALSHOOLARKA LIQUID**

Composition

Anise oil	0.00012 ml.
Caraway oil	0.00012 ml.
Dill water conc.	0.006 ml.
Sodium Bi-carbonate	12 mg.
Chloroform spirit	0.048 ml.
Alcohol content	4% v/v

***Product Name*: BRENTO TABLETS**

Composition: Each prepared from dry powder of aqueous:

Extract	100 mg.
Derived from:	

Shankhapushpi	100 mg.
Brahmi	100 mg.
Ashwagandh	100 mg.
Yastimadhu	100 mg.
Kath	50 mg.
Vacha	25 mg.
Sarpagandha	25 mg.
Jathiphala	20 mg.
Chandroday	5 mg.
(sugar coated)	

Dosage: 1-2 tablets, 3 times a day.

How Supplied: 50 tabs., 130 tabs.

Uses: Absent mindedness, Loss of memory, nervine tonics.

***Product Name*: CAMPHO CODI VASAKA COUGH SYRUP**

Composition: Each 5 ml. contains:

Terpin hydrate	6.65 mg.
Camphor	0.8375 mg.
Menthol	0.8375 mg.
Codeine phosphate	8.375 mg.
Ephedrine HCl	1.675 mg.
Syrup tolu	0.8375 ml.
Extract adhatoda vasica	0.4125 ml.
Alcohol content	2% v/v

***Product Name*: CORAZAN CAPSULES**

Composition

Extract of Maha sudarshan churna	300 mg.
Hingual	10 mg.
Tankan	10 mg.
Sunthi	10 mg.
Maricha	10 mg.
Pippali	10 mg.
Pippali moola	10 mg.
Vatsanabh	2.5 mg.

Dosage: 1-2 capsules, 23 times a day.

Uses: Body aches, Common cold, Flu, Nasal congestion, Respiratory congestion, Sinusitis, Sneezing.

***Product Name*: GESTONE GRANULES**

Composition

Ashagandha	40 mg.
Shatavari	40 mg.
Nagkeshar	40 mg.
Yashtimadhu	40 mg.
Sunthi	40 mg.
Balamool	30 mg.
Gokshuru	30 mg.
Pippali	20 mg.
Draksha	64 mg.
Loha bhasma	16mg.
Praval bhasma	16 mg.
Swarna makshik bhasma	10 mg.
Rasa sindur	4 mg.
Banga bhasma	10 mg.

***Product Name*: K-4 TABLETS**

Composition

Chandraprabha	120 mg.
Extract of Guduchi	120 mg.
Haridra	20 mg.
Kanyalohadi	40 mg.

Bhavna of bilvapatra rasa and Karela rasa.

Dosage: 2 tablets, 2 times a day with water or milk.

How Supplied: 75 tabs.

Uses: Enlarged prostate, Renal stones, ureteritis, Urinary tract infections.

***Product Name*: LIVOTRIT LIQUID**

Composition: Each 5 mlk. contains:

Bhringraj	100 mg.
Guduchi	200 mg.
Kurchi	100 mg.
Kalmegh	100 mg.
Punarnava	200 mg.

Katuki	100 mg.
Vidanga	75 mg.
Rakta rohida	75 mg.
Nishoth	75 mg.
Daru haridra	75 mg.
Chitramoola	75 mg.
Kalipath	75 mg.

Dosage: 1-2 teaspoonful, 3 times a day with water and glucose.

How Supplied: 100 ml.

Uses: Infective hepatitis, Liver dysfunction, Enlarged a fatty liver.

***Product Name*: PANCHARISHTA LIQUID**

Composition: Each 10 ml. contains:

Draksha, Kumari	2.5 g. each
Dashmoola	2 g.
Ashwagandha, Shatavari	1 g. each
Trifala	0.6 g.
Amruta Bala, Yashtimadhu	0.5 g. each
Trikatu, Trijat	0.3 g. each
Arjuna, Lodhra, Manjishta	0.2 g. each
Ajmoda, Dhanayaka, Haridra, Gandhshathi, Jaraka, Lavang	0.1 g. each
Contains self generated Alcohol not more than	11% v/v.

***Product Name*: OVOUTOLINE LIQUID**

Composition: Each 5 ml. contains:

Aqueous Extract derived from

Ashok	250 mg.
Lodhra	250 mg.
Cuduchi	100 mg.
Shatavari	100 mg.
Tagar	50 mg.
Kurchi	50 mg.
Yashtimadhu	300 mg.

***Product Name*: RHUMASYL LINIMENT**

Composition: Each 10 ml. contains:

Maha mash taila	2.5 ml

Voishagarbha taila	2.5 ml
Narayan taila	2.5 ml
Gandhapuro taila	2.5 ml

***Product Name*: RHUMAYOG TABLETS**

Composition

Banga Bhasma	5 mg.
Nag bhasma	5 mg.
Loha bhasma	5 mg.
Makshik bhasma	5 mg.
Mandur bhasma	5 mg.
Abhrak bhasma	5 mg.
Rasa sindur	5 mg.
Yog raj guggul	30 mg.
Maha rasnadi quath	235 mg.

Uses: Ankylosing spondilitis, Back ache and weakness in ladies, Fibrositis, Frozen shoulders, Leg cramps, Lumbago, Muscle spasms, Post delivery pelvic aches and pains.

***Product Name*: STRENEX TABLETS**

Composition

Ashwagandha	100 mg.
Kauncha	100 mg.
Chandrodaya	100 mg.
Manikya bhasma	100 mg.
Praval bhasma	100 mg.
Abhrak bhasma	50 mg.
Shilajit	50 mg.
Nux vomica	25 mg.
Kantaloha	20 mg.
Nutmeg	15 mg.
Manikya rasa	10 mg.
Borneol	5 mg.
Amber	5 mg.

***Product Name*: TRIBANG SHILA TABLETS**

Composition

Tribang bhasma	30 mg.
Gymnema sylvestre	80 mg.

Melia azadirachta linn	80 mg.
Shilajit	40 mg.
Solid extract enicostemalittorale blume	40 mg.
Solid extract Eguenia-jambolana linn	40 mg.

Dosage: 2-4 tablets, 2 times a day before meals with water/milk/honey/turmeric juice.

Uses: Diabetes melitus.

***Product Name*:** **VIGOREX TABLETS**

Composition

Rasa sindur	10 mg.
Abrak bhasma	10 mg.
Loha bhasma	10 mg.
Shilajit	50 mg.
Makshik bhasma	10 mg.
Vidanga	10 mg.
Musali	25 mg.
Guduchi churna	25 mg.
Kauncha	50 mg.
Gokshurak	25 mg.
Shalmali	25 mg.
Amalak	25 mg.
Bhallatakbij	25 mg.
Ashwagandha	50 mg.
Jathiphala	10 mg.
Lavanga	0.003 ml.
Kapur baras	5 mg.
Vishtinduk	10 mg.

Dosage: 1-2 tablets, 2 times a day with milk.

Uses: Unsatisfactory erection, Functional impotence, Decreased libido, sexual neurasthania, Sexual weakness, tiredness, Unsatisfactory sexual performance, Loss of vitality.

***Product Name*:** **ZANDU BALM OINTMENT**

Composition

Menthol	20% w/w
Oil Gaultheria	10% w/w
in base q.s.	

Product Name: ZANDUZYME TABLETS

Composition

Pippalimool	15 mg.
Dantimool	15 mg.
Ajwan	15 mg.
Aconite	15 mg.
Aconite	15 mg.
Tamarind bark-ash	15 mg.
Asafoetida	15 mg.
Gulvel	15 mg.
Nux vomica	15 mg.
Kajjali	15 mg.
Chitrak	20 mg.
Trikatu	60 mg.
Yavakshar	10 mg.
Sajikshar	10 mg.
Suryakshar	10 mg.
Shankh bhasma	30 mg.
Carica papaya	30 mg.

Dosage: 2 tablets, 2 times a day after meals.

How Supplied: 40 tabs., 300 tabs.

Uses: Digestive disorders, Colonic dyspepsia, Flatulence, Gaseousness, Indigestion.

Product Name: ZEFS COUGH SYRUP

Composition: Each 5 ml. contains Ext. of:

Vasaka	200 mg.
Kanatakari	200 mg.
Chavak	10 mg.
Karkat shrungi	10 mg.
Dhamasa	10 mg.
Bharangmoola	10 mg.
Rasna	10 mg.
Kachura	10 mg.
Chitrakmoola	10 mg.
Musta	10 mg.
Suthi	10 mg.
Maricha	10 mg.

Pippli	10 mg.
Yastimadhu	200 mg.

Dosage: ½-2 teaspoonful, 2-3 times a day.

How Supplied: 100 ml.

Uses: Bronchial asthma, Bronchiectasis, Bronchitis, Common cold, Cough, influenza, laryngitis, Naso respiratory allergy, Rhinopharyngitis, Tubarcular cough, Whooping cough.

***Product Name*:** **KESARI JIVAN**

Composition: Each 10 g. contains:

Ginger	20 mg.
Black pepper	20 mg.
Long pepper	20 mg.
Cinnamon	20 mg.
Cinnamomum tamala	20 mg.
Cardamom	20 mg.
Messua ferrea	20 mg.
Clove	20 mg.
Sandalwood	20 mg.
Pyrethrum	20 mg.
Nutmeg	20 mg.
Terminalia chebula	10 mg.
Terminalia belerica	10 mg.
Phyllanthus emblica	10 mg.
Hygrophilia spinosa	10 mg.
Mucuna pruriens gum	10 mg.
Abutilon indicum seeds	10 mg.
Withania somnifera	10 mg.
Tribulus terrestris	10 mg.
Asparagus ascendens	10 mg.
Embeli ribes	10 mg.
Saffron	25 mg.
Abhrak bhasma	3.7 mg.
Rasa sindur	3.7 mg.
Javantri	3.7 mg.
Pulp fresh amla (Phyllanthus emblica)	3000 mg.
Ghee (Clarified butter)	370 mg.
Flavour & sugar	q.s.

***Product Name*: RHUMASYL OINTMENT**

Composition

Narayan taila sh. M.ch.	18% v/w
Vishagarbha traila ni.R.	18% v/w
Maha mash taila Bh.R.	18% v/w
Gandhapuro taila (Oil of gaultheria) in Ointment base	18% v/w

Dosage: To be massaged gently into skin over the affected areas.

How Supplied: 25 g.

Uses: Lumbago, Sciatica, Sprains, Stiff-neck and other muscular pains.

11

Project Profiles

HAIR OIL

Cost Calculation

1.	Rated Planted 1000 Litres Hair Oil/day 5000 Nos. Bottles of 100 ml. Capacity 1000 Nos. Bottles of 150 ml. Capacity 500 Nos. Bottles of 500 ml. Capacity		
2.	Land Building	Rs.	9,25,000
3.	Plant and Machinery Required	Rs.	4,25,000
4.	Other Fixed Expenses	Rs.	3,25,000
5.	Fixed Capital Required	Rs.	16,75,000
6.	Raw Material/Month	Rs.	22,45,450
7.	Salary Wages/Month		
	(i) Salary Wages	Rs.	70,000
	(ii) Overheads Utility	Rs.	1,20,000
8.	Working Capital Required	Rs.	24,15,450
9.	Total Capital Required	Rs.	89,21,350
10.	Production Cost/Annum	Rs.	3,07,46,368
11.	Turnover/Annum	Rs.	3,45,00,000
12.	Profit/Annum	Rs.	37,53,632
13.	Fixed Cost/Annum	Rs.	26,72,968
14.	B.E.P.	41.5%	

For exhaustive informations ask to NIIR for **Market Survey cum detailed Techno Economic Feasibility Report** on **Hair Oil**.

National Institute of Industrial Research,
106-E, P.B. No. 2162,
Kamla Nagar (Near Delhi University),
Delhi-7 (India).

Ph.: 2923955, 3935654, 2945886
Fax: 91-11-2941561
E-mail: niir@vsnl.com

BATH AND MASSAGE OIL

Cost Calculation

1. Rated Plant: 200 kg bath oil/massage oil/day of 100 ml bottles
   Working Hours/day-8
   Working days/annum-300
   Working days/month-25

2.	Land and Building Required	Rs.	4,20,000
3.	Plant and Machinery Required	Rs.	2,15,000
4.	Other Fixed Expenditure	Rs.	2,45,000
5.	Fixed Capital Required	Rs.	8,80,000
6.	Raw Material Required/Month	Rs.	10,02,400
7.	Salary Wages/Month	Rs.	29,500
8.	Overheads and Utility/Month	Rs.	1,75,000
9.	Working Capital Required/Month	Rs.	12,06,900
10.	Total Capital Required	Rs.	45,00,700
11.	Production Cost/Annum	Rs.	1,53,80,476
12.	Turnover/Annum	Rs.	1,80,00,000
13.	Profit/Annum	Rs.	26,19,524
14.	Fixed Cost/Annum	Rs.	18,76,276
15.	B.E.P.	41.73%	

NEEM OIL

Cost Calculation

1.	Rated Plant: 500 kg. Neem oil/day		
	Working hours 16 hours/day		
	Working day/annum 300		
	Working days/month 25		
2.	Land and Building Required	Rs.	9,25,000
3.	Plant and Machinery Required	Rs.	9,10,000
4.	Other Fixed Expenditure	Rs.	4,55,000
5.	Fixed Capital Required	Rs.	22,90,000
6.	Raw Material Required/Month	Rs.	7,08,000
7.	Salary Wages/Month	Rs.	57,000
8.	Overheads and Utility/Month	Rs.	1,60,000
9.	Working Capital Required/Month	Rs.	9,25,000
10.	Total Capital Required	Rs.	50,65,000
11.	Production Cost/Annum	Rs.	1,22,93,075
12.	Tournover/Annum	Rs.	1,32,00,000
13.	Profit/Annum	Rs.	9,06,925
14.	Fixed Cost/Annum	Rs.	22,34,675
15.	B.E.P.		71.13%

VICKS LIKE COMPOUNDS

Cost Calculation

1.	Rated Plant: 200 kgs Vicks like Compound/day Working hours/day 8 Working days/month 25 Working days/annum 300		
2.	Land and Buidling Required	Rs.	3,00,000
3.	Plant and Machinery Required	Rs.	8,00,000
4.	Other Fixed Expenditure	Rs.	5,00,000
5.	Fixed Capital Required	Rs.	25,00,000
6.	Raw Material Required/Month	Rs.	11,94,750
7.	Salary Wages/Month	Rs.	70,000
8.	Overheads and Utility/Month	Rs.	5,00,000
9.	Working Capital Required/Month	Rs.	17,64,750
10.	Total Capital Required	Rs.	77,94,250
11.	Production Cost/Annum	Rs.	2,27,92,465
12.	Turnover/Annum	Rs.	2,55,00,000
13.	Profit/Annum	Rs.	27,07,535
14.	Fixed Cost/Annum	Rs.	43,51,465
15.	B.E.P.	61.64%	

SUNCARE/SKIN LIGHTENING COMPOUNDS

Cost Calculation

1.	Rated Plant: 100 kg. Sun Care Ointment/day Working Hours/day 8 Working days/annum 300 Working days/month 25		
2.	Land and Building Required	Rs.	4,50,000
3.	Plant and Machinery Required	Rs.	2,50,000
4.	Other Fixed Expenditure	Rs.	2.70.000
5.	Fixed Capital Required	Rs.	9,70,000
6.	Raw Material Required/Month	Rs.	1,38,672
7.	Salary Wages/Month	Rs.	38,500
8.	Overheads and Utility/Month	Rs.	1,02,500
9.	Working Capital Required/Month	Rs.	18,09,016
10.	Total Capital Required	Rs.	18,09,016
11.	Production Cost/Annum	Rs.	37,76,937
12.	Turnover/Annum	Rs.	45,00,000
13.	Profit/Annum	Rs.	7,23,063
14.	Fixed Cost/Annum	Rs.	10,97,673
15.	B.E.P.		60.28%

EYE DROPS

Cost Calculation

1. Rates Plant: 6000 numbers of drops, 15 ml capacity containers/day

   Working Hours/day 8

   Working days/annum 300

2.	Land and Building Required	Rs.	7,20,000
3.	Plant and Machinery Required	Rs.	12,00,000
4.	Other Fixed Expenditure	Rs.	5,80,000
5.	Fixed Capital Required	Rs.	25,00,000
6.	Raw Material Required/Month	Rs.	4,00,000
7.	Salary Wages/Month	Rs.	60,000
8.	Overheads and Utility/Month	Rs.	1,50,000
9.	Working Capital Required/Month	Rs.	6,10,000
10.	Total Capital Required	Rs.	43,30,000
11.	Production Cost/Annum	Rs.	84,44,500
12.	Tournover/Annum	Rs.	12,00,00,000
13.	Profit/Annum	Rs.	38,55,500
14.	Fixed Cost/Annum	Rs.	21,32,500
15.	B.E.P.	37.49%	

HERBAL LIVER TONIC

Cost Calculation

1.	Rated Plant: 10,000 Bottles of 100 ml. Tonic/day Working days/month 25 Working days/annum 300 Working hours/day 8		
2.	Land and Building Required	Rs.	8,00,000
3.	Plant and Machinery Required	Rs.	12,00,000
4.	Other Fixed Expenditure	Rs.	3,55,000
5.	Fixed Capital Required	Rs.	23,55,000
6.	Raw Material Required/Month	Rs.	3,85,000
7.	Salary Wages/Month	Rs.	35,500
8.	Overheads and Utility/Month	Rs.	7,89,000
9.	Working Capital Required/Month	Rs.	12,09,500
10.	Total Capital Required	Rs.	59,83,500
11.	Production Cost/Annum	Rs.	1,59,31,780
12.	Turnover/Annum	Rs.	3,00,00,000
13.	Profit/Annum	Rs.	1,40,68,220
14.	Fixed Cost/Annum	Rs.	47,11,200
15.	B.E.P.	25.09%	

LAL TOOTH POWDER

Cost Calculation

1. Rated Plant: 2 Tons Tooth Powder/day of which 50 gm pack of 1 Ton

   100 gm pack of 500 kg.

   200 gm pack of 500 kg.

2.	Land and Building Required	Rs.	17,75,000
3.	Plant and Machinery Required	Rs.	11,10,000
4.	Other Fixed Expenditure	Rs.	7,40,000
5.	Fixed Capital Required	Rs.	36,25,000
6.	Raw Material Required/Month	Rs.	14,19,250
7.	Salary Wages/Month	Rs.	69,000
8.	Overheads and Utility/Month	Rs.	5,32,000
9.	Working Capital Required/Month	Rs.	20,20,250
10.	Total Capital Required	Rs.	96,85,750
11.	Production Cost/Annum	Rs.	2,63,56,810
12.	Turnover/Annum	Rs.	3,60,00,000
13.	Profit/Annum	Rs.	96,46,190
14.	Fixed Cost/Annum	Rs.	49,98,610
15.	B.E.P.	34.13%	

SHAMPOO

Cost Calculation

1.	Rated Plant: 500 Litres/day Working Hours/day 8 Working days/month 25 Working days/annum 300		
2.	Land and Building Required	Rs.	9,25,000
3.	Plant and Machinery Required	Rs.	7,40,00
4.	Other Fixed Expenditure	Rs.	5,25,000
5.	Fixed Capital Required	Rs.	21,90,000
6.	Raw Material Required/Month	Rs.	9,00,000
7.	Salary Wages/Month	Rs.	3,30,000
8.	Overheads and Utility/Month	Rs.	3,30,000
9.	Working Capital Required/Month	Rs.	12,89,000
10.	Total Capital Required	Rs.	60,57,000
11.	Production Cost/Annum	Rs.	1,67,97,135
12.	Turnover/Annum	Rs.	1,87,50,000
13.	Profit/Annum	Rs.	19,52,865
14.	Fixed Cost/Annum	Rs.	31,94,335
15.	B.E.P.	62.05%	

12

Machinery Section

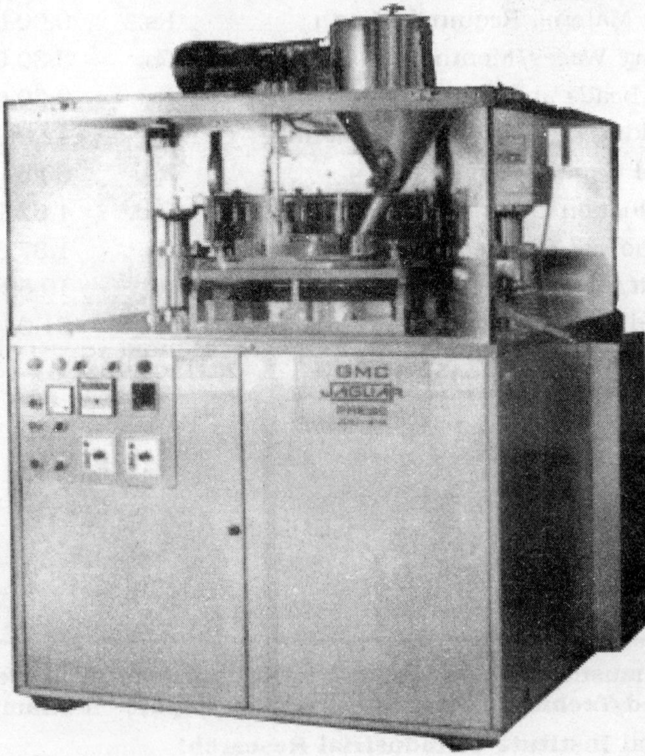

A Versatile Tablet Press

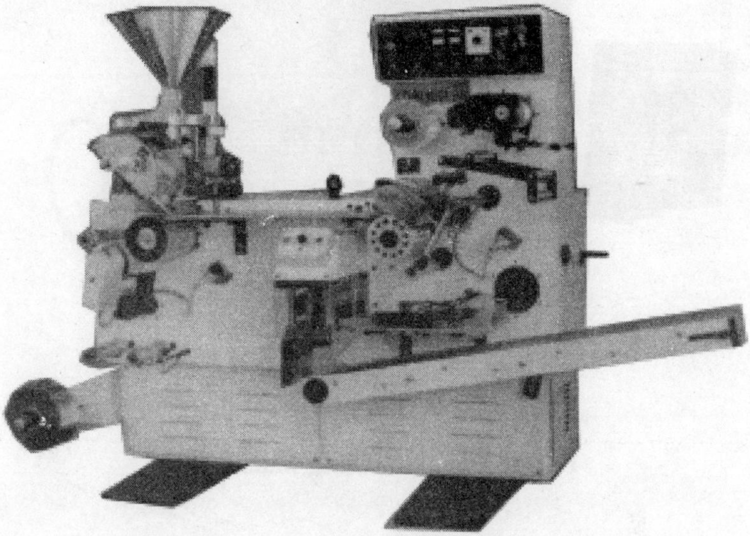

100-150-240 CH-CW Blisterpack Machine

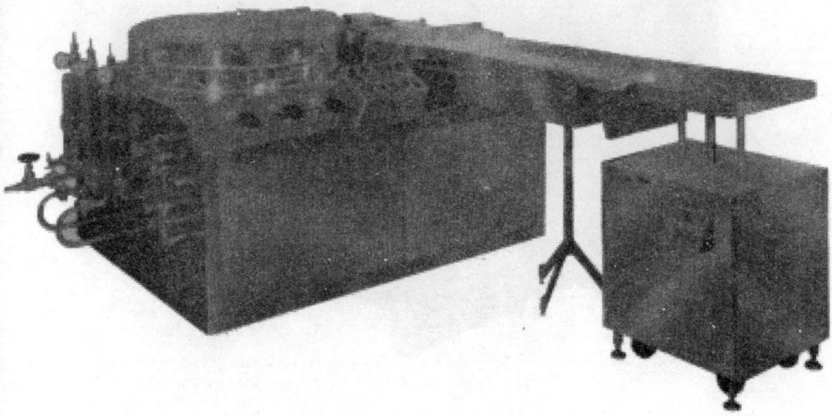

Automatic Rotary Vial Washing Machine

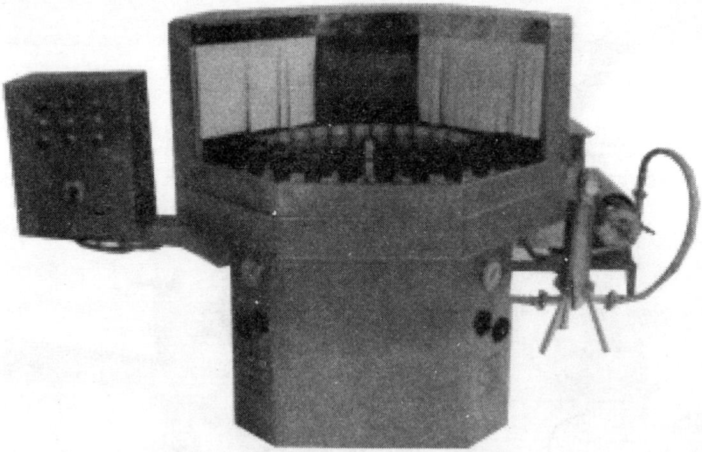

Rotary Bottle Washing Machine

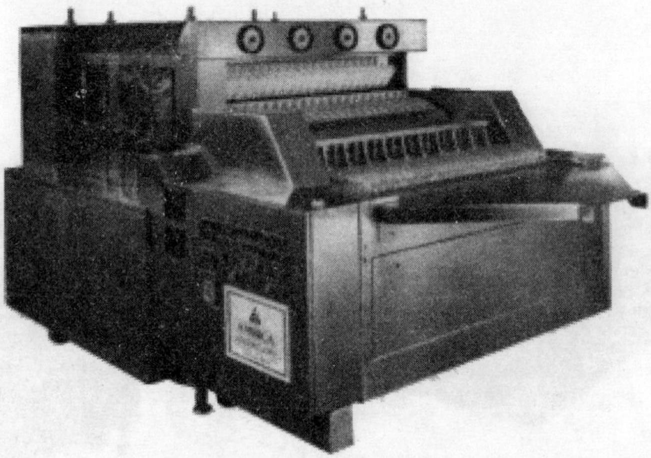

Automatic High Speed Linear Vial / Bottle Washing Machine

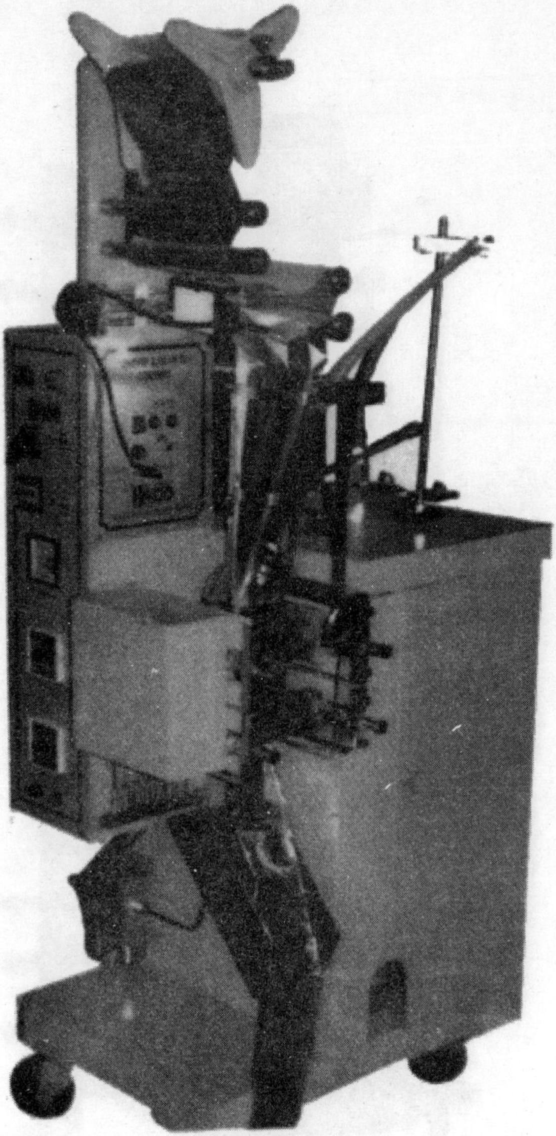

Automatic Packing of Liquid and Paste Substances

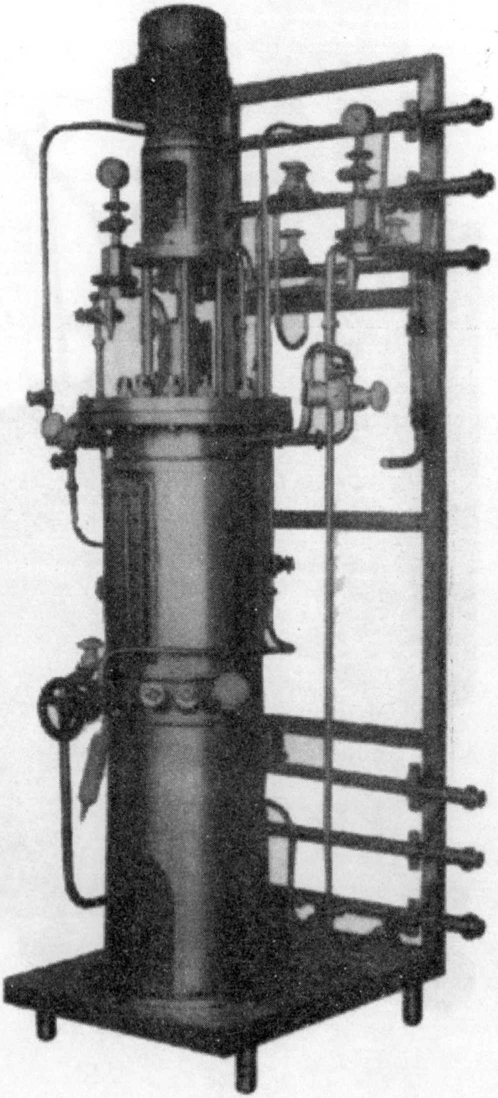

Fermenter

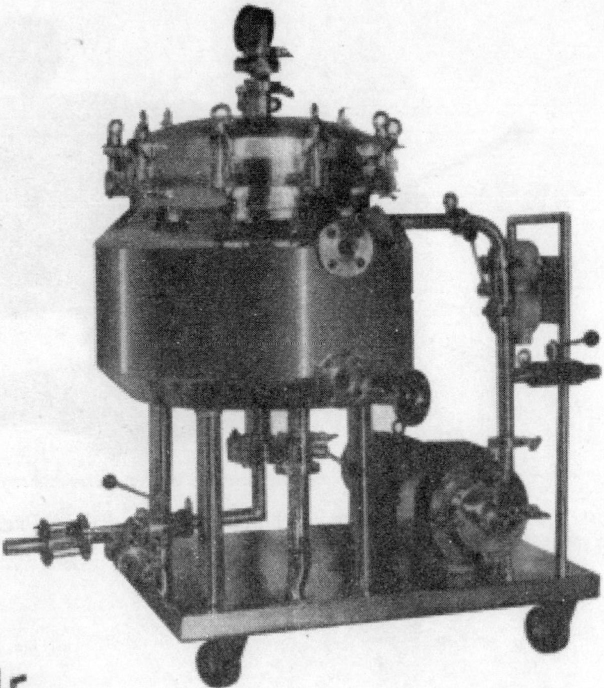

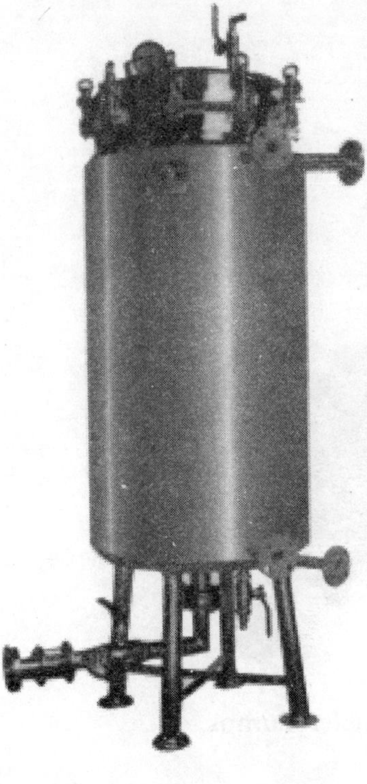

Horizontal Plate Type Filter Press

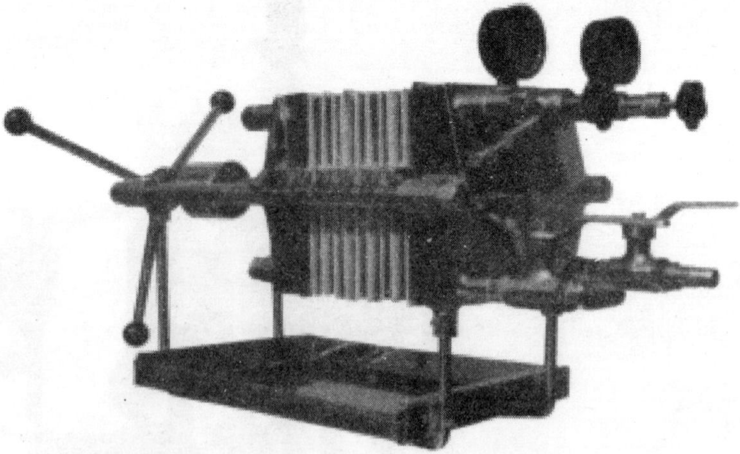

Plate and Frame Type Filter Press

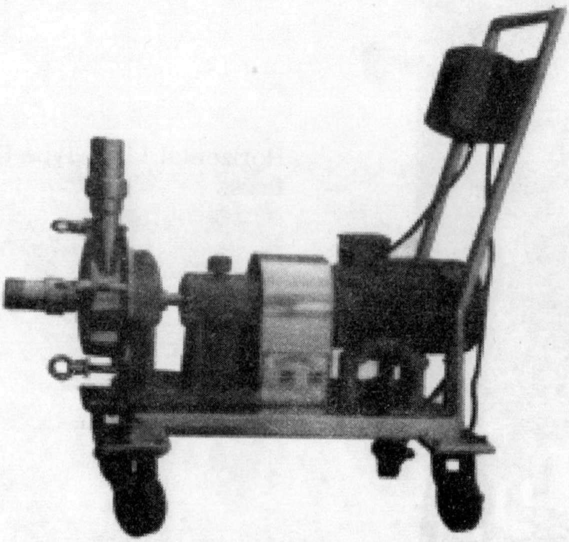

Centrifugal Type Transfer Pumps

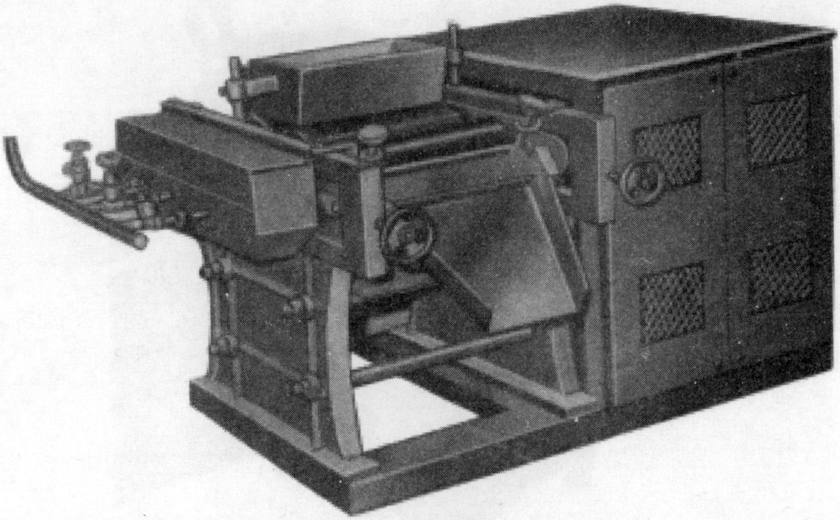

Roll Mill

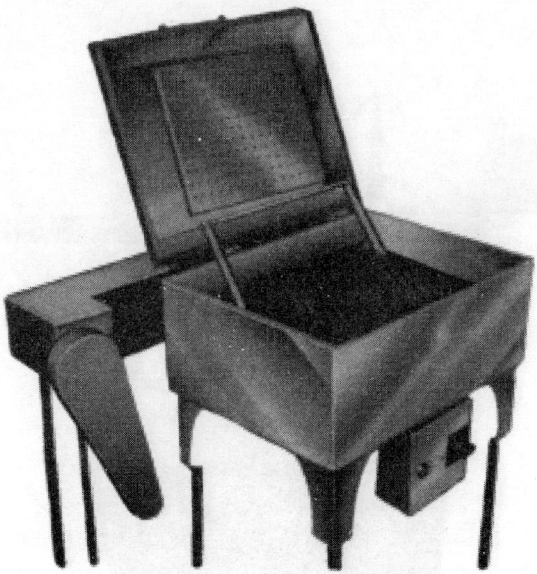

Ampoule Washing Machine

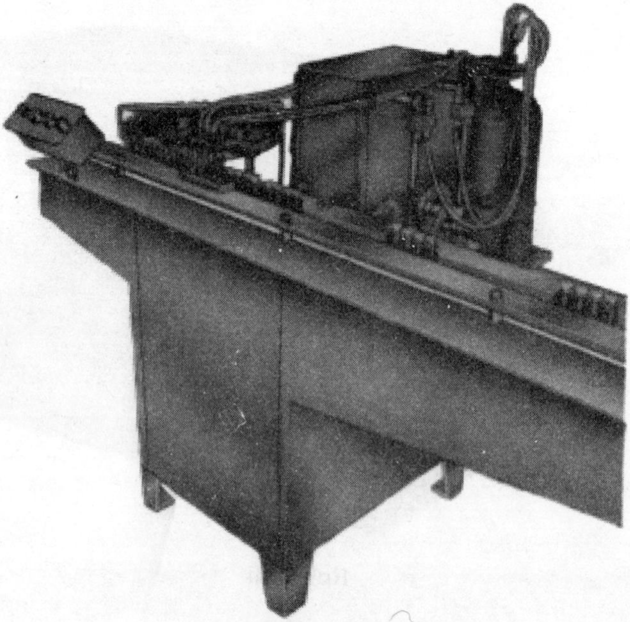

Automatic Four Head Vial Filling Machine

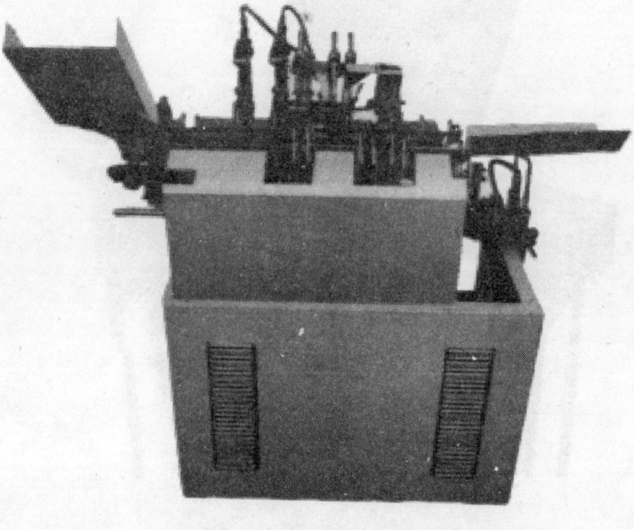

Automatic Double Head Ampoule Filling & Sealing Machine

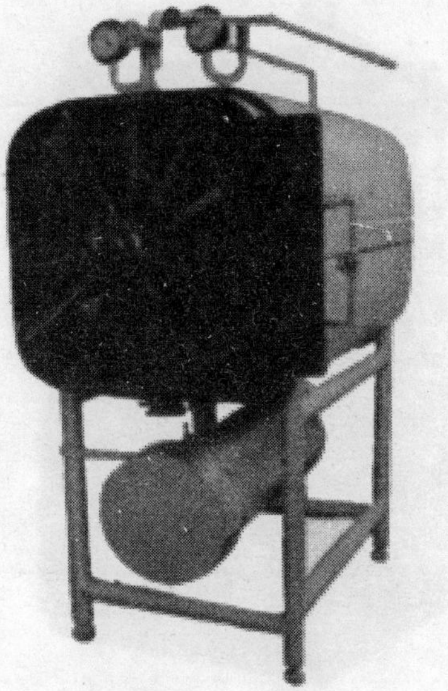

High Pressure Autoclave

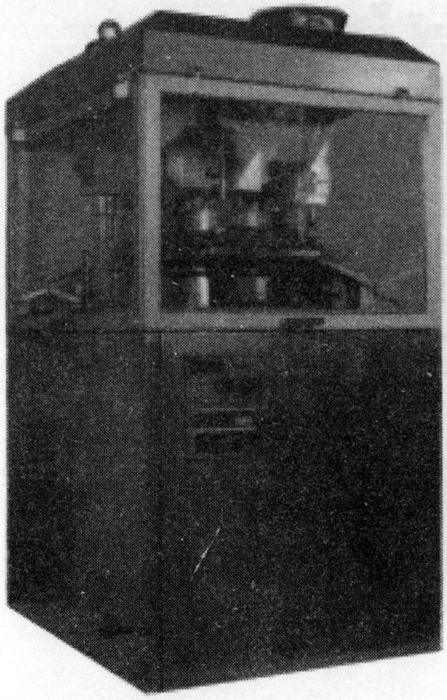

Tablet Press

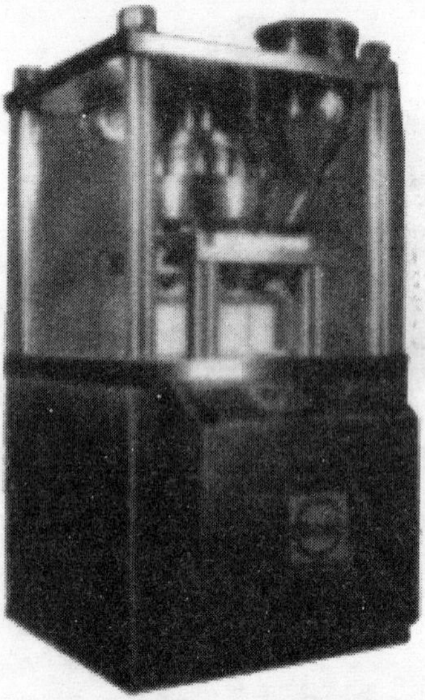

Tablet Press - Mini Press

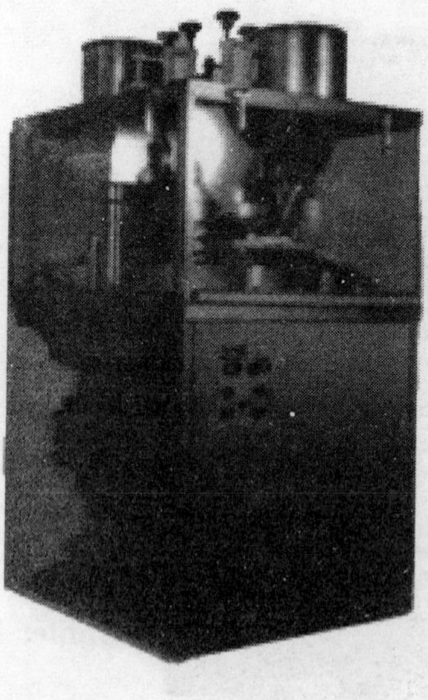

Double Sided Square Model GMP Tablets Press

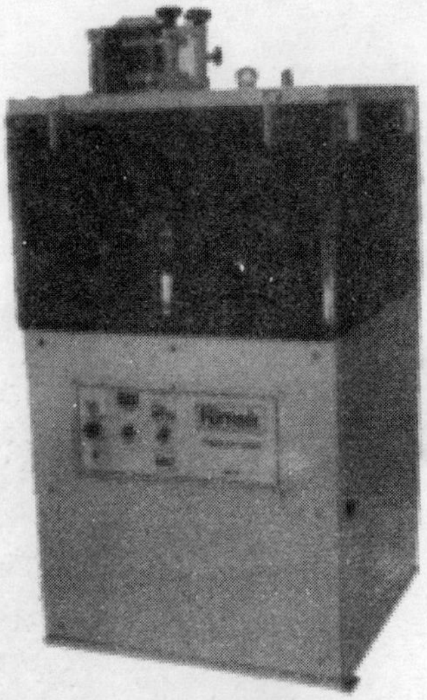

Single Sided Rotary Square Model GMP Tablet Press

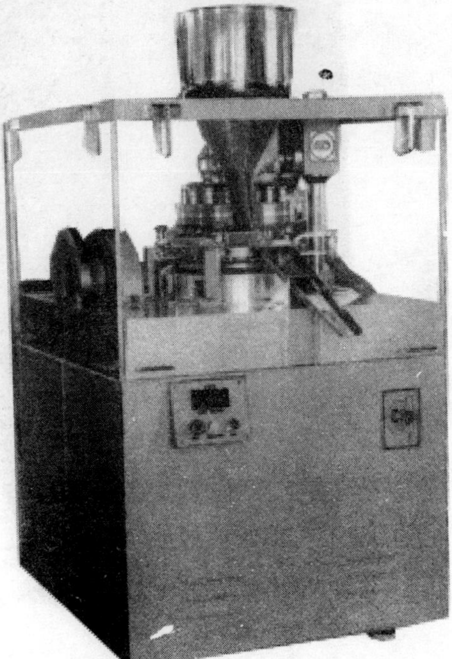

Rotary Tableting Machine

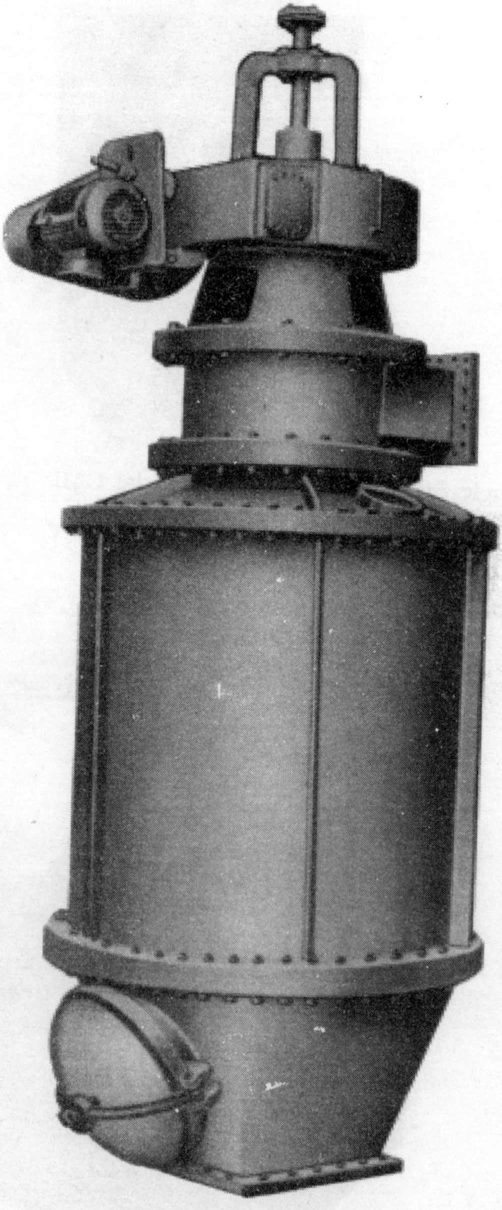

Vacuum Spraying Unit

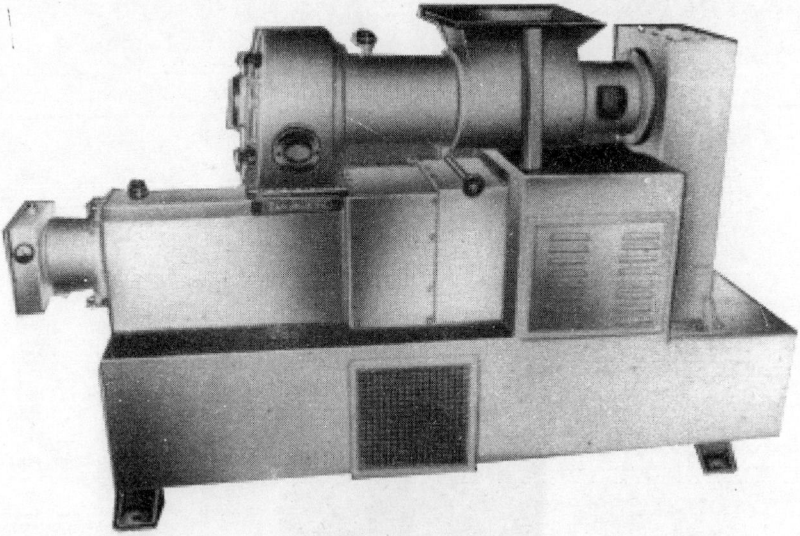

Plodder

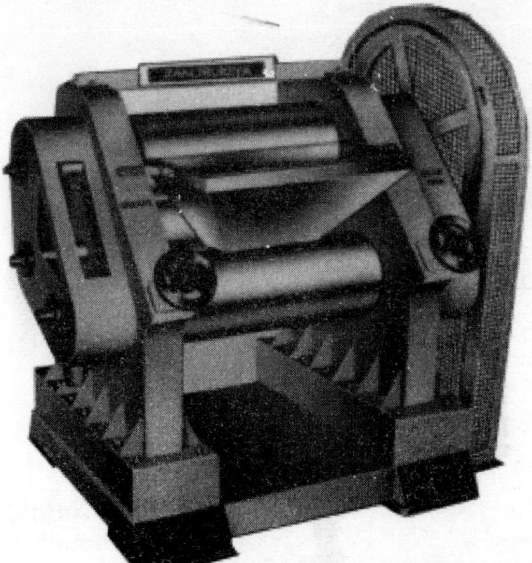

Three Roll Milling Machine

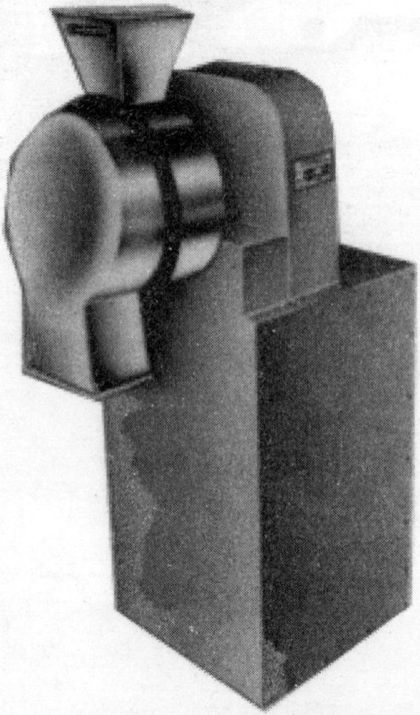

Soap Chips Making Machine

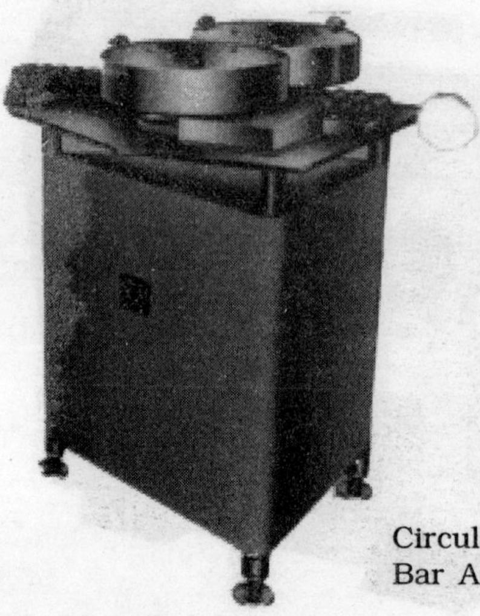

Circular Cutting Machine for Bar Automatic

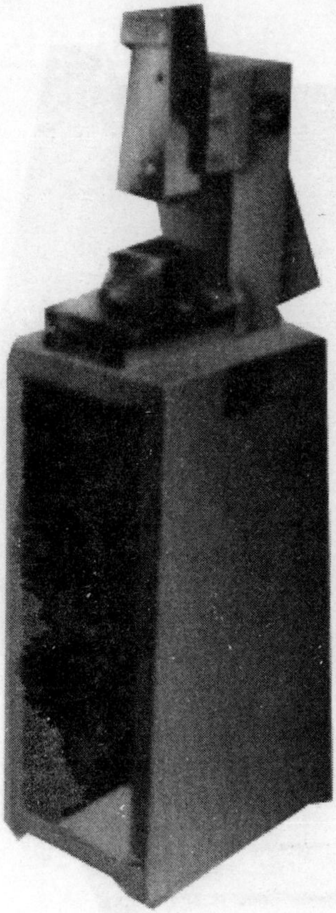

Foot Operated Stamping Machine

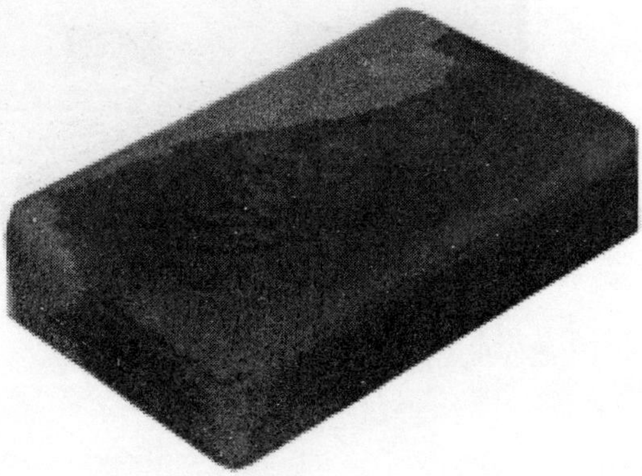

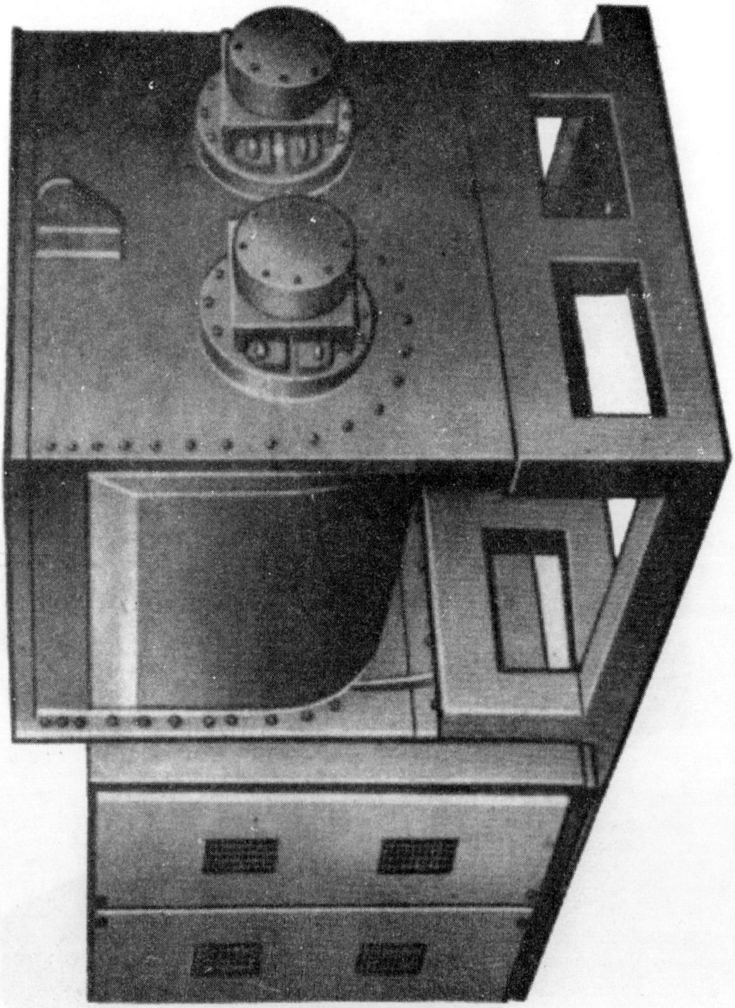

Mixer

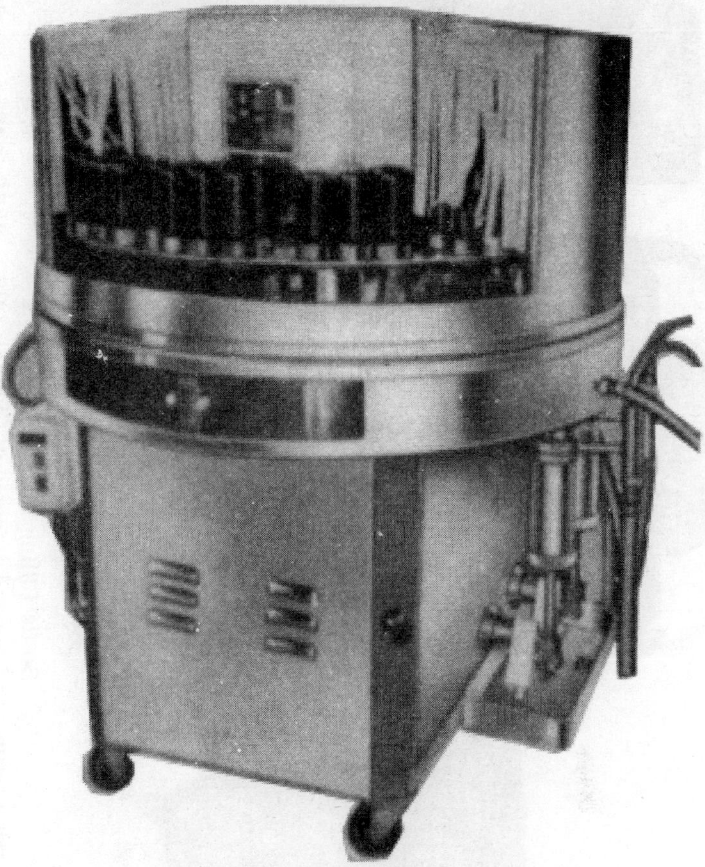

Rotary Bottle Washing Machine
Output - 60 to 80 per minute

Approx. Dimension :
Length 45" - Width 48" - Height : 62"

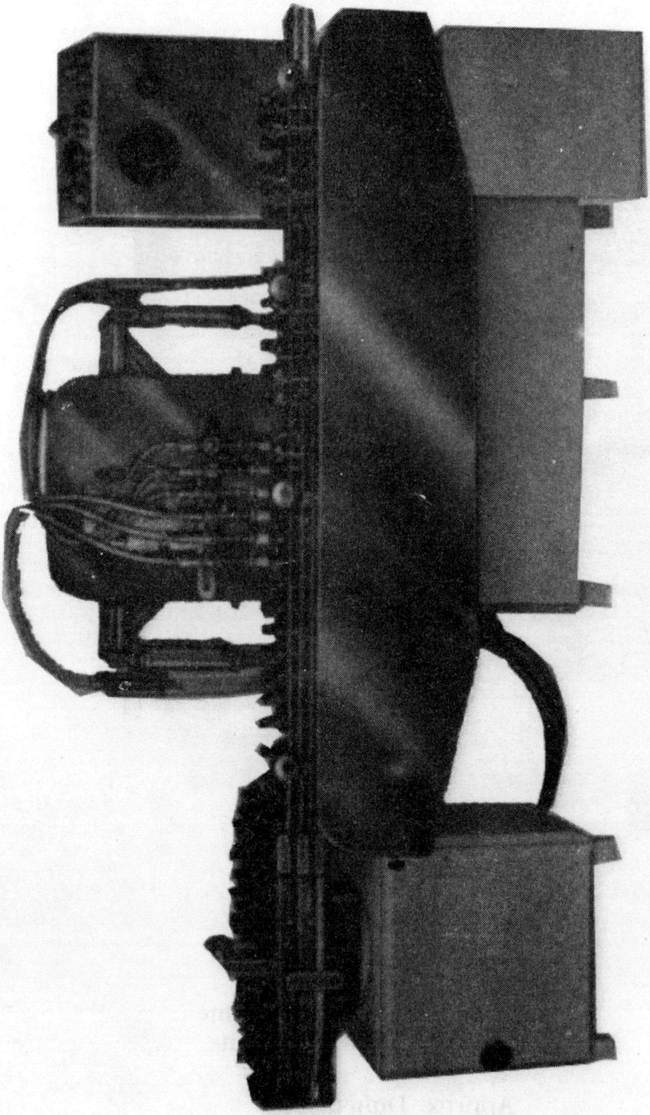

Bottle Filling Machine

Approx Dimensions : Length : 96" Width : 42" - Height 54"

Speed : 60 to 80 bottles per minute

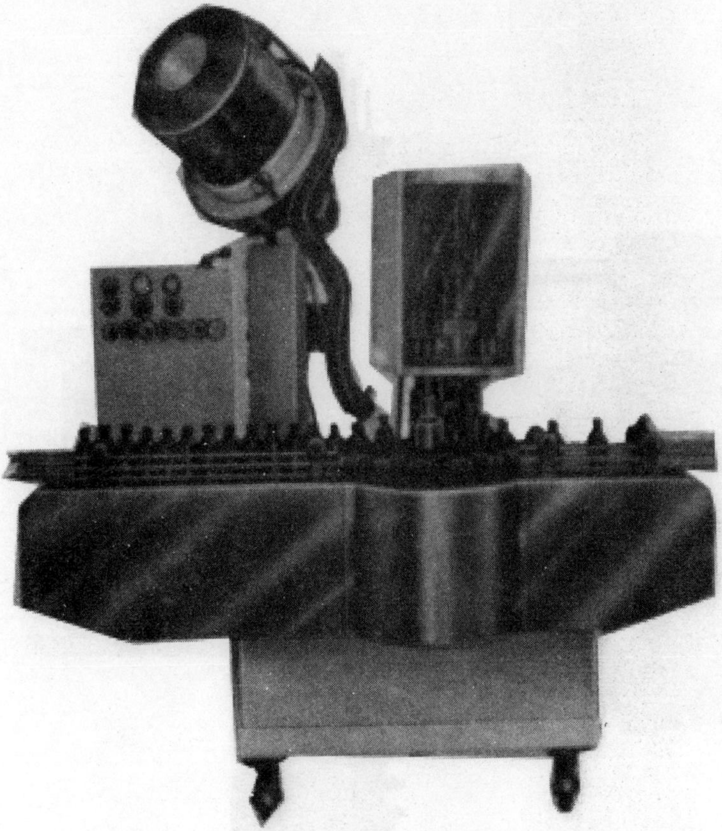

ABS - SSC Capping Machine
Speed - 60 - 80 bottles per minute

Approx Dimensions :
Length 84"
Width : 40"
Height : 72"

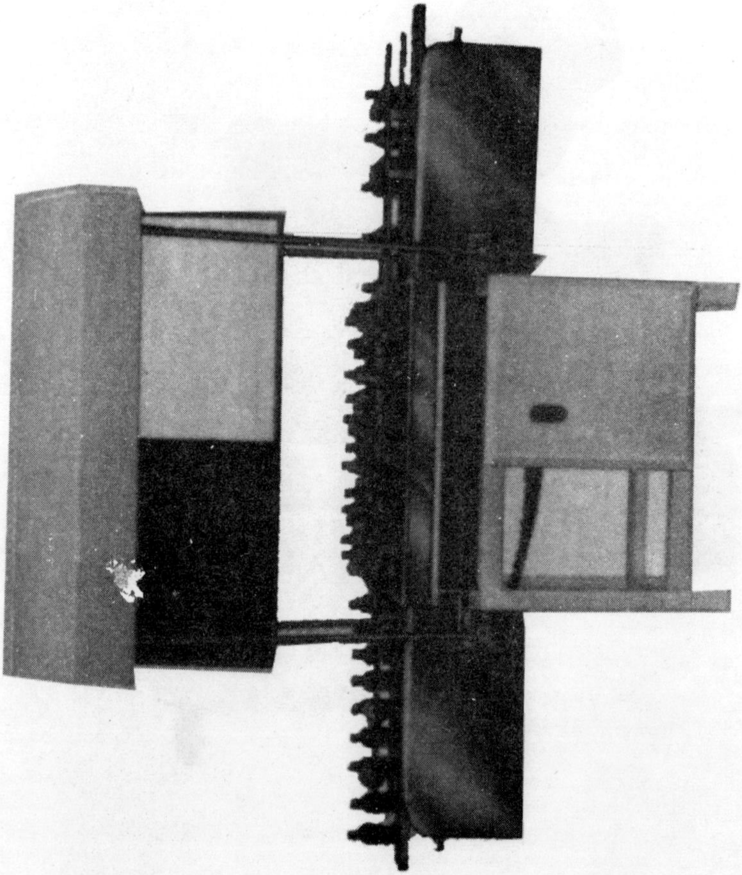

Bottle Checking Machine

Approx. Dimensions : Length : 72" - Width : 30" - Height : 66"

Speed - 60 to 80 bottles per minute

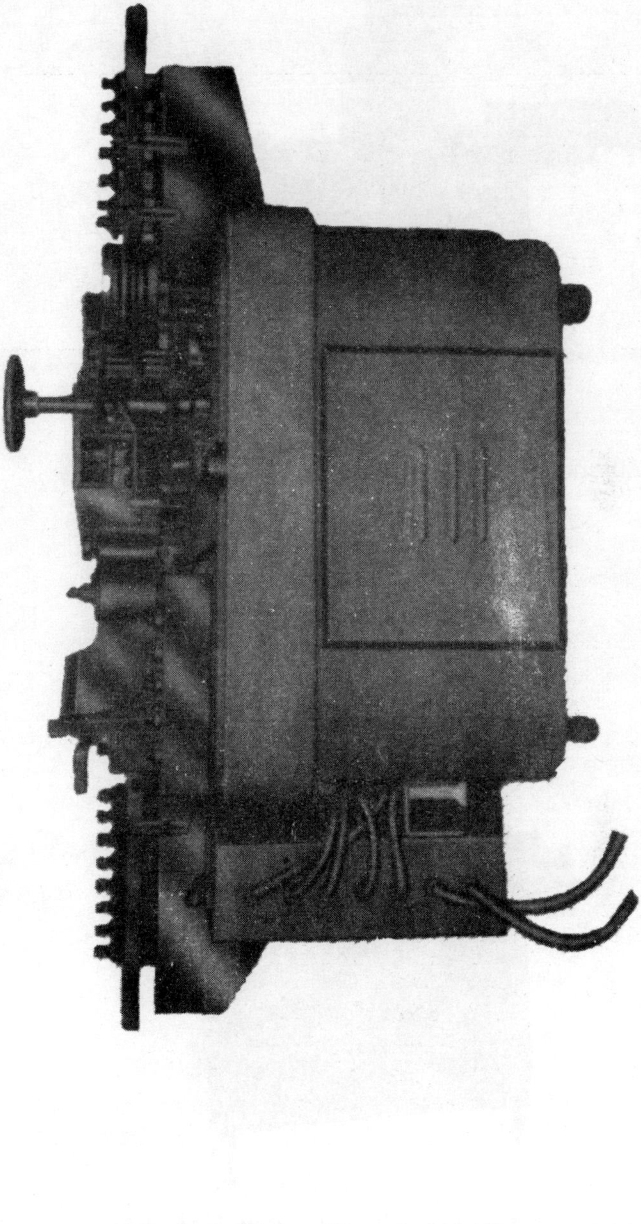

Bottle Labelling Machine
Speed - 80 to 100 bottles per minute.
Approx Dimensions : Length : 84" Width 40" Height : 40"

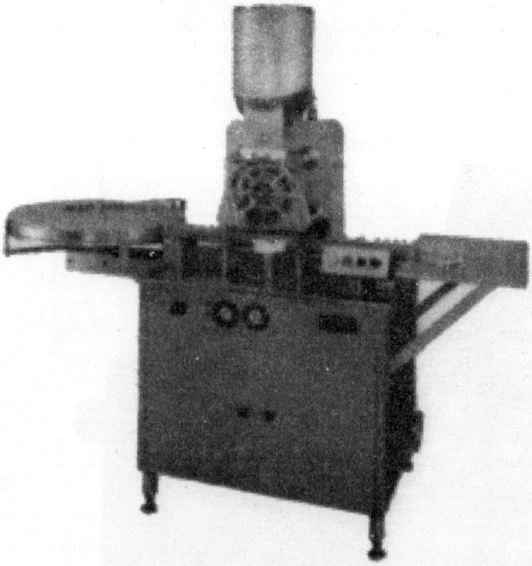

Automatic Injectable Powder Filling Machine

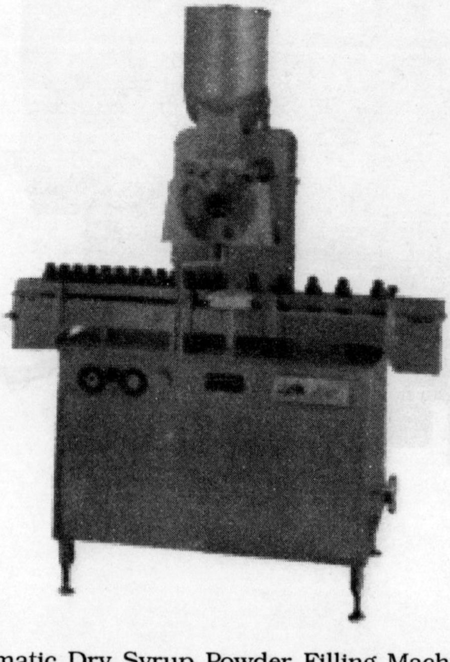

Automatic Dry Syrup Powder Filling Machine

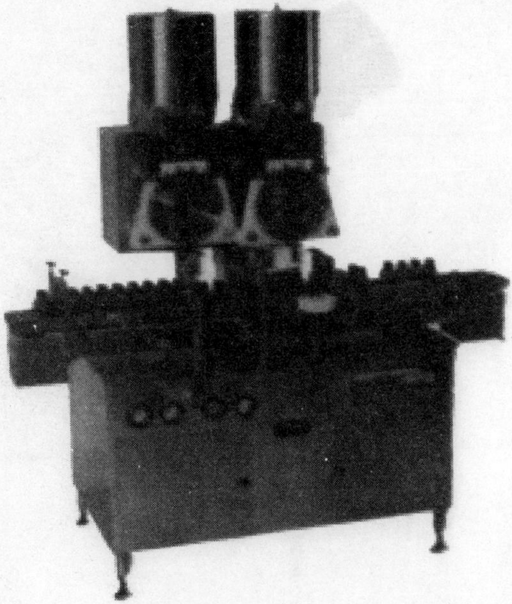

Automatic High Speed Dry Syrup Powder Filling Machine

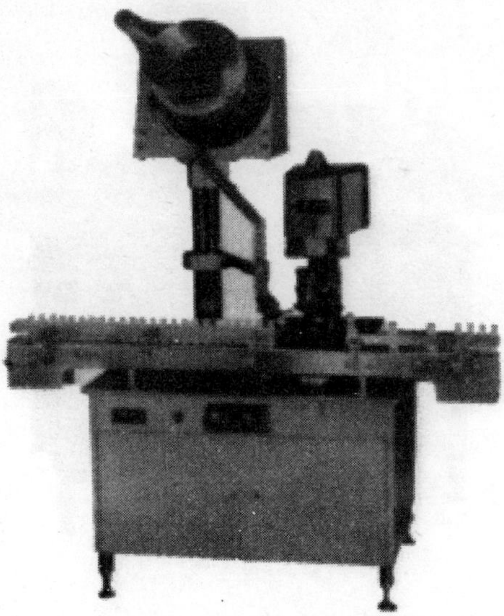

Automatic Single Head ROPP Cap Sealing Machine

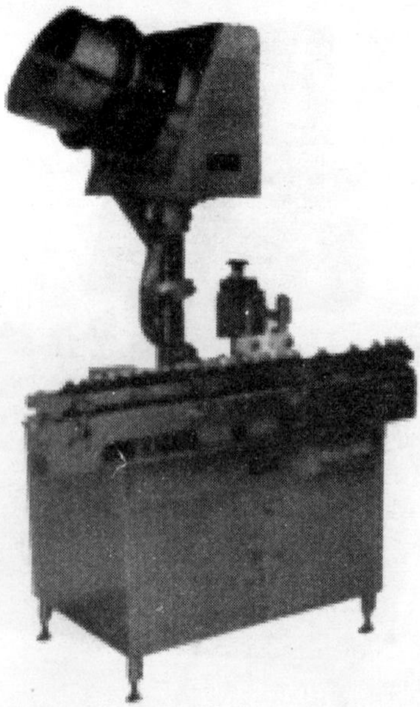

Automatic Measuring Cup Placement and Pressing Machine

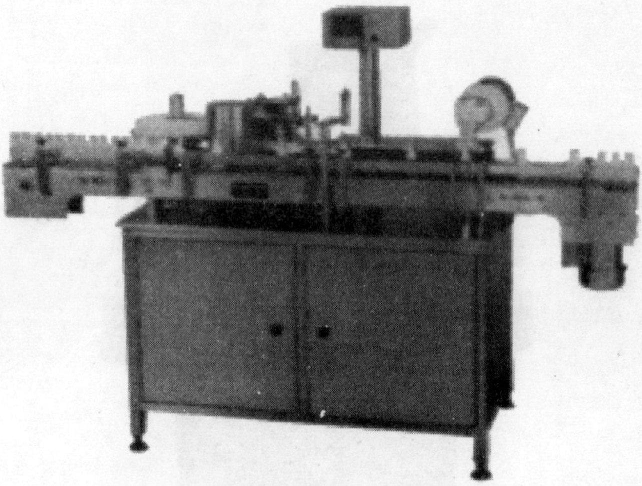

Auto Self Adhesive Vertical Labelling Machine

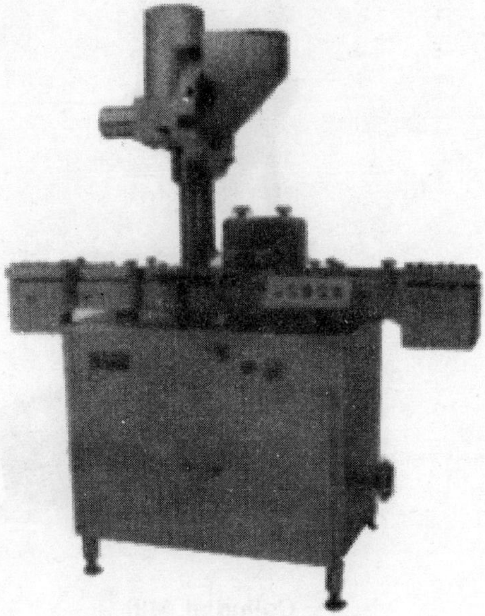

Automatic High Speed Rubber Stoppering M/C

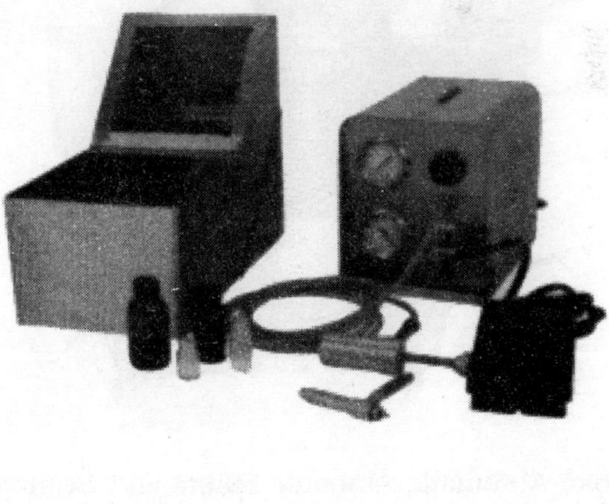

Semi Automatic Powder Filling Unit

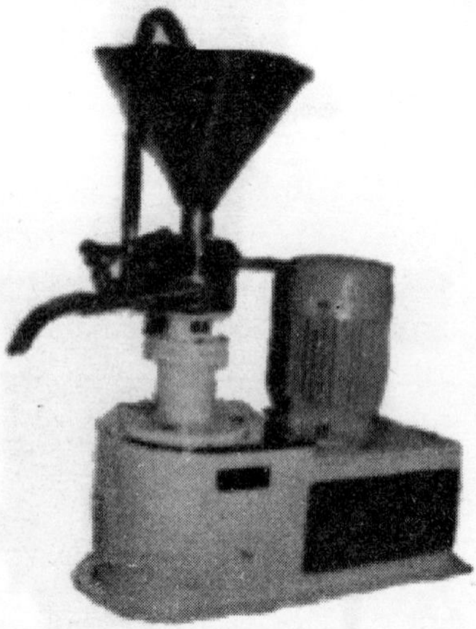

Collodial Mill

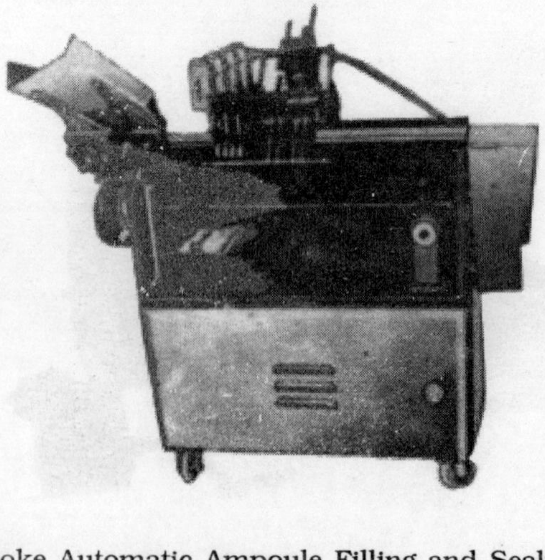

Four Stroke Automatic Ampoule Filling and Sealing Machine

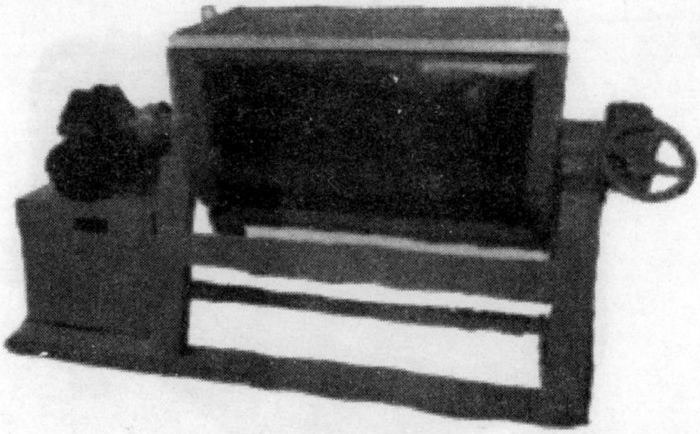

Mass Mixer

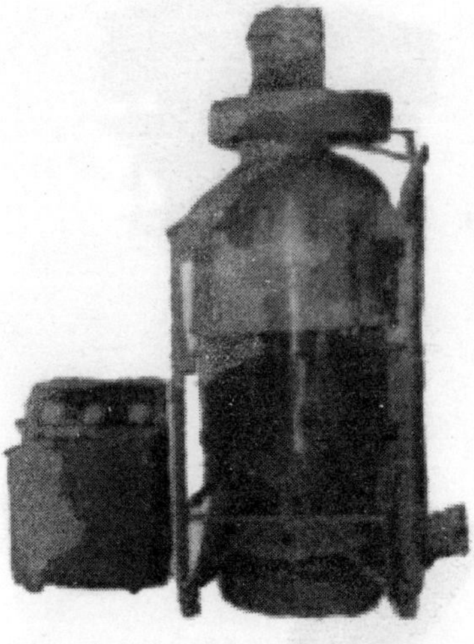

Fluid Bed Dryer

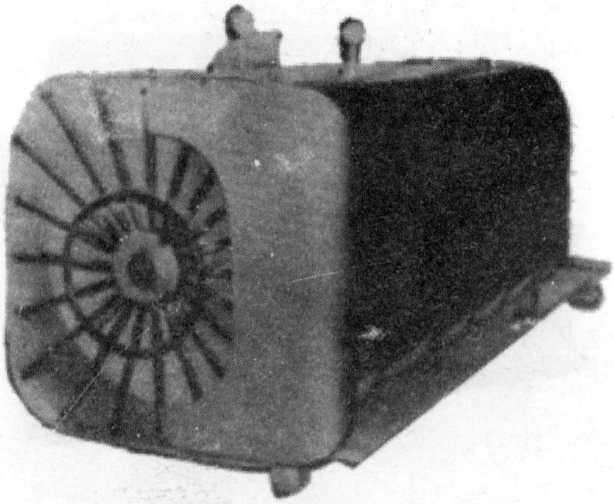

Autoclave

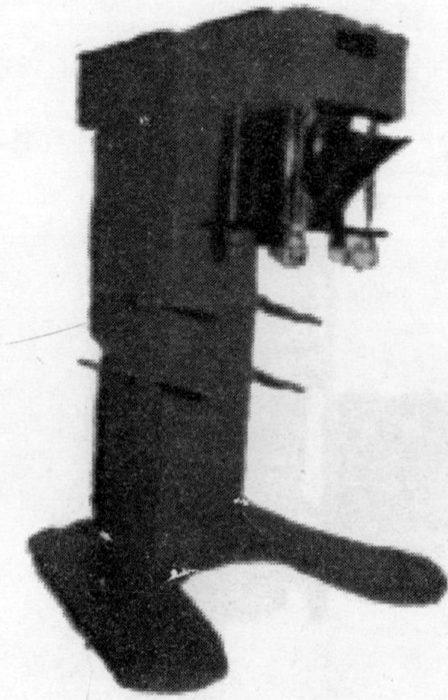

Granulator

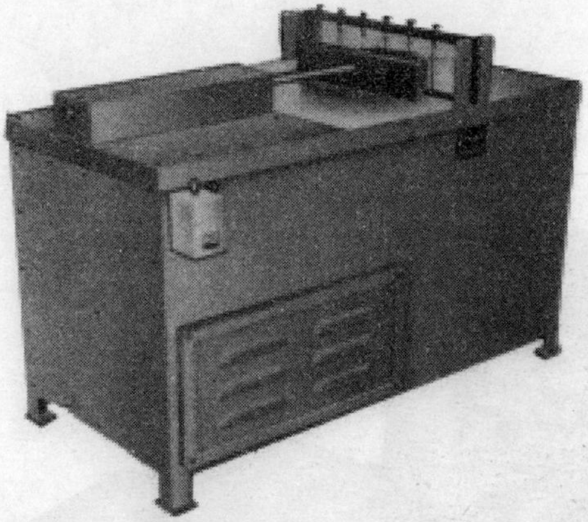

Cube Cabe Cutting Machine

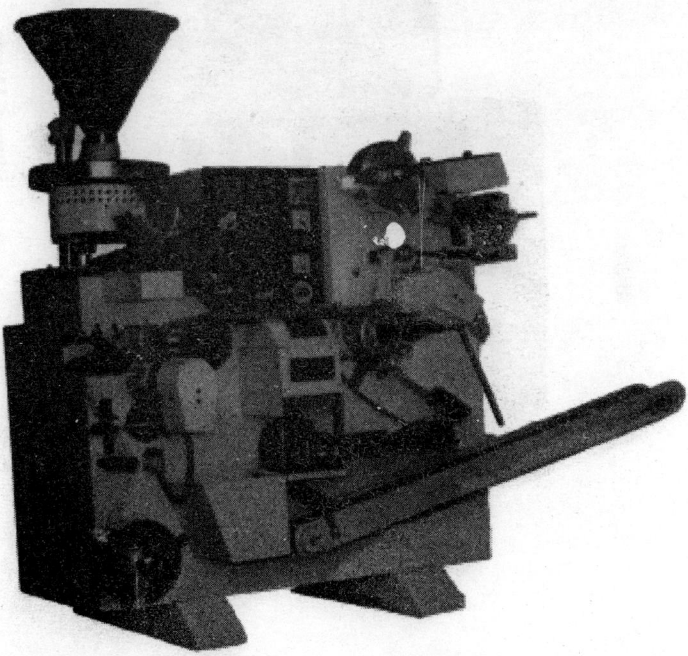

Blister Technology

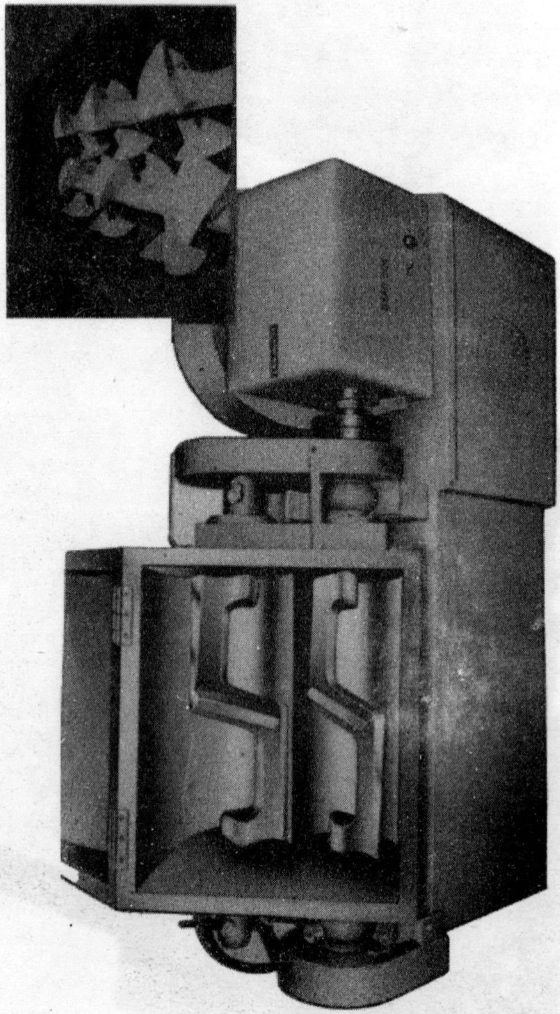

Sigma Mixer

13

Name of the Suppliers of Raw Material

For Tobacco

1. M/s. Chourasia Tobacco Industries
   B-27, Industrial Area, Jhilmil
   Shahdara, Delhi-110 032
   Phone : 2283212

2. M/s. Jagan Nath Dalip Singh
   526, G. T. Road, Ghaziabad
   Phones : 717226, 716725

3. M/s. Kalpana Chemicals
   303/307, Samual Street
   34 Abhishek Mumbai- 400003
   Phones : 022-3428402, 3439681
   Fax: 91-22-3436965

4. M/s Shree Sidh Nath Industries
   73-74, Vishal Nagar society,
   Adajan Road, New Water tank
   Surat-395009
   Phones : 0261-682109, 687810
   Fax : 0261-686109

5. M/s Bharat Jyoti
   22-S,Gandhi Marg (Princess Street)
   P.B. No. 2715, Mumbai- 400002
   Phone : 022-2012116,2064950
   Fax : 022-2053945, 2085977

6. M/s Kripa Chemicals Ltd
   Royal Chambers S. No.47
   Paud Road, Pune - 411038
   Phones : 212-333245, 331825
   Fax : 212-337191

7. M/s V. V. Deepa Aromatics Pvt. Ltd
20, Kastari Building Jamshedji Tata Road,
Churchgate, Mumbai- 400020
Phones : 233041, 233081

8. M/s R.A. Company Sayadwara,
Budaun-243601
Phones : 200,499

9. M/s. D.V. Deo, Post Box No. 135,
Cochin-682002
Phones : 24196, 26903, 802248

10. M/s. Creative Fragrance, 304, AVG Bhawan,
M-3,Connaught Circus, New Delhi-110001
Phones : (011) 3324100, 3324200
Fax : 91-11- 3317776

11. M/s Destilacione Berdas Chinchurreta s.a.
Oficinas Y Fabrica, Carretera De Carmona 30,
Fax : (95) 4417152
Phone : 449000 (11 Lines)
41008 Sevilla Apartado N-11

12. M/s Golden Sun Manufacturing Company,
70, Princes Street, Mumbai- 400002
Phones : 318054

Mentha Crystal

13. M/s Mentha and Allied Products Ltd.
Rahe- Raza, Civil lines Rampur, (U.P) Ind a
Phones : 24855, 24923
Fax : (0595) 34046

14. M/s. Rajshree Agro Chem.
T-4/56, Phase-1,
Mangalpure Industrial, Delhi- 110085
Phone : (011-07165916
Fax : (011) 7254944

15. M/s. Arihant Chemicals I.T.I. Road,
Aligarh- 202001 (U.P)
Phones : (0571) 402053, 402210

16. M/s . Everest Flavours and Fragrances
46, Wadia Building, 2nd Floor
9 B, Cowasji Patel Street, Fort
Mumbai-400001
Phones : 2873357, 2834726
Fax : 2872315

Mentha Oil

17. M/s. Procter and Gamble India Ltd.
Tiecicon House, Dr. E. Moses Road
Mumbai- 400011
Phones : 4925700
Fax : 91-22-4942115

18. M/s. Balsara Hygiene Product Ltd.
12A, Jorawar Bhawan
Maharshi Karve Road, Mumbai-400020
Phones : 022-256241, 295469
Fax : 91-22-942222

19. M/s. Central Institute of Medicinal and Aromatic Plants
Post Bag No. 1
Post Office : R.S.M. Nagar,
Lucknow

20. M/s. Alchem International (Pvt.) Ltd.
201 Empire Plaza
Mehrauli- Gurgon Road, Sultanpur,
New Delhi-30
Phones : 91-11-6803500/01/02/03
Fax : 91-11-6802101/C802423

22. M/s. Active Organics 11230 Cruder Street,
Dallas, Texas- 75238, USA
Phone : 214-348-2015
Fax : 214-348-1557

23. M/s. International Biochemicals
498, Kingston Road, Satellite,
Beach-FL - 32937, USA
Fax : (407) 777-4235, Phone:(407) 773-7457

Name of the Plant & Machinery Suppliers

For Mixing Vessel

1. M/s. Harrisons's Pharma Machinery Pvt. Ltd.
4648/21, Shedumal Building
Darya Ganj, New Delhi-110 002
Phones : 3275631, 3278924
Fax : 91-11-3285585

2. M/s. Chemical Engineering Corporation
Chandra Building, Kalkaji Temple
Post Bag No. 8, New Delhi-110 019
Phones : 6439427, 6439318, 6435318

3. M/s. Air Flow Pvt. Ltd.
13/1090, Hardhian Singh Road
Karol Bagh, New Delhi-110 005
Phone : 5721236

4. M/s. Indo-German Pharma Chem. Equipments
Kothan House, Plot A, B,
Off Cross Road, B-Street-5
M.I.D.C. Andheri (E)
Mumbai-400 093
Phones : 8342338, 8323615
Fax : 91-22-8374426

5. M/s. Pharma Mach
10, Chaupatty Road, Beliaghata
Calcutta-10
Phones : 3502567, 4756187

6. M/s. Sehgal Industrial Works
T-1698, Malkaganj Road, Subji Mandi
Delhi-110 007
Phone : 233823
Fax : 252038

For Drier

7. M/s. S.S.P. Private Ltd.
13, Mathura Road
Faridabad-121 003
Phones : (0129) 277442,, 277730, 275968
Fax : (0129) 277441

For Disintegrator

8. M/s. Kirloskar Brothers Ltd.
Udyog Bhawan, Tilak Road
Phune-411 002
Phone : 431056
Telex : 0145-247 KBPN IN

9. M/s. Air Flow Private Ltd.
13/1090, Hardhian Singh Road
Karol Bagh, New Delhi-110 005

10. M/s. Sanosil Chemicals (India) Pvt. Ltd.
VBC Warden House, Sir P.M. Road
Bumbai-400 001
Phones : (022) 2930186, 2872295
Fax : (022) 2873475

Packing Machine

1. M/s. Samarpan Fabricator Ltd.
plot No. A-182-183, Lane -Z
Road No. 16, Wagle Industrial Estate
Thane-400604
Phones : 505373, 505630, 505653

2. M/s. Crystal Engineeing Co. India
WZ-2 C/1, Basai Darapur,
Near Shiv Mandir
Delhi
Phone : 591628

3. M/s. Bakubhai Ambalal
Divsion of Sarabhai Machinery Ltd.
3. Marwah Estate, Sakivihar Road
Saki Naka
Mumbai-400072
Phone : 022-8501706, 8501753, 850805
Fax : 91-22-8503413

4. M/s. Gansons Engineers Pvt. Ltd.
118-121, Swastik Chambers
Office : Sion-Trombay Road, Chembur
Mumbai- 400071
Phones : 524548, 524967

5. M/s Ajay & Abhay Pvt. Ltd.
B-84/1, Okhla Industrial Area, Part - 11
New Delhi-110020
Phone : (011) 6831215, 6913010
Fax : (011) 6830190, 6833207

16. M/s. Bukubhi Ambalal
Division of Sarabhi Machinery Ltd.
3, Marwash Estate
Sakivihar Road, Sakinaka
Mumbai- 400072
Phone :8901706, 8501753
Fax :91-22- 8503413

17. M/s. Indogerman Pharma Chem. Equipments
Kothar Hopuse, Plot A, B Off Cross Road
B Street 5, M.I.D.C. Andheri (E)
Mumbai- 400093
Phone : 022-8342338, 8323615
Fax : 91-22-8374426

18. M/s. Sehgal Industrial Works
T- 1698, Malkaganj Road,
Subji Mandi
Delhi- 110007

19. M/s. Rollon Packaging (P) ltd.
Plot No. 329, Sector- 24
Faridabad- 121005
Phone : (011) 8-232603

20. M/s. Bakubhai Ambalal
Division of Sarabhai Maachinery Ltd.
3, Marwah Estate, Sakivihar Road, Sakinaka
Mumbai- 400072
Phones : 022-8501706, 8501753
Fax : 91-22-8503413

21. M/s. Mixofil India
H. No. 2869, Bulbuli Khana, Bazar Sitaram
Delhi - 110006
Phones : 011-3270735, 2263362

Evaportor, Extractor Manufcturer/ Fabricator

22. M/s. Industrial Service Company
Chemical Plant and Equipment Divsion
546, Marshall house, 33/1, Netaji Subhash Road, Calcutta-
Phone. Office : 033-220-4905/3566
Fax :91-33-330/3566

For Airfiltration

23. M/s. Pharama Mach
10, Chaulpatty Road, Beliaghata
Calcutta- 10
Phone : 3502567, 4756187

24. M/s. Ready Engineering works
Hall No. 8-9, D.S.I.D.C. Sheds
Raghubir Ngar
New Delhi- 27
Phone : 011-541037

25. M/s. Indogerman pharma Chem. Equipments
Kothari House, Plot A, B Off Cross Road
B- Street- M.I.D.C. Andheri (E)
Mumbai- 400093
Phones : 022-8342338, 8323615
Fax : 91-22-8374426

26. M/s. Sehgal Industrial Works
T- 1698, Mlaka Ganj Road, Subji Mandi
Delhi-110007
Phone :011-233823
Fax : 011-252038

27. M/s. Krishna Engineering Corporation
D-1/64, Dwarkesh Park
Near Bhatia School, Saibaba Nagar
Bonisli (W)
Mumbai- 400092
Phones :(022) 8610985, 8190200
Fax : 91-22-8195840

28. M/s. Sukhras Machines
145, Adarsh Induatrial Estate
Sahar Road, Chakala, Andheri (East)
Mumbai- 400099
Phones : 8322721, 8325957, 8325764

29. M/s. Richard Engineering (Bombay) Pvt. Ltd.
25, M.I.D.C. Chemical Zone, Ambarnath-421501
Phone: (0251) 582513, 583272
Fax : 91-0251-582785

30. M/s. Kotari Pharma
C/11, M.K. Brass Industrial Estate
Jaimari, Andheri Kurla Road, Andheri (E)
Mumbai-72
Phones : 851-0837/2794/3584
Fax : 91-22-8389961

31. M/s. Pragat Engineering Works
Plot No. W-B Shed No. W 88 (A)
Chinkhaloli-H.I.D.C. Ambernath- 421501
Phone :(0251) 582961
Fax : (0251)585054

32. M/s. Amin Machinery Instrument Manufacturers
C-1/12, G.I.D.C Esate
Vithal Udoyog Nagar-389121, Gujarat
Phone : (02692) 46029
Fax : (02692) 47443, 46439

33. M/s. Parishram Engineering works
115, Marol Co-operative Industrial Esate
Mathurdas Vasanji Road
Near Saki Naka,
Mumbai-400059
Phones : (022) 8504786/88, 8508662
Fax : (022) 8505979
Product Detail : Herbal Tonic

14

Foreign/Buyers/Sellers Processors/Manufacturers of Herbal/Traditional Single and Compound Medicinal Materials

1. M/s. A. Natterman and CIE GMBH
Nattermannallee 2, D-5000
Koln 30, Germany
Tel. : (49) 22150901
Fax : (49) 2215092711
Product Detail : Herbal Medicines and Herbal Teas

2. M/s. A Nelson and Co. Ltd.
5 Endeavour Way
Wimbeldon, London, SW5 9SX
U.K.
Tel. : (81) 94685527
Fax : (81)9466202
Product Detail : Homoeopathic Remedies and
OTC Products

3. M/s. A Strofali and Co. Ltd.
Meandrou Poleos 4
11524 Ambelokipa 1, Athens, Greece
Tel. : (30) 16420944
Product Detail : Herbal Remedies and
Food Supplements

4. M/s. Abkit INC
1160 Park Avenue, New York
NY 101128, U.S.A.
Tel. : (212) 8608358
Fax. : (212) 8600761
Product Detail : Hair and Body Care Product
and Homoeopathic Remedies

5. M/s. Aboca SRL
Frazione Aboca 20
52037 Sansepolcro (AR), Italy
Tel. : (575) 733509/735544/735454
Fax. : (575) 736185
Product Detail : Herbal Medicines, Food Supplements, Natural and Fruit Juice

6. M/s. Acta Pharmacal Co.
1131 N. Fair Oaks Ave
Sunnyvale, CA-94089
U.S.A.
Tel. : 408-734-1148
Fax : 308-734-1149
Product Detail : Cranberry/Kava/Echinacea/Ginseng/Golden/Seal/Green Tea/Saw Palmetto/Valer

7. M/s. Air Mancur
Jalan Raya Solo Seragen, KM7 Palur Solo
PO Box PT3, Sola-Fa Central jawa
Indonesia
Tel. : (62) 214240177
Product Detail : Traditional medicines & Natural Cosmetics

8. M/s. Alnoroil Co. Inc
70 East Sunrise Highway
Suit 418, Valley Stream
New York-11581
U.S.A.
Tel. : (516) 5616146
Fax. : (516) 5166123
Product Detail : Castor Oil, Tung Oil

9. M/s. Amax Industries INC
California, U.S.A.
Tel. : 909-869-7728
Fax. : 909-869-0986
Product Detail : Botainical Extracts/Pueraria/Stevia/Dhea Bilerry/Ginseng/Wild Yam/Ginkgo E

10. M/s. Arax Co. Ltd.
2-26 Marunocuchi, 3-Chome
Naka-KU, Nagoya 460
Japan
Tel. : (81) 529517211
Fax : (81) 529615005
Product Detail : Herbal & Folkloric Medicies and Pharmaceutical Products

11. M/s. Arkopharma (UK) Ltd.
6 Redlands Centre, redlands, Coulsden
Surrey, CR5 2HT, U.K.
Tel. : (81) 7631414
Fax : (81) 7632124
Product Detail : Herbal Medicine

12. M/s. Arokopharma Inc.
918 Gravenstein Avenue
Sebastopol, CA 95472, U.S.A.
Tel. : (707) 8290890
Fax : (707) 8291609
Product Detail : Herbal Remedies

13. M/s. Arno Wole's Nature System
P.B. No. 1014, Buesovej 19
Kattinge, DK-4000 Roskilde
Denmark
Tel. : (45) 02402867
Product Detail : Herbal Medicines

14. M/s. Arrowmed Ltd.
4 Pyramid House, 59 Winchester Road
Four Marks, Alton, Hampshire GU34 5HR
U.K.
Tel. : (420) 564300
Fax. : (420) 563564
Product Detail : Natural Products

15. M/s. Ashland
Fine Ingredients, Distribution Dept.
464, Box 2219, Colombus, OH 53216
U.S.A.
Tel. : (614) 7904343
Fax : (614) 7903465
Product Detail : Caffeine, Citrates, Colours
Dyes, Natural Gums

16. M/s. Asia Pharmaceutical Product
SDN BHD, 24 Lorang Mak Mandin Dua
Mukim 14, Butterworth, 13400 Penang
Malaysia
Tel. : (60) 4348488/542
Fax : (60) 4324566
Product Detail : Pharmaceutical Products and
Herbal Remedies

—

17. M/s. Asta Medica
Weissmullerstrasse 45
Po Box 100105, D, 6000 Frankfurt
Germany
Tel : (49) 6940010
Fax : (49) 6940012741
Product Detail :Herbal Medicine And ethical Pharmaceuticals

18. M/s. Ban Choon Tong SDN BHD
85 HUGH LAW ST, 30000 IPON
Perak Darnl Ridzuan
Mallaysia
Tel : (60) 5549648
Fax : (60) 5501215
Product Detail : Herbal Medicines, Medicianal

19. M/s. Beaufour Ipsen
42, Rue Du Docteur Blanche
75016 Paris
France
Tel : (33) 144304343
Fax :(33) 144304321
Product Detail : Natural Medicinal Products And Vasoactive Medications

20. M/s. Beeking (Thailand) Ltd.
1011-1013 Mangkorn Road,Chaikkawad
Samphantawong
Bangkok, Thailand
Tel :(66) 2229286
Fax :(66) 22558268
Product Detail : Bee Product

21. M/s. Bio- Strang AG
Muhlebachstrasse 25
Postfach 8032, Zurich
Switzerland
Tel : (41) 12518151
Fax : (41) 12624326
Product Detial : Herbal Tonics And Remedies

22. M/s. Biobotanica Inc.
75 Commerce Drive, Happauge,NY 11788
U.S.A.
Tel : (516)2315522
Fax :(516) 2317332
Product Detail : Herbal Extracts, Homeopathic Creams And Herbal Remedies, Botanical Extract.

23. M/s. Bioforce (UK) Ltd.
Olympic Business Park, Dundonald
DA2 9BE
U.K.
TEl : (563) 851177
Fax : (563) 851173
Product Detail : Herbal and Homoeopathic Remedies

24. M/s. Bioforce AG, Postfach 76
CH-9325 Roggmil TG
Switzerland
Tel : (41) 71483101
Fax : (41) 71481968
Product Detail : Herbal and Homoeopathic Medicine

25. M/s. Bioforce of America Ltd.
PO Box 507, Kinderhook
NY 12106
U.S.A.
Tel : (518) 7586060
Fax : (518) 7589500
Product Detail :Herbal and Homoeopthic Remedies

26. M/s. Biona
Endustreprike Ni
4800 Neukubihg F
Denmark
Product Detail : Herbal Medicines

27. M/s. Bionorica GMBH
Kerschshensteinerstr 11-15
Postfach 67
D-8430 Newmarkt 10 PF
Germany
Tel : (49) 918123190
Fax : (49) 9181231265
Product Detail : Ethical Herbal Medicines

28. M/s. Bolak CO. Ltd
San 60-1 Songsan-RI
Yangham- Myun Hwasumg- Kun
Kyungki-DO
Korea
TEl : (0339) 524341
Fax : (0339) 5264558
Product Detail : Pharmaceutical Products and Traditional Herbal Medicines

29. M/s. BO Ryung Pharmaceutical Co. Ltd
5th Floor, Eun-Seok Bldg.
1-30 Yonji- dong, Chongro-Ku
Korea
Tel : (020 7638981-90
Fax : (02) 7440682
Product Detial : Traditional Herbal Medicines and Pharmaceuticals Product

30. M/s. Boehringer Ingelheim GMBH
Postfach 200
D-6507 Ingrlheim-AM-Rhein
Germany
Tel : (49) 6132770
FAx : (49) 613277383
Product Detail : Herbal Medicines and Ethical Pharmaceuticals

31. M/s. Boericke And Tafel
2381 Ciradian Way
Santa Rosa CA 95407
U.S.A
Tel : (707) 5718202
Fax : (717) 5718237
Product Detail : Homoeopathic Remedies

32. M/s. Boiron
20 RUE DE LA Liberation
69110 Sainte Foye Lyon
France
Tel : (33) 72324020
Fax : (33) 78596916
Product Detail : Homeopthic and Herbal Remedies

33. M/s. Bon Cho
595-39 Jinchun-Dong
Talseo-Ku, Daegu
Korea
Tel : (53) 633-115-7
Product Detail : Korean Traditional Medicine and
Pharmaceutical Product

34. M/s. Bonusan Bv
Groeneweg 25
3281 XB Numansdrop
Netherlands
Tel : (31) 18651022/1646
Fax : (31) 18654221
Product Detail : Herbal and Homoeopathic Medicines

35. M/s. Boots Healthcare International
Castle Quay, Castle Boulevard
Nottingaham, NG2 3AA
U.K.
Tel :(602) 688622
Fax ;(602) 498312
Product Detial : Otc Pharmaceuticals

36. M/s. Botanical Interantional
2550 El Presidio Street,
Long Beach, CA 90810
U.S.A.
Tel : 310-637-9566
Fax : 310-637-3644
Product Detail : Botanical Extracts, powders, Solids,
Fluids, Standardized Extracts

37. M/s. Brewhurst Health Food Supliers
Abbot Close, Oyster lane, Byfleet
Surrey, KT14 7JP
U.K.
Tel : (932) 354211
Fax : (932) 336235
Product Detail : Herbal Remedies, Health food, Pharmacies

38. M/s. Bu Kwang Pharm Ind.
398-1 Daebang- Ding
Kongjak- Ku, Seoul
Korea
Tel : (02) 8123251-60
Fax : (02) 8123251-60
Product Detail : Traditional Herbal Medicines and Pharmaceutical Products

39. M/s. Camden Industries(M) SDN BHD
998 Solok Pernsahaan Tiga
Kawasan Miel, prai Indl. Estate
13600 prai penang
Malaysia
Tel : (60) 4307319
Fax : (60) 4397234
Product Detail : Traditional Chinese Medicines, Haie & Oral Product

40. M/s. Camstar Berahal products Ltd.
Chesnut farm Eye
Suffolk IP23 7HN
U.K.
Tel : (01379) 870669
Fax : (01379) 870683
Product Detail : Growers, processors of fresh Herbs, Air Dried, Freze Dried and Herbs in

41. M/s. Carlo Sesso Spa
Viale gramsci 212, 20099 Sesto San Giovanni (Mi)
Italy
Tel : (02) 26222227
Fax : (02) 2428070
Product Detail : Herbal Medicines, Health Foods, Natural Cosmetics

42. M/s. Carls- Bergh
Biokeemiska AB, Box 47076
40298 Goteborg
Swden
Tel : (46) 31480010
Fax : (46) 31432571
Product Detial : Herbal Medicines

43. M/s. Casa Santiveri Sa
Calle, Barcelona
Spain
Tel. : (34) 32230099
Fax : (34) 30030295
Product Detail : Herbal & Dietetic Products

44. M/s. Cedar Health Ltd.
Peppar Raod, Hazel Grove
Cheshire, SK7 5BW
U.K.
Tel. : (61) 4831235
Fax : (61) 45664321
Product Detail : Herbal Products

45. M/s. Cederroths
International AB, Pox 715
S-19427 Upplands Vasby
Sweden
Tel. : (46) 859086080
Fax : (46) 859092795
Product Detail : Herbal Medicines

46. M/s. CelestialSeasonings Inc.
4600 Sleepytime Drive
Boulder, CO 80301
U.S.A.
Tel. : (303) 5305300
Product Detail : Herbal and Medicinal Teas, Health Food Products

47. M/s. Cha Krom Pion
229 Chakanati Road, Bangkok
Thailand
Tel. : (66) 2113272
Product Detail : Traditional Thai Medicine

48. M/s. Charles Gordon Assoc. Ltd.
Littlemead Indl. Estate, Gordon House
Cranleigh Surrey, G48 8ND
U.K.
Tel. : (01483) 267707
Fax : (01483) 267783
Product Detail : Mustards

49. M/s. Chart Corporation Inc.
787, East 27th ST
Paterson, NJ 07504
U.S.A.
Tel. : 201345-5554
Fax : 201-345-2239
Product Detail : Botanical Extracts, Food, Flavour, Health care, Cosmetics Products

50. M/s. Chief Foods & Chemicals Inc.
7th Floor, Sam-Sung Bldg.
50 Eulchi--RO 1-GA
Chung-Ku, Seoul
Korea
Tel. : (02) 7758751
Fax : (02) 7734915
Product Detail : Traditional Herbal Medicines and Pharmaceutical Products

51. M/s. Chia Shin Trading Co. Ltd.
RM712, 152 Sung Chiang Road
7th Floor Hung Tai sungkiang Bldg.
Taipei, Taiwan
Tel. : (886) 25641700
Fax : (886) 25426694
Product Detail : Chinerse Traditional Medicines, Cosmetics and Health Food

52. M/s. Cho Dang Pharm Co. Ltd.
44 Kuro-5 Dong
Kuro-Ku, Seoul, Korea
Tel. : (02) 8690181
Fax : (02) 8690181
Product Detail : Traditional Herbal medicines and Pharmaceutical Products

53. M/s. Cho Seon Pharm & Trading Co. Ltd.
339--1 Daebang-Dong
Dongjak-Ku, Seoul
Korea
Tel. : (02) 8172011
Fax : (02) 8133133
Product Detail : Traditional Herbal Medicines and Pharmaceutical Products

54. M/s. Christaens
Chausee De Gent 615, 1080 Bruxelles
Belgium
Tel. : (32) 24640611
Fax : (32) 24640698
Product Detail : Herbal Teas

55. M/s. Chun He Pharm. Co. Ltd.
246-47 Dodang-Dong
Bucheon-City, Kyungki-Do
Korea
Tel. : (032) 6766320
Product Detail : Traditional herbal Medicines and
Pharmaceutical Products

56. M/s. Chun Il Pharmaceutical Co. Ltd.
173-14 Dongkyo-Dong
Mapo-KU, Seoul, Korea
Tel. : (02) 3351001
Fax. : (02) 3321001
Product Detail : Traditional Herbal Medicies

57. M/s. Chung Gei Pharm Co. Ltd.
94-69 Youngdeungpo-Dong
7-GA, Youngdeungpo-Ku, Seoul, Korea
Tel. : (02) 6772828
Fax : (02) 6775911
Product Detail : Traditional Herbal Medicines and
Pharmaceutical Products

58. M/s. Commerciale Winter SRL
Via Albisola 51, 16163 Genova
Bolzaneto, Italy
Tel.: (010) 720154/720215/720244
Fax. : (010) 720241
Product Detail : herbal Medicines, Food Supplements,
Propolis and Sports Nutrition Product

59. M/s. Cornucopia Natural Foods Inc.
260 Lake Road
Dayville, CT 06241, U.S.A.
Tel. : (203) 7792800
Fax : (203) 7792812
Product Detail : Health Food, Herbs and
Natural Medicines

60. M/s. CPL
Rue De L'Industrie
Zone Industrielle, 3895 Foetz-GR D
Luxembourg
Tel. : (352) 556066
Product Detail : Herbal Products

61. M/s. Creeer
Rua Da Madalena 171--2, 1100 Lisbon
Portugal
Tel. : (351) 1872165
Product Detail : Herbal Medicines

62. M/s. D Ulrich
Via Pisacane 9, 10042 Nichelinao (TO)
Italy
Tel. : (011) 625824
Fax. : (011) 625893
Product Detail : Herbal Medicines, Health Foods and Herbal Extracts

63. M/s. Dae Do Pharm Co. Ltd.
167-1 Nae-Dong, Chung-Ku
Bucheon, Kyungki-Do
Korea
Tel. : (032) 6748023
Fax. : (032) 6719058
Product Detail : Traditional Herbal Medicines and Pharmaceutical Products

64. M/s. Dae He Pharmaceutical Co. Ltd.
8-48 Kalwol-Dong
Yongsan--Ku, Seoul
Korea
Tel. : (02) 7540631
Fax. : (02) 7756165
Product Detail : Traditional Herbal Medicines and Pharmaceutical Products

65. M/s. Dae IL Pharm.Co. Ltd.
742-5 Banpo-Dong
Seocho-Ku, Seoul, Korea
Tel. : (02) 5492164
Product Detail : Traditional Herbal Medicines and Pharmaceutical Products

66. M/s. Dae Lim Pharm Co. Ltd.
164-98 Anyoung-RI
Teahn-Myun, Hwasung-Kum
Kyungki-Do, Korea
Tel. : (0331) 321819
Fax : (0331) 327018
Product Detail : Traditional Herbal Medicines and Pharmaceutical Products

67. M/s. Dai Wang Pharmaceutical Co. Ltd.
7 Bongrae-Dong, 1-GA
Chung-Ku, Seoul, Korea.
Tel. : (02) 7525871
Fax : (02) 7510937
Product Detail : Traditional Herbal Medicines and Pharmaceutical Products

68. M/s. Daischi Yakuhin Kogyo Co. Ltd.
Toyama 930
Japan
Tel. : (81) 764328571
Fax : (81) 764528626
Product Detail : Kampo and Pharmaceutical Medicines

69. M/s. Daisho Pharmaceutical Corp.,
168 Koka-Cho, Oharaichiba
Koka County, Shiga-Pref (520-34)
Japan
Tel. : (81) 748884181
Fax : (81) 748882181
Product Detail : Herbal and Folkloric Medicines

70. M/s. Danske Droge A/s
DK 2635 Ishoj, Industrieskellet 20
Denmark
Tel. : (45) 43542444
Fax : (45) 43540102
Product Detail : Herbal Medicines

71. M/s. Dawood Trading Co.
10 Palm Street No. 4, Old Anarkali
P.O. Box 1277, Lahore
Pakistan
Tel. : (92) 42251986
Product Detail : Unani, Herbal Medicines

72. M/s. Denolin
152 Rue Des Cogons, Bruselles 1070
47 Rue Du Chateau
1400 Braine l'Allende, Belgium
Tel. : (32) 25210105
Fax : (32) 23850257
Product Detail : Herbal Teas, Combinations and Powdered Herbs

73. M/s. Dietisa Sa
C/Ventuka Plasa 9, 08028 Barcelona
Spain
Tel. : (34) 34224100
Fax : (34) 34319050
Product Detail : Herbal Remedies, Dietary Supplements

74. M/s. Diplan Sa
Avda De Laredo Nave 8D
Polig Industrial "El Alamo"
Fuenlabrada (Madrid), Spain
Tel. : (34) 16154592
Fax : (34) 16158787
Product Detial : Health Fods, Dietary Supplements

75. M/s. Distribourg
217 Chemin Du Grand--Revoyet
69561 Saint-Genis-Laval, Cedex
France
Tel. : (33) 72399797
Fax. : (33) 72399456
Product Detail : Herbal Products

76. M/s. Dolisos Sa
62 Rue Beaubourg
F-75003, Paris 03, France
Tel. : (33) 142719616
Product Detail : Homoeopathic Remedies

77. M/s Dong Koo Pharmaceutical Co. Ltd.
195-2 Kocheok-Dong
Kuro-Ku, Seoul, Korea
Tel. : (02) 6845421-5
Fax : (02) 6811880
Product Detail : Traditional Herbal medicines and Pharmaceutical Products

78. M/s. Dong Kook Pharmaceutical Co. Ltd.
997-8 Dae Chi-3 Dong
Kang Nam-Ku, Seoul
Korea
Tel. : (02) 55311671/5
Fax : (02) 5668542/7812
Product Detail : Traditional Korean Medicines
Pharmaceutical and Oral Hygiene Product Heal

79. M/s. Dong Shin Pharm Co. Ltd.
884-3 Daechi-Dong
Kangnam-Ku, Seoul
Korea
Tel. : (02) 5569966
Fax : (02) 5578898
Product Detail : Traditional Herbal Medicines and
Pharmaceutical Products

80. M/s. Dong Sung Pharm. Co. Ltd.
234-20 Nonhyun-Dong
Kangnam-Ku, Seoul
Korea
Tel. : (02) 5490921-6
Fax : (02) 5444192
Product Detail : Traditional Herbal Medicines and
Pharmaceutical Products

81. M/s. Dong Wha Pharm. Ind. Co. Ltd.
5 Soonwha-Dong
Chung-Ku, Seoul
Korea
Tel. : (02) 7784331
Fax : (02) 7574677
Product Detail : Traditional Herbal Medicines and
Pharmaceutical Products

82. M/s. Dong Yang Pharmaceutical Co. Ltd.
7-281 Pongcheon-Dong
Kwanak-Ku, Seoul
Korea
Tel. : (02) 8731617
Product Detail : Traditional Herbal Medicines and
Pharmaceutical Products

83. M/s. Donmar Health and Beauty Product
210-Denison Street
Markham, On L3R 1B6, Canada
Tel. : (416) 4756530
Fax : (416) 4759698
Product Detail : Herbs and Natural Medicines

84. M/s. Dr. Reckeweg and Co. GMBH
Berliner Ring 32, 6140 Bessheim, Germany
Tel : (49) 625110970
Fax : (49) 62513342
Product Detail : Homoeopathic Remedies

85. M/s. Dr. Willmar Schwabe GMBH
Willmar Schwabe Strasse 4
Box 410925,D7500 Karlsruge, Germany
Tel. : (49) 72140050
Fax : (49) 7214005202
Product Detail : Herbal Medicines, Homoeopathic Remedies

86. M/s. Eagle and Pagoda Brand
Teck Aun med. Fty
486-489 Jin Sungai Rambai
14000 Bukit Mertajam, Penang, Malaysia
Tel. : (60) 4511533
Fax : (60) 4593675
Product Detail : Traditional Chinese Medicines and Pharmaceutical

87. M/s. Earthrise Trading Co. Inc.
424 Payran Street, Petaluma, CA 44952
U.S.A.
Tel. : (707) 7789078
Fax : (707) 7789028
Product Detail : Herbal Remedies, Food Supplements and Primary Algai Production

88. M/s. Eastern Pharmaceutical Co. Ltd.
547-9 Seungdoo-Ri
Gongdo-Myun, Ansung-Kum
Kyungki-Do, Korea
Tel. : (033) 532319
Fax : (033) 530829
Product Detail : Traditional Herbal Medicines and Pharmaceutical Products

89. M/s. Eclectic Institute Inc.
14385 Se Lusted Road
Sandy, OR 97055, U.S.A.
Tel. : (502) 6684420
Fax : (503) 6683227
Product Detail : Herbal Extracts, Freezze Dried Herbas and Nutritional Supplements

90. M/s. English Grains Health Care
Swains Park, Industrial Estate
Park Road, Overseal
Burton-on-Trent, Staffs, DE12 6TT
U.K.
Tel. : (283) 221616
Fax : (283) 550185
Product Detail : Herbal Medicines, Health Supplements

91. M/s. Enzymatic Therapy
825 Challenger Drive, Green Bay
Wislonsin, W1 54311
U.S.A.
Tel. : (414) 4891313
Fax : (414) 4374087
Product Detail : Herbal Extracts, Herbal Capsules, Nutritional Supplements

92. M/s. Erba Vita BLF
Piazza Immacolata 1-CP
241-88074 Crotone (CZ)
Italy
Tel. : (0962) 2414025472
Product Detail : Herbal Teas and Natural Cosmetics (Shampoos)

93. M/s. Erabavita
Del Dr. Carlo Bollini
Via selve Dei Baudi 20
47031 Murata-Rep San Marino
Italy
Tel. : (0549) 999163
Fax : (0549) 999163
Product Detail : Herbal Teas, Natural Cosmetics
Herbal Medicines

94. M/s. Erola
Viale Dell Industria 49
20037 Paderno, Dugnano (MI)
Italy
Tel. : (02) 9105217
Fax : (02) 99040945
Product Detail : Herbal Medicines, Herbal Teas, Health Foods and Propolis

95. M/s. Eurosalus Srl
Piazzale Dei Legnami 1
34145 Trieste, Italy
Tel. : (040) 824777/380322
Fax : (040) 828944
Product Detail : Health Foods, Heral Medicines and Chinese Herbal Teas

96. M/s. Ever Honor Industries Inc.
9F-3203 Ho-Ping East Road
Sec. 2, Taipei, Taiwan
Tel. : (886) 27043326/7082366
Fax : (886) 27050736
Product Detail : Traditional Chinese Medicines, Natural Herbal Nutritional Supplements

97. M/s. Extracts Plus
2770 Loker Avenue West
Carlsbad Ca 92008
U.S.A.
Fax : 6194318610
Product Detail : Steria

98. M/s. Farga
Rua Cidade De
Manchester 15, 1100 Lisbon
Portugal
Tel. : (351) 1825544
Product Detail : Natural Product

99. M/s. Ferrosan
Sydmarken 5, DK-2860, Soeborg
Denmark
Tel. : (45) 39692111
Fax: (45) 39696518
Product Detail : Herbal Medicines

100. M/s. Firma Gooderd
Zoning Hirebusch, L--8320 Capellen
Luxebourg
Tel. : (352) 3124311
Fax : (352) 312431828
Product Detail : Herbal Teas

101. M/s. Flora Distributors
396 Deerhurst Drive
Brampton, Ontario, L60 5H9
Canada
Tel. : (416) 7913111
Fax. : (416) 7911773

102. M/s. Florina
Ettau, 49670 Valanjou
France
Tel. : (33) 41454330
Fax : (33) 41454995
Product Detail : Supply of Bulk Herbs

103. M/s. Fmali Herb Co.
831 Almar Avenue
Santa Cruz, CA 95060
U.S.A.
Tel. : (408) 4237913
Fax. : (408) 4295173
Product Detail : Herbal Remedies, Herbal Teas

104. M/s. Fukudarya Co. Ltd.
5-11 NishiTenma
1-Chome, Kita-Ku, Osaka 530
Japan
Tel. : (81) 63645861-3
Product Detail : Herbal Extracts and
Raw Materials, Japanese and Chinese Crude Drugs And
spic

105. M/s. Galia Herbs Inc.
62 Old Littleon Road
Harvard, MA 01451
U.S.A.
Tel. : (508) 4563049
Fax : (508) 4569154
Product Detail : Fresh Plant Extracts

106. M/s. GB Tre Spa
Via Seganitini 31/A
20092 Cinisello Balsamo, Italy
Tel. : (02) 6188697/6121413
Fax : (02) 6128950
Product Detail : Herbal Medicines, Herbal Teas, health Food Natural Cosmetics and Food Supply

107. M/s. Gerard House Ltd.
Mulberry Court, Stour Road
Christchurch Dorset, BH23 1PS U.K.
Tel. : (202) 487733
Fax : (202) 488333
Product Detail : Herbal Remedies, Cosmetics, Dietary Supplements

108. M/s. Good N'Natural
90 Orville Drive
Bohemia, NY 11716 U.S.A.
Tel. : (516) 2442034
Fax : (516) 2440230
Product Detail : Herbal Medicines

109. M/s. Goodness Foods
South March, Daventry
Northants, NN11 4PH
U.K.
Tel. : (327) 706611
Fax : (327) 300437
Product Detail : Natural Food Wholesaler

110. M/s. Gowiro Srl
Via Roma 13, 34132 Trieste
Italy
Tel. : (040) 61000
Fax : (040) 62540
Product Detail : Herbal Remedies

111. M/s. Gr Lane Health Products Ltd.
Sisson Road, Gloucester GLI 3OB
U.K.
Tel. : (452) 524012
Fax : (452) 300105
Product Detail : Herbal Remedies, Health Foods, Cosmetics

112. M/s. Green Foods Corp.
620 Maple Avenue, Tarrance
CA 90503-5001, U.S.A.
Tel. : (310) 6180678
Fax : (310) 6189246
Product Detail : Herbal Tonic Drinks, Food Supplements

113. M/s. Groupe Limagrain Holding
BPI, 63720 Chappes, France
Tel. : (33) 73634284
Fax : (33) 73624080
Product Detail : Food Supplements

114. M/s. Ha Won Pharm Corp.
2nd Floor, Dae-Shin Bldg.
140-6 Samsung-Dong, Kangnam-Ku
Korea
Tel. : (02) 5542012
Fax : (02) 5544557
Product Detail : Traditional Herbal Medicines and
Pharmaceutical Products

115. M/s. Hae Dong SS Pharmaceutical Co. Ltd.
157-3 Dodang-Dong
Iucheon City, Kyungki-Do, Korea
Tel. : (032) 6785771--5
Fax : (032) 6753385
Product Detail : Traditional herbal Medicines and
Pharmaceutical Prouducts

116. M/s. Hae Kong Pharm. Ind. Co. Ltd.
704 Noweon-Dong
Bukogu, Daegu, Korea
Tel. : (053) 326460
Fax : (053) 6689
Product Detail : Traditional Herbal Medicines and
Pharmaceutical Products

117. M/s. Hae Woi Pharm. Ind. Co.
114-15 Sungsan Dong
MAPO-KU, Seoul, Korea
Tel.: (02) 3393992-5
Fax. : (02) 3383294
Product Detail : Traditional Herbal Medicines and
Pharmaceutical Products

118. M/s. Hamdard Laboratories
(Waqf) Pakistan, Hamdard Centre
Nazimabad, Karachi-18
Pakistan
Tel. : (92) 21616001-5
Product Detail : Unani Medicine

119. M/s. Han Dok Remedia Ind. Co. Ltd.
344 Sangbang-1 Dong
Choongrang-Ku, Seoul
Korea
Tel. : (02) 4901000
Fax : (02) 4923197
Product Detail : Traditional herbal Medicines and Pharmaceutical Products

120. M/s. Han Il Corp. Ltd.
120 Sungsu-Dong 1-GA
Sungdong-Ku, Seoul
Korea
Tel. : (02) 4640511
Fax : (02) 4680518
Product Detail : Tradtional herbal Medicines and Pharmaceutical Prouducts

121. M/s. Han Kook Sin Yak Pharmaceutical Co.
610-7 Kwanjeo-Dong
Seo-Ku, Dajeon
Korea
Tel. : (42) 3253031
Fax : (042) 5412349
Product Detail : Traditional Herbal Medicines and Pharmaceutical Products

122. M/s. Han Kun Pharma. Co. Ltd.
251 Namjungori, Shindun-Myun
Icheon-Ku, Kyungki-Do
Korea
Tel. : (0336) 327422/7505
Product Detail : Traditional Herbal Medicines and Pharmaceutical Products

123. M/s. Han Poong Pharm Co. Ltd.
333-24 Palbok-Dong
1GA Duckjin-Ku
Jeonju City, Chunbuk-Do
Korea
Tel. : (0652) 2110254
Fax : (0652) 2511490
Product Detail : Traditional Herbal Medicines and Pharmaceutical Prouducts

124. M/s. Han Yang Pharm. Co. Ltd.
405-1 Seokyo-Dong
Mapo-Ku, Seoul
Korea
Tel. : (02) 332176-7
Fax : ()2) 3230680
Product Detail : Traditional Herbal Medicines and Pharmaceutical Products

125. M/s. Han Young Co. Ltd. Remedy
1056-16 Namhyun-Dong
Kwanak-Ku, Seoul
Korea
Tel. : (02) 5877921
Fax : (02) 5877928
Product Detail : Traditional Herbal Medicines and Pharmaceutical Products

126. M/s. Harasawa Pharmaceutical
3-19-17 Takanawa
Minato-Ku, Tokyo 108
Japan
Tel. : (81) 334415791
Product Detail : Home Remedies, Feet Care and Health Food Proudcts

127. M/s. Health & Diet Food Co. Ltd.
Europa Park, Stoneclough Road
Radcliffe, Manchester, M26 238
U.K.
Tel. : (602) 866615
Fax : (602) 861559
Product Detail : Herbal Medicines and Herbal Food Products

128. M/s. Health Stores (Wholesale) Ltd.
Queens Road
Nottingham, NG12 3AS,
U.K.
Tel. : (602) 866615
Fax : (602) 861559
Product Detail : Herbal Products

129. M/s. Healthcrafts Ltd.
Beaver Hourse, York Close
Byfleet, Surey, IT 14 7HN
U.K.
Tel. : (932) 336366
Fax : (932) 336095
Product Detail : Herbal Remedies and Food Supplements

130. M/s. Healthlife Ltd.
Charles Town House, Basildon
Shipley, West Yorkshire, BD17 5BR
U.K.
Product Detail : Herbal Remedies

131. M/s. Heca Pharm.
Import/Export Division
DK-3230, Graested
Denmark
Tel. : (45) 42292800
Fax : (45) 42292311
Product Detail : Herbal and Homeopathic Medicines

132. M/s. Heel GMBH
PO Box 729
D-7570 Baden-Baden
Germany
Tel. : (49) 722150100
Fax : (49) 7221501210
Product Detail : Homeopathic Remedies and Natural Cosmetics

133. M/s. Herba Kos NV
Elektronikallan 9, 2610 Wilrijk
Belgium
Tel. : (32) 38301495
Fax : (32) 3301408
Product Detail : Herbal Medicines and health Food Products

134. M/s. herbal Pharm Proc. & Mfg. Plant
Cotabato, Regional Hosp. Compound
Rosary Heights, Cotabato City
Philippines
Tel. : (63) 212193
Product Detail : Herbal Medicines

135. M/s. Herbion Pakistan Pvt. Ltd.
8, Ruksana Bldg.
E-2, Block 7 & 8
Shaheed E Millat Road, Karachi
Pakistan
Tel. : (92) 21449575
Fax : (92) 212620823
Product Detail : Herbal Unani Medicines

136. M/s. Heumann harma GMBH
Heideloffstr 18-20
D-3500 Nuernberg 1
Germany
Tel. : (49) 91143021
Product Detail : Herbal Medicines, Herbal Teas
And ethical Pharmaceuticals

137. M/s. Hind Pharmaceutical Co. Ltd.
33 2-Chome, Doshomachi
Higashi-Ku, Osaka 541
Japan
Tel. : (81) 62315847
Fax : (81) 62317309
Product Detail : Kampo Medicines, Medicinal Heabs
and Spices

138. M/s. Hisaya Daikokudo Co.
1-19 Kitahama
2-Chrome, Chuo-Ku, Osaka 541, Japan
Tel.: (81) 62640521
Product Detail : Herbal and Japanese Folkloric Medicines

139. M/s. Hiya Paharmaceutical Co. Ltd.
4-11 Temma 1-Chome
Kita-Ku, Osaka 530, Japan
Tel. : (81) 63513031
Fax : (81) 63542252
Product Detail : Herbal Medicines and Tonics

140. M/s. Ho Yan Hor Pharmaceutical Sdn Bhd
121 Jalan Kuala Kangsar
30010 IPOH Perak
Malaysia
Tel.: (60) 4414929/5549690
Fax : (60) 5501215
Product Detail : Herbal Tea, Medicinal Oil, Health Supplements

141. M/s. Holistica International
6 Parc Des Jalassieres
13510 Eguilles, France
Tel. : (33) 42951717
Fax (33) 42951718
Product Detail : Health and Food Supplements

142. M/s. Homeoropa
7 Zwarte Land 21
3825 ZG, Scherpenzeel
Netherlands
Tel. : (31) 34974575
Product Detail : Herbal Products

143. M/s. Hoyu Co. Ltd.
501 Tokugawa 1-Chome
Higashi-Ku, Nagoya 461, Japan
Tel. : (81) 529 359556
Fax : (81) 529 373186
Product Detail : Traditional Medicines, Hair Cosmetics and Dyes

144. M/s. IK SU Pharmaceutical Co. Ltd.
250-8 Jamsil-Dong
Sangpa-KU, Seoul, Korea
Tel. : (02) 4161112-7
Fax : (02) 4161118
Product Detail : Traditional Herbal Medicines and Pharmaceutical Products

145. M/s. IL Dong Pharmaceutical Co. Ltd.
45 Sinseol-Dong
Dongdaemun-Ku, Seoul, Korea
Tel.: (02) 9230081
Fax : (02) 9252044
Product Detail : Traditional Herbal Medicines and Pharmaceutical Products

146. M/s. IL Flor DI Loto
Via Don Caustico 131
10095 Grugliasco (TO), Italy
Tel. : 011-4054527
Fax : 011-4054612
Product Detail : Health Food and Herbal Medicines

147. M/s. IL Hwa American Corp.
401B 5th Avenue
NYC, NY 10016
U.S.A.
Tel. : (212) 2960130
Fax : (212) 7790493
Product Detail : Herbal Remedies and Korean Ginseng

148. M/s. IL Hwa Co. Ltd.
437 Sutaeg-Dong
Kuri-City, Kyungki-Do
Korea
Tel. : (02) 433-6141-7
Fax : (02) 7453327
Product Detail : Traditional Herbal medicines and Pharmaceutical Products

149. M/s. IL Yang Pharm. Co. Ltd.
24-5 Hawolgog Dong
Sungbug-Ku, Seoul,
Korea
Tel. : (02) 9125291
Fax :(02) 9127875
Product Detail : Traditional Herbal Medicines and Pharmaceutical Prouducts

150. M/s. Illingworth Health Foods Ltd.
York House, York Street
Bradfort, BD8 OHR, U.K.
Tel. : (274) 488511
Fax : (274) 541121
Product Detail : Herbal Products

151. M/s. IM International
2-10 Ramkhamhaeng 24 Road
Huamak, Bangkok, Thailand
Tel. : (66) 23143279
Fax : (66) 23143279
Product Detail : Health Foods

152. M/s. Indonesian Herbs
Menteng Dalam, B-B RT 008/01 No. 30
Pancoran Tebet, Jakarata, Selatan
Indonesia
Tel. : (62) 218293219
Fax : (62) 218298521
Product Detail : Traditional Jamu Medicine

153. M/s. Inno-Vite Inc.
196 Wildlat Road
Downsuiew on M3J 2N5
Canada
Tel. : (416) 6618272
Fax : (416) 6615992
Product Detail : Herbs and Natural Medicines

154. M/s. Intregral Sa
Rue De Strassbourg 95-99
Level Appie
Luxembourg
Tel. : (352) 485656
Product Detail : Herbal Medicines

155. M/s. Interpharm APS
Kirke Vaerlosevej 14
DK-3500 Vaerlose, Denmark
Tel. : (45) 4248180
Fax : (45) 41481285
Product Detail : Natural Product and Homoeopathic Remedies

156. M/s. Inveroni Della Beffa
Group SPA
Via Ripamonti N 99, 20141 Milano, Italy
Tel. : 02-574961
Product Detail : Botanical Derivativea & Pharmaceuticals Cosmetics

157. M/s. Isola IBI
Viale Pio VII
50-106 R, 16148 Genova, Italy
Tel. : (010) 395310/3922355/392309
Fax : (010) 3771530
Product Detail : Herbal Medicines, Natural Cosmetics and Herbal Extracts

158. M/s. Jacoby Pharmazeutika
A-5400 Hallein,
Kaltenhausen
Austria
Tel. : (43) 624525510
Fax : (43) 62452568
Product Detail : Herbal Medicines and Teas

159. M/s. Jin Ro Pharm. Co. Ltd.
302 Noryangjin-Dong
Dongjag-Ku,
Seoul,
Korea
Tel. : (02) 8123101-3
Fax : (02) 8177083
Product Detail : Traditional Herbal Medicines and Pharmaceutical Products

160. M/s. Joong Gyung Pharm. Co. Ltd.
259 Hangang-RO
1-GA, Yongsan-Ku, Seoul,
Korea
Tel. : (02) 7926663
Fax : (02) 7920588
Product Detail : Traditional Herbal Medicines and Pharmaceutical Products

161. M/s. JPS Pharmaceuticals Co. Ltd.
4-42-22 Higashiyamada
Kohoku-Ku, Yokohama City
Kanagawa-Pref 223
Japan
Tel. : (81) 455932050
Fax : (81) 455932070
Product Detail : Herbal and Kampo Medicines

162. M/s. Jung Ang Pharm.
813-1 Jegi-2 Dong
Dongdaemun-Ku, Seoul
Korea
Tel. : (02) 9686340
Fax : (02) 9686349
Product Detail : Traditional Herbal Medicines and Pharmaceutical Products

163. M/s. Jung Woo Pharmaceutical Co. Ltd.
Dodang-Dong, Bucheon City
Kyungki-Do, Korea
Tel. : (02) 56933216
Fax : (02) 5579914
Product Detail : Traditional Herbal Medicines

164. M/s. Kabi Pharmacia AB
Kai Pharmacia, Self Care
S11287 Stockholm, Sweden
Tel. : (46) 86958000
Fax : (46) 8831006
Product Detail : Ethical Pharmaceuticals, Food Supplements

165. M/s. Kaiser Pharmaceutical Co. Ltd.
8 Hwan Kung Road
Yung Kang Industrial Park
Yung Kang Tainan 71020, Taiwan
Tel. : (886) 62336681
Fax : *886) 62321021
Product Detail : Chinese Medicines and Chinese Herbs Concentrate

166. M/s. Kali Chemie AG
Postfach 220, D-3000 Hannover 1
Germany
Tel. : (49) 5118571
Fax : (49) 51282126
Product Detail : Ethical Herbal Medicines

167. M/s. Kanebo Pharmaceuticals Division
1-3-12 Motoakasaka
Minato-Ku, Tokyo 10, Japan
Tel. : (81) 35411350
Fax : (81) 354113568
Product Detail : Kampo Medicines and Pharmaceutical Products

168. M/s. Kanoldt Arzeneimmittel GmbH
Postfach 220, Hans-Bockler-Allee 20
3000 Hannover 1, Germany
Tel. : (49) 90745080
Fax : (49) 9074376
Product Detail : Ethical Pharmaceuticals for Prostratre Problems

169. M/s. Karder Trading Co. Ltd.
440 FU Hsing N Road
Taipei, Taiwan
Tel. : (886) 25028554
Product Detail : Chinese Medicines

170. M/s. Kelkin Nature Products Ltd.
Whitestown Industrial Estate
Tallaght, Dublin 24, Ireland
Tel. : (353) 1520377
Fax : (353) 1519111
Product Detail : Herbal Medicines

171. M/s. Kernpharm BV
Rooseveltillan 6, 5460 AA Veghel
Netherlands
Tel. : (31) 413041492
Fax : (31) 713067919
Product Detail : Herbal Products

172. M/s. Keum Kang Pharm. Co. Ltd.
404-1 Sohyun-RI
Daeduk-Myun, M
Ansung-Kun, Kyungki-Do, Korea
Tel. : (0334) 720221
Fax : (0334) 720222
Product Detail : Traditional Herbal Medicines and Pharmaceutical Products

173. M/s. Khao-La-Or Laboratories Ltd.
146/22 Group 3, Suksawad Road
T Pakklong-Bangplakod
A Pharasamutjadee Samutprakarn
Thailand
Tel. : (66) 24258531/4259036/4259037
Fax : (66) 24258332
Product Detail : Herbal Medicines, Health Food Herbal Drinks and Tea

174. M/s. Ki Wha Pharmaceutical Co. Ltd.
313-5 Sandae-Dong
Chinju-City, Kyungnam-Do, Korea
Tel. : (0591) 557401
Fax : (0591) 531270
Product Detail : Traditional Herbal medicines and Pharmaceutical Products

175. M/s. Kiluva SA
Avda San Ramon
Nanato 22, 08028 Barcelona, Spain
Tel. : (34) 3349054
Fax : (34) 3349399
Product Detail : Herbal Remedies, Plant Extracts
Herbal Teas

176. M/s. Kingdom Pharmaceutical Co.
4th Floor 267 Tun-HWA
South Road, Sec 2, Taipei, Taiwan
Tel. : (886) 27362236
Fax : (886) 27357004
Product Detail : OTC Chinese Medicines,
Pharmaceutical Preparations

177. M/s. Klinge Pharma GMBH
Berg-Am-Laim STR 129
D-8000 Munch 80, Germany
Tel. : (49) 89454401
Fax : (49) 894544329
Product Detail : Ethical Herbal Medicines

178. M/s. Kneipp-Werke
Steinbachtal 43, PO Box 5960
D-8700 Wurzburg 1, Germany
Tel. : (49) 93180020
Fax : (49) 9318002104
Product Detail : Herbal Remedies

179. M/s. Robatashi Pharmaceutical Co. Ltd.
25-5 Chome, Doshomachi
Higashi-Ku, Osaka-541, Japan
Tel. : (81) 62220184
Fax : (81) 62311785, 1749
Product Detail : Home Remedies, House hold
Product and Pharmaceutical Products

180. M/s. Kokando Co. Ltd.
92-Chome
Umezawacho, Toyama 930
Japan
Tel. : (81) 764242271
Fax : (81) 764242271
Product Detail : Pharmaceutical Tonics, Herbal Products

181. M/s. Korea Central Pharmaceutical Co. Ltd.
466-8 Seokyu-Dong
Mapo-Ku,
Seoul
Korea
Tel. : (02) 3351122
Fax : (02) 3351129
Product Detail : Traditional Herbal Medicines and Pharmaceutical Products

182. M/s. Korea Eundan Pharm. Co. Ltd.
31-6 Jangchoong-Dong 1 GA
Jungwon-Ku,
Seoul
Korea
Tel. : (02) 2770006
Fax : (02) 2775829
Product Detail : Traditional Herbal Medicines and Pharmaceutical Products

183. M/s. Korea Green Pharm Co. Ltd.
903-4 Sansgsin-RI, Hyangnam-Myun
Hwasung-Kum, Kyungki-Do
Korea
Tel. : 0339-526671
Fax : 02-5796675
Product Detail : Traditional Herbal Medicines and Pharmaceutical Products

184. M/s. Korea Pharmacy Co. Ltd.
754-7 Yongdu-2 Dong
Dongdaemun-Ku, Seoul
Korea
Tel. : (02) 9251277
Fax : (02) 9233298
Product Detail : Traditional Herbal Medicines and Pharmaceutical Products

185. M/s. Kali Tobacco and Ginseng
100 Pyongchon-Dong
Taedong-Ku, Taejeon
Korea
Tel. : (042) 9328048
Fax : (042) 9328048
Product Detail : Traditional Herbal Medicines

186. M/s. Korean Drug Co. Ltd.
95 Hangang-RO, 2-GA
Yongsan-Ku, Seoul, Korea
Tel. : (02) 7976321
Fax : (02) 7975076
Product Detail : Traditional Herbal Medicines and Pharmaceutical Products

187. M/s. Koshiro Co. Ltd.
Doshomachi 2-5-8 Chuo-Ku
Osaka 541, Japan
Tel. : (81) 62311803
Fax : (81) 62270187
Product Detail : Herbal Extracts and Medicinal Herbs

188. M/s. Kwang Dong Pharmaceutical Co. Ltd.
212-13 Kuro-Dong
Kuro-Ku, Seoul, Korea
Tel. : (02) 8623439
Fax : (02) 8623439
Product Detail : Traditional Herbal Medicines and Pharmaceutical Products

189. M/s. Kyoei Pharmaceutical Co. Ltd.
4576 Nakada, Takaoka City,
Toyama Pref 939-12
Japan
Tel. : (81) 766 361116
Fax : (81) 766 361607
Product Detail : Home Remedeis and Eye Care Products

190. M/s. Kyung Jin Pharmaceutical Co. Ltd.
1-8 Kwayinm-Dong
Sihung-City, Kyungki-Do
Korea
Tel. : (02) 7627459
Product Detail : Traditional Herbal Medicines and Pharmaceutical Products

191. M/s. Kyushin Seiyaku Co. Ltd.
No. 21-7-1 Chome Wada
Suninamu-Ko, Tokyo
Japan
Tel. : (81) 353 853211, 338 46063
Fax : (81) 353 853210, 333846063
Product Detail : Plant Based Health Tonic

192. M/s. L'arca
Prodotii Natural Sas
Via Fontant 10, 14100 ASTI
Italy
Tel. : (0141) 33351
Fax : (0141) 437146
Product Detail : Herbal Medicines and Food Supplements

193. M/s. La Maison De M
Messague Italia
Z Art Localita S Igaro
25010 San Felice,
Del Benaco (B)
Italy
Tel. : (0356) 520528
Fax : (0356) 520527
Product Deetail : Herbal Medicines and Natural Cosmetics

194. M/s. Laboratoire Ardeval
29 Rue M Cachin
94200 LVRY Sur Seine, France
Tel. : (33) 146584807
Fax : (33) 146587782
Product Detail : Herbal Remedies

`195. M/s. Laboratorie Fuca
IBIS Rue de Plaisance
BP 40, 94732 Nogent Sur Marne
France
Tel. : (33) 48711053
Fax : (33) 48721806
Product Detail : Herbal Remedies

196. M/s. Laboratories Arkopharma
1st Avenue
2709M LID Cerres Le Broc
Oeste Canoo Cedex
France
Tel. : (33) 93291128
Fax : (33) 93291162
Product Detail : Herbal Medicines, Especially slimming Products, Herbal Teas and Tonics

197. M/s.
5/7 Rue Salvador Allende
91127 Palaiseau, Cedex
France
Tel. : (33) 69302182
Fax : (33) 69305740
Product Detail : Herbal Medicines, Medicinal Herbal Teas Homoeopathic Remedies, Ethical

198. M/s. Laboratories Monot
Impasse Des Boussenarts
BP7, F-21801 Quetigny, Cedex
France
Tel. : (33) 80636200
Product Detail : Medicinal Herbal Teas

199. M/s. Laboratorium Biohorma BV
Industriestraat 5, 8081 HH Elburg
Netherlands
Tel. : (31) 52507200
Fax : (31) 52503932
Product Detail : Homoeopathic Medicines

200. M/s. Larkhall Natural Health Ltd.
225-229 Putney Bridge Road
SW15 2PY, London
U.K.
Tel. : (81) 8741130
Fax : (81) 8711130
Product Detail : Herbal Remedies, Dietary Supplements and Special Diet Foods

201. M/s. Lehning Laboratories
1 Plasee Arsene Vigeant
BP 326, 47007 Metz
France
Tel. : (33) 87654444
Product Detail : Homoeopathic Medicines

202. M/s. L:ichtwer Pharma GmbH
Wallenroder STR 8-10
D-1000, Berlin 26, Germany
Tel. : (49) 3040370112
Fax : (49) 3040370103
Product Detail : Herbal Medicines

203. M/s. Lichitwer Pharma. US Inc.
Foster Place 10, 680 Anderson DRI E
Pittsburgh, PA 15220-2700, U.S.A.
Tel. : (412) 9289334
Fax : (412) 9289655
Product Detail : Herbal Products

204. M/s.Lifeplan Products Ltd.
Elizabethan Way, Lutterworth
Leicestrershire, LE17 4ND
U.K.
Tel. : (455) 556281
Product Detail : Herbal Medicines

205. M/s. Lizofarm
WIV D Millelire 13
20147 Milano
Italy
Tel. :. (02) 48707760
Fax : (02) 4040986
Product Detail : Herbal Medicines

206. M/s. Lobelin Ltd.
6 Chhryssmyrnis Street
Akgyroupolis, 16452 Athens
Greece
Tel.: (30) 19917220
Fax : (3)) 19925991
Product Detail : Herbal Medicies and Food Supplements

207. M/s. Lumen Naturae BV
Van Deventer Straat 27
3910 AA Rhenen
Netherlands
Tel. : (31) 837612450
Product Detail : Herbal and Homoeopathic Medicines

208. M/s. Madaus AG
Ostmerheimerstrasse 198
5000 Koln 91
Germany
Tel. : (49) 22189981
Fax : (49) 2218998305
Product Detail : Herbal medicines Homoeopathic Remedies and Pharmaceuticals Products

209. Madaus Murdock
10. Mountain Springs, Parkway
Springville, Utah 8463
U.S.A.
Tel. : (801) 4893631
Fax : (801) 4893639
Product Detail : Herbal Remedies

210. M/s. Makers of Kal
6415 De Soto Avenue
Woodland Hills, CA 91365--4023
U.S.A.
Tel.: (818) 3403035
Fax : (818) 7029956
Product Detail : Herbal Medicines

211. M/s. Marathon Natural Foods Ltd.
1375 Commercial Way
Penticton BC, V2A 3H4
Canada
Tel. : (604) 4937887
Fax : (604) 4938993
Product Detail : Herbs & Natural Medicines

212. M/s. Marcor Development Corp.
108, John Street, Hackensack
NJ 07601-4103, U.S.A.
Telex : 7109905131 Marcorde Hak
Fax : 201-489-7357
Product Detail : Papain, Boswellia Silymarin, Inulin

213. M/s. Martins Y Costs LDA
R Pereira Henriques 6-12
1900 Lisbon, Portugal
Tel. : (351) 18583899
Fax : (351) 18584784
Product Detail : Foods and Dietary Supplements

214. M/s. Matas A/S
Ryttermarken 11
Postbokds 205, DK-3520 Farum
Denmark
Tel. : (45) 42957000
Fax : (45) 42951087
Product Detail : Health Products

215. M/s. MCM Klosterfrau
Vertreibsgesselschaft
Gereonsmuhlengasse 1-11
5000 KOLN 1, Germany
Tel. : (49) 2216520
Fax : (49) 2211652474
Product Detail : Herbal Medicines

216. M/s. Mcsand Herbal Inc.
PO Box 5312, Santa Monica
California, CA 90409, U.S.A.
Tel. : (213) 3920404
Fax : (310) 8221050
Product Detail : Herbal Medicines & Extracts

217. M/s. Medic Herb AB
Frokottegatan 10
Box 30060, S-40093 Goteorg
Sweden
Tel. : (46) 31490195
Fax : (46) 31497390
Product Detail : Herbal Medicines

218. M/s. Medice GmbH
Kuhloweg 37-39
Postfach 20653
5860 Iserlohn/West Falen
Germany
Tel. : (49) 23713511
Fax : (49) 237135`1329
Product Detail : Herbal Medicines, Homoeopathic Remedies, Ethical Pharmaceuticals

219. M/s. Mezina Natur Produkter APS
Energivej 2, 6700 Esbjerg
Denmark
Tel. : (45) 75181611
Fax : (45) 75138172
Product Detail : Herbal and Homeopathic Medicines and Dietary Supplements

220. M/s. Mikuni & Co. Ltd.
25, 2-Chome, Doshomachi
Higashi-Ku, Osaka 541
Japan
Tel. : (81) 6232357
Product Detail : Herbal Extracts and Kampo Medicine

221. M/s. Ministar International Inc.
PO Box 1057, Walnut, C-91789
U.S.A.
Tel. : 818-8108532
Fax : 818-913-8387

222. M/s. Morishita Jintan Co. Ltd.
1-1-30 Tamatsukuri
Higashi-Ku, Osaka 540, Japan
Tel. : (81) 67611131
Product Detail : Kampo Medicines Breath Freshners Health Food and OTC Drugs

223. M/s. Motherland International Inc.
13840 Magnolia Avenue
Chino, CA 91710, U.S.A.
Tel. : 909-590-5471
Fax : 909-590-5470
Product Detail : Botanical Extracts, Angelica, Astragalus Atractylodis, Codonopsis, Pilos

224. M/s. Much Pharma AG and
Ostfach 1349
6232 Bad Soden/TS
Germany
Tel. : (49) 6196202226
Fax : (49) 6196/62016
Product Detail : Herbal Medicines Pharmaceuticals

225. M/s. Murdock Health Care
10 Mountain Springs
Parkway Springville, Utah 84663
U.S.A.
Tel. : (801) 4891500
Fax : (801) 4891700
Product Detail : Herbal and Homoeopathic Medicines

226. M/s. MYP Son Bho
9-9A Jalan Petaling
Larking Ind. Area
80350 Johore, Bahru, Johore
Malaysia
Tel. : (60) 7371509
Fax : (60) 7373593
Product Detail : Traditional Malaysian Medicines

227. M/s. Nam Chang Pharmaceutical Co.
7-6 Munhwa-Dong
Chung-Ku, Daegu
Korea
Tel. : (053) 4244456
Product Detail : Traditional Herbal Medicines

228. M/s. Nam Ganj Pharm Co. Ltd.
656-670 Sungsu-Dong
Sungdong-Ku, Seoul, Korea
Tel. : (02) 4635701
Fax : (02) 4623251
Product Detail : Traditional Herbal Medicines and Pharmaceutical Products

229. M/s. Natiris-Centro Dietetico Ltd.
R Santo Antonio A
Estrela 31-B, Lisbon, Portugal
Tel. : (351) 13976061
Fax : (351) 1603908
Product Detail : Herbal Medicines, Cosmetics and Food Supplements

230. M/s. Natur Drogeriet
Nydamswej 13-15, 8362 Horning
Belgium
Tel. : (45) 86923333
Fax : (45) 86923343
Product Detail : Herbal Medicines and Herbal Teas

231. M/s. Natura Holding
Via Cavour 20
10048 Vinova (TO), Italy
Tel. : (011) 9652384
Fax : (011) 9653763
Product Detail : Health Foods, Natural Cosmetics, Homeopathic Remedies, Ginseng

232. M/s. Natural Medicine Co. Ltd.
Stroughan, Blessington Co.
Wicklow,
Ireland
Tel. : (353) 4565575
Fax : (353) 4565727
Product Detail : Herbal Medicines

233. M/s. Nature Works Inc.
5431 Derry Avenue, Eagoura Hills
California, Ca 91301, U.S.A.
Tel. : (818) 3891602
Fax : (818) 8894041
Product Detail : Herbal Tonics and Teas

234. M/s. Nature's Apothecary
997 Dixon Road
Boulder, CO 80302, U.S.A.
Tel. : (303) 440742
Fax : (303) 4400440
Product Detail : Herbal Medicines & Extracts

235. M/s. Nature's Bounty
90 Orville Drive
Bohemia, NY 11716, U.S.A.
Tel. : (516) 2442042
Fax : (516) 5670230
Product Detail : Herbal Medicines, Ethical Pharmaceuticals

236. M/s. Nature's Herbs
1113 N Industrial
Park Drive, Orem, UTAH 84057
U.S.A.
Tel. : (801) 2254443
Fax : (801) 2256790
Product Detail : Herbal Medicines

237. M/s. Nature's Store Ltd.
Linley Road
Talke, Stoke-on-Trent
Staffs, ST7 1XS, U.K.
Tel. : (782) 785255
Fax : (782) 774015
Product Detail : Health Food Products

238. M/s. Nature's Sunshine Products Inc.
PO Box 1000, Spanish Fork
Utah-84660,
U.S.A.
Tel. : (801) 7984200
Fax : (801) 7982730
Product Detail : Herbal Supplements

239. M/s. Nature's Way
Hebron Industrial Estate
HebronRoad, Kolienny, Ireland
Tel. : (35) 35665402
Fax : (35) 35665140
Product Detail : Herbal Remedies

240. M/s. Naturwaren OHG
Marktplatz 12, Postfach 1559
6850 Homburg/Sarr, Germany
Tel. : (49) 68416907-0
Fax : (49) 68416907-65
Product Detail : Herbal Medicines health Food Products

241. M/s. New Century Pharmaceutical Co. Ltd.
8th Floor Sae-dae Bldg.
11-3 Heohyun-Dong
3GA, Chungku, Seoul, Korea
Tel. : (02) 7555823
Fax : (02) 7546732
Product Detail : Traditional Herbal Medicines

242. M/s. Nihon Herb Medicine Lab. Ltd.
2-327-2 Shimo Suketo Cho
Tokushmia City, Tokushima 770
Japan
Tel. : (081) 886540323
Product Detail : Herbal Medicines, Herbal Tea, Dietary and Supplementary Foods

243. M/s. Nippon Shinyaku Co. Ltd.
14 Nishinosho-Monguchi-Cho
Kisshoin, Kyoto 601,
Japan
Tel. : (81) 75321 11111
Fax : (81) 75321 0678
Product Detail : Herbal and Pharmaceutical Medicines, Ethical and OTC & Food Additives

244. M/s. Norgine Ltd.
116-120 London Road
Headington, Oxford, OX3 9BA,
U.K.
Tel. : (86) 5750717
Product Detail : Herbal Medicines

245. M/s. Nuova Linnea
Via Cantonale
CH-6595 Riassino, Switzerland
Tel. : (41) 92642578
Fax : (41) 92641840
Product Detail : Herbal Medicines, Extracts, Otc Products

246. M/s. Nuovo Centro Erboristico
Via Agrte 21
20049 Concorezzo (MI), Italy
Tel. : (039) 6041607
Fax : (039) 647454
Product Detail : Aromatherpay Oils, Health Foods, Vitamin and Food Supplements & Herbal Medicines

247. M/s. Nutana
Ringstedvej, DK-4632 Bjaeverskov
Belgium
Tel. : (45) 53670019
Fax : (45) 53671919
Product Detail : Health Foods, Dietary Supplements, Herbal Medicines

248. M/s. Nutrix Iberica SL
Plaza Eryes Magos 9
28007 Madrid, Spain
Tel. : (34) 15523984
Product Detail : Herbal Products

249. M/s. Ohta's Isan Co. Ltd.
3-2 Sengoku 2-Chome
Bunkyo-Ku, Tokyo 12, Japan
Tel. : (81) 339441 311
Fax : (81) 33947 8322
Product Detail : Herbal and Folkloric Medicines and Pharmaceutical Product

250. M/s. Orbiselora
Erboristeria Aromatica E
Medicinale
Industria E Commercio Import-Export
Corso Pemponte 2
10099 SAN, Mauro Torino
Italy
Tel. : (011) 2735324, 2735525, 2735458

251. M/s. Orits of Belgium
B-4750 Elsenborn
Belgium
Tel. : (32) 80445786
Fax : (32) 80444280
Product Detail : Herbal Medicines and Cosmetics

252. M/s. Padma AG
Dammstrasse 29, CH-8702 Zollkon
Switzerland
Tel. : (41) 1391955
Fax : (41) 13919818
Product Detail : Tibetan Medicines

253. M/s. Pakistan Pharmaceutical Product Ltd.
5th Floor, Nelson Chambers
11 Chundrigar Road, Karachi
Pakistan
Tel. : (92) 212 637905
Fax : (92) 212 635851
Product Detail : Unani Medicines

254. M/s. Pep Products Inc.
3130 N Commerce Court
Castle Rock, CO 80104, U.S.A.
Tel. : (303) 6886633
Fax : (303) 6881591
Product Detail : Herbal Remedies

255. M/s. Perran Distributors
North Road, Finglas
Dublin 11,
Ireland
Tel. : (353) 1342233
Fax : (353) 1362271
Product Detail : Herbal Medicines

256. M/s. Perusahaan Sri Kandi
No. 100 Bangunan PKNM
JLN Bung Tanjung, Taman Maju
77000 Jasin Melaka
Malaysia
Tel. : (60) 6592639
Product Detail : Herbal Remedies

257. M/s. Pfluger KG
Bielefelder Strasse 17
4840 Rheda-Wiedenbruck
Germany
Tel. : (49) 52422081
Product Detail : Homoeopathic Remedies

258. M/s. Pharma Vinci A/s
Undalsvej 6
DK 3300 Freriksvaerk
Belgium
Tel. : (45) 42121723
Product Detail : Herbal Medicines and Food Supplements

259. M/s. Pharmaton SA
PO Box CH6903, Lugano
Switzerland
Tel. : (41) 91503111
Fax : (41) 915003209
Product Detail : Herbal Medicines and Major Supplier of Ginseng

260. M/s. Piere Fabre Sante
29 Avenue Du Sidobre
81106 Castres, Cedex
France
Tel. : (33) 63714600
Fax : (33) 63714676/97
Product Detail : Health and Beauty Products

261. M/s. Planta Medica
Locahia Mocaie 44/B
52031 Anghiari (AR)
Italy
Tel. : (0575) 749988
Fax : (0575) 749891
Product Detail : Natural Cosmetics, Herbal Extracts and Growers of Herbs

262. M/s. Plantes Et Medicines
Le Payrat
Begoux, 46000 Cahors, France
Tel. : (33) 65223256
Fax : (33) 65226787
Product Detail : Plant Based Products

263. M/s. Plantorgan GmbH & Co. OHG
Hornbuxch 1
D-2903 BAD, Zwischenahn
Germany
Tel. : (49) 44036020
Fax : (49) 440360220
Product Detail : Herbal Medicines and Pharmaceuticals

264. M/s. Potters (Herbal Suplies) Ltd.
Leyland Mill Lane
Wigan, Lancs, WN1 2SB
U.K.
Tel. : (942) 34761
Fax : (942) 820255
Product Detail : Herbal Remedies

265. M/s. Power Health Hellas
40 Messologiou Str.
14231 N Lonia,
Athens
Greece
Tel. : (30) 127960801
Fax : (30) 12758619
Product Detail : Herbal Remedies

266. M/s. Power Health Products Ltd.
10 Central Avenue, Airfield Estate
Pocklington York, YO4 2NR
U.K.
Tel. : (759) 302595
Fax : (759) 304286
Product Detail : Herbal Medicines

267. M/s. Prasat Thong Osoth Co. Ltd.
268 Plapplachi Road, Bangkok
Thailand
Tel. : (66) 2226663
Product Detail : Traditional Thai Medicine

268. M/s. Procordia Health Food AB
Box 14, S--16126 Bromma
Sweden
Tel. : (46) 87041995
Fax : (46) 31497390
Product Dentail : Ethical Pharmaceuticals Herbal Medicines

269. M/s. Prodient (Productor Dieticos Sa)
PO Box 423
Carretera Igoalada a La
Pobla 2, 08700 Igualada
Spain
Tel. : (34) 38042161
Product Detail : Herbal Remedies,
Dietary Supplements, Health Foods

270. M/s. Prosperita SNC
Via Edison 27, 40027 Castel S
Pietro Terme (BO)
Italy
Tel.: (051) 946204
Fax : (051) 943621
Product Detail : Aromatherapy Oils, Cosmetics, Anrohikha
Perfume Oils, Ayurvedic Medicines

271. M/s. Pt Darya-Varia Laboratoria
Wigo Building 4th Floor
JL Tendean 39,
Jakarta 12790
Indonesia
Tel. : (62) 217974510
Fax : (62) 21326071/520021
Product Detail : Ethical Pharmaceutical & Curcuma Perparation

272. M/s. Pt Mustika Ratu
Mustika Centre, Penthouse Floor
Ji Gatot Subroto Kav 7475
Jakarta 212870
Indonesia
Tel. : (62) 218306754, 218711291
Fax: (62) 218306760
Product Detail : Herbal Medicines and Health Drinks

273. M/s. Pt Nyona Meneer
Chase Plaza Building
18th Floor JI Jend Sudirman Kav 21
Jakarta
Indonesia
Tel. : (62) 215206902
Fax : (62) 215704170
Product Detail : Herbal Medicines, Cosmetics and Beverages

274. M/s. Purity Life Inc
100 Elgin Street
Action, Ontario
Canada
Tel. : (519) 8533511
Product Detail : Health Food and Herbal Products

275. M/s. Quest Vitamin
1781 West 75th Avenue, Vancouver
Canada
Tel. : (604) 2610611
Product Detail : Herbal Medicines and Food Supplements

276. M/s. Rainbow Light Nutritional Systems
207 Mcpherson Street
Santa Cruz, California, CA 95060, U.S.A.
Tel. : (408) 4299089
Fax : (408) 4290189
Product Detail : Herbal Remedies, Distary Supplements and Vitamins

277. M/s. Reckkit & Coleman
Dansom Lane
Hul, HU8 7DS, U.K.
Tel. : (482) 26151
Product Detail : Ethical Pharmaceuticals, OTC Products and Herbal Mediciens

278. M/s. Regina Health Ltd.
2A Alexandra Grove
Finchley,
London, N12 8NU, U.K.
Tel. : (81) 4466644
Fax : (81) 4454551
Product Detail : Herbal Medicines and Health Food

279. M/s. Ricola AG
Basel Str. 31
CH-4242 Laufen
Switzerland
Tel. : (41) 617654121
Fax : (41) 617654122
Product Detail : Herbal Medicines

280. M/s. Rio Trading Co. (Health) Ltd.
Rio House, 2 Eaton Place
Brighton, BN2 1EH
U.K.
Tel. : (273) 570987
Fax : (273) 691226
Product Detail : Herbal Medicines

281. M/s. Rohto Pharmaceutical Co. Ltd.
8-1 Tatsumi Nishi 1-Chome
Ikyno-KU, Osaka 544
Japan
Tel. : (81) 67581231
Fax : (81) 67575155
Product Detail : Traditional Medicines, Eye Care, Health Food and Pharmaceutical

282. M/s. Rok Sung Pharmaceutical Co.
3rd Floor, Jung-Lim Building
1443--3 Seocho-Dong
Seocho-Ku,
Seoul
Korea
Tel. : (02) 5855511
Fax : (02) 5218134
Product Detail : Traditional Herbal Medicines and Pharmaceutical Products

283. M/s. Ryukakusa Co. Ltd.
5-12 Higashi-Kand--2 Chome
Chiyod--KU, Tokyo 101
Japan
Tel. : (81) 38661177
Fax : (81) 338661177
Product Detail : Traditional Chinese medicines, Cough Medicines, Cosmetics, Balm

284. M/s. Sa Homeoden NV
Kasteellaan 75, B-9000 Gent
Belgium
Tel. : (32) 91258733
Fax : (32) 91230076
Product Detail : Herbal Products and Dealers of Homoeopathic Medicines

285. M/s. Sae Han Pharm. Co. Ltd.
376-11 Sokyo-Dong
Mapo-KU, Seoul
Korea
Tel. : (02) 3364221
Fax : (02) 3364771
Product Detail : Traditional Herbal Medicines and Pharmaceutical Products

286. M/s. Salues Haus
Bahnofstassse 24, Postfach 1180
D-8206 Bruckmuhl (088)
Germany
Tel. : (49) 80629010
Fax : (49) 80629197
Product Detail : Herbal Tonics, Herbal Remdies, Herbal Teas nd Food Supplements

287. M/s. Sam Chun Dang Pharm. Co. Ltd.
94-97 Youngdeungpo
Dong 2-GA, Youngdeungpo-Ku
Seoul
Korea
Tel. : (02) 6790146-9
Fax : 02) 6715673
Product Detail : Traditional Herbal Medicines and Pharmaceutical Products

288. M/s. Sam Ik Pharm. Co. Ltd.
5th Floor Dong-BO Bldg.
1253 Soongin-Dong
Chongro-KU, Seoul, Korea
Tel. : (032) 924196
Fax : (032) 9233749
Product Detail : Traditional Herbal Medicines and Pharmaceutical Products

289. M/s. Sam Jin Pharmaceutical
338-8 Seokyo-Dong
Mapo-Ku, Seoul, Korea
Tel. : (02) 3347091
Fax : (02) 3925312
Product Detail : Traditional Herbal Medicines and Pharmaceutical Products

290. M/s. Sam Sung Pharm. Ind.
19-6 Mojin-Dong
Sungdong-Ku, Seoul, Korea
Tel. : (02) 4571241-5
Fax : (02) 4536292
Product Detail : Traditional Herbal Medicines and Pharmaceutical Products

291. M/s. Sam Young Pharm Co.
287-2 Sajik-Dong
Chunan-City, Choongnam-Do
Korea
Tel. : (0417) 624300
Fax : (0417) 56755446
Product Detail : Traditional Herbal Medicines

292. M/s. Sandox Nutrition Ltd.
118 Monbijoustrasse, CH-3000 Bern
Switzerland
Tel. : (41) 31466968
Fax : (4) 31455211
Product Detail : Herbal Medicines, Otc Productions, Nutritional Supplements and Health Foods

293. M/s. Sato Yukuhin Kogyo Co. Ltd.
9-2 Kannonji-Cho
Kashihar-Shi, Nara--Pref 634, Japan
Tel. : (81) 744280021
Fax : (81) 744280030
Product Detail : Herbal and Japanese Folkloric Medicines

294. M/s. SB Fink
Benzstrasse 25
7033 Herrenberg, Germany
Tel. : (49) 703220020
Fax : (49) 70325221
Product Detail : Herbal Medicines and Pharmaceuticials

295. M/s. Schaper & Brummer
Postfach 611160
D3320 Salzgitter 61
Germany
Tel. : (49) 53413070
Fax : (499) 6341307124
Product Detail : Herbal Medicines

296. M/s. Scotia Holdings PLC
Woodbridge Meadows, Guildford
Surrey, Gul1 1BA
U.K.
Tel. : (283) 574949
Fax : (483) 506682
Product Detail : Herbal Medicines and Ethical Pharmaceuticals

297. M/s. Se Mo Co. Ltd.
RM1401 Sung-Ji Bldg.
538 Dohwa-Dong
Mapo-Ku,
Seoul
Korea
Tel. : (02) 7023535
Fax : (02) 7029873
Product Detail : Traditional Herbal Medicines and
Pharmaceutical Products

298. M/s. Selerbe Srl.
Amm Via Savigliano 15
12060 Roreto Di, Cherasco (CN)
Italy
Tel.: (0172) 495594
Fax : (0172) 495860
Product Detail : Herbal Extracts

299. M/s. Seoul Pharm. Co. Ltd.
RM 608 Ha-Na Bldg.
Voido-Dong, Youngdeungpo-Ku,
Seoul
Korea
Tel. : (02) 7857347
Fax : (02) 7827783
Product Detail : Traditional Herbal Medicines and
Pharmaceutical Products

300. M/s. Seven Seas Ltd.
Hedon Road, Marfleet
Hull, HU9 5NJ
U.K.
Tel. : (482) 75234
Fax : (482) 74345
Product Detail : Herbal and Homoeopathic Remedies

301. M/s. Shaklee Corporation
Shaklee Terraces, 444 Market Street
San Francisco, CA 94111, U.S.A.
Fax : (415) 9542098
Product Detail : Herbal Products

302. M/s. Sheng Chang Pharmaceutical Co. Ltd.
591 Yuan San Road
Chungho, Taipei Hsien, Taiwan
Tel. : (886) 22234195/6
Fax : (886) 22237007
Product Detail : Chinese Medicines, Single herbal Extract Powder, Import and Export of Chine

303. M/s. Shin Hwa Pharmaceutical Co.
152-4 Sangin-Dong
Salseo-Ku, Daegu, Korea
Tel. : (053) 6327666
Fax : (053) 6327667
Product Detail : Traditional Herbal Medicines

304. M/s. Shin Seong Pharm Co. Ltd.
943-7 Dogok-Dong
Kangnam-Ka, Seoul, Korea
Tel. : (02) 5537328
Fax : (02) 5528869
Product Detail : Traditional Herbal Medicines and Pharmaceutical Products

305. M/s. Shing Chang Pharmaceutical
RM 504 Dong-Bou Bldg.
1256 Sungin-Don, Chongro-Ku, Seoul
Korea
Tel. : (02) 9244541
Fax : (02) 9254524
Product Detail : Traditional Herbal Medicines and Pharmaceutical Products

306. M/s. Siam Algae Co. Ltd.
Central Chidlow Tower 16 Floor
22 SOI Somkit Ploenchit Road
Pathumwan, Bangkok 10330
Thailand
Tel. : (66) 22547101-2
Fax : (66) 225471103
Product Detail : Spirulina Dried Powder

307. M/s. Similasan AG
Alte Obfelderstrasse 68
e8910 Affoltern AA
Switzerland
Te. : (41) 17611961
Fax : (41) 17612419
Product Detail : Homoeopathic Remedies

308. M/s. Solaray Inc.
2815 Industrial Drive
Ogden, Utah 84401, U.S.A.
Tel. : (801) 6215631
Fax : (801) 6212961
Product Detail : Herbal and Food Supplements

309. M/s. Solime
Via Ca Dalla Chiesa 10
42025 Cavriago (RE), Italy
Tel. : (0522) 577347/57498
Fax : 0522) 575996
Product Detail : Single and Compound Herbal
Medicine and Herbal Extracts

310. M/s. South African Essential Oil
PO Box 16, Goudo 6821
South Africa
Tel. : 236-320429
Fax : 236-320429
Product Detail : Bochu Leaf

311. M/s. Sovex
Rua Dos Anjos 71-1 ESQ
11000 Lisbon, Portugal
Tel. : (35) 1537787
Fax : (351) 1531852
Product Detail : Herbal Products

312. M/s. Specchiasol Vita Verde SRL
Via F Da Levanto 7, 37138 Verona
Italy
Tel. : (045) 574611
Fax : (045) 574188
Product Detail : Natural Cosmetics, Vitamins Supplements,
Herbal Medicines etc.

313. M/s. Standard Homeopathic Co.
210 W 131ST Street
PO Box 61067
Los Angeles, CA 90061, U.S.A.
Tel. : (213) 3214284
Fax : (310) 5168579
Product Detail : Homoeopathic Remedies

314. M/s. Steigerwald Arzneimittalwerk GmbH
Havelstrasse 5, D-6100 Darmstrot
Germany
Tel. : (49) 61513305-0
Fax : (49) 6151317832
Product Detail : Ethical Herbal and Homoepathic Medicines

315. M/s. Stevia Pacific Distributor
87-87A, Frankel Avenue
Singapore 1545, Singapore
Tel. : (65) 4495319
Fax : (65) 2416779
Product Detail : Liquorice Sweetner, Liquorice Antioxidants, Natural Preservative Stevia

316. M/s. Su Do Pharm. Ind. Co. Ltd.
168-9 Yeomri-Dong
Mapo-Ku, Seoul, Korea
Tel. : (02) 7184211-6
Fax : (02) 7182569
Product Detail : Traditional Herbal Medicines

317. M/s. Sunsource Health Products Inc.
4731, W. Atlantic Avenue
Suite 13, Delray Beach, Florida 33445
U.S.A.
Tel. : (407) 4993113
Fax : (407) 4987557
Product Detail : Herbal Products

318. M/s. Suzuki Nippondo Co. Ltd.
15, 4 Chome, Nihonbashi-Honcho
Chuo-Ku, Tokyo 103, Japan
Tel. : (81) 332412122
Fax : (81) 352556630
Product Detail : Especially Medicated Plasters, Liniments for Muscular Pains, Medical Heal

319. M/s. Swedish Herbal Institute
Viktoriagatan 15, 41125 Goteborg
Sweden
Tel. : (46) 31116779
Fax : (46) 3117147
Product Detail : Herbal Medicines & Extracts

320. M/s. Taiko Pharmaceutical Co. Ltd.
34-14 Uchihonmachi, 3-Chome
Suita, Osaka 564, Japan
Tel. : (81) 63821021
Fax: (81) 63192185
Product Detail : Herbal Japanese Folkloric Medicines for Gastro-Intestinal Disorders

321. M/s. Taisho Pharmaceutical Co. Ltd.
24-1 Takata 3-Chome
Toshima-Ku, Tokyo 171, Japan
Tel. : (81) 303985111
Product Detail : Kampo Medicines

322. M/s. Teikoku Seiyaku Corp. Ltd.
567 Santonmatsu
Onchi-Cho, Okawa-Gun
Kagawa 769-26, Japan
Tel. : (81) 879 252221
Fax : (81) 879 241555
Product Detail : Kampo Medicines, Especial Plaster and Plastices, Anti inflamatory

323. M/s. Teras Perkasa SDN BHD
19 Ji 11A/133, Sri Sentosas
58000 Kuala Lumpur, Malaysia
Tel. : (60) 37941782
Fax : (60) 27941793
Product Detail : Herbal Products

324. M/s. Tiger Medicals Ltd.
2 Chia Ping Road, hex 0900
Haw Par Tiger Balm Bldg.
Singapore
Tel. : (65) 2652777
Fax : (65) 2654703
Product Detail : Natural Product

325. M/s. Tokko Koshin Co. Ltd.
Kamiuma Central Bldg.
2-5 Kamiuma, 4 Chome
Setagaya-Ku, Tokyo 154, Japan
Tel. : (81) 334143156
Fax : (81) 334143180
Product Detail : Whole Ground Herbs

326. M/s. Tong IL Trading
Via Trento 22/B
24035 Curno (BG), Italy
Tel. : (035) 61276
Fax : (035) 610426
Product Detail : Natural Cosmetics and Food Supplements

327. M/s. Tong-IL SL
Doctor Gomez Ulla 8
28028 Madrid, Spain
Tel. : (34) 17262185
Fax : (34) 17266780
Product Detail : Herbal Medicines

328. M/s. Traditional Medicinal Inc.
4515 Ross Road
Sebastopol, CA 95472, U.S.A.
Tel. : (707) 8238911
Fax : (707) 8231599
Product Detail : Herbal and Medicinal Teas, Kwai Garlic and Recycled Pepper Products

329. M/s. Tree of Life Inc.
1750 Tree Boulevard
St. Augustine, Floride 32086, U.S.A.
Tel. : (904) 8248181
Fax : (904) 8252009
Product Detail : Herbal and Homoeopathic Remedies, Vitamins and Minerals

330. M/s. Trophic Canada Ltd.
260 Okanagan Avenue E
Penticton BC, V2A 3JT,
Canada
Tel. : (604) 4928820
Fax : (604) 4925066
Product Detail : Herbal Medicines

331. M/s. Tsumura & Co. Ltd.
12-7 Niban-Cho
Chiyoda-Ku, Tokyo-102, Japan
Tel. : (81) 33221001
Fax : (81) 332215282
Product Detail : Kampo Medicines, Herbal Tea, Cosmetics and Chiyota Herbs

332. M/s. Unda SA-NV
Rante De Lorce 16
4920 Harce, Belgium
Tel. : (32) 041845901
Fax : (32) 846655
Product Detail : Homeopathic Medicines nd Phytomedicines

333. M/s. United Medical Plants.
26. Rue Du Mont Roti
78550 Houdan, France
Tel. : (33) 130596006
Fax : (33) 130595292
Product Detail : Herbal Remedies and Herbal Teas

334. M/s. Vepro
Via Val Saviore, 25100 Brescia, Italy
Tel. : (030) 320387/320389
Fax : (030) 320389
Product Detail : Herbal Medicines and Food Supplements

335. M/s. Vitalmina Ltd.
Agamemnonos 18
15561 Holargos, Athens, Greece
Tel. : (30) 16526581
Fax : (30) 16522039
Production Detail : Herbal Remedies and Herbal Cosmetics

336. M/s. VSM Geneesmiddelen BV
Berenkoog 35, 1800 GH Alkmaar, Netherlands
Tel. : (31) 72661122
Fax : (31) 72623883
Product Detail : Homoeopathic and Herbal Products

337. M/s. W Spitzner Arzneimittel Fabrik GmbH
Bunsenstr 6-10, 7505 Ettlingen, Germany
Tel. : (49) 724310610
Fax : (49) 7243106333
Product Detail : Herbal Products Especially Nasal Decongestant

338. M/s. Wakunaga of America Co. Ltd.
23501 Madero
Mission Viejo, CA 92691
U.S.A.
Tel. : (714) 8552776
Fax : (714) 4582764
Product Detail : Herbal and Homoeopathic Remeides

339. M/s. Wakunaga Pharmaceutical Co. Ltd.
2-14 Fushimi, 4-Chome
Chuo-Ku, Osaka 553
Japan
Tel. : (81) 62058901
Fax : (81) 62058920
Product Detail : Kampo Medicine

340. M/s. Weider Nutrition
2875 Bates Road
Montreal PQ, H3S 1B7
Canada
Tel. : (514) 7312783
Fax : (514) 7317082
Product Detail : Herbs and Natural Medicines

341. M/s. Weleda
544 Arlesham
Switzerland
Tel. : (41) 61014141
Fax : (41) 617014115
Product Detail : Homoeopathic and Natural Cosmetic Products

342. M/s. Weleda UK Ltd.
Heanor Road, Likeston
Derbyshire, DE7 8DR,U.K.
Tel. : (602) 303151
Fax : (602) 440349
Product Detail : Herbal and Homoeopathic Medicines

343. M/s. Woelm Pharma GmbH & Max Woelm Stras
Postfach 840
D-3400 Eschwege
Germany
Tel. (49) 565180101
Fax : (49) 5651801384
Product Detail : Herbal Medicines, Pharmaceuticals

344. M/s. Woo Chun Pharm Co. Ltd.
1337-25 Seocho-Dong
Seocho-Ku, Seoul
Korea
Tel. : (02) 5669956-7
Fax : (02) 5661150
Product Detail : Traditional Herbal Medicines and
Pharmaceutical Products

345. M/s. Woo Kwang Pharm. Co. Ltd.
379-3 Singhyun-RI
Opp Myun, Kwangju-Kun, Kyungki-Do
Korea
Tel. : (0342) 447835
Product Detail : Traditional Herbal Medicines

346. M/s. Yamamoto Yakuhin Kogyo Co. Ltd.
3 Nihonbashi Honcho
4-Chome, Chuo-Ku, Tokyo-103, Japan
Tel. : (81) 32416111
Product Detail : Herbal Extract and Raw Material

347. M/s. Yomeishu Seizo Co. Ltd.
16-25 Nanpidai-Cho
Shibuya-Ku, Tokyo-150, Japan
Tel. : (81) 334628132
Fax : (81) 334628339/8492
Product Detail : Herbal Tonic

348. M/s. Young Jin Pharm Co. Ltd.
656-230 Sungsoo-Dong
1-GA, Sungdon-Ku, Seoul
Korea
Tel. : (02) 4638131
Fax : (02) 4642257
Product Detail : Traditional Herbal Medicines and
Pharmaceutical Products

349. M/s. Zyma Sa (Inc. Valverde)
Route De L-Etrax
1260 Nyon-Ch
Switzerland
Tel. : (41) 223632111
Fax : (41) 223621744
Product Detail: Ethical Pharmaceutical and Herbal Medicines

15

Directory of Perfumes & Flavours

Manufacturers/Distributors/Suppliers/Traders/Exporters/Importers

CENTRAL REGION

Name of Address	*Phone/Fax Telex Nos.*	*Business Activities*
ABC Enterprises C-101, Jumbo Darshan 2nd Koldongri, Andheri (East) Bombay-400 069 *Chief: S.N. Niduja* *Alternate: C.S. Hiduja*	Est.: 1980 Tel.: 8341364 8382122	Dealers : Essential Oils and Aromatic Chemicals
A.A. Attarwala 5, Commercial Chambers Yusuf Maherali Road Opp. Zakaaria Masjid Bombay-400 003 *Chief: Abdul S.A. Attarwala* *Alternate: Mohd. F.A. Attarwala*	Estd.: 1953 Tel.: 3438763 3447306	Dealers : Perfumes, Perfumery Agarbatti Spary Perfume
A.A. Attarwala & Co. Pvt. Ltd. 82-84, Clare Road Agarbathes Bombay-400 008 *Chief: Mohd. Yunus Ahmernoor* *Alternate: Mohammed Rizwan*	Est.: 1980 Tel.: 3086252 3085795, 309104 Fax: 3076660	Manufacturers : Perfumers, Perfumery Campounds, Attars, Scent & Cosmetics

Directory of Perfumes and Flavours–Manufacturers/ Distributors/Suppliers/Traders/Exporters/Importers

Name & Address	Phone/Fax Telex Nos.	Business Activities
A.A. Attarwala & Sons 295 Janjikar Street Opp. Jumma Masjid Bombay-400 002 *Chief: Mohammed Yusuf*	Estd.: 1977 Tel.: 3425677	Dealers : ACOS & RIKOS Brand Scent & Spray
A.H. Chemist & Sons 293, Ebrahim Rahimtuila Road Patka Manzil Bombay-400 003 *Chief: A.H. Siddiqui*	Est.: 1957 Tel.: 3437893	Manufactures : Industrial Perfumary Compounds, Flavouring Essence, Edible Food Colours, Rose water etc.
A.R. Attarwala 325, Sheikh Memon Street Juma Masjid Bombay-400 002 *Chief: Abdul Rehman*	Est.: 1985 Tel.: 3429923 3426261	Manufacturers : Perfumery Compounds Dealers : Agarbatties, Aromatic Chemical, Attars etc.
A.S. Attarwala & Sons 160, Abdul Rehman Street Bombay-400 003 *Chief: Ismail M. Attarwala*	Estd.: 1880 Tel.: 3423974 Fax.: 3420376	Manufacturers : Rose Water Kevda Water etc.
A. Hami Bros. 71-C, Mohamedali Road P.O. Box 3488 Bombay-400 003 *Chief: Gulam abbas Hami* *Alternate: Ahsan Hami*	Estd.: 1939 Tel.: 3445082 3435440 3433996 Fax: 3715207 Fax: 3741848	Manufacturers : Perfumery Compounds Indian Absolutes Attars, Sandalwood Oil, Agarwood Oil, Hair Oils & Dyes
ACME Synthetic Chemicals 308, Veer Savarkar Marg. Dadar Bombay-400 028 *Chief : Rajiv R. Kallianpur* *Alternate: Vijay C. Kallianpur*	Estd.: 1970 Tel. Off.: 4465127 4452706 Fax: 8724258 8722581 Fax: 4440282	
Ajmal & Sons 99-CD, Mohammedali Road Bombay-40 003 *Chief: Sirajuddin Ajmal* *Alternate: Mohibul Haque*	Estd. 1977 Tel.: 34279082 3427030 2856976 Telex:011-84304 MUSK IN Fax: 2856609	Manufacturers : Exporters & Dealers: All kinds of Indian Perfumers, Perfumery Compounds, Esential Oils, Agaroudh & Agarbatti

Name & Address	*Phone/Fax Telex Nos.*	*Business Activities*
Chimanal Maganlal & Co. 1-A, IInd Floor, Chamen Chambers Cinema Road, Dhobi Talao Near Metro Bombay-400 020 *Chief: Mahendra Ajmera*	Estd.: 1938 Tel.: 2018945 2015250 2090028 Fax: 2019064	
Clovex Aromatics 68/4, Tarun Bharat Chakala, Andheri (E) Bombay-400 099 *Chief: P.R. Pendarkar*	Estd.: 1987 Tel.: Off.: 8368647 Fac.: 02145- -321189	Manufacturers : Essential Oils and Chemicals Aroma Chemicals
Concorde Chemical Corporation 205, Pinky Palace No. 750, S.V. Road, Bombay-400 052 *Chief: Shekhar Parekh* *Alternate: H.V. Parekh*	Estd.: 1980 Tel.: 6463601 6463597 Fax: 6463940	Traders : Importers of Aromatic Chemicals, Essential and Pharmaceuticals
Cosmair Products 101, Centre Point, Julibhai Lane, Lalbaug Bombay-400 012 *Chief: Sudhir Kapadia* *Alternate: Anjum Samel*	Estd.: 1985 Tel. : Off.: 4123214 4122144 Fac.: 0252-355770 Fax: 4148226	Manufacturers: Perfumery Compounds
D.D. Shah & Company Damodar Building 105, Princess Street Bombay-400 002 *Chief: Shailesh D. Shah* *Alternte: S.B. Bansi*	Estd.: 1955 Tel. : Off.: 2850577 (4 lines) Fax.: 2850581 Tlx: 011-85732 DDS IN	Manufacturers : Aroma Chemicals Essential Oils and Fragrances
D.G. Boys & Co. Mohamedi House 79, Mohamedali Road Bombay-400 003 *Chief: S.K. Hatimbhai* *Alternate: S.K. Abbasbhai*	Estd.: 1947 Tel.: 3424327	Manufacturers : Indian Perfumery Compounds Non Alcoholic

Name & Address	*Phone/Fax Telex Nos.*	*Business Activities*
D.G. Gore 31,Mangaldas Road Bombay-400 002 *Chief: Y.J. Gore* *Alternate: D.V. Gore/A.Y. Gore*	Estd.: 1917 Tel.: 2080909 2066346 Fax: 2083408	Manufacturers : Fragrances
D.L. Dhane 24, Prarthana Apts. S.K. Bole Road N.M. Kale Marg, Dadar Bombay-400 029 *Chief: A.D. Dhane*	Estd.: 1989 Tel.: 4372690	Manufacturers : Natural Essential Oils
Dayalji Shamji 14, Deepak Niwas Cardinal Gracious Marg, Chakala, BOmbay-400 099 *Chief: Bharat Kumar*	Estd.: 1968 Tel.: 8381670 8381455	Dealers: Aroma Chemicals Natural Essential Oils and Resinods
Devi Prasad Aromatics 13, Mahendra Mansiori 28, Babu Genu Road Bombay-400 002 *Chief: B.N.V. Pai* *Alternate: G.V. Kamath*	Estd.: 1986 Tel.: 2091301 2069544	Dealers : Essential Oils, Aromatic Chemicals and Perfumery Compounds
Deevien Agencies 6, Pitha Street, Off. P.M. Road, Bombay-1 *Chief: Aswin Nadkami* *Alternate: Nitin S. Nadkami*	Estd.: 1979 Tel.: 2047991 2824773 Fax: 2873811	Agents : For Aroma Chemicals Fragrances, Flavours & Ess. Oils
Deep Deep Niraj Chemicals Pvt. Ltd. E-26, M.I.D.C., Nagpur-28 *Chief: S.K. Mehta* *Alternate: M.V. Gadgil*	Estd.: 1987 Tel.: 01704-36715 Fax: 07104-37734	
Dhiraj & Company 7, Hiranandaji Indl. Estate Opp. Kanjurmarg, Rly. Stn. Kanjurmarg (W) Bombay-400 078 *Chief: Govind Bahroos*	Estd.: 1967 Tel.: 5782352 5785812 Fax: 5779075	Manufacturers : Distillation jobwork of Aroma Chemicals and Essential Oils, Aromatic Pepperment & Spearmint Oils, Clove oil, orange oils, Eugenol etc.

Name & Address	*Phone/Fax Telex Nos.*	*Business Activities*
Dujodwala Industries 814, 815 Tulsiani Chambers 212 Nariman Point Bombay-400 021 *Chief: Shyamsunder V. Dujodala*	Estd.: 1967 Tel.: 2822502 2822503 2822492 Fax: 2854095 Telex: 84752 DIBY IN	
Dujodwala Resins & Terpenes Pvt. Ltd. 812, Tulsianai Chambers 212 Nariman Point Bombay-400 021 *Chief: O.R. Dujodwala* *Alternate: P.R. Dujodwala*	Estd.: 1978 Tel.: 2824089 5 lines Fax: 2841284 2841281	Manufacturers : Camphor, Terpene Chemicals, Rosin & Synthetic Resins
Eastern Agencies 301, Mangal Simran 28th Road, Off. turner Road Bandra (West) Bombay-400 050 *Chief: J.L. Bhatia* *Alternate: Sushil Bhatia*	Estd.: 1956 Tel.: 6433242 6453958 Fax: 6435189 Telex: 11-76387 AJAY IN	Dealers : Aromatic Chemicals Essential Oils, Resinoids Sodium Saccharin etc.
Eastern Aromatics Pvt. Ltd. Datta Mandir Road Bhandup (West) Bombay-400 078 *Chief: Yashawant M. Kale* *Alternate:* *Dr. Mrs. Saroj Y. Kale*	Estd.: 1968 Tel.: Off.: 5600396 5619797 Fax: 5680260	Manufacturers : Aromatic & Perfumery Chemicals
Emmco Perfumers 17/19, New Bengalipura St. Bombay-400 003 *Chief: Abdul Majid A. Kazi* *Alternate: Shabbir Ahmed Kazi*	Estd.: 1948 Tel.: 3711370 3741978	Manufacturers and Exporters : Cosmetics & Perfumery Compounds
The Enamdar Trading Corporation 63, Devkaran Mansion S.G. Marg Bombay-400 002 *Chief: Prakash V. Rane*	Estd.: 1991 Tel.: 2010305	Manufacturers : Industrial Perfumes

Name & Address	*Phone/Fax Telex Nos.*	*Business Activities*
Esofaly Mahomedaly & Co. 102/104, Sarang Street Post Box No. 3177 Bombay-400 003	Estd.: 1845 Tel.: 3425633	Dealers : Flavouring Essences and all requirements of aerated water trade
FFC Aromas Pvt. Ltd. Plot No. A-42, Street No. 2 Marol Indl. Area (MIDC) Andheri (East) Bombay-400 093 *Chief: N.A. Nimbalkar* *Alternate: Arun Nimbalkar*	Estd.: 1962 Tel. Off.: 8375234 8301524 Fax: 7686993 Fax: 8364491 Telex: 011-78490 FFC IN	Manufacturers : Fragrances & Aroma Chemicals
Floral Fragrance No. 3 Railway Shopping Centre Vidyavihar (E) Bombay-400 077 *Chief: Paras Daftary*	Estd.: 1991 Tel.: 5130389	Traders : Aromatic Chemicals and Essential Oils
Bhagat Impex Pvt. Ltd. 164, Sitaram Poddar Marg Bombay-400 002 *Chief: Praveen Biyani*	Estd.: 1989 Tel.: Off.: 2086587 2086828 Fax: 89-58613 89-28727 Fax: 2057084	Manufacturers : Mentha Oil Basil Oil & Other Essential Oils
Foreign Scent Supplying Syndicate Scent House, Station Road Goregaon (West) Bombay-400 062 *Chief: Yogesh Jain*	Estd.: 1948 Tel.: 8721444 8722612 8722280 Fax: 8720818 Telex: 01170038 FAIS IN	Manufacturers and Exporters : Perfumes Essential Oils etc.
Fragrance & Aroma 305, Swasti House 70, Kazi Sayed Street Bombay-400 003 *Chief: Pravin Makwana* *Alternate: Suresh G. Vora*	Estd.: 1981 Tel.: 3435424 3444434 (711) 473684	Dealers : Aromatic Chemicals Natural Essential Oils Perfumery Compounds etc.

Name & Address	Phone/Fax Telex Nos.	Business Activities
Fragrochem 311, Anant Deep Chambers 3rd Floor, 273/77 Narsi Natha Street Bombay-400 009 *Chief: Bhupen Thakkar* *Alternate: Niranjan Thakkar*	Estd.: 1980 Tel.: 3757039 3765378	Manufacturers : Industrial Perfumery Compounds
Gajanan Rajaram Kshetramade 34, anamika,10th Gulmohar Cross Road, J.V.P.D. Scheme Bombay-400 049 *Chief: Gajanan R. Kshetramada*	Estd.: 1983 Tel.: 6210011 6241956	Agent : For Laxmi Chemicals
Garden Chemical Works Shiv Krupa Indl. Estate Unit No. 113, Ist Floor L.B.S. Marg, Vikhroli Bombay-400 083 *Chief: Motila Chawla*	Estd.: 1968 Tel.:	Manufacturers : Flavouring Compounds and Synthetic Colours
Garodia Trade & Agency 504, Lotus Vasant Valley Film City Road, Malad (East) Bombay-400 097 *Chief: Vijay Garodia*	Estd.: 1991 Tel.: 8410834 8410836	Agents : For Citronella Oil
General Additives Pvt. Ltd. E124, Ansa Indl. Estate Sakivihar Road, Sakinaka Bombay-400 072 *Chief: J.P.Wanchoo*	Estd.: 1984 Tel.: 5783326 5785381 Fax: 5774952	Manufacturers : Flavours & Perfumery Compounds
The General Import Co. (India) 102, Princess Street Keshav Bagh Bldg. Bombay-400 002 *Chief: Srichand Talreja* *Alternate: Gopal Talreja*	Estd.: 1948 Tel.: 2014497 2057958 Fax: 2088614	Dealers : Aromatic Chemicals Solvents, Food Colours etc.

Name & Address	*Phone/Fax Telex Nos.*	*Business Activities*
Girish Enterprise Govind Bld. (Parshwadeep) 12A, 128/142, S.G. Marg Bombay-400 002 *Chief: Girish J. Vajani*	Estd.: 1985 Tel.: Off.: 2083258 2060561 Fax: 4946128 4923601 Fax: 4939019	Manufacturers : Perfumery Compound Agent of: M/s F Chauvet S.A., France for Aromatic Chemicals Essential Oils and Resinoids
Gohil Chemicals 211, 'Anand' 82/84 Kazi Sayed Street Bombay-400 003 *Chief: Naresh Gohil* *Alternate: Viren Gohil*	Estd.: 1974 Tel.: 3424515 3446191 Fax: 3400992 Telex: 076325 GDCIN	Agents : For Robin Chemicals Pvt. Ltd. Madras Dealers : Flavouring Essences
Golax Industrial Perfumes A/4, Vimal Udyog Bhavan Opp. Badal Cinema, Mahim Bombay-400 016 *Chief: D.N. Nankani*	Estd.: 1961 Tel.: 4307525 4302307 4302307 Fax: 4363160	Manufacturers : Industrial Perfumery Compounds
Goldem Aroma 48, Ranvir Building 70, Princess Street Bombay-400 002 *Chief: Anup Shah* *Alternate: Jyotin Shah*	Estd.: 1976 Tel.: Off.: 2052745 2054930 Fac.: 3079599 Fax: 2018054	Manufacturers : Perfumery Compounds Aromatic Chemicals and Flavours
Goldensun Laboratories 421, Parekh Market Opera House Bombay-400 004 *Chif: Jyotin Shah*	Estd.: 1976 Tel.: 2052745 2054930 Fax: 2018054	
Goldensun Manufacturing Co. 48, Ranvir Building 70 Princess Street Bombay-400 002 *Chief: Jyotin Shah*	Estd.: 1962 Tel.: Off.: 2052745 2054930 Fac.: 8734066 8732696 Fax: 2018054	Manufacturers : Aromatic Chemicals Essential Oils, Resinoids Perfumery Compounds etc.

Name & Address	*Phone/Fax Telex Nos.*	*Business Activities*
Goldfield Fragrances Ltd. 17/1, Prabhadevi Estate Veer Savarkar Road Prabhadevi Bombay-400 025 *Chief: Ravi Mullick* *Alternate: G.H. Kamat*	Estd.: 1992 Tel.: Off.: 4934634 4951825 4960314 Fax: 4934634	Manufacturers : Fragance Compounds & Aroma Chemicals
Govindji Khimji Thakkar 13, Maturesh Building 3rd Floor, V.P. Cross Road No. 1, Opp. Sharon School, Mulund (W) Bombay-400 080 *Chief: Govindji K. Thakkar*	Estd.: 1956 TEl.: 5614926	Broker : Aromatic Chemicals Essential Oils etc.
Grover Brothers 79-E, Shamaldas Gandhi Marg Bombay-400 002 *Chief: Kulbhushan Grover* *Alternate: Somdutt Grover*	Estd.: 1972 Tel.: 2013207 2055517	Dealers : Perfumery Compounds Aromatic Chemicals Agarbatti & Spray Requisites
Gujrat Essence Mart Pvt. Ltd. 124/126 Shamaldas Gandhi Marg Bombay-400 002 *Chief: M.C. Kathrani* *Alternate: J.C. Kathraja*	Estd.: 1947 Off.: 2017214 2011449 Fax: 8341112 8221658 Fax: 8380164 Telex:011-79124 ACWB IN	Dealers : Essence Dry Flavours Food Colours (ISI) Motor Brand Sacchann (ISI) Perfumery Compounds Mustard Oils Vanillin Pure, Essential Emulsions etc. Agents Asian Chemical Works (Bombay) Pvt. Ltd.
Gwalior Chemical Industries Ltd. 1&2 Western India House Sir P.M. Road, Fort Bombay-400 001 *Chief: Harisingh Shyamsukha* *Alternate: N. Nair*	Estd.: 1977 Tel.: Off.: 2870415 2873541 2833028 Fax: 2851809 Tlx.: 011-86554 MINA IN	

Name & Address	*Phone/Fax Telex Nos.*	*Business Activities*
H.K. Daftary 39, Shamaldas Gandhi Marg Near Ndrabhuvan Hotel Bombay-400 002 *Chief: Kiran H. Daltary*	Estd.: 1954 Tel.: 2061335 3820352	Manufacturers : Perfumery Compounds and Agarbatti
H.V. Parfumerie 2, Savitha 58/59 Chedda Nagar Bombay-400 089 *Chief: K.P. Balakrishanan*	Estd.: 1983	Manufactures : Perfumery Compounds
Haji Atiq and Sons 178, Sherif Devji Steet Bombay-400 003	Estd.: 1976 Tel.: 3441098 3414558 3441675 Fax: 3401422	Manufacturers : Indian Attars, Perfumery Compounds, Agarbathies Sandalwood oil etc.
Hami and Company Ismail Building, 1st Floor New Cutlery Market Juma Masjid Bombay-400 002 *Chief: Tayebli E. Attarwala* *Alternate: Mohsin Attarwala*	Estd.: 1935 Tel.: 3424879 3449027 3400240 Fax: 3410920	Manufacturers : Indian Perfumes and Attars
Harish J. Vajani 1/13, Mani Bhavan 9, Pathakwadi Bombay-400 002 *Chief: Harish Vajani*	Estd.: 1992 Tel.: 2052239 Fax: 2069749	Traders : Perfumery Raw Materials
Harisons Chemicals 51, Popatwadi, 1st Floor Kalbadevi Road Bombay-400 002 *Chief: G.H. Desai* *Alternate: Ms. Sheetal Desai*	Estd.: 1971 Tel.: 2058691 4093899 40777476 Fax: 4071419	Dealers : Aromatic & Essential Oils, Organic & Inorganic Chemical, Drugs, Vitamins etc.

Name & Address	*Phone/Fax Telex Nos.*	*Business Activities*
Harsha Aromatics G-4, Riddhi Siddi Apt. Mahagar 'X' Road, Mulund (E) Bombay-400 081 *Chief: Uday L. Shah* *Alternate: Kishore L. Shah*	Estd.: 1978 Tel.: Off.: 5611063 5673676 Fac.: 5605490 Fax: 5649415	Manufacturers : Perfumery Compounds and Aromatic Chemicals
Hasanali Kamroodin 820, Bhavani Peth G.R. Sathe Memorial Complex Near Bhavani Mata Mandir Pune-411 002 *Chief: Imteaz Bhagat*	Estd.: 1888 Tel.: 644876 Fax: 091-212-644876	Manufacturers : Perfumery Compounds Ayurvedic Medicines Essential Oils & Aromatic Chemicals
Hemani Aromatics Minerva Estate Bunder Road, Sewri (East) Bombay-400 015 *Chief: Girish Hamani*	Estd.: 1959 Tel.: 4124605 4154401 Fax: 4076425	Manufacturers : Industiral Perfumery Compounds & Rectified Natural Essential Oils
Hemani Brothers 108, Himalaya House 79, Pilton Road Bombay-400 001 *Chief: Viraj M.Hemani* *Alternate: Anil P. Hemani*	Estd. : 1964 Tel.: 2615902 Fax: 2611580 Telex: 11-80039 CPCO-IN	Traders : Aromatic Chemicals & Essential Oils
Herdillia Chemicals Ltd. **Air India Bldg.** 13th Floor, Nariman Point Bombay-400 021 *Chief: Rajiv M. Pandia* *Chief: Rajiv M. Pandia* *Alternate: S.K. Chan*	Estd.: 1968 Tel.: Off.: 2024224 Fac.: 7681153/54 Fax: 7671891	Manufacturers : Commodity and Speciality Chemicals Including Aroma Chemicals
Himalaya Agencies Chamber Bhavan, 3rd Floor 226, Kalbadevi Road Bombay-400 002 *Chief: Madhusudan Nevathia* *Alternate: Ram Niranjan Nevatia*	Estd.: 1972 Tel.: 2011458 2015301 Fax: 2011458	Dealers : Distilled Turpentine Dipentine, Pine Oil Terpeneol, Rosin etc.

Name & Address	*Phone/Fax Telex Nos.*	*Business Activities*
Himanshu Aromatics Mahalaxmi Indl. Estate Unit No. 11, 2nd Floor Gandhi Nagar, Lower Parel Bombay-400 013 *Chief: Himanshu B. Desai* *Alternate: Rajni B. Desai*	Estd.: 1983 Tel.: 4937877 4927105	Manufacturers : Industrial Fragrances
Hindustan Aromatics 166, Ebrahim Rehmatullah Road Bombay-400 003 *Chief: Mushtaq Husain* *Alternate: Aziz*	Estd.: 1972 Tel.: Off.: 3762194 2018005 Fac.: 3746409 3093416 Fax: 3738075	Manufacturers : Aromatic Compounds
Hindustan Lever Ltd. Chemicals Division I.C.T. Link Road Andheri (East.) Bombay-400 099 *Chief: Ulhas Vairagkar*	Estd. 1933 Tel.: 8221696 8329471 Fax: 8225708 Tlx.: 79437 HLCD IN	Manufacturers : Aroma Chemicals
Hitesth Chemicals Works Shankar Niwas Maskasath Nagpur-440 002 *Chief: Kirikumar H. Chandama*	Estd.: 19709 Tel.: Off.: 43610 Fac.: 43620 Fax: 43487	Manufacturers : Perfumes
IDL Chemicals Ltd. 'Nirmal' 15th Floor, Nariman Point Bombay-400 021 *Chief: B. Srinivas Reddy*	Estd.: 1964 Tel.: 2026946 2025318 2041267 Fax: 2041167 Telex: 011-82539 IDLB IN	Manufacturers/Agents Aromatic Chemicals Inbrosan, Timbrone Cyclogalbanate, Allyl Phenoxy Acetate Estergam etc.
(The) INA Trading Company 107, Damodar Bldg. Princess Street Bombay-400 002 *Chief: Rakesh C. Jani*	Estd.: 1863 Tel.: 2081979	Manufacturers : All kinds of Aromatic Compounds

Name & Address	*Phone/Fax Telex Nos.*	*Business Activities*
Indian Organic Chemicals Ltd. Chemtex House, 2nd Floor Main Street, Sector 12 Hiranandani Gardens, Powai Bombay-400 076 *Chief: S.G. Makim* *Alternate: R.M. Adhyapak*	Estd.: 1960 Tel.: 5780625 5780232 Fax: 5793924 Telex: 71970 IOCL IN	
Indo Nippon Chemical Co. Ltd. Maker Bhavan No. 2 18,New Marine Lines Bombay-400 020 *Chief: P.I. Bhuva* *Alternate: K.B. Kukami*	Tel.: 2051723 Fax: 2053488 Tlx.: 118-2081 INCC IN	Estd.: 1960
Industrial Aromatics 2/32, Verma Nagar Old Nagardas Road Bomby-400 069 *Chief: B.K. Parikh* *Alternate: H.B. Parikh*	Estd.: 1982 Tel.: Off.: 8349352 Fac.: 8720132	Manufacturers : Perfumery Compounds and Aromatic Chemicals
Industrial Perfumes Ltd. Hay Bunder Road Tank Road P.O. Bombay-400 033 *Chief: A.C. Malik*	Estd.: 1957 Tel.: 3711001 3711003 3711004 Fax: 3739313 Tlx.: 11-76695 INPF IN	Manufacturers : Aromatic Chemicals Fragrance Compouds Natural Ess. Oils, Resinoids, Spice Oils and Oleoresins
Interchemie 243/3-B, Mangaldas Bldg. Mangaldas Road Bombay-400 002 *Chief: Natin Parekh* *Alternate: Rajan Parekh*	Estd. 1971 Tel.: 2017409 2053823 2064673 Fax: 2064688	Traders : Chemical, Pharma Ceutical Raw Materials Perfumeries Essential Oils, Menthol etc.
Ishwarlal Jethalal Mul Ratna, 3rd Floor, No. 7 334 Narsi Natha Street Katha Bazar Bombay-400 009 *Chief: Arvindbhai* *Alternate: Jitendrabhai*	Estd.: 1965 Tel.: 3425632 3446157	Dealers : Menthol, Thymol Camphor, Aromatic Chemicals Natural Essential Oils etc.

Name & Address	*Phone/Fax Telex Nos.*	*Business Activities*
IVY Fragrances Unit No. 108 Creative Indl. Estate N.M. Joshi Marg Bombay-400 011	Estd.: 1981 Tel.: 3088302	Manufacturers : Flavouring Compounds and Perfumery Compounds
J.B. Patel & Co. 133, New Apollo Estate Mogra Road, Andheri (E.) Bombay-400 069 *Chief: J.B. Patel* *Alternate: P.B. Patel*	Estd.: 1984 Tel.: 8322631 8320989 Fax: 8378156	Agents : Universal Food Flavours Dealing in Speciality Seasonings for Snack Foods like potato chips Extruded/Directly expanded snacks etc.
J.D. Savant & Co. Govardhandas Khimji Bldg. 1st Floor, 35, Vithaldas Road S.G. Marg Bombay-400 002 *Chief: A.J. Savant* *Alternate: B.A. Savant*	Estd.: 1963 Tel.: Off.: 2017456 Fac.: 6243558 6207969 Fax: 6249780	Dealers : Industrial Perfumery Compounds, Aromatic Chemicals, Ess Oils Resinoids etc.
Jupiter Trading Co. 18, Devkaran Mansion Chowk 20, Mangaldas Road Bombay-400 002 *Chief: Ashesh* *Alternate: Rajesh*	Estd.: 1960 Tel.: Off.: 2054710 6153338 Fac.: 8385129	Dealers : Natural Essential oils
James Wright Ltd. 909, Embassy Centre Nariman Point Bombay-400 021 *Chief: K.G. Jhajharia*	Estd.: 1941 Tel.: 2047593 Fax: 2840645	Manufacturers : Java Citronella oil
K.H. Dhamdhere 45/47, Shamaldas Gandhi Marg Bombay-400 002 *Chief: Amol Dhamdhere*	Estd.: 1928 Tel.: 2081683	Traders : Essential Oil, Aromatic Chemicals Perfumery Compounds etc.
K.K. Enterprises 16-A Mulchand Mansion Ist Floor, S.G. Marg Bombay-400 002 *Chief: Kaushik Doshi*	Estd.: 1969 Tel.: Off.: 2058495 3345466 Fac.: 4226527	Manufacturers and Dealers : Aromatic Compounds & Chemicals, Natural Essential Oils

Name & Address	*Phone/Fax Telex Nos.*	*Business Activities*
Kanta Flavouring Industries A-15 & 16, Royal Ind. Estate 5--B Naigaum Cross Road Wadala (West) Bombay-400 031 *Chief: Sharad Sejpal* *Alternate: Devendra Sejpal*	Estd.: 1972 Tel.: Off.: 4123165 4124347 Fac.: 4126784 4136154	Manufacturers : Flavouring Compounds Flavouring Emusions Food Colours and Saccharin
Kavas N. Petigara 801, Citadel, 18-B Ruparel Marg Bombay-400 006 *Chief: Kavas N. Pabgara* *Alternate: D.B. Billimona*	Estd.: 1979 Tel.: Off.: 3632889 Fac.: 4360425 Fax: 3632889	Agents : Berje Inc. USA Oxford Chemicals, UK Fragrance Resources Inc. USA Dealers: Aroma Chemicals Flavours Flavour Chemicals etc.
Keva Fragrances Ltd. Devkaran Mansion ented 36, Mangaldas Road Bombay-400 002 *Chief: Ramesh V. Vaze*	Estd.: 1980 Tel.: Off.: 2069609 2019198 Fac.: 5645273/74 Fax: 5645271 2081204 Tlx: 011-71939 KEVA IN	Manufacturers : A 100% Export Ori- Unit, Perfumery Compounds and Flavouring Essences for Exports only No domestic sales
Khanna Aromatics Sharaf Mansion, 2nd Floor 32 Princess Street Bombay-400 002 *Chie: Bhishma Khanna* *Alternate: Pankaj Khanna*	Estd.: 1988 Tel.: Off.: 2012853 Fac. 8211931	Manufacturers : Industrial Fragrances
Krupa Scientific & **Industrial Apparatus Co.** 113/115 Shivam Indl. Estate Station Road, Govandi Bombay-400 088 *Chief: P.V. Karnik* *Alternate: J.V. Harshe*	Estd.: 1981 Tel.: 5563702 5569881 Fax: 5562781	Manufacturers : Aromatic Chemicals

Name & Address	*Phone/Fax Telex Nos.*	*Business Activities*
Kushal Chand Sons Devkaran Mansion Room No. 07/3 Block No. 1, 2nd Floor Bombay-400 002 *Chief: Lalit Hirani* *Alternate: Amit Hirani*	Estd.: 1922 Tel.: 2052190 2080937 Fax: 2084265	
L.B. Aroma & Chemicals Pvt. Ltd. 4, Omex Chamber, Gr. Floor Rajashree Shahu Marg Andheri (E) Bombay-400 069 *Chief: Gopalbhai Ghoghan*	Estd.: 1990 Tel.: 8326277 Fax: 6107700	Dealers : Natural Essential Oils & Aromatic Chemicals
L. Liladhar & Company 257-259 Samuel Street Vadgadi Bombay-400 003 *Chief: Madhusudan Mody*	Estd.: 1992 Tel.: Off.: 3422988 3447690 Fac.: 7670396 7671102	Manufacturers : Dyes, Food Colours, Food Flavours etc. Food Flavours etc.
Laboratory Suppliers A/10, New Life Co. Op. Hsg. Society, Shivsrishti Kurla (E) Bombay-400 024 *Chief: V.S. Mahajan* *Alternate: Parag Mahajan*	Estd.: 1982 Tel.: Off.: 5227439 5220865 Fac.: 7682060 Fax: 5231709	Manufacturers : Aromatic Chemicals
Lalit & Vijay 115, Mangaldas Bldg., No. 2 Mangaldas Road Bombay-400 002 *Chief: Lalit Vigh* *Alternate: Vijay Vigh*	Estd.: 1979 Tel.: 2055060	Manufacturers : Perfumery Raw Materials
Lalji Lakhamshi Chemicals (P.) Ltd. Mani Bhavan, 15 Pathak Wadi, Lohar Chawl Bombay-400 002 *Chief: Sanjay Pandya* *Alternate: Manish Chheda*	Estd.: 1985 Tel.: 2081923 2052513 Fax: 2084212 Telex: 011-83935 LALU IN	Dearlers : Aromatic Chemicals

Name & Address	Phone/Fax Telex Nos.	Business Activities
Lana Floressens Pvt. Ltd. 13, Swastik Indl. Estate 178, C.S.T. Road, Kalina Bombay-400 098 *Chief: K.L. Narayan* *Alternate: Ms Kusum Ballal*	Estd.: 1967 Tel.: 6122928 6127440	Manufacturers : Industrial Flavours and mgrances
The Laxmi Chemicals 84, Industrial Estate Kopargaon Ahmednagar *Chie: Bhaskar D. Hon*	Estd.: 1984 Tel.: 23154/23354 23265 Fax: 91-62423 23145	Manufacturers : Aromatic Chemicals Diethyl Phthalate
Laveesha Enterprises 216/217 Anjani Complex 2nd Floor, Pereira Hill Road Opp. Guru Nanak Petrol Pump Andheri Kurla Road, Andheri (E) Bombay-400 099 *Chief: Lalit Vigh*	Estd.: 1986 Tel.: 8216159 Fax: 8216261	Dealers : Aroma Chemicals Essential Oils and Perfumery Compound
Leela Aromatics Room No. 2, 1st Floor 24, Mangaldas Road Devkaran Mansion Princess Street Bombay-400 002 *Chief: Jagdish Pal*	Estd.: 1983 Tel.: 2050558 2057314	Manufacturers : Eseential Oils Dealing in Aroma Chemicals
Lovely Research Chemical (India) 2/6, Anand Bhawan 17, Babu Genu Road Bombay-400 002 *Chief: P.C. Jain*	Estd.: 1980 Tel.: 2017150 2066418 Fax: 2016509	Manufacturers : Exporters of Natural & Synthetic Perfumery Compounds
Mac Industry A/6, Harsha Apartment Bhakti Marg, Mulund (W) Bombay-400 080 *Chief: Ashok V. Shah*	Estd.: 1992 Tel.: 5641463 5646164 5603929	

Name & Address	*Phone/Fax Telex Nos.*	*Business Activities*
M.C. Davar & Company Sai Bhavan, 2nd Floor 143, Princess Street Bombay-400 002 *Chief: Ashit M. Patel* *Alternate: Ramesh R. Shah*	Estd.: 1968 Tel.: 2085752	Dealers : Chemicals, Fragrances and Naturals
M.D. Tolia Corporation 29, Mangaldas Road 192, Mangaldas Bldg., No. 3B Bombay-400 002 *Chief: Devendra Tolia* *Alternate: Narendra Tolia*	Estd.: 1970 Tel.: 2069099 2053470 Fax: 2061366	Dearlers : Aroma Chemicals, Essential Oil and Resinoids
M.M. Nabikhan & Co. 135, Bhandra Road Ganja Khet Nagpur-440 002 *Chief: Ale Nabikhan* *Altrnate: Habib Nabikhan*	Estd.: 1976 Tel.: 44460	Dealers : Aromatic Compounds Perfumes, Agarbaties Empty bottles, Corks etc.
M.R.Mody 3B/29, Mangaldas Road Bombay-400 002 *Chief: H.R. Thakker* *Alternate: J.H. Thakker*	Estd.: 1939 Tel.: 2019724 2087571	Dealers : Aromatic Chemicals Natural Essential Oils and Resinoids
M. Rawji Brothers Gulabi House, 4th Floor 111/115, Jazu Styed Street Bombay--400 003 *Chief: Lalit Rawji* *Alternate: Kumarpal Rawji*	Estd.: 1977 Tel.: 3429598 3445455 3448769 Fax: 3410694	Manufacturers : Aromatic Fine Chemicals and Fragrances
Madhura Concentrates Kothrud Post Office Bldg. Pune-411 029 *Chief: A.A. Vyas* *Alternate: M.A. Vyas*	Estd.: 1983 Tel.: C/o 338232 Fax: C/o 348904	Manufacturers : Flavours, Perfumes Fragrances, Aroma Raw Materials etc.
Maharashtra Aromatics 72, Haroon Cottage Opp. Ashok Nagar Vakola Pipe Line (Santacruz (E) Bombay-400 055 *Chief: N.N. Inamdar*	Estd.: 1986 Tel.: 6147616	Manufacturers : Aromatic Chemicals

Name & Address	*Phone/Fax Telex Nos.*	*Business Activities*
Malve Chemicals "SHABRI" Building, Kopar Road Ahead of Santoshi Mata Bldg. Dombivli (W)-421 202 *Chief: Datta Malve* *Alternate: Suhas Malve*	Estd.: 1984 Tel.: Off.: 452336 Fac.: 590846 Fax: 452636	
Manak Citrus Products Pvt. Ltd. At & Post: Ultran, Tal, Erandol Distt. Jalgaon-425 117 *Chief: Satish Sanghavi*	Estd.: 1975 Tel.: (02576)-40070	Manufacturers : Lime Juice, Lime Oil, Pectin and other Citrus Products
Maneklal & Bors. 61/A, Devkaran Mansion S.G. Marg (Princess Street) Bombay-400 002 *Chief: Bharat Mehta* *Alternate: Nilesh Mehta*	Estd.: 1919 Tel.: 2011671	Dealers : Aromatic Chemicals Perfumery Compounds Soda Water Requisites
Mangal Perfumers 304, Prabhadevi Unique Indl. Estate Bombay Dyeing Compound V.S. Marg, Prabhadevi Bombay-400 025	Estd.: 1981 Tel.: 4303680	Manufacturers : Perfumes
Mayur Corporation 2/11, Arondekar Bhavan 14, H.F. Society Road Jogeshwari (East) Bombay-400 060 *Chief: K.G. Satoskar* *Alternate: K.V. Shah*	Estd.: 1987 Tel.: 2062868 8328699	Dealers : Aromatic Chemicals & Essential Oils
Mayur Enterprises 45, Mangaldas Bldg. No. 1 2nd Floor Mangaldas Road Above Grindlays Bank Bombay-400 002 *Chief: Kaushik V. Shah*	Estd.: 1983 Tel.: 2088051 2088057	Dealers : Aromatic Chemicals & Essential Oils Agent : Ms. Amruta Industries Nasik

Name & Address	*Phone/Fax Telex Nos.*	*Business Activities*
Meenakshi Kemicals & Trading Co. 113, Maganlal House S.V. Road,Malad (West) Bombay-400 064 *Chief: J.K. Talati*	Estd.: 1985 Tel.: 8881513 8828262 Telex: 70076 PCOX IN Fax.: 8822757 MTD 62	Traders/Indentors Exporters : Raw Materials of Cosmetics, Agarbattis Perfumes, Soaps- Detergents
Megha Enterprises 197/1, Sion (West) Post Box No. 6554 Bombay-400 022 *Chief: Suresh L. Meghani*	Estd.: 1970 Tel.: 3759950 Fax: 3737064	Manufacturers and Traders : Natural Essential Oils Flavours & Fragrances Attars, Oleoresins Perfumes spice oils etc.
The Mercantile Essential Oil Co. 101, Centre Point Jilibhai Lane, Lalbaugh Opp. Parel Post Office Bombay-400 012 *Chef: Sudhir Kapadia* *Alternate: Ketan Sheth*	Estd.: 1947 Tel.: 4123214 4124208 Fax: 4148226	Manufacturers : Non Alcoholic Perfumes Talcum Powder
Min Chem India 117, Loha Bhavan P D'Mello Road, Masjid (E.) Bombay--400 009 *Chief: Pravin V. Parekh*	Estd.: 1986 Tel.: 3400515 3439045 Telex: 011-76603 MICI IN Fax: 3401619	Traders : Aromatic Chemical & Natural Essential Oils
Mody & Co. Engineer Building 265 Shamaldas Gandhi Marg Bombay-400 002 *Chief: P.M. Banker* *Alternate: S.L. Mehta*	Estd.: 1985 Tel.: Off.: 2013463 2084785 Fac.: 5321468 5320593	Manufacturers : Viola Flavouring Essences and Food Colours Chameli Agarbattis
(The) Mohini Agency 309, Hill View Industrial Estate Amrut Nagar, Ghatkopar (W) Bombay-400 086 *Chief: Madhu Assar*	Estd.: 1911 Tel.: 5170125 5173420 Fax: 5169733	Manufacturers : Perfumery & Agarbatti Compounds

Name & Address	Phone/Fax Telex Nos.	Business Activities
Mohini Perfumers P. Ltd. 13, Krishnakunj 144/145 M.G. Road, Ghatkopar Bombay-400 077 *Chief: V.B. Assar*	Estd.: 1992 Tel.: Off.: 5133092 Fac.: 7685454 7685643 Fax. 5160729	Manufacturers : Perfumery Compounds
Mukesh Industries 7, Anjirwadi, 2nd Floor Champsi Bhimji Road Mazagaon, Bombay-400 010 *Chief: Jayantilal Gada*	Estd.: 1968 Tel.: 3750896 3739557 Fax: 3738484	Manufacturers : Agarbatties, Camphor Tablets, Perfumery Compounds Dearlers : Aroma Chemicals
Multiflora 72, Mangaldas Road Dwarkadas Building Lohar Chowl Bombay-400 002 *Chief: Jetha L. Bhatia*	Este.: 1981 Tel.: 2080666 Fax: 6400128	Manufacturers : Perfumery Compounds Agents : Nippon Zeon Co. Ltd. Tokyo Japan
Muralidhar Chemical Industries 364, Kaliandas Udyog Bhavan Near Century Bazar, Prabhadevi Bombay-400 025 *Chief: M. Venkatraman* *Alternate: M. Shridhar*	Estd.: 1975 Tel.: Off.: 4225432 4226853 Fac.: 7686369 Telex: 011-71154 BAKE IN Fax: 4309294	Manufacturers : Food Chemicals & Industrial Chemicals
Musks & Fragrance 11, lankar, 2nd Floor Above Nadco Stores S.V. Road, Andherei (W) Bombay-400 058 *Chief: Mukesh No. Patel*	Estd.: 1965 Tel.: Off.: 6244121 6249902 6703348 Fax: 6249842 2060992	Manufacturers : Cinnamic Alcohol Yara Randarom, Rasinoid Olebanum, Resinoid Banzoin Agents : M/s. Kuraray Co. Ltd. Japan M/s. FFC Aromas Pvt. Ltd. Bombay M/s. Riddhi Intermediates Chemicals P. Ltd. Panolt

Name & Address	*Phone/Fax Telex Nos.*	*Business Activities*
Mysore Dhoop & Agarbatti Works E-2/2, Bharat Nagar Bombay-400 007 *Chief: Mohanial K. Kataria* *Alternate: Manoj M. Kataria*	Estd.: 1958 Tel.: Off.: 3082405 3084866 Fax: 3080773	Manufacturers : Agarbatti & perfumery Agarbatti & Perfumery Compounds
Mysore Fine Agarbatti Factory 711, Raheja Centre Nariman Point Bombay-400 021 *Chief: Anil M. Ahuja* *Alternate: Sunil M. Ahuja*	Estd.: 1958 Tel.: Off.: 2844597 2832128 Fac.: 8329506 Telex: 011-86517 Fax: 2830710	Manufacturers Agarbatties
Mysore Sugandhi Dhoop Factory Pvt. Ltd. 208, Embassy Centre Nariman Point Bombay-400 021 *Chief: K.K. Luthria* *Alternate: M.K. Luthria*	Estd.: 1980 Tel.: Off.: 3424584 2833858 2832006 Fac.: 335283 Tlx.: 86288 MSDF IN Fax: 2028213/ 3870142	Manufacturers : Indian Incense Sticks (Agarbatties) Cones & Dhoops
Mysore Y.S. Agarbathi Works 6, Arab Lane Bombay-400 008 *Chief: Mohd. Yusuf* *Alternate: Asif Yusuf*	Estd.: 1980 Tel.: 3082444	Manfacturers : Perfumery Compounds and Agarbatties
NEC Petro Chemie Fine Enterprise A/10, Ness Baug, 5th Floor Nana Chowk Bombay-400 007 *Chief: E.H. Mistry* *Alternate: C.H. Mistry*	Estd.: 1980 Tel.: 3876528 Fax: 3850566	Agent : Dealing in Aromatic Chemicals Manufactured by Bruno Court Eurovanillin

Name & Address	*Phone/Fax Telex Nos.*	*Business Activities*
N.R. Shah & Co. 4B, Ranvir Building 70, Princess Street Bombay-400 002 *Chief: Mukund R. Shah*	Estd.: 1953 Tel.: 2052745 2054930 Fax.: 2018054	Traders : Perfumery Raw Materials
N. Chimanlal & Company Post Box No. 2574 160 Princess Street Chikhal House Bombay-400 002 *Chief: Narendra C. Suvarnkar* *Alt: Chandravadan C. Suvarnkar*	Estd.: 1942 Tel.: Off.: 2012010 2019890 Fac.: 427877 Fax.: 2012010	Manufactures : Perfumery Raw materials Natural Essential Oils Aromatic Chemicals perfumery Compounds Corks Alluminium Bottles, etc.
N. Girdharlal & Co. 146-A Chikhal House Princess Street Bombay-400 002 *Chief: Suryakant N.Bhuta*	Estd.: 1948 Tel.: 2061476	Traders : Flavour, Fragrance & Food Colour
Nagpur Chemicals W-36, M.I.D.C. Indl. Area Hingna Road Nagpur-440 016 *Chief: Vinod Shankar Gan.*	Estd.: 1981 Tel.: Off.: (07104)-	Manufacturers : Aromatic Chemicals and Methyl Anthrandate, Alpha ACA etc. & Industrial Perfumes
National Arochem Labs National House 13/14/15 Sahra Road, Vile Parle (W) Bombay-400 057 *Chief: Sudhir Choksey* *Alternate: Jagdish Thakkar*	Estd.: 1967 Tel.: Off.: 20919724 2087571 Fac.: 8342407	Manufacturers : Aromatic Chemicals & Rectified Natural Ess. oils
National Essence Supply Co. 12, Shalimar, Gulmohar Cross Lane, 10, Juhu Scheme, Juhu Bombay-400 049 *Chief: Pravin Jain*	Estd.: 1958 Tel.: 6206831	Manufacturers & Dealers : Soap Perfumes & Other Essences
National Polymers Sibibal Trust Building 14/16, Bhandari X Lane H.No. 23, II Floor Bombay-400 003 *Chief: Kiran N. Agrawal*	Estd.: 1986 Tel.: 3435041 3435042 Fax.: 3435046	Traders & Agents : Flavour & Perfumery Raw Material and other related products

Name & Address	Phone/Fax Telex Nos.	Business Activities
Nemat Enterprises Devloaran Mansion 2nd Floor, 43 Princes Street Bombay-400 002 *Chief: Anis I Attarwala* *Alternate: Ismail M. Attarwala*	Estd.: 1984 Tel.: Off.: 2019816 2068917 Fac.: 6324650 Fax: C/o 2085977	Manufacturers : Indian Perfumes Attars & Agarbattis
New Barouliya Aromatics Co. 14, Dhanlaxmi Chambers II Floor Opp. Khandelwal Mithaiwala Thane-400 601 *Chief: Pradeep Barouliya* *Alt: Jalnarayan K. Barouliya*	Estd.: 1977 Tel.: Off.: 5332280 5331208 5429076 Fac.: 542 Fax.: 5331208	Manufacturers : Perfumery Compounds
New India Aromatics Co. Mukund Madhav Udyog Nagar Unit No. 2, Plot No. 142 Village Navghar, Vasai (E) Distt. Thane *Chief: Ashit Patel* *Alternate: Ramesh Shah*	Estd.: 1945 Tel.: (712) 326280	Manufacturers : Industrial Perfumes
Niranjan & Company Zakaria Building 7, Chakla Street Bombay-400 003 *Chief: M.M. Bhuta*	Estd.: 1952 Tel.: 342882` 3428822 Fax: 4147261 Tlx.: 11-76109 ROSE IN	Dealers : Natural Essential Oils Aromatic Chemicals
Odhawji Lawji & Co. Gold Mohur Building 1st Floor, R. No. 4 174 Shamakdas Gandhi Marg Bombay-400 002 *Chief: Pradip Arvindkumar Bhuta* *Alternate: Ashok A. Bhuta*	Estd.: 1930 Tel.: 2050273	Traders : Flavouring Essences, Food, Colours, Essential Oils, Aromatic Chemicals & Compounds Saccharine & Chemicals Agents: Bush Boake Allen (I) Ltd. Duckworth Flavour (I) Pvt. Ltd.

Name & Address	*Phone/Fax Telex Nos.*	*Business Activities*
Omega Polycoats 'Nirmal' Near Khare Town P.O. Dharampeth Nagpur-440 010 *Chief: Dilip Pandharpukar*	Estd.: 1987 Tel.: Off.: 0712-531006 Fac.: 07104-36667	Manufacturers : Benzyl Acetate-FFC Eugenol, Isoeugenol
Opal Products 2/9, Three View Building Opp. Century Bazar, Prabhadevi Bombay-400 025 *Chief: Dr. V.V. Devasthale* *Alternate: D.B. Pandit*	Estd.: 1962 Tel.: 4221595	Manufacturers : Atomatic Chemicals Shynthetic Essential Oil, Perfumery bases and Compounds
Oriental Aromatics Pvt. Ltd. Sion Trombay Road, Govandi Bombay-400 088 *Chief: Anil K. Bodani* *Alternate: Dharmil a. Bodani*	Estd.: 1972 Tel.: 5563613 5559837 Telex: 011-61013 OA IN Fax: 5560708	Manufacturers : Perfumes & Flavours
P.A. Lodha & Sons 1617 Shukrawar Peth. Subhansha Road Pune-411 002 *Chief: Kishore P. Lodha* *Alternate: Dilip P. Lodha*	Estd.: 1931 Tel.: 474409	Agents Avon Flavours in Trishul Food Colours, Raj Foods Traders : Food Flavours, Colours and Food Chemicals
P.M. Rathod & Co. Pvt. Ltd. Chikhal House, 1st Floor 453, Kalbadevi Road Bombay-400 002 *Chief: Suresh T. Mehta* *Alternate: Jitendra T. Mehta*	Etd.: 1954 Tel.: Off.: 2010103 2089160 Fac.: 5611688 Fax.: 5670598	Manufacturers : Industrial perfumery Compounds
P.M. Vora and Co. Ramesh Chamber, 1st Floor 14, Rabibdas Street, Vadgadi Bombay-400 003 *Chief: Gunvantbhai Bora* *Alternate: Sanjay Bora*	Estd.: 1972 Tel.: 3438487 3445367 Fax: 3446013	Dealers : Natural Essential Oils Food Colours Aromatic Chemicals Flavours Food Chemicals
P. Muncherji & Company 10, Ambalal Doshi Marg Old Hamam Street Bombay-400 023 *Chief: R.D. Mullan* *Alternate: Mrs. N.E. Taleyarkhan*	Estd.: 1895 Tel.: 2654865 2653837	Agents : Perfumery Compounds & Aromatic Chemicals

Name & Address	*Phone/Fax Telex Nos.*	*Business Activities*
P.R.S. Narayanan Flat No. 21, II Floor Jayanti Apartments J.S. Dossa Road, Mulund (W) Mombay-400 080 *Chief: P.R.S. Narayanan*	Estd.: 1956 Tel.: 5684376	Agents : Commission Cum Canvassing Agent in Indian Natural Essential Oils Spice Oils and Oleoresins
Pankaj Aero Chemicals 203, Himalaya House, II Floor 79, Palton Road Bombay-400 001 *Chief: Pankaj Anil Hemani* *Alternate: Manhar P. Hemani*	Estd.: 1978 Tel.: Off.: 2619182 Fac.: 7681131 Telex: 11-80039 CPCO-IN Fax: 2611580	Manufacturers : Aromatic Chemicals & Essential Oils
Parekh Perfumery Works 128, Bhuleshwar Road Kabutarkhana Bombay-400 002 *Chief: Harkishan R. Parekh*	Estd.: 1958 Tel.: Off.: 3739711 3739712 Fac.: 3727052 Fax: 022-3739711	Manufacturers : Indian Perfumed Agarbatties and Non-Alcoholic Perfumery Compounds
Passion Aromatics 12-A, Laxmanrao Kirloskar Road Opp. K.O.E.L., Khadki Pune-411 003 *Chief: Dilip Resiklal Shah*	Estd.: 1982 Tel.: Off.: 311234 Fac.: 31778 Fax: (0212)-435253	Manufacturers : Aroma Chemicals & Essential Oils i.e. Benzyl Acetate Benzyl Group products Iso Amyl Alcohol, Amyl Acetate Terpinyl Acetate Phenyl Ethyl Methyl Ether, Citronella Oil Derivatives, Alpha Amyl Cinnamic Alehyde etc.
Perfine Chemical Industries Date Bungalow, Thanawala Lane Vileparle (E) Bombay-400057 *Chief: Ashok Bhatia* *Alternate: Pradeep Datar*	Estd.: 1979 Tel.: Off. : 8341332 Fac.: 461492	Manufacturers : Dihydroisojasmine Hydratropic Aldehyde Olibanum Resinoid Geranyl Nitnle
Perfume Centre 94-C Mohamedali Road Bombay-40 003 *Chief: Aliasgar I. Attari* *Alternate: Ibrahim I. Attari*	Estd.: 1964 Tel.: 3443049 Fax.: 3420551	Traders : Perfumery Compounds Agarbatties & Allied items

Name & Address	*Phone/Fax Telex Nos.*	*Business Activities*
Perfumatics Plot NO. 42, Sector, 24 G.E. Scheme Behind Gupta Weigh Bridge Turbhe New Bombay-400 705 *Chief: IBV Raghavan*	Estd.: 1983 Tel.: 7682323 7681322 Tlx.: 1311281 PERF IN Fax.: 7672537	Traders : Perfumery Chemicals & Essential Oils Agents : Sairex Chemie Gmbh Germany
Pharm Aromatic Chemicals 507, Nain Krupa 118/122, Kazi Syed Street Bombay-400 003 *Chief: Madhu L. Thakkar*	Estd.: 1978 Tel.: 3432526 3448032 Fax: 3401805	Traders : Aromatic Chemicals, Natural Essential Oils Baisam Toki Baisam Peru, Baisam Copaiba Agents : Calabrian Citrus Centre Italy
Pharmaco 101, Saraf Mansion, 1st Floor 32, Princess Street Bombay-400 002 *Chief: Kishore D. Pansare*	Estd.: 1987 Tel.: 2083309 2055741 Fax: 2055741	Impoters-Traders : Aromatic Chemicals & Pharmaceutical Raw Materials
Planters International Company 16A, 2nd Floor Double View Bldg. 52, Mint Back Road, Fort Bombay-400 001 *Chief: K.S. Nanjappa*	Estd.: 1987 Tel.: Off.: 2626203 Telex: 011-82426 PIC IN Fax: 2611635	Agents : Essential Oils & Aroma Chemicals
Poonam International 45/49 Babu Genu Road Balkrishna Krupa Co-op. Hsg. Soc. Ltd. Office No. 81A, Ground Floor Kalbadevi Bombay-400 002 *Chief: Manubhai D. Pandya*	Estd.: 1981 Tel.: 2057131 2086559	Traders & Agents : Aromatic Chemicals
Prabhat General Agencies 154/6, Mittal Tower, B Wing Nariman Point Bombay-400 021 *Chief: V.T. Chudiwala* *Alternate: J.P. Singh*	Estd.: 1947 Tel.: 2823680/ 8182 2825055 Fax.: 2842147 Telex: 11-84164 PGA IN	Manufacturers : Terpineol Extra Pure Terineol BP Terpmyl Acetate, Beta Pinene ISO longifolene, Acetyl Longifolence, Acetyl Longifolence fine Oil Drentene Turpentine IPDC Estergum BG etc.

Name & Address	*Phone/Fax Telex Nos.*	*Business Activities*
Praful J. Parkesh 45, Mangaldas Bldg. No. 1 Mangaldas Road Above Grindlays Bank Bombay-400 002 *Chief: Praful Parekh*	Estd.: 1981 Tel.: 2088051 2088057	Broker : Aromatic Chemicals, Natural Essential Oils Resinoid & Perfumery Compounds, etc.
Pragati Aroma Oil Distillers Pvt. Ltd. 2/6, Anand Bhavan,17 Babu Genu Road Princess Street Bombay400 002 *Chief: Pankaj Jain*	Estd.: 1992 Tel.: Off.: 2017150 2066418 Fax: 2016509	Manufacturers : Essential Oils Concretes & Absolutes
Pranav Perfumers 61/A, Devkaran Mansion Princess Street Bombay-400 002 *Chief: Bharat Mehta* *Alternate: Uday Mehta*	Estd.: 1986 Tel.: 2011671	Traders : Aromatic Chemicals & Perfumery Compounds
Pravinkumar Hiralal 35, Kazi Sayed Street Bombay-400 003 *Chief: Pravin H. Khurana*	Estd.: 1991 Tel.: 3450620 3438431 Fax: 3737064	Traders : Aromatic Chemicals Natural Essential Oils Perfumery Compounds Resinoids etc.
Privi Organics Pvt. Ltd. 205, Princess Street Bombay-400 002 *Chief: Mahesh Babani* *Alternate: D.B. Rao*	Estd.: 1989 Tel.: 2062626 (6 Lines) Fax.: 2080282	Manufacturers : Aromatic Chemicals and Rectified Processed Essential Oils
Procter & Gamble India Ltd. Godrej Soaps Administration Bldg. Pirojshahnagar Eastern Express Highway Vikhroli (East) Bombay-400 079 *Chief: L.N. Prasad*	Estd.: 1966 Tel.: 5173082 Fax.: 5173080 Telex: 11-73827 RICH IN	Manufacturers : Pharmaceuticals and Consumers Products

Name & Address	*Phone/Fax Telex Nos.*	*Business Activities*
Pushpak Chemicals Pvt. Ltd. Harikrupa, Plot No. 30 Kamala Nehru Cross Road No. 3, Kandivli (West) Bombay-400 067 *Chief: Rajnikant D. Ghelani*	Estd.: 1985 Tel.: 8051552 8060998 Fax: 8051444	Manufacturers : Fine Aromatic Chemicals
Quest International India (A division of Pond's (India) Ltd.) Plot No. 6, Saki Vihar Road Sakinaka Bombay-400 072 *Chief: V. Sankaran* *Alternate: S.B. Sule*	Estd.: 1948 Tel.: 5782305/ 06/07/08 Telex: 11-72162 QUEST IN Fax: 5787787	Manufacturers : Interalia Flavouring Compounds, Fragrance Compounds
R.C. Aromatics & Chemicals 69, Narayan Rao Koli Marg (Bhansari Street), Koliwada Mandvi, Near Vadgadi Bombay-400 003 *Chief: Anil R. Shah* *Alternate: Vikram R. Shah*	Estd.: 1962 Tel.: Off.: 3432235 Fac.: 624735 6246809	Manufacturers : Aromatic (Perfumery) Chemicals such as Aldehyde C14 Aldehyde C16, Dimethyl Hydroquinone, Paracresyl Acetute Phenyl Ethyl Methyl Ethet Yara Yara Terpinyl Acetate etc.
R.D. Corporation 42/44 Babu Genu Road 2nd Floor, Room No. 5 Princess Street Bombay-400 002 *Chief: Paresh G.K. Khakhar* *Alternate: Mukund G. Khakhar*	Estd.: 1980 Tel.: 2061122 2068961 2089459 Fax.: 2068961	Traders : Aromatic Chemicals Perfumery Compounds & Natural Essential Oils
R.K. Shapurji & Co. Prospect Chambers, 4th Floor R.No. 8, 319, Dr. D. Naoroji Road Bombay-400 001 *Chief: Miss Jinee R. Icewalla*	Estd.: 1943 Tel.: 2047408 Fax: 3865951	Traders & Agents : Aromatic Chemicals Essential Oils, Aldhydes Perfumes Raw Materials
R. Jayantilal & Co. 190, Samuel Street Khoja Gali, 1st Floor Bombay-400 009 *Chief: Jitendra J. Gandhi*	Estd.: 1993 Tel.: 3759383 3762523 Fax.: 3736915 6109780	Traders : Aromatic Chemicals Essential Oils, etc.

Name & Address	*Phone/Fax Telex Nos.*	*Business Activities*
R. Sureshchandra & Co. Kshamalaya, 3rd Floor 37 New Marine Lines Bombay-400 020 *Chief: Vinoobhai U. Shah* *Alternate: Navin U. Shah*	Estd.: 1948 Tel.: 2009397 2003533 2004272 Telex: 011-83617- RSCO IN Fax: 2005238	Traders & Agents : Aromatic Chemicals, Fine Chemicals, Bulk Drugs & Pharmaceutical Raw Materials
Radhakishan Rajaram & Co. 141, Shamaldas Gandhi Marg Bombay-400 002 *Chief: Shashi Valavalkar*	Estd.: 1932 Tel.: Off.: 2091094 Fac.: 4936450 Fax: 2081094	Manufacturers : Perfumery Compounds
Rajasthani Trading Co. 349 Samuel Street 4th Floor, Indu Chambers Bombay-400 003 *Chief: Mahesh Khandelwal* *Alternate: Ashish Khandelwal*	Estd.: 1969 Tel.: Off.: 3441981 3411807 3442875 Fax: 3411806	Manufacturers : Flavours, Pastes & Emulsions, Fragrances Essential Oils etc.
Ram and Company 73, Princess Street Devakaran Mansion Bombay-400 002 *Chief: Ketan R. Chande* *Alternate: Avunish R. Chande*	Estd.: Tel.: 2069996	Traders : Aroma Chemicals & Perfumery Compounds
Rayon Industries 21, Yayyug Mansion N. Bharuca Marg Near Grant Road Station (W) Bombay-400 007 *Chief: Shivananda V. Shendy*	Estd.: 1948 Tel.: 3878801	Manufacturers : perfumes & Flavours
Reliance Sales B-33, Nandjyot Ind. Estate Kurla Andheri Road Safed Pool Bombay-400 072 *Chief: Mrs. Pushpal R. Mantn*	Estd.: 1984 Tel.: 5121820 Fax.: 6210924	Indenting Agents : Henkel KGaA, Grau Aromatics GmbH Aroma Chemie Pual Kaders GmbH

Name & Address	*Phone/Fax Telex Nos.*	*Business Activities*
Remlin Laboratories 39 Nand Bhuvan 59, Babu Genu Rd. Bombay-400 002 *Chief: Linesh N. Shah*	Estd.: 1981 Tel.: 2069885 7670551 Fax.: 2051593	Agents : K.L. Koh Enterprise Pte Ltd. Singapore Dealers : Perfumery Chemicals and Compounds
Ronak Fine Industries 18-20 Ghanshyam Indl. Estate Veera Desai Rad, Andheri (W) Bombay-400 053 *Chief: Narendra Pandya* *Alternate: Ashok Pandya*	Estd.: 1969 Tel.: 6292543 3424338 3435142 Fax.: 6267298	Manufacturers : Menthol, Peppermint Oil and Fine Chemicals
Roshanlal & Sons Gopal Niwas 1st Floor 133 Princess Street Bombay-400 002 *Chief: Ashok Jhingan* *Alternate: Surender*	Estd.: 1962 Tel.: 2084579 2031798	Agents : Bush Boake Allen (I) Ltd. Hackson & Dadajee ltd. Corn Products Co (I) Ltd. Dealers : Flavours Food Colours Aroma Chemicals and Essential oils
Rupin Chemicals 30, Hari Market, Khar (W) Bombay-400 052 *Chief: P.H. Mehra* *Alternate: Ravi Mehra*	Estd.: 1925 Tel.: 6491331 6041691 Fax: 6464076	Manufacturers : Flavours, Pastes, Soft Drinks Concentrates Wine Flavours
S.B. Bhagade L 2/3 Sunder Nagar S.V. Road, Malad West Bombay-400 064 *Chief: S.B. Bhagade*	Est.: 1984 Tel.: Off.: 8725866 Fac.: 5150777 5166986 Fax: 8737185	Dealers : Aromatic Chemicals and Consulting Engineers
SB Bhgade L 2/3, Sunder Nagar, S.V. Road, Malad West Bombay 400 064 Chief: S.B. Bhagade	Estd. 1984 Tel: Off.: 8725866 Fac.: 5150777 5166986 Fax: 8737185	Dealers: Aromatic Chemials and Consulting Engineers

Name & Address	*Phone/Fax Telex Nos.*	*Business Activities*
S.H. Kelkar & Co. Ltd. Devkaran Mansion 36 Mangaldas Road Bombay-400 002 *Chief: G.D. Kelkar* *Alternate: S.V. Vcze*	Estd.: 1955 Tel.: Off.: 2069609 2019130 Fac.: 5642242/43 5642245 Telex: 011-83450 011-71960 Fax: 5647334	Manufacturers : Fragrances, Flavours Resinoids, Aroma Chemical Natural & Chemical Natural & Synthetic Essential Oils
S.H. Mokashi & Co. 401, Rakhi Apartments Tilak Road Dombivli (E)-421 201 *Chief: Swapnil Mokashi*	Estd.: 1990 Tel.: (711)470489 Fax: (711)470489	Manufacturers : Aromatic Chemicals Aldehyde C_9, C_{10}, C_{11}, C_{12}, C_{14}, Citronellol Geraniol, Cinnamic aldhyde etc.
S. Flavours & Fragrances of India 109, Nav Vivek Indl. Estate Mogul Lane, Mahim Bombay-400 016 *Chief: Sudhir A. Hitani*	Estd.: 1980 Tel.: Off.: 6152323 6152324 6153998 Fac.: 4466671 4467983 Fax: 6118141	Traders : Aroma Chemicals & Perfumery Compounds
S. Zhaveri and Co. 109 Shiv Smriti Chambers 49, Dr. Annie Besant Road Bombay-400 018 *Chief: Mrs. Uma R. Javeri*	Estd.: 1951 Tel.: 4932949 4932044 Tlx. 11-76264 ALOK IN Fax: 4930300 4952742	Manufacturers : H.E. Daniel Ltd. U.K. ROEHM GmbH Germany for Natural Essential Oils. Balsams, Film Coating Resins, etc.
S. Kushal Chand & Co. B/1/B-2, Jay Apartments Service Road, Opp. Western Highway, Vile Parle (E) Bombay-400 057 *Chief: Anil K. Hirani* *Alternate: Sunil A. Hirani*	Estd.: 1922 Tel.: Off.: 6152324 6152324 Fac.: 4466671 4467983 Fax.: 6118141	Dealers : Chemicals Aromatic Chemicals, Natural Essential Oils Pharmaceutical Raw Materials etc.

Name & Address	*Phone/Fax Telex Nos.*	*Business Activities*
(The) Sahyadri Trading Co. 22-A, Dawood Baug Road Andheri (West) Bombay-400 058 *Chief: Prashant R. Savant* *Alternate: Raghunath J. Savant*	Estd.: 1062 Tel.: 6246318 6208918	Manufacturers : Perfumery Compound, Aromatic Chemicals Natural Essential Oils Resinoids
Sai Aromas Pvt. Ltd. 223/224, Sanjay Bldg. No. 3 Mittal Indl. Estate Kurla Andheri Road Bombay-400 059 *Chief: Ajay M. Patel* *Alternate: Apoorva M. Patel*	Estd.: 1979 Tel.: 8340013 8388992 Fax: 8364711	Manufacturers : Industrial Perfumes
Saiba Industries Pvt. Ltd. 129/131, Kazi Sayed Street Bombay-400 003 *Chief: Avinash Marathe*	Estd.: 1960 Tel.: Off.: 3446395 Fac.: 8321242 8329049	Manufacturers : Solubdised Spices Flavours, Blended Essential Oils, Oleoresins and total Extracts of Medicinal Plants
Sambhav Interchem P. Ltd. 301 Gokul Arcade Swami Nityanand Marg Vile Parle (E) Bombay-400 057 *Chief: Amit Shah*	Estd.: 1989 Tel.: 8301673 8344884 Fax.: 8326171	Traders : Importers of Chemicals & Solvents
Sanrad Chemicals & Essential Oils 302, Shivdarshan Shopping Centre, Opp. Rly. Station Santacruz (W) Bombay-400 054 *Chief: Satish Nair*	Estd.: 1985 Tel.: 6493260 6487218 6050978 Fax: 6050464	Agents : Bush Boarke Allen London, Siva Essential Oil & Chemicals, Delhi Bush Boarke Allen, Madras Devi Industries Madurai for Aromatic Chemicals & Natural Essential Oils

Name & Address	*Phone/Fax Telex Nos.*	*Business Activities*
Sarigon Organics Ltd. Khanna Construction House 44, A.G. Khan Road, Worli Bombay-400 018 *Chief: Ashok Kumar Goenka* *Alternate: G.P. Mittal*	Estd.: 1986 Tel.: 4930795 4932943 Fax: 4935856	Manufacturers : Dl Ethyl Phthalate (DEP) Dl Methyl Phthalate (DMP) & Other Plasticizers
Satish Perfumers 12-B, Shalimar Industrial Estate, Near Tata Power House Matunga Labour Camp, Matunga Bombay-400 019 *Chief: Vasant M. Kalkar* *Alternate: Dr. Satish V. Kelkar*	Estd.: 1950 Tel.: Off.: 4016706 Fac.: 4092539	Manufacturers : Industrial Perfumes Flavours, Aroma Chemicals and Agarbatties
Sesu Trading Corporation Sai Chambers 367/369 Narai Natha Street Bombay-400 009 *Chief: V. Subramaniam* *Alternate: K. Jayaraman*	Estd.: 1974 Tel.: 3426402 3414444 Fax: 3420832 Telex: 01172247 SESU IN	Traders : Perfumery Compounds Aromatic Chemicals & Natural Essential Oils
Seth Brother (Perfumers) Pvt. Ltd. 6 Souri Buidling, 1st Floor 74/80, Babu Genu Road Bombay-400 002 *Chief: V.N. Dave* *Alternate: S. Kapoor*	Estd.: 1949 Tel.: 2053297 2057108	Manufacturers : Industrial Perfumes
Setty & Shah 105, Princess Street Damodar Bldg., Ist Floor P.B. No. 2593 Bombay-400 002 *Chief: Hiralal Shah* *Alternate: Sanjay Shah*	Estd.: 1961 Tel.: 2068066 2067560 2090010 Fax: 2090011 Telex: 11-83018 SETY IN	Traders : Aromatic Chemicals Essential Oils & Resinoids

Name & Address	Phone/Fax Telex Nos.	Business Activities
Shah Agarbatti & Co. Prestige Chambers 66/68 Kalyan Street Danabunder Bombay-400 009 *Chief: K.N. Shah* *Alternate: A.N. Shah*	Estd.: 1953 Tel.: 3765514 Fax: 3744239	Manufacturers : Agarbattis and Perfumery Compounds
Shaivi Agencies Sai Bhuvan, 1st Floor 141 Princess Street Bombay-400 002 *Chief: Mrigendra Jain*	Estd.: 1974 Tel.: 2066657 2091104 Fax: 2068906	Indenting Agent & Traders : Aromatic Chemicals Industrial Perfumes & Natural Essential Oils
Snehnil Sheri House, 6th Floor Cawasji Patel Street, Fort Bombay-400 001 *Chief: R.D. Mullan* *Alternate: N.E. Teleyarkhan*	Estd.: 1977 Tel.: 2654865 2653837 Tlx: 011-48	Manufacturers : Agarbatties, Perfume Compounds, Shampoos Aromatic Chemicals
Shiel ICE & Chemicals Pvt. Ltd. Dharma Patil Compound Opp. Mahalaxmi Dyeing Mills Kalyan Shil Road MIDC Phase I Dombivli (E)-421 203 *Chief: Ramesh KJhandelwal*	Estd.: 1991 Tel.: Off.: (711)470753 (711)470533	Manufacturers : Aroma Chemicals
Shivom Company 20, Kitchen Garden Lane 6, Mangaldas Market Bombay-400 002 *Chief: Bhagwandas G. Mehta* *Alternate: Beharilal B. Dhameja*	Estd.: 1964 Tel.: 2017597 2014616 Fax: 2091527	Agents : Quest International India Bush Boake Ailen (I) Ltd. RCE Ltd. Roha Dye-Chem Ltd. Dealers : Flavouring Essence Fragrance Compounds Food Colours etc.

Name & Address	*Phone/Fax Telex Nos.*	*Business Activities*
Shree Mangalam Pharma Pvt. Ltd. 292, Princess Street 2nd Floor, Ner Flyover Bombay-400 002 *Chief: G.M. Dhoot* *Alternate: K.E. Krishnan*	Estd.: 1977 Tel.: 2087969 2087411 2087489 Tlx.: 011-84643 MRPL IN Fax: 2087074	Manufacturers : Aromatic Chemicals Phenyl Ethyl Alcohol
Soofi Enterprises 1317 Dalamal Tower 211 Nariman Point Bombay-400 021 *Chief: Dr. Ashok K. Manghnani*	Estd.: 1970 Tel.: 2045748 2043044 2833074 Tlx.: 011-84187 SUFI IN Fax.: 2047657	Agents : Dealing in Aroma & Perfumery Chemicals Essential Oils Resin Oils etc.
Spac Aromas 206/208, Planet Indl. Estate Subhash Road, Vile Parle (E) Bombay-400 057 *Chief: Jagdish H. Thakker* *Alternate: Bhadresh H. Thakker*	Estd.: 1960 Tel.: Off.: 2087571 2019794 Fac.: 8345574 8340543 Fac.: 8345574	Manufacturers : Industrial Fragrances & Flavouring essences
Standard Synthetics Pvt. Ltd. 302, Pujit Plaza, Sec-11 CBD Belapur New Bombay-400 614 *Chief: Ravi Nangia*	Estd.: 1976 Tel.: Off. 7570521 7570104 Fac.: 7681614 7683368 Fax: 7570212	Manufacturers : Aroma Chemicals
Sudhir Aromatics 103, Princess Street Oawawala Builindg Bombay-400 002 *Chief: Shantilal V. Vasani* *Alternate: Sameer S. Vasani*	Estd.: 1961 Tel.: Off.: 2069726 Fac.: 3726962	Manufacturers : Aromatic Compounds Aromatic Chemicals Essential Oils etc.
Sugand Aromatics No. 12, First Floor Above Bombay Mercantile co-op. Bank 69, Mohammadali Road Bombay-400 003 *Chief: L. Sugand*	Estd.: 1983 Tel.: 3400310 3412942	Manufacturers & Traders : Aromatic Chemicals Essential Oils, Flavours & Perfumery Compounds

Name & Address	Phone/Fax Telex Nos.	Business Activities
Sugandha Enterprises 424 Milan Indl. Estate off. T.J. Road Cottongreen Bombay-400 033 *Chief: Ramakant harlalka*	Estd.: 1983 Tel: Off.: 4139058 4125565 4121431 Fax: 4146502	Manufacturers : Aroma Chemicals Essential Oils Concretes & Absulutes
Suman Enterprises 220/224, Kalbadevi Road Harbilas Building, 1st Floor Bombay-400 002 *Chief: G.K. Gupta* *Alternate: Manoj Gupta*	Estd.: 1987 Tel.: 2019208 2063809 Fax: 7669910	Manufacturers : Natural Menthol Peppermint Oil Essential Oils & Chemicals
Pinnacle Flavours and Chemicals Pvt. Ltd. 60, 1st Floor Raja Industrial Estate P.K. Road, Mulund (W) Bombay-400 080	Estd.: 1993 Tel.: 5689803 Fax: 5689802	Manufacturers : Flavours and Blends Agents : PFW Aroma Chemicals BV Holland, Tastemaker, Holand
Synoflor Company 32, S.G. Marg Bombay-400 002 *Chief: Mansoor H. Calcuttawala* *Alternate: Toffique H. Calcuttawala*	Estd.: 1956 Tel.: 2018099 2065882	Manufacturers : Industrial Perfumes
Synthetics & Aromatics 1/CKulsum Terrace 7, Wealton Road, Colaba Bombay-400 039		Dealers : Aromatic Chemicals and Perfumery Compounds
Swastika Industries Bageshree, Dr. Deodhar Compound Markandi, Chiplun Distt. Ratnagiri-415 605 *Chief: Suresh D. Sathe*	Estd.: 1981 Tel.: 52547	Manufacturers : Aromatic Raw Materials Perfumery Compounds Pure Perfumes
T.P. Haran 2/5 Kastur Kunj Sri Bhalchandra Rd Matunga Bombay-400 019 *Chief: T.P. Haran*	Estd.: 1982 Tel.: 4141664 5170334	Dealers : Aromatic Chemicals Essential Oils and Perfumery Compounds

Directory of Perfumes and Flavours–Manufacturers/ Distributors/Suppliers/Traders/Exporters/Importers

Name.& Address	*Phone/Fax Telex Nos.*	*Business Activities*
T. Ali Mahomed & Co. 144-146, Sarang Street Bombay-400 003 *Chief: Taiyeb Mulla Hasanally*	Estd.: 1924 Tel. 3427131 3426663 Fax.: 3425230	Dealers : Essential Oils Flavours
T.S. Abdulla Bhoy & Co. 290/92, Abdul Rehman Street Bombay-400 003	Estd.: 1939 Tel.: 3425133 343803	Traders & Agents : Essences, Perfumes, Saccharin, Food Colours & Annatto Butter Colour Quest International India, Bombay Bush Boake Allen (I) Ltd. Madras Kanta Flavouring Industries Bombay The Vesco Products Co. Calcutta
Tapan Chemicals 402, Ramniwas G.B. Indulkar Rd Vile Parle (E) Bombay-400 057 *Chief: Narendra Shah* *Alternate: Rasesh Shah*	Estd.: 1983 Tel.: Off.: 8345150 Fac.: 079-5890925	Manufacturers : Aromatic Chemicals e.g. Bencyl Acetate Benzyl Benzoate Benzyl Alcohol etc.
Tej Chemicals Pvt.Ltd. 23/24, Siddhi Vinayak Apartment, Mithagar X Road Bombay-400 081 *Chief: Uday L. Shah* *Alternate: Kishore L. Shah*	Estd.: 1984 Tel.: 5611063 45673676 Fax.: 5649415	Manufacturers : Industrial Perfumes
Tradex Impex 103, Princess Street 3rd Floor, Sancheti Bhavan Sancheti Bhavan Bombay-400 002 *Chief: Ram Sitani* *Alternate: Amit Masand*	Estd.:1984 Tel.: 2066160 2064492 Telex : 84982 TRIM IN Fax: 2012508	Agents : Charabot, France, Sanghi Organics & Phytochem Ltd., Indore D.D. Shah & Co. Bombay Triveni Chemical, Bombay Arofine Chemical Inds. Bombay

Name & Address	*Phone/Fax Telex Nos.*	*Business Activities*
Trescho Incorporation 2/3 SarafKasakr Indl. Estate Rear Wing, S.V. Road Oshiwara Jogeshwari (W) Bombay-400 102	Estd.: 1972 Tel.: 6284462	Manufacturers : Perfumes and Cosmetics
Triveni Chemicals Trimbak Ashish Society Gandhi Nagar Dombivli (E)-421 204 *Chief: Dr. D.M. Phatak* *Alternate: K.G. Satoskar*	Estd.: 1980 Tel.: Off.: 711472920 Fac.: 711-472520	Manufacturers : Aromatic Chemicals Fragrance and Flavour Chemicals
Twenty First Century Chemicals Pvt. Ltd. 260, Samuel Street, Vadgadi Bombay-400 003 *Chief: Dr. Tushar Mavani* *Alternate: Dr. Prakash Pradhan*	Estd.: 1987 Tel.: Cff.: 3422960 Fac.: 7668288 Fax.: 3425532	Manufacturers : Aromatic Chemicals Aldehyde C16 Hydroxy Citronellal Geraniol
U.A. Attarwala 72, Jail Road North Opp. J.J. Hospital Gate No. 6 Bombay-400 009 *Chief: Mohd. Usman*	Estd.: 1979 Tel.: 3726361 3766163 Fax: 3719508	Manufacturers : Attars, Perfumery Compounds, Scent Sprayers, Cosmetics and Agarbathies
U.K. Aromatics & Chemicals 8, Kailashu Krupa, First Floor Sion Fort Raod, Sion East Bombay-400 022 *Chief: Shabd Krishnakant Mehta* *Alternate: Krishnakant B. Mehta*	Estd.: 1992 Tel.: Off.: 4071155 Fac.: 7682359	Manufacturers :- Aromatic Chemicals, Esters, Distillation Essential Oils and Perfumery Compounds
Uday Traders 1399 Sadashiv Peth Pune Vidyarathi Graha Road *Chief: Shailesh N. Godbole* *Alternate: P.N. Godbole*	Estd.: 1969 Tel.: 475539	Agents : Sati Kelkar & Co. Ltd. Bombay, K.V. Arochem Ltd. Vapi

Name & Address	*Phone/Fax Telex Nos.*	*Business Activities*
Udaipur Phosphates & Fertilisers Ltd. 53/57, Laxmi Insurance Building Sir P.M. Road, Fort Bombay-400 001 *Chief: Dillip P. Goculdas*	Estd.: 1980 Tel.: 2660578 2661680 Tlx.: 0118-2527 KOSN-IN Fax: 2662366	Manufacturers : Natural Menthol Peppermint Oil Rectified, Menthone Ex-Mint Oil, Mint Linalool Ex-Basil Eucalyptus Oil Diphenyl Methane (D.P.M.) and Benzophenone
Unisons 231, Dr. D.N. Road, 4th Floor Commissariat Bldg. Fort Bombay-400 001 *Chief: Bipinkumar V. Udani*	Estd.: 1959 Tel.: 2614316 2653407 Fax: 2653408	Dealers : Aromatic Chemicals & Industrial Chemicals
United Chem Exim Industries 46, Adhta Bldg., 2nd Floor 9-B, Cawasji Patel Street, Fort Bombay-400 001 *Chief: Anand R. Ladsariya* *Alternate: Kamal R. Ladsariya*	Estd.: 1983 Tel.: 2873357 2834726 Tlx.: 85566 MTCL IN Fax: 2872315	Traders : Menthol, Peppermint Natural Essential Oils etc.
VV Deepa Aromatics Pvt. Ltd. 20, Kasturi Bldg., J. Tata Road Churchgate Bombay-400 020 *Chief: Mrs. Padma Varadan* *Alternate: Miss Varadan*	Estd.: 1977 Tel.: Off.: 2833041 2833081 2044907 Fax: 2044907	Manufacturers : perfumery Compounds and Retail Personal Perfume Packs
V.V. Parekh & Sons A/109, Gokul Aracade Swamy NItyananda Marg Vile Parle Bombay-400 057 *Chief: Pravin Parekh* *Alternate: Mahul Parekh*	Estd.: 1967 Tel.: 6292658 6294028	Traders : Aromatic Chemicals & Solvents
V. Harkishandas & Co. 32, Shamaldas Gandhi Marg Princess Co-op. Housing Society Ltd. Bombay-400 002 *Chief: C.T. Parekh* *Alternate: M.T. Parekh*	Estd.: 1947 Tel.: 2057294	Traders : Perfumery Compounds and Aromatic Chemicals

Name & Address	*Phone/Fax Telex Nos.*	*Business Activities*
Vaishali Aromatics (India) Pvt. Ltd. Ayodhya, 256, N-3, CIDCO Aurangabad-431 210 *Chief: Vijay Madhukar Joshi* *Alt.: Mahendra Madhukar Joshi*	Estd.: 1986 Tel.: Off.: 0240-482807 0240-484385 Fac.: 0240-484120 0240-484193 Telex: 0745238 VPL In Fax: 0240-482078	Manufacturers : Essential Oils Aromatic Chemicals Flavours & Fragrances, Perfumery Compounds etc.
Vasu Preservatives Pvt. Ltd. 1 Nimish Apartment Juhu Scheme, Road No. 5 Vile Parle (W) Bombay-400 056 *Chief: Parag Vinod Jhaveri* *Alternate: Nilesh Vinod Jhaveri*	Estd.: 1985 Tel.: Off.: 6112014 6146892 fax: 6112014	Manufacturers : Clove Oil (Rect) & their derivatives
Vijayam Varadan & Co. 20, Kasturi Bldg., J. Tata Road Chuachgate Bombay-400 020 *Chief: Mrs. Padma Varadan* *Alternate: Mr. V. Chari*	Estd.: 1962 Tel.: 2833041 2833081 Fax: 2044907	Agents : Marketing Agents for: Viva Collection Perfume Sprays
Vikuvima Chemicals A3-16, Margao Industrial Estate St. Jose De Areal Goa-403 730 *Chief: Hari M. Sudakar*	Estd.: 1973 Tel.: 0834/735032	Traders : Benzophenone
Vipul Products Corporation Kanakia Park, II, C/213 Thakur Complex Kandivli (East) Bombay-400 101 *Chief: Bakul B. Patel* *Alternate: Vipul B. Patel*	Estd.: 1975 Tel.: Off.: 8873061 8874034 Fac.: 4458644	Manufactures : Aromatic Compounds for Soaps, Cosmetics and Agarbathies
Vital Additives 8/4 Surya Niwas, Sion (West) Bombay-400 022 *Chief: Raju Apte* *Alternate: Shyam Apte*	Estd.: 1983 Tel.: 5515982 Fax.: 5515982	Manufacturers : Flavouring Compounds & Perfumery Compounds

Name & Address	*Phone/Fax Telex Nos.*	*Business Activities*
Vithal Vaman Muthye 11, Shamshet Street Chhipi Chawl Bombay-400 002 *Chief: Rajendra J. Muthye*	Est.: 1923 Tel.: 3425700 3442463 5320350	Agents: S.H. Kelkar & Co.Ltd. Bombay and K.V. Arochem Ltd. Vapi
Alka Aromatics 87/A, Bombay Talkies Compound Near Joshi Electricals Malad (West) Bombay-400 064 *Chief: Babubhai S.Jani*	Estd.: 19 Tel.: 8810198	Manufacturers : Perfumery Compounds

Associate Members

Flower Valley Perfumes Pvt. Ltd. 4/13, Kamal Mansion Arthur Bunder Road, Colaba Bombay-400 005 *Chief: Mohd. Sirajuddin Ajmal* *Alternate: Mohd. Baruddin Ajmal*	Estd.: 1994 Tel.: 2856976/77 2044077 Fax: 2856609 Tlx.: 011-84304 MUSK IN	Manufacturers : Perfumery Compounds Natural Ess Oils, Aromatic Chemicals etc.
Suprabharath Exports Pvt. Ltd. E-107, Ansa Indl. Estate Saki Vihar road, Sakinaka Bombay-400 072 *Chief: K.S. Balkrishna Setty* *Alternate: Vijay Kumar*	Estd.: 1994 Tel.: Off.: 5793592 5793355 Fac.: 5784920 Fax: 5780555	Manufacturers & Exporters : Agrbattis, Essential Oils & Perfumes
Tribal Co-op. Marketing Development Federation of India Ltd. Unit No. 8, 11th Floor Centre 1, World Trade Centre Cuffe Parade Bombay-400 005 *Chief: M. Bhav Singh*	Estd.: 1987 Tel: 2182159 2182337 2151309 Tlx.: 86539 Fax: 2182337	Dealers : Procurement, Processing and Marketing of all Tribal (Agriculture and Forest) Produce

Name & Address	Phone/Fax Telex Nos.	Business Activities

Individual Members

Prof. Jagdish S. Pal Professor Department of Chemical Technology, University of Bombay Bombay-400 019	Telx.: 4115616 Fax: 4145614	Researcher and Consultant
Prof. V.G. Pangarkar Professor of Chemical Department of Chemical Technology, University of Bombay Bombay-400 019	Tel.: 4145616 Fax: 4145614	Researcher and Consultant

Northern Region

A.S. Industries A-17, Lawrence Road Industrial Area Delhi-110 035 *Chief: Amarjeet Singh Khanna*	Estd.: 1952 Tel.: 7185958	Manufacturers : Alcoholic Essences under Govt. Bond Emulsions Essences etc.
Aggarwal Impex 75, Civil Lines Rampur (UP)-244 901 *Chief: Neeraj Gupta* *Alternate: L.N. Gupta*	Estd.: 1991 Tel. (0595) 25064 24161 Fax.: (0595)25056 (011) 576243 Tlx.: (5701)216 GUPT IN	Manufacturers : Menthol, Liquid Menthol, Rectified Shivalik, All Grades Peppermint of Minthyl Acetate Thymol & Perfumery Compounds
Ajit Traders 6629, 1st Floor Main Bazar Khan Baoli Delhi-110 006	Estd.: 1975 Tel.: 235146 2919242 Fax: 2919242	Dealers : Aromatic Chemicals Natural Essential Oils Agents: Pankaj Aero Chemicals K. Kar, Calcutta
Anand Trading & Mfg. Co. 133/148 Block 'O' Kidwainagar Kanpur-208 023 *Chief: V. Kumar* *Alternate: Anand Kumar*	Estd.: 1986 Tel.: (O) 319288 (F) 273177 Fax.: 270164	Manufacturers : Sandalwood Oil Nagar Motha Oil Rooh Khus & All kind of Essential Oils Natural & Indian Attars

Directory of Perfumes and Flavours–Manufacturers/ Distributors/Suppliers/Traders/Exporters/Importers

Name & Address	*Phone/Fax Telex Nos.*	*Business Activities*
Aroma Industries DSIDC Shed No. 111 Okhla Indl. Area Phase-II New Delhi-110 020 *Chief: Manorma Gogia* *Alternate: Rohil Gogia*	Estd.: 1986 Tel.: 6841353 6914573 Fax: 6840763	Manufacturers : Essential Oils & Aromatic Chemicals
Aromatic & Allied Chemicals B-8, Industrial Area C-8, Ganj Bareilly-243 502 *Chief: Brijesh Mittal* *Alternate: Rjeev Agrawal*	Estd.: 1983 Tel.: 576906 Fax: 476906 Tlx.: 0577-227	Manufacturers : Indian Basil Oil Mentha Oil, Menthol Crystal, Methyl Acetate Lead Alcohol Leaf Acetate etc.
Aromatic Essential Oil Co. Naaz Cinema Road Khiyaliganj Lucknow-226 018 *Chief: Rakesh Suri* *Alternate: Sanjeev Suri*	Estd.: 1973 Tel.: 230159 Fax.: 242182	Manufacturers : Industrial Perfumes & Attars
Aromatika 4797/23, Bharat Ram Road Daryaganj New Delhi-110 002 *Chief: Atul Anadn* *Alternate: Kailash Anand*	Estd.: 1978 Tel.: 3261075	Dealers : Benzyl Acetate Alcohol Benzoate DEP etc.
Arun Chemical Industries 4/61 Punjabi Bagh New Delhi-110 026 *Chief: Arun Dev Bhardwaj* *Alternate: Vam Dev Bhardwaj*	Estd.: 1972 Tel.: (O)573606 (F) 5131615 Fax: 5475776 5132564	Manuracturers : Culinary Food Essence Baking Powder, Food, Colours etc.
Arun Minerals & Chemical Co. 19577, Partap Nagar Delhi-110 007 *Chief: Arun Kumar* *Alternate: Achal Kumar*	Tel.: 523511 7513079 Fax: 7524403 Telx: 031-62267 HCK IN	Estd.: 1973 Agents : For Aromatic Chemicals

Name & Address	*Phone/Fax Telex Nos.*	*Business Activities*
Azad Bharat Chemical Co. 2127, Tialk Bazar Delhi-110 006 *Chief: Kanwal Jit Singh* *Alternate: Raminder Pal Singh*	Estd.: 1958 Tel.: 2528825	Dealers : Aromatic Chemicals Perfumery Compounds Essence of Food Colours
Banarsi Dass Bholanath Khattri Subzi Mandi Road Kannauj-209 725 *Chief: Arun Kumar Mehrotra* *Alternate: Lalit Kumar Mehrotra*	Estd.: 1976 Tel.: 34460	Manufacturers : Essential Oils, Indian Attars, Concretes and Absolutes
Bhai Ji Attar Wale 39 Kutab Road Delhi-110 009 *Chief: Maninder Pal Singh*	Estd.: 1879 Tel.: (O) 7519531 7770722 (F) 7437974 7245578	Manufacturers : Perfumery Compounds, Agaribatties etc.
Bhai Ji Attar Wale Attari Bazar Jalandhar City-144 001 Punjab *Chief: Inder Pal Singh* *Alternate: Jaspreet Singh*	Estd.: 1878 Tel.: (O) 281563 Fax.: (F) 254927	Manufacturers : Hair Dyes, Hair Oils & Perfumes Dealers : Fragrances & Chemicals
Bombay Perfumery Company 1997, Gali Nilawali Bazar Sita Ram Delhi-110 006 *Chief: Sunil Kumar Goel* *Alternate: Sudhir Kumar Goel*	Estd.: 1952 Tel.: 730217	Manufacturers : Perfumery Compounds for Industrial use
Brisbane Chemical Research Co. 2317/25 Nanak Market Gali Hinga Beg. Tilak Bazar Dehi-110 006 *Chief: Chander Mohan*	Estd.: 1989 Tel.: 2915808 2925808	Dealers : Aromatic Chemicals Natural Essential Oils Perfumery Compounds Resinoids, etc.

Name & Address	Phone/Fax Telex Nos.	Business Activities
Camphor & Allied Products Ltd. Universal Bldg. 1st Floor 2/2A, Asaf Ali Road New Delhi-110 002 *Chief: Elich Mendiratta* *Alternate: Amit Varma*	Estd.: 1961 Tel.: 3278778 3275684 3275679 Fax.: 3282331 Tlx.: 031-63131 CAPL IN	Manufacturers : Aromatic & perfumery Chemicals, Industrial Solvents, Resins and Phamaceutical & Camphor Products
Camphor & Allied Products Ltd. P.O. Clutterbuckganj Bareilly-243 502 *Chief: Dr. A.P. Singh*	Estd.: 1962 Tel.: (0581)470088 473624 Fax: (0581)472810 Tlx: 0577-208 CAPL IN	Manufacturers : Camphor, Thymol, CP Resins, Astrolide & Terpene Chemicals
Capri De Conias 1702/103, 1st Floor Shrinath Market Bhagirath Palace Delhi-110 006 *Chief: Satish Kharbanda* *Alternate: Ramesh Sharma*	Estd.: 1992 Tel.: (O) 2967502 2965302 (F) 7294956 Fax: 2956850	Manufacturers & Exporters : Essential Oils & Aroma Chemicals
Charanjilal & Sons Iqbalganj Road Ludhiana *Chief: Prem Sagar*	Estd.: 1968 Tel.: (O)400007 (F) 32520	Traders : Milk Powder Essences & Chemicals
Chunnamal Ram Dayal Aminabad Road Lucknow-226 018 *Chief: V. Vijayvergiya*	Estd.: 1890 Tel.: 246160 221748 Fax: 212621	Manufacturers : Attars, Perfumes Perfumery Compounds Dealers : Essential Oils, Aromatic Chemicals Essences
Creative Fragrances 304, AVG Bhawan M-3, Cannaught Circus New Delhi-110 001 *Chief: Mrs. Asha Sanganeria* *Alt.: Ms. Bhuvana Nageshwaran*	Estd.: 1975 Tel.: 3324100 3324200 Fax: 3317776 Telex: 031-61558 SANG IN	Manufacturers : Flavours & Fragrances Perfumes Oils, Flower & Fruit Oils, Perfumery Raw Materials, Aromatic Chemicals & Essential Oils

Name & Address	*Phone/Fax Telex Nos.*	*Business Activities*
D.S. Chemicals Subash Road, Tapovan Chandausi-202 412 *Chief: Dinesh Agrawal*	Estd.: 1985 Tel.: (O) 50802 50822 (F) 50809 Fax. 05921-50345	Manufacturers : Menthol Peppermint Essential Oils & Aromatic Chemicals
Dev Chemicals Siddhi Sadan Tiraha Tube Well Colony Moradabad-24 001 *Chief: Subodh Kumar* *Alternate: Sudhir Gupta*	Estd.: 1984 Tel.: 314365 314364 Fax: 0591-311208	Manufacturers : Mentho,, Linalool Peppermint Oil Thymol, Anethil etc.
Elpee Enterprises B-3/114, Janakpuri New Delh-110 058 *Chief: I.K. Gakhar*	Estd.: 1985 Tel.: 5592961 5507718 Fac.: 5598399 Fax: 5591202	Manufacturers : Natural Ess, Oils & Aromatic Chemicals
Fab Flavours & Fragrances Pvt. Ltd. B--16, Phase-II Industrial Area, S.A.S. Nagar Mohali-160 055 (Punjab) *Chief: Sohinder Singh* *Alternate: Mrs.Harmeet Chhabra*	Estd.: 1985 Tel.: (O)5451142 5431556 (F) 673521 672305 Fax: 2913599	Manufacturers : Flavours, Fragrances Emulsions, Cloudyfying Agents
Fakirchand & Sons Lohar Gali Agra-282 003 *Chief: Purshotamdas* *Alternate: M.K. Mittal*	Estd.: Tel.: 75840	Manufacturers : Perfumes and Dealers in Agarbathies Scents and Flavouring Essences
Fragrance Laboratories Chowk Bazar Mathura-281 001 *Chief: Pratap Singh Verma* *Alternate: Smt. Pushpa Verma*	Estd.: 1984 Tel.: 405186	Manufactures : Industrial Perfumes and Flavorus Concentrates
Fragrance Specialities 1028 Mahadeo Street Mandi Ram Das Mathura-281 001 *Chief: R.K. Singh* *Alternate: N.K. Singh*	Estd.: 1992 Tel.: 409279 408572	Manufacturers : Fragrances, Flavours and Related Products

Directory of Perfumes and Flavours–Manufacturers/ Distributors/Suppliers/Traders/Exporters/Importers

Name & Address	Phone/Fax Telex Nos.	Business Activities
Glorious Perfumes Centre Pvt. Ltd. 609, 6th Floor 'City Centre' 53/2 The Mall Kanpur-208 001 *Chief: Obaidul Rab Raufi*	Estd.: 1961 Tel.: (O) 354528 317343 (F) (0669)- 34392/34393 Fax.: (0512)- 313957 311627 Tlx.: 32585 SKY P AL OBAID IN	Manufacturers : Non Alcoholic Perfumery Compounds & Essential Oil
Goel Traders Ganj Road Sambhal-244 302 *Chief: Navneet Goel* *Alternate: Vineet Goel*	Estd.: 1962 Tel.: (O)(05924)- 4330 (F)(05924) 4331 Fax: (05924)4751	Dealers : Mentha Oil, Menthol De Mentha Oil & All Essential Oils
Gogia Chemical Industries Pvt.Ltd. A-127, Okhla Indl. Area Phase-II New Delhi-110 020 *Chief: Mohit Gogia*	Estd.: 1967 Tel.: 6836007 69120329 Fax.: 684063	Manufacturers : Synthetic Flavours Essential oils & Perfumery Compounds
Gulab Singh Johrimal 320 Dariba Kalan Delhi-110 006 *Chief: Praful Gandhi*	Estd.: 1816 Tel.: 3271345 Fax.: 3283643	Manufacturers : Indian Attars Perfumes, Agarbathies & cones
Gulati & Company 1487, S.P. Mukherjee Marg Delhi-110 006 *Chief: Pradeep K. Gulati* *Alternate: H.L. Gulati*	Estd.: 1983 Tel.: 2512986 2516310 2940931	Dealers : Aerated Water, Ice Cream, Bakery Confectionery Perfumery Compounds etc. Agents :Classic Aromat- ics, Madras

Name & Address	Phone/Fax Telex Nos.	Business Activities
Gupta & Company Ltd. XIV/294-95, Gali Mandi Pan Sadar Bazar Delhi-110 006 *Chief: Sudhir Jain*	Estd.: 1928 Tel.: (O)7774742 528923 (F) 5472468 Fax: 7519215 Tlx: 031-66075	Manufacturers : Aromatic Chemicals Natural Essential Oils Synthetic Essential Oils Industrial Fragrances and Glavour Concentrates
Guptaji Gopalji & Co. Aminabad Road Lucknow *Chief: Davesh Gupta*	Estd.: 1908 Tel.: 247491 Fax: (522)2199470	Manufacturers : Perfumatic Compounds Essential Oils Attars, and Aromatic Chemicals
Gyan Aromatics Hari Chand Mela Ram Farm Wazirabad Road Delhi-110 094 *Chief: Vijay Raj Rastogi*	Estd.: 1988 Tel.: 2113719	Manufactures : Aromatic Chemicals Menthol, Rectified Peppermint Oil Anethol, Linalool Menthone & Terpenes
H.B. Chemicals 10 Tilak Bazar 2nd Floor Delhi-110 006 *Chief: Anil Mehta*	Estd.: 1980 Tel.: 2913551 2529071 Fax: 2941346	Traders : Aromatic Chemicals
Hafiz-ji-ki Mashoor Qadimi Dookan 33/220, Moolganj Kanpur	Estd.: 1963 Tel.: 261169 248935	Dealers : Perfumery Compounds
Hargovind Das & Sons Deeparganj, Chhipatti Kannauj-209 725 *Chief: Pushpraj jain* *Alternate: Atul Jain*	Estd.: 1928 Tel.: 34114 34614 Fax.: (05694) 34617	Manufacturers : Perfumery Compounds Attars & Distillers of Sandal Wood oil & Natural Ess Oils
Hari Industries Baggi-175 027 Mandi (HP) *Chief: Surender Mohan* *Alternate: Manoj Gupta*	Estd.: 1980 Tel.: (01906)71232 71132 Fax: 01905-22831	Manufacturers : Natural Essential Oils Resinoids and Absolutes

Name & Address	*Phone/Fax Telex Nos.*	*Business Activities*
Hari Om Distillers V & P.O. Shivrajpur Distt. Kanpur (Dehat) *Chief: Raghu Nandan P. Verma* *Alternate: Vikash Chandra*	Estd.: 1990 Tel.: 87214 87215	Manufacturers : Sandalwood Oil Nagar Motha Oil
Harish C. Khosla & Co. Zinat Mahal Lalkuan Bazar P.O. Box No. 1328 Delhi-110 006 *Chief: Satya Pal* *Alternate: Arun Kumar*	Estd.: 1948 Tel.:7524804 733160 Fax: 7524803 Tlx: 031-62267 HCK-IN	Commission Agents : Dealers in Perfumery Compounds Essential Oils Aromatic Chemicals Saccharin Essences etc.
Harish C. Khosla & Co. Pvt. Ltd. Zinat Mahal, Lalkuan Bazar Delhi-110 006 *Chief: Satyapal* *Alternate: Arun Kumar*	Estd.: 1968 Tel.: 7524403 733160 Fax: 7524403 Tlx: 031-62267 HCK-IN	Agents: Quest International India Dealers in Essences, Perfumery Compounds, Essential Oils, Aromatic Chemicals etc.
Hindustan Chemicals & Allied Industries Barehseni Street Chandausi-202 412 *Chief: Phool Prakash*	Estd.: 1976 Tel.: (O)(0582)- 50550 (F) 51274 Fax: 50074	Manufacturers: Natural Menthol Crystals, Essential Oils & Aromatic Chemicals
Hitesh Aromatics P.O. Baggi-175 027 Via-Walsar Distt. Mandi (HP) *Chief: Rajender Mohan* *(Associate Member)*	Estd.: 1995 Tel.: 71241 Fac.: 71288	Manufacturers Natural Essential Oil & Resinods
Indo Organics 75, Mohkampur Indl. Complex, Phase-I Delhi Road, P.B. No. 409 Meerut-250 002 *Chief: Dr. Shiromani Sharang* *Alternate: Dinesh Kumar*	Estd.: 1988 Tel.: 27049 Fac.: 511663	Manufacturers : Aromatic Chemicals

Name & Address	*Phone/Fax Telex Nos.*	*Business Activities*
Indo Vanillon Chemicals Ltd. K1/131 Chittaranjan Park EPDP, New Delhi-110 019 *Chief: P.P. Khanna* *Alternate: Vivek Khanna*	Estd.: 1992 Tel.: 6445547 6474217 Fax: 6474217	Manufacturers : Ethyl Vanillin
Indian Fragrances & Chemical Works Mahatma Gandhi Road Kannauj-209 725 (UP) *Chief: Krishna Narain Kapoor*	Estd.: 1974 Tel.: 34716 34297 Fax: 34286	Manufacturers : Sandal Wood Oil, Natural Essential Oils, Indian Flower Attars, Absolutes and floweral Water
Industrial Chemical Enterprise P.O.Box No. 3597 New Delhi-110 024 *Chief : Amar Lal*	Estd.: 1977 Tel.: 8524500 8555400 Fax: 8523104	Manufacturers : Menthol, Dementholised Oil, Mentha Oil and Peppermint Oil
J.K. Aromatics & Perfumers 2187/13, Beri Market Gali Hinga Beg. Tilak Bazar Delhi-110 006 *Chief: Subhash Chand Gupta*	Estd.: 1989 Tel.: 2930437 2518179	Manufacturers : Industrial Perfumery Compounds & Synthetic Essential Oils
J.K. Industrial Perfumers A-7/7 Krishna Nagar Delhi-110 051 *Chief: Jitendra Gupta*	Estd.: 1964 Tel.: Off.: 2243454 Fac.: 8525092	Manufacturers : Industrial Perfumes and Synthetic Essential Oils
J.K. Perfumery Company 1st Floor, Sapna Market 2308, Gali Hinga Beg Delhi-110 006	Estd.: 1988 Tel.: 2927470 2512645	Manufacturers : Perfumes & Synthetic Essential Oils
J. Kanti Bhai Company Perfumes Kannauj-209 725 *Chief: Ashok Jain* *Alternate: Kishore Jain*	Estd.: 1975 Tel.: (O) 34375 (F) 34255	Manufacturers : Soap, Agarbatti Perfumes all Indian Attars and Natural Ess Oils

Name & Address	*Phone/Fax Telex Nos.*	*Business Activities*
Jagat Aroma Oils Distillery Mannauj-209 725 *Chief: J.N. Kapoor* *Alternate: Pradeep Kapoor*	Estd.: 1973 Tel.: 34401 Fax: 34335 Tlx: 31-65376	Manufacturers : Sandalwood Oil Cypriol, Celeryseed Oil, Calamus Oil Carroseed Oil Attars and Perfumery Compounds
Jain Aromatics A-53 Gandhi Nagar Moradabad-244 001 (UP) *Chief: Ajit Jain* *Alternate: Rajat Jain*	Estd.: 1974 Tel.: 0591-312142 313348 Fax: 0591-3109	Manufacturers : Menthol & Essential Oils
Japan Bottle House 312,Tilak Bazar Delhi-110 006 *Chief: Mohd. Sualeh* *Alternate: Mohd. Rizwan*	Estd.: 1936 Tel.: 2513057 Fax: 2930582	Manufacturers : Perfumes, Essential Oils, Aromatic Chemicals, Solvents etc.
Jay Kay Aroma A-733, Rajendra Nagar P.O. Izart Nagar Bareilly-243 122 *Chief: Jayesh H. Haswani*	Estd.: 1987 Tel.: 77746	Manufacturers : Natural Essential Oils Mentha Products & Aroma Chemicals
Jindal Exports Ltd. C-54/2 Wazirpur Indl. Area Delhi-110 052 *Chief: J.P. Jindal*	Estd.: 1974 Tel.: 7219693 7130397 7436908 Fax: 7135328 7244405 Tlx: 31-79063 JIND IN	Manufacturers : Mentha oil, Spearmint Oil, Mentha Pipenta Oil, Indian Basil Oil Sandalwood Oil, Russian Origin Ess. Oils, Natural Mint. Oil etc.
K.K. Aromatics "Shree Ram Kunj" Indra Nagar Bareilly-243 122 (UP) *Chief: Kamlesh K. Mittal*	Estd.: 1992 Tel.: (0581)474188 Fax: (0581)450147	Traders : Natural Essential Oils & Aromatic Chemicals

Name & Address	*Phone/Fax Telex Nos.*	*Business Activities*
Kanpur Sandalwood Oil Distillery Pvt. Ltd. 54/27 Naya Ganga Kanpur-208 001 *Chief: Mahesh Chandra Gupta*	Estd.: 1987 Tel.: Off.: 310362 363726 363585 Fac.: 81224 Fax.: 363483	Manufacturers : Sandalwood Oil, Natural Ess. Oils, Spice Oil
Kanta Chemical Co. 133, Tilak Bazar Delhi-110 006 *Chie: Jugal Kishore Gupta* *Alternate: Alok Kumar Gupta*	Estd.: 1971 Tel.: 2528650 2529163 Fax: 2914267 Tlx.: 31-78073 KCCO IN	Manufacturers : Aromatic Chemicals Resinoids, Natural Essential Oils & Perfumery Compounds
Khattri Perfumers (P) Ltd. Khattri House Tikat Rai Talab Lucknow-226 004	Estd.: 1986 Tel.: 63232 63535 62789 Fax: 62119	Manufacturers : Industrial Perfumes Kimam
Khushboo Essential Oils 15, Navrang Bldg. Professor Colony Budaun-243 601 *Chief: Rakesh Kumar Vaish* *Alternate: Manoj Kumar Vaish*	Estd.: 1989 Tel.: 54624 55049 Fax: 54796	Traders : Mentha Oil, Menthol Othr Essential Oils and Aroma Chemicals
Krips Consultants 16-E, Community Centre Basant Lok, Vasant Vihar New Delhi-110 057 *Chief: Ravi Bahl*	Estd.: 1978 Tel.: 676871/72 Fax: 672017 Tlex: 31-63179 KRIP IN	Agents : For Expression Perfumes, France Molinard, France Fontarome, USA Tournaire, France
Kulu Aromatics Shamshi-175 126 Kulu (HP) *Chief: Nand Lal Seth*	Estd.: 1979 Tel.: 91-1902-5179 Fax: 91-1902-2720	Manufacturers : Natural Ess. Oils Resinoids & extracts

Name & Address	*Phone/Fax Telex Nos.*	*Business Activities*
Kumud Products Bara Bazar Kannauj-209 725 *Chief: Pankaj Kumar Mehrotra* *Alternate: Neeraj Mehrotra*	Estd.: 1973 Tel.: 34294 34460 34735 Fax: 091-05694 34894	Manufacturers : Indian Attars, Essential Oils, Concretes & Absolutes
L.D.G. International Plot No. 1, 2 & 3 Khasra No. 43/2/5 Village Badli Delhi-110 042 *Chief: M.P. Gandhi*	Estd.: 1982 Tel.: 7291539 7291540 Fax: C/o 5734343	Manufacturers : Industrial Perfumes Synthetic Essentical Oils, Resinoids
Lala Pragdutt & Co. Perfumers, Makrandnagar Kannauj-209 726 *Chief: M.D. Saini* *Alternate: Vinod Saini*	Estd.: 1969 Tel.: 34209 34459 Fax: (05694)- 34234	Manufacturers : Indian Attars and Distillers of Essential Oils
Lalji Aromatics (Pvt.) Ltd. 253/44, Nadan Mahal Road Lucknow-226 004 *Chief: Narendra Nath Mehrotra*	Estd.: 1988 Tel.: Off.: 266650 265165 265171 Fac.: 256864 Fax: 265165	Manufacturers : Perfumes, Perfumery Compounds, Synthetic Essential Oils Tailor Made exclusive perfumes etc.
M.L. Shukla & Company 66, Turner Road Cantt. Kanpur-208 004 *Chief: Amit Shukla*	Estd.: 1954 Tel.: 366062 367344 Fax: 367344	Manufacturers : Natural Ess. Oils Aromatic Chemicals Oleoresins etc.
Madras Chemical Works 315 Tilak Bazar Delhi-110 006 *Chief: Vijay Gambhir* *Aternate: Rakesh Gambhir*	Estd.: 1951 Tel.: 2529374 2929332 Fax: 2511729	Dealers : Essences & Flavours
Magnum Perfumers (P) Ltd. 3/6013, Gali No. 1 Dev Nagar, Karol Bagh New Delhi-110 005 *Chief: Jayant Gandhi* *Alternate: Jaideep Gandhi*	Estd.: 1990 Tel.: 5733747 5732485 Fax: 5134343	Manufacturers : Industrial Fragrance

Name & Address	Phone/Fax Telex Nos.	Business Activities
Malayagiri Sandalwood Oil Distllery 105/696, Kalpi Road (Bhannana Punwa) Kanpur-208 003 (UP) *Chief: V.K. Tandon* *Alternate: Vipul Tandon*	Estd.: 1958 Tel.: Off.: 546579 313680 Fac.: 295730 297708 Fax: (0512) 319556	Manufactures : Sandalwood Oil Agmarked quality & other Essential Oils
Manohardas Sewakram Perfumers Kannauj-209 725	Estd.: 1908 Tel.: 34334 39434	Dealers : Aromatic Chemicals Essential Oils and Petroleum Products
Mehta Bros. (India) 1482, S.P. Mukherjee Marg (Behind Novelty Cinema) Delhi-110 006 *Chief: Krishan Kumar*	Estd.: 1965 Tel.: 2514361 2519672	Dealers : Aerated Soda Water materials, Bakery, Ice Cream, Food Colours, Saccharin, Essences, Bottles, Corks etc.
Mehta Jee & Co. 1484, S.P. Mukherjee Marg Behind Novelty Cinema Delhi-110 006 *Chief: V.N. Seth* *Alternate: Satish Kumar*	Estd.: 1970 Tel.: 2513290 2527007	Dealers : Food Colour, Essence Sacchrine, Soda Water requisities and Chemicals
Mehtha & Allied Products Ltd. "Munshi Niketan" 1/10, Asaf Ali Road New Delhi-110 002 *Chief: Arvind Nanda*	Estd.: 1977 Tel.: 731355 731356 730614 Fax: 7521189 Tlx: 031-66058 MINT IN	Manufacturers : Menthol, Peppermint Oil, Menthone, Basil Oll, Mentha Piperita Brucine, Strychnine etc.
Mohan Perfumery Co. 144A, Tilak Bazar Khari Baoli Delhi-110 006 *Chief: Chander Mohan*	Estd.: 1993 Tel.: 2915808 2925808	Traders : Perfumery Compounds & Essential Oils

Name & Address	*Phone/Fax Telex Nos.*	*Business Activities*
Mohanlal Pyarelal 5594, Gandhi Market Sadar Bazar Delhi-110 060 *Chief: Prakash C. Dhingra*	Estd.: 1950 Tel.: Off.: 7517228 7528184 Fac.: 7512683 Fax: 7772807	Manufacturers : Industrial Perfumes
Mohit Chemicals Shakuntla Bhawan Mal Godam Road Budaun-243 601 (UP) *Chief: D.K. Agarwal* *Alternate: S.K. Agarwal*	Estd.: 1985 Tel.: 54331 54883 Fac.: 54922 54507 Fax.: 55085	Manufacturers : Natural Essential Oils Menthol, Anethol Linalool etc.
Mool Chand Nanak Chand W/9.MIG Juhi Gaushala P.O.Kanpur-208 014 *Chief: Nanak Chand Jain*	Estd.: 1960 Tel.:271973 277010	Manufacturers : Zarda, Panmasala Agarbatti, Toilet Soap & Perfumery Compounds
Mysore Sales International Ltd. C-4, 2nd Floor Baba Kharak Singh Marg New Delhi-110 001	Estd.: 1966 Tel.: 343863 Tlx.: 031-63403 MSIL IN	Agents : For Karnataka Saops & & Detergents Ltd. Bangalore and Encee Aromatics Ltd. Mattupalayam
Naresh Chand & Co. 497, Katra Ishwar Bhawan Khari Baoli Delhi-110 006 *Chief: Naresh Chand*	Estd.: 1978 Tel.: 2529122 Fax: 2914800 Tlx.: 31-78079 DEEPA IN	Manufacturers : Sandal wood oil and other Essential oils
National Aromatics 98-Y-1 Block Kidwai Nagar Kanpur-208 011 (UP) *Chief: Rahul Jain* *Alternate: D.K. Jain*	Estd.: 1990 Tel.: 276829	Manufacturers : Natural and Synthetic Perfumes
Northern Agencies 1417/7 Gali Telian Tilak Bazar Delhi-110 006 *Chief: Rajesh Seth*	Estd.: 1989 Tel.: 2931622	Agents : Shree Mangalam Pharma Pvt. Ltd. Bombay

Name & Address	Phone/Fax Telex Nos.	Business Activities
Northern Aromatics Pvt. Ltd. 8/1-B Site IV Sahibabad Indl. Area Gaziabad (UP) *Chief: R.K. Sharma*	Estd.: 1981 Tel.: 770536 770583	Manufacturers : Aromatic Chemicals Flavouring and Perfumery Compounds
Okhla Chemicals Ltd. Paharpur Business Centre 21 Nehru Place New Delhi-110 019 *Chief: Kamal Meattla* Tlx: 31-62979	Estd.: 1971 Tel.: Off.: 6461287 6474701 Fac.: 8770487 etc. PCTD IN	Manufacturers : Alevritic Acid, Dewaxed Bleached Shellac ISO Ambretolide Natural Rose Water
Prakash Chand Khanna 2139 Tilak Bazar Kari Baoli Delhi-110 006 *Chief: K.K. Khanna*	Estd.: 1951 Tel.: 2526606 2528575	Agents : Bush Boarke Allen (I) Ltd. for Essences & Food Colours
Perfumers (India) P. Ltd. 4, Nanpara House P.O. Box No. 87 B.N. Road Lucknow-226 001 *Chief: S.K. Suri* *Alterrnate: Kiran Suri*	Estd.: 1952 Tel.: 224244 248804 Fax: 218090	Manufacturers & Exporters : Natural Essential Oils Synthetic Essential Oils, Oriental Perfumes Floral Water and Attars
Perfumes & Essential Oils Co. facturers : 47-48 New Market P.O. Box NO. 165 Kaiserbagh, Lucknow *Chief: Rajneesh Kumar* *Alternate: Nischal Suri*	Tel.: 272309 242040 371361 Fax: 234927	Estd.: 1979 Manu- Pure Attars, Perfumery Compounds, Natural and Synthetic Essential Oils, Floral Absolutes
Prakash Chemicals Anaj Mandi Budaun-243601 *Chief: Prakash Chandra Gupta* *Alternate: Prateesh Kumar Gupta*	Estd.: 1986 Tel.: (O)54642 (F) 55331	Manufacturers : Essential oils, Aroma Chemicals & Menthol

Name & Address	*Phone/Fax Telex Nos.*	*Business Activities*
Prayag Dutt Sunderlal Perfumers Kannauj-209 725 (UP)	Estd.: 1900 Tel.: 34258	Manufacturers : Natural Essential Oils Perfumes, Sandal Wood Oils, Synthetic Compounds, Aromatic Chemicals Indian Attars
Premprakash Gupta & Bros. (P) Ltd. P.O. Box No. 109 11, 4th KM Bareilly (UP) *Chief: Premprakash Gupta*	Estd.: 1979 Tel.: 475482 475487 Fax: 474280 450140 Tlx.: 577227 GREL IN	Manufacturers : Anethole, Estragole Aromatic Chemicals
Progressive Enterprises Shastri Nagar P.O. Bazpur (Distt. Naintal) Uttar Pradesh-262 401 *Chief: Subhash Chandra Mittal* *Alternate: Ramesh Chandra Gupta*	Estd.: 1976 Tel.: 88359 88489 88030 Fax.: (05949)	Manufacturers : Natural Essential Oils Mentha Oil, Peperita Oil Citrata Oil and Basil
R.A. Chemicals Sayadwara Budaun-243 601 *Chief: Ashok Kumar Rastogi*	Estd.: 1989 Tel.: Off.: (05832)-54200 Fac.: (05832)-55305 Fax:)5832)-54135	Manufacturers : Essential Oils Piperita, Basil, Spear mint, Tagets, Jamrosa and Extracts of Flowers
R.S. Silk Agency 49/72, Naughara Kanpur-208 001 (UP) *Chief: Mohanlal Maheshwari* *Alternate: S.K. Maheshwari*	Estd.: 1968 Tel.: Off.: 318473 356228 Fac.: 821261 Fax: (0512)-256010	Manufacturers : Sandal Wood Oils Natural Essetial Oils, Dehydrated Onion Flacks and Pltato Dehydrated Flacks

Name & Address	*Phone/Fax Telex Nos.*	*Business Activities*
Radha Sales Corporation 304 AVG Bhawan M-3, Connnaught Circus New Delhi-110 001 *Chief: Sant Sanganeria* *Alternate: P. Majumdar*	Estd.: 1971 Tel.: 3324100 3324200 Fax : 031-61558 SANG IN	Agents and Traders : Flavours & Fragrances, Perfume Oils, Perfumery Raw Materials, Essential Oils Flower & Fruit Oils Aromatic Chemicals etc.
Rahul Aroma M-4 Sai Bhawvan A-10 Commercial Complex Ranjit Nagar New Delhi-110 008 *Chief: R.P. Chhibbar*	Estd.: 1988 Tel.: 5709740 5709750 5709600	Dealers : Perfumery Compound Aroma Chemicals Essential Oils etc. Agents : Sai Aromas Pvt. Ltd. Bombay, Nishant Aromas Bombay
Rajhans Aromatics 201, IInd Floor Inderprastha Tower Commercial Complex Wazirpur Indl. Area Delhi-110 052 *Chief: Prem K. Varma* *Alternate : Harbans Lal*	Estd.: 1994 Tel.: 7134004 7417637 Fax: 7254501	Dearlers : Essential Oils Mentha Oils Aroma Chemicals All Mint Products Menthol Bold Crystals etc.
Rakesh Sandal Industries 7/177-A Swaroop Nagar Kanpur-208 002 (UP) *Chief: Yogesh Dubey*	Estd.: 1972 Tel.: Off.: 214071 210236 294693 Fac.: 277211 Fax: 294675 214993 Tlx: 325-484 RSIK IN	Manufacturers : Natural Ess. Oils Spice Oils, Sandal Wood OPil Products Indian Attars, Perfumery Compound Aromatic Chemicals etc.
Ram Krishna Gupta and Brothers 33/107, Gaya Prasad Lane Kanpur-208 001 *Chief: Ram Krishna Gupta* *Alternate: Ankur Gupta*	Estd.: 1970 Tel.: 314091 314987	Manufacturers : Perfumery Compound Aromatic Chemicals and Attars

Name & Address	*Phone/Fax Telex Nos.*	*Business Activities*
Rasiklal Hemani Agencies Pvt. Ltd. 506, Khari Baoli Delhi-110 006 *Chief.: Rasiklal Hemani*	Estd.: 1975 Tel.: 238389 2940757 Fax: 29330582 Tlx.: 31-78046 RHA IN	Agents for North India: For S.H. Kelkar & Co. Ltd. Bombay K.V. Arochem Ltd. Vapi K.L. Koh Ent. P. Ltd. Singapore
Rasiklal Hemani Agencies Pvt. ltd. 29, Prince Complex 2nd Floor Navalkishore Road Hazratganj Lucknow-226 001 *Chief: Kishore Hemani*	Estd.: 1987 Tel.: 232080	Agents : For S.H. Kelkar & Co. Ltd. Bombay
Red Club Flavours Pvt. Ltd. C-75, Kirti Nagar New Delhi-110 015 *Chief: Gumish Singh Chhabra* *Alternate: Mrs. Manmohan Kaur*	Estd.: 1965 Tel.: 5431556 5451142 Fax: 2913599	Manufacturers : Flavours & Flavouring Compounds & Soft drink Concentrates
S.K. Florescences B-1711, Shastri Nagar Delhi-110 052 *Chief: B.L. Sharma* *Alternate: B.R. Sharma*	Estd.: 1983 Tel.: 7533560 521337	Manufacturers : Cheetah Brand Flavours Fragrances, Natural Essential Oils
S.N. Traders 33/211, Gaya Prasad Lane Kanpur-208 001 *Chief: Sheo Narayan Agarwal* *Alternate: Amar Nath Agarwal*	Estd.: 1978 Tel.: 365834 315606 Fax: 364023	Traders : Synthetic Essential Oils, Aromatic Chemicals etc.
S. Mohd Ayub Mohd Yaqub Mohallah Pansaryan Kannauj-209 725 *Chie: Abdul Malik* *Alternate: Abdul Akhir*	Estd.: 1896 Tel.: Off.: 34204 34267 Fac.: 34303 Fax.: 34417	Manufacturers : Non Alcoholic Attars

Name & Address	*Phone/Fax Telex Nos.*	*Business Activities*
Sachee Fragrances & Chemicals Ltd. D-11 & 12 Sector 2 Noida-201 301 *Chief: Rakesh Arora* *Alternate: Manoj Arora*	Estd.: 1982 Tel.: 85-36111 8536222 8520134 Fax: 011-8524643	Manufacturers : Perfumery Compounds Aromatic, Chemicals & Essential Oils
Sachendi Farms Imperial Cinema 14/125 Parade Kanpur-208 001 *Chief: Manoj Garg* *Alternate: V.N. Garg*	Estd.: 193 Tel.: 353224	Manufacturers : Essential Oils Mentha Oils Aroma Chemicals All Mint Products Menthol Bold Crystals etc.
Sarman Industries A-37, Gandhi Nagar Moradabad-244 001 *Chief: Arvind Gupta*	Estd.: 1976 Tel.: 0591-312544 Fax.: 0591-312187	Manufacturers : Peppermint Oil Piperata Oil, Basil Oil, Mentha Citrata Oil Jamrosa Oil etc.
Satyanarain Sudarshanlal & Co. 11, Khun Khunji Road Chowk, Lucknow-226 003 *Chief: Harish P. Digamber*	Estd.: 1961 Tel: 269176	Dealers : Perfumery Raw Material and Chemicals
Seth Brothers (Perfumers) Pvt. Ltd. C-197, Naraina Indl. Area Phase-I New Delhi-110 028 *Chief: Vinod Kumar Seth*	Estd.: 1949 Tel.: 535228 2528659 2918000	Manufacturers : Industrial Perfumery Compounds
Seth Brothers (Perfumers) Pvt. Ltd. K-62/98, Sapta Sagar Varanasi-221 001 *Chief: Raghuwansh Seth* *Alternate: Vinod Kumar Seth*	Estd.: 1949 Tel.: 63385	Dealers : Perfumery Compounds Aromatic Chemicals Resinoids and Flavouring Essences

Directory of Perfumes and Flavours–Manufacturers/ Distributors/Suppliers/Traders/Exporters/Importers

Name & Address	*Phone/Fax Telex Nos.*	*Business Activities*
Shaivi Industries P.B. No. 50 42/2 Saket Palli Lucknow-226 001 (UP) *Chief: Shailendra Jain* *Alternate: Aditya Jain*	Estd.: 1968 Tel.: Off.: 225694 213847 Fac.: 267689 Fax.: 213847	Manufacturers : Industrial Perfumes
Sharp Menthol India (P) Ltd. C-15 SMA, Co-op, Indl. Estate Delhi-110 033 *Chief: Sanjay Singhal*	Estd.: 1989 Tel.: 7214362 7226846 7131325 Fax: 7226406 Tlx.: 031-79070 SMI IN	Manufacturers : Menthol & Ess.Oils
Sheetal Chemicals Opp. Police Parade Ground Civil Lines Budaun UP *Chief: Vishnu Gupta*	Estd.: 1980 Tel: Off.: 54257 54827 Fac.: 54179 Fax: 54068	Manufacturers : Natural Ess. Oil & Menthol D.M.O. Anethole etc.
Shivam Marketing Co. 233/1, Tilak Bazar Khari Baoli Delhi-110 006 *Chief: Jagmohan Bajaj*	Estd.: 1889 Tel.: 2925515 2935515 2936700	Traders : All kinds of Perfumery Chemicals & Compounds
Shree Associates Sunanda House 17/10, Old Rajinder Nagar New Delhi-110 060 *Chief: Mrs. Shashi Lal* *Alternate: Rajiv Lal*	Estd.: 1971 Tel.: 5716850	Agents & Traders : Essential Oils Aromatic Chemicals Flavours, Perfumery Compounds and Agarbathies
Shree Veer Chemicals 23/3 East Patel Nagar New Delhi-110 008 *Chief: Ajay Kumar Jain* *Alternate S.K. Jain*	Estd.: 1987 Tel.: Off.: 5730485 5755209 Fac.: 2269721 Fax: 5755209 Tlx.: 031-77352 VRAT IN	Manufacturers : Essential Oils Aroma Chemicals Perfumery Raw Materials etc.

Name & Address	Phone/Fax Telex Nos.	Business Activities
Siva Essential Oils & Chemicals Dua Complex 24, Veer Savarkar Block Shakarpur, Delhi-110 092 *Chief: S.C.Varshney* *Alternate: Sanjay Varshney*	Estd.:1973 Tel.: Off.: 2244035 2247928 Fac.: 8551012 8520739 Fax.: 2204284 2456772 Tlx.: 031-62434	Manufacturers : Essential Oils & Isolates
Sohan Singh Attarwala & Son 903, Chowk Qutab Road Delhi-110 006 *Chief: Amarjit Singh* *Alternate: Jagtar Singh*	Estd.: 1919 Tel.: Off.: 7777771 7512171 Fac.: 2912063 2932063 Fax.: 2932064 Tlx: 31-78298 SSAS IN	Manufacturers & Exporters Perfumes, Incense sticks Incense cones Heena Powder Perfumery Compounds Hair Oil, Cosmetics etc.
Sona Products Pvt. Ltd. B-180 Okhla Insustrial Area, Phase-I New Delhi-110 020 *Cheif: Kishore K. Mittal* *Alternate: Vijay Mittal*	Estd.: 1993 Tel.: 6811313 6811314 Fax.: 6811317	Manufacturers : Terpenless Menthol Crystal, Essential Oils & Aromatic Chemicals
Suman Industries 46, Diamond Dairy Kabir Marg Lucknow-226 001 *Chief: Vijay Acharya* *Alternate: Rakesh Sharma*	Estd.: 1981 Tel.: 44158 46363	Manufacturers : Aromatic Chemicals
Supreme Enterprises Perfumers Makrand Nagar Kannauj (UP) *Chief: Rakesh Narain Gupta*	Estd.: 1989 Tel.: 34573 34179	Manufacturers : Indian Attars and Natural Ess. Oils

Name & Address	*Phone/Fax Telex Nos.*	*Business Activities*
Thakar Dass & Company 20, Ansari Market Darya Ganj New Delhi-110 002 *Chief: S.K. Kapoor* *Alternate: H.K. Kapoor*	Estd.:1959 Tel.: 3278040 3275491 3271457 Fax: 3280977 Tlx: 031-62234 TDC IN	Agents : Bayer (Inida) Ltd. Bombay Indian Organic Chemicals Ltd. Bombay Corpn. Ltd. Baroda Herdillia Unimers Ltd. Bombay
Thakur Bros. 1479 S.P.Mukherjee Marg (Behind Novelty Cinema) Delhi-110 006 *Chief: Rattan Kumar Thakur* *Alternate: Parmod Kumar Thakur*	Estd.: 1979 Tel.: 2493635 2529911	Dealers ; Essence, Saccharin Crown Corks, Ice Cream and Soda Water requisites
Ultra International Pvt. Ltd. 304 AVG Bhawan M-3 Connuaught Circus New Delhi-110 001 *Chief Sant K. Sanganena* *Alt: Ms. Bhuvana Nageshwaran*	Estd.: 1989 Tel.: 3324100 3324200 Fax: 3317776 Tlx.: 03161558 SANG IN	Manufacturers : Perfumery Raw Materials, Aromatic Chemicals, Flavours & Fragrances, Perfume Flower Oils & Essential Oil
United Perfumers P. Ltd. 66/188, Bhusatoli Road Kanpur-208 001 *Chief: S.K. Shukla*	Estd.: 1945 Tel.: 366584 350217 350347	Manufacturers : Aromatic Chemicals Essential Oils, and oleoresins
Vardhman Arochem 229, 1st Floor Shiv Market 2221-22 Gali Hinga Beg Tilak Bazar, Delhi-110 006 *Chief: A.K. Jain* *Alternate: N.K. Jain*	Estd.: 1991 Tel.: 2920536	Dealers : Aromatic Chemicals Perfumery Compounds Natural Ess. Oils Resinoids etc.
Vishal Chemicals Sneh Bhawan Professors Colony Budaun-213 601 *Chief: Vishal Rastogi* *Alternate: Subhash Rastogi*	Estd.: 1992 Tel.: 54560 54103	Manufacturers : Natural Essential Oils

Name & Address	*Phone/Fax Telex Nos.*	*Business Activities*
Southern Region		
A.P. Vivekananda 43, (Old No. 9), First Main Road Gandhi Nagar, Adyar Madras-600 020 Nadu, *Chief: A.P. Vivekananda*	Estd.: 1075 Tel.: 415628	Agents : For Arofine Chemical Industries, Bombay for Andhra, Tamil Kerala and Pondicherry
AVM Aromatics G-1, Industrial Estate Machuvadi Pudukkottai-622 004 Tamil Nadu *Chie: M. Nalliah*	Estd.: 1989 Tel.: 21973 Fax.: 04322-21973	Manufacturers : Aromatic Fine Chemicals & Flavours
A. Gowrishankar Post Box No. 447, No. 2/2 Patalamma Temple Street Armugam Circle, Basavanagudi Bangalore-560 004 *Chief: A. Gowrishankar*	Estd.: 1984 Tel.: 6612835 606455	Agents : Sub Agent for CMA International, France Kao Corp, Japan, and E. Flachsman AG, Switzerland
ACE Arcmatics Pvt. Ltd. 108/109, Swiss Complex 33 Race Course Road Bangalore--560 001 *Chief: M.T. Srivasta* *Alternte: M.a. Dattal*	Estd.: 1988 Tel.: Off.: 2205455 2250118 Fac.: 3351626 Fax.: 2202875	Manufacturers : Aldehyde C-11 (Undecylenic)
Agro Extracts Limited Plot No. 16, Phase II Peenya Industrial Area Bangalore-560 058 *Chief: Praveen Jaipuria*	Estd.: 1975 Tel.: 8394216 8394922 8395928 Fax: 8392134	Manufacturers : Non Edible Vegetable Oils, De Oiled Cakes & Agarbathi Chemicals like Di Ethyl Phthalate
Amreli Industrial Aromatics 301., Royal Plaza, 3rd Floor Kandaswamy Lane, 4-4-933/35 Sultan Bazar Hyderabad-500 195 *Chief: S.K. Mehta* *Alternate: K.B. Mehta*	Estd.: 1982 Tel.: Off.: 516880 592323 Fac.: 501080	Traders & Agents : U.K. Aromatics & Chemicals, Bombay for Perfumery Compounds Flavours Aromatic Chemicals, Solvents, Glycols, Glycerine Essential Oils, etc.

Directory of Perfumes and Flavours–Manufacturers/ Distributors/Suppliers/Traders/Exporters/Importers

Name & Address	*Phone/Fax Telex Nos.*	*Business Activities*
Aromaco 459, Ashoka Pillar Road Jayanagar, 2nd Block Bangalore-560 011 *Chief: K.L. Ngendra* *Alternate: R. Srinivas*	Estd.: 1987 Tel.: 6639344 642472 Fax.: 6639344	Agents : ACE Agencies, Bombay Bombay Oil Inds. Ltd. Bombay CAPL, Bareilly DEP DOP Niraj Chemicals
Aromatic Agencies 36, K.V. Temple Street Bangalore-560 053 *Chief: M.V. Sathish*	Estd.: 1968 Tel.: Off.: 2870238 Fac.: 605484	Manufacturers and Agents : Perfumery Comounds
The Aromatic Chemical & Oil Co. Ponpadi R.S. & P.O. Pin-631 213, Chengai MGR Distt. Tamil Nadu *Chief: A. Prabhakar*	Estd.: 1946 Tel.: Off.: 04118-88322 04118-88344 Fax: 91-44- 5341011	Manufacturers : Food Flavours Fragrances, Natural Essential Oils & Viscose Bottle Seals
Aromatic Chemical & Oil Co. Pvt. Ltd. D-7-8, Industrial Estate Visakhapatnam-530 007 *Chief: A. Vijayam*	Estd.: 1986 Tel.: 559039 Fax.: 556014	Manufacturers : Natural Essential Oils, Aromatic Chemicals Synthetic Food Colours Food Flavours & Fragrances
Aromatik (India) 28 (46) III Cross Kumarapark West Bangalore-560 020 *Chief: N.R. Gawankar* *Alternate: S.A. Kelekar*	Estd.: 1954 Tel.: Off.: 3363692 Fac.: 8395799 Tlx.: 0845/8848 ITBG IN Fax: 8397352	Manufacturers : Industrial Perfumes Flavours
Aswathi Chemicals Pvt. Ltd. 56, Bommasandra Industrial Area, Hosur Road Bangalore-562 158 *Chief: K. Venkataramani*	Estd.: 1985 Tel.: Off.: 2268238 2268239 Fac.: 8422241 Tlx.: 845-3202 JENE IN Fax: 22058240	Manufacturers : Musk Ambrette Musk Ketone, Musk Xxylol

Name & Address	*Phone/Fax Telex Nos.*	*Business Activities*
Benson Co. 167, Chamarajpet Bangalore-560 018 *Chief: B.N. Prahlada Rao* *Alternate: P. Ravindra*	Estd.: 1949 Tel.: Off.: 605228 6621402 Fac.: 6621034 6612329 Tlx.: 0845-8576 Fax: 6602697	Agents : Bush Boake Allen (I) Ltd. Madras Manufacturers : Perfumry Compounds
Bhadrinath Trading Co. No. 77, Merlecha Mansion Nagarihpet Bangalore-560 002 *Chief: Ananth Kumar Bhadrinath*	Estd.: 1981 Tel.: 2239299 2239072 2239048	Dealers and Intending Agents :
Bhandya Narasimha Vaman Pal 190/V High School Road P.B. No. 26 Kundapura-576 201 (DK) *Chief: B.N.V. Pai* *Alternate: P.S. Nayak*	Tel.: 20621 21426	Estd.: 1974 Dealers : Essential Oils and Aromatic Chemicals
Bharani Agencies No. 40, 1st 'A' Cross, R.M.V. Extn. V.V. Raman Avenue Mekhri Circle Bangalore-560 080 *Chief: Ramani Arun Kumar*	Estd.: 1958 Tel.: 3347556 3345533 Tlx: 0845-8101 RAKA IN Fax: 3349993	Agents : For Natural Concretes Absolutes and Flavours (Food Grade)
Bharani Chemical Co. 30, Watkins Street, Perambur Madras-600 011 *Chief: R.R. Kumar* *Alternate: V. Nagarajan*	Estd.: 1984 Tel.: 619542 619858	Manufacturers : Flavouring Essences, Food Colour Preparations and Milk Flavour Concentrates
Bharat Bottle Stores Afzal Gunj Hyderabad-500 012 *Chief: B. Sudershan Rao*	Estd.: 1966 Tel.: 4619064 6365612	Traders : Perfumery Compounds and Natural Essential Oils

Name & Address	*Phone/Fax* *Telex Nos.*	*Business Activities*
Bush Boake Allen (India) Ltd. Seven Wells Street St. Tomas Mount Madras-600 016 *Chief: Arun Bewoor* *Alternate: G.S. Ranade*	Estd.: 1931 Tel.: 2341131/2/3 Fax: 2346017 2346158	Manufacturers : Flavours, Fragrances and Aroma Chemicals
C.M Ahuja & Co. 11/9, Maldarpet, Nagarthpet Cross Bangalore-560 002 *Chief: Ravi G. Ahuja* *Alternate: Rajesh G. Ahuja*	Estd.: 1957 Tel.: 2213297 2258558	Agents : D.D. Shah & Co. Bombay, For Industrial Perfumery Raw Materials Aromatic Chemicals etc.
Charu Incense India No. 211, Cottonpet Bangalore-560 053 *Chief:Bharath S. Shah*	Estd.: 1989 Tel.: Off.: 600813 6601793 Fac.: 3359183 Fax: 6613082	Manufacturers : Aromatic Chemicals & Perfumery Chemicals
Chemifuture No. 2, 4th Cross, 6th Street Surendranagar, Adambakkam Madras-600 088 *Chief: S.M. Gadre* *Alternate: M.M. Gadre*	Estd.: 1993 Tel.: 2346099	Traders : Aromatic Chemicals Natural Essential Oils Perfumery and Flavouring Compounds
Chemixil Corporation D-102, Industrial Estate Rajajinagar Bangalore-560 044 *Chief: B.S. Garuraj* *Alternate: T.A.S. Murthy*	Estd.: 1986 Tel.: 3300221 3341247 Fax: 3300221	Agents : Sarigon Organics Ltd. Pankaj Aero Chemicals Krupa Scientific, Vikram Enterprises
Chillies Export House Limited 35, M.C. Chidambara Nadar Street Virudhunagar-626 001 *Chief: A.P. Murugan*	Estd.: 1963 Off.: 04562-43315 Fac.: 04562-43345 Tlx.: 0449-202 CHEX IN Fax: 04562-45089	Manufacturers : Spice Oils & Oleoresins

Name & Address	Phone/Fax Telex Nos.	Business Activities
Chunilal Dayaldas Batliwala 15-5-97, Atzal Ganj Hyderabad-500 012	Estd.: 1970 Tel.: 524998 557001	Dealers : Aromatic Chemicals Perfumery Compounds Flavours, Essential Oils and Resinoids
Circars Lakshmi Engineering Company Convent Street Vijayawada-520 001 *Chief: B.S. Subrahmanyam* *Alternate: Suryam S.B.*	Estd.: 1986 Tel.: 0866-424642 (4 lines) Tlx: 0475-6321 Fax: 0886-423562	Manufacturers and Exporters : Palmarosa Oil
Chloro Organics 826/1, Ranilaxmibai Rad Near Vaccine Depot Tilakwadi (W) Belgaum-590 006 *Chie: Ajit Surendra Doddarnavar* *Alt.: Vinod Surendra Doddanavar*	Estd.: 1990 Tel.: Off.: 425934 Fac.: 771228 Fax: 0831-421730	Manufacturers : Aromatic Chemicals like Citronellol, Di Methyl Octanol, Geraniol Hydroxy Citronellal, Alpha Amyl Cinnamic Aldehyde Styrallyl Acetate etc.
D.J. Industries 3, Mandapam Road Kilpauk Garden Madras-600 010 *Chief: Jagdish J. Ajani* *Altrnate: Mrs. Damayanti J. Ajani*	Estd.: 1982 Tel.: 617153 618186	Manufacturers : Flavouring Essences, Traders in Aromatic Chemicals & Food Colours
D.V. Deo V/1084, Pandit Road Corner Cochin-682 002 *Chief: Dhananjai D. Deo* *Alt.: Chandra Pràkash D. Deo*	Estd.: 1946 Off.: 224196 226903 373809 Fac.: 422248 Tlx.: 885-7041 Fax: 373780	Manufacturers : Palmarosa Oil Cinnamonleaf Oil Lemongrass Oil, Citronella Oil, Spice Oils, Black Pepper, Celery Seed Oil, Paprika, Curcumin & Oleoresins
Deccan Bottle Stores Maharani Jhansi Road, Afzalgunj Hyderabad-500 012 (AP) *Chief: A. Ravinder* *Alt.: A. Padmanabhan*	Estd.: 1942 Tel.: 500237	Traders : Perfumes, Essences, Empty Bottles, Synthetic Food Colours, Aerated Water requisites

Name & Address	*Phone/Fax Telex Nos.*	*Business Activities*
Deccan Chemical & Essence Mart 15.9.382/5, Maharani Jhasni Road, Afzalgunj Hyderabad-500 012 *Chief: J.K. Dhawan* *Alternate: Anil Dhawan*	Estd.:1962 Tel.: 500970	Traders : Aromatic Chemicals Perfumery Compounds Essential Oils & Resinoids
Desaraj Natural Essential Oils 15, Netaji Road Kuppam-517 425 (AP) *Chief: v. Hemraj*	Estd.: 1971 Tel.: 55035 Fax: 080-6612845	Manufacturers : Essential Oils such as Davana Oil Palmarosa oil, Ginger gas oil, Eucalyptus Citriodora Oils etc.
Devson Organics No. 38, 6th Cross Pipeline, Chelurpalya Vijaynagar, Magadi Rd. Bangalore-560 023 *Chief: G.D. Kantharaj*	Estd.: 1981 Tel.: 3300076 3350104 Fax: 3350562	Manufacturers : Agaratti Compounds Dealers : Aromatic Compounds & Allied Chemicals
Devi Industries 2/176, Subbiah Naidu Industrial Complex Y. Pudupatti Arumbanur, Post 625 107 Madurai North *Chief: S. Rajagopal* *Alternate: R. Rajamannar*	Estd.: 1968 Off.: 0452-832731 0452-832823 Fac.: 0452-832631 Tlx.: 0445-310 SSP IN *Fax: 602455*	Manufacturers : Cardamom Oil
Dinamit Enterprises 12, 11th A Cross II Stage West of Chord Road Bangalore-560 086 *Chief: Prakash Gandhi* *Alternate: Dhiren Gandhi*	Estd.: 1989 Tel.: 3323132 3321799 Tlx.: 0845-3261 MDDP IN Fax: 3326621	Manufacturers : Perfumes & Flavour Compounds, Spary Perfumes
Drachem Speciality Chemicals Ltd. 8, Cathedral Road Madras-600 086 *Chief: C.G. Sethuram* *Alternate: Ravi Subrahmanyam*	Estd.: 1991 Tel.: 8273333 Tlx: 041-8479 GEON IN Fax: 8269359	Manufacturers : Speciality Aroma Chemicals

Name & Address	*Phone/Fax Telex Nos.*	*Business Activities*
Encee Aromatics Limited 14-1-68 & 69, Main Road Mettupalayam-641 301 *Chief: N.Krishnaswamy*	Estd.: 1978 Tel.: Off.: 23204/ 23863 Fac.: 22326 Tlx.: 08506-205- ENCE IN Fax: 91-04254- 22596	Manufacturers : Floral Concretes, Absolutes, Essential Ois, and Synthetic Aromatic Chemicals
Enjayes Spices & Chemical Oils Pvt. Ltd. Spices Hill, Vallicode Kottayam Pathanamthitta-689 656	Estd.: 1980 Tel.: 2980 Tlx.: 885-7047 EMJS IN	Manufacturers : Essential Oils, Spice Oleoresins and Natural Food Colours
Esthapanose Sons Synam Church Road Post Box No. 9 Alwaye-683 101 *Chief: K.S. Tomy*	Estd.: 1978 Tel.: 24044 24344 23330	Traders : Essential Oils Lemongrass Oil, Vitivrt Oil, Citronella Oil, Cinnamon Leaf Oil
Flora Cosmetics Pvt. Ltd. 509, Topaz Bldg. 5th Floor Amruta Hills, Panjagutta Hyderabad-500 482 (AP) *Chief: Dr. Anil Kumar Jaswal*	Estd.: 1991 Tel.: 314116	Manufacturers : Perfumery Compounds
Florale (India) Pvt. Ltd. 1768, 15th Main, 34th Cross Banashankari II Stage Bangalore-560 070 *Chief: Dr. K.W. Gopinath* *Alternate: Ms. Seems Sibbal*	Estd.: 1983 Tel.: Off.: 6610108 Fac.: 642141 Fax: 6610474	Manufacturers : Flavours, Perfumes & Essential Oils
Food Ingredient Specialities (P) Ltd. Al-111, Anna Nagar Madras-600 040 *Chief: B. Raghuramaiah*	Estd.: 1990 Tel.: 6211346 6211305 Fax: 6264839	Manufacturers : Flavouring Essences

Directory of Perfumes and Flavours–Manufacturers/ Distributors/Suppliers/Traders/Exporters/Importers

Name & Address	*Phone/Fax Telex Nos.*	*Business Activities*
Fragrance P.B. No. 3220, Shenoi Niwas M.G. Road, Ernakulam Cochin-682 035 *Chief: R. Vinod Kumar* *Alternate: R. Sudhir Shenoy*	Estd.: 1989 Tel.: 366887 363696 Tlx.: 0885--6344 FRAG IN Fax.: 362073	Manufacturers : Aromatic Chemicals Perfumery Materials and Essential Oils
G.R. Associates V/905, G.K. Avenue Cochin-682 002 *Chief: P.S. Gore* *Alternate: Mrs. Mrinalini P. Gore*	Estd.: 1981 Tel.: 226081 Fax.: 0484- 226081	Manufacturers : Perfumery Compounds Aromatic Chemicals & Essential Oils
Gogia Chemical Industries 133, Walltax Road Madras-600 005 *Chief: O.A. Vijayakrishnan*	Estd.: 1982 Tel.: 562653 Fax.: 567735	Manufacturers : Flavours, Essential Oils Aromatics Compounds and Fragrances
Guru Agencies 1676/33, Eastend 'A' Main Road, 39th Cross 9th Block, Jayanagar Bangalore-560 009 *Chief: T.N. Raghavendra Rao*	Estd.: 1981 Tel.: 2259819	Agents : Goldensun Mfg.Co. for Aromatic Chemicals & Perfumery Compounds
Hawarden Traders 50, South Masi Street Post Box No. 170 Madurai-625 001 *Chief: K.R. Satish Bapu* *Aalternate: K.R. Ramesh Bapu*	Estd.: 1955 Tel.: 24002 25764	Manufacturers : Perfumes, Aromas Essential Oils Dealing in Spice oils
High Tech. Flavours & Fragrances C-133, Peenya Indl. Area 2nd State Bangalore-560 058 *Chief: T.S. Gulhati*	Estd.: 1989 Tel.: Off.: 839389 Fac.: 8394804 Tlx.: 845-8848 IIBG-IN Fax.: 3334802	Manufacturers : Flavours & Fragrances
Hyderbad Zarda Works 22-6-183 Pathergatty Hyderabad-500 002 (AP) *Chief: Surendra Prasad* *Alternate: Shailendra Prasad*	Estd.: 1975 Tel.: 523294 522966	Manufacturers : Zarda, Quiwam, Attars Perfumes, Agarbathi etc.

Name & Address	*Phone/Fax Telex Nos.*	*Business Activities*
IDL Chemicals Limited P.B. No. 1, Sanatnagar (IE) PO Hyderbad-500 018 *Chief: T.S.P. Sarathy*	Estd.: 1964 Tel.: Off.: 264161 270742 Fac.: 260671 Tlx.: 0425-6864 Fax: 270772	Indenting Agents/ Stockists: Copenhagen Pectin Denmark, for Fragrance and Flavour Chemicals
Indfrag Pvt. Ltd. S-913, Manipal Centre Dickenson Road Bangalore-560 042 *Chief: Philip Samuel*	Estd.: 1987 Tel.: 5589521 Fax: 5589521 5560594	Manufacturers : Natural Floral Extracts (Concretes & Absolutes) Essential Oils Botanicals & Herbal Extracts
Indian Aromatics (Bangalore) 2, KMK Building Magadi Main Road Bangalore-560 023 *Chief: Aamod V. Gavankar*	Estd.: 1979	Manufacturers : Non-Alcoholic Industrial Perfumes and Flaours
Indian Essential Oil Plantations Gopalkrishna Pai Compound Talour Post-576 230 Kundapur Taluk *Chief: S.J. Thomas*	Estd.: 1989 Tel.: 21127 Fax.: 21127	Manufacturers : Essential Oils
Indian Flavours & Fragrances Ltd. 5/82, P.G. Pudur K. Vadamathural Post Combatore-641 017 *Chief: Mrs. Sivaramakrishnan S.* *Alternate: C. Sethuraman*	Estd.: 1979 Tel.: (0422)- Fax.: 447819 213800	Manufacturers : Floral Concretes Absolutes and Musk Ambreltolide
Jasmine Concrete Exports Pvt. Ltd. 19, Josier Street Nungumbakkam Madras-600 034 *Chief: A.K. Venkatasamy* *Alternate: S. Natarajan*	Estd.: 1991 Tel.: 8279451 Tlx.: 41-6381 OHM IN Fax.: 8259270	Manufacturers & Exporters : Jasmine Concretes Jasmine Absolutes Mimosa Concretes, Absolutes Jasmin Sambac Concrete and Absolutes

Name & Address	*Phone/Fax Telex Nos.*	*Business Activities*
K.B. Perfumeries 17, Rasappa Chetty Street Madras-600 003 *Chief: Kishore B. Bhatt* *Alternate: Hemant K. Bhatt*	Estd.: 1955 Tel.: Off.: 58-1857 Fac.: 4340417	Manufacturers : Perfumery Compounds Dealers : Perfumery Raw Materials
K.K. Viswanathan & Co. 9/37, Library Road Alwaye-683 101 *Chief: K.K. Viswanathan* *Alternate: V. Reghu*	Estd.: 1975 Tel.: 24449	Agents : For S.H. Kelkar & Co. Ltd. K.V. Arochem Ltd. in Kerala
K. Rajiah M.L. Narayana 1402 (1-5-91), General Bazar Secunderabad-500 003 *Chief: K. Nagender Rao* *Alternate: B. Dhanam Jaya*	Estd.: 1920 Tel.: 812058 843641	Traders : Aerated water trade and Pharmacauticals Materials
Kancor Flavours & Extracts Ltd. Bazar Road, Mattanchery Cochin--682 002 *Chief: J.J. Negandhi* *Alternate: Geemon Korah*	Estd.: 1991 Tel.: Off.: 223551 223661 227037 Tlx.: 880-5204 KANA IN Fax: 0484-225844 04856-52662	Manufacturers : Spice Oils, Oolressins Essential Oils, Natural food colours
Karnataka Soaps & Detergents Limited KS&DL, P.B. No. 5531 Bangalore Pune Highway Bangalore-560 005 *Chief: Dr. K.B. Pabi*	Estd.: 1918 Tel.: 3371103-06 Tlx.: 0845-2656/ 8236 Fax: 3370498	Manufacturers : Sandalwood Oil, Toilet Soaps, Detergents Glycerine, Stearic Acid, and Agarbatties
Karthik Agencies Karthikeya, 500, 9th Main Road 47th Cross, 5th Block Jayanagar Bangalore-560 041 *Chief: C.V. Jagannathan* *Alternate: R. Jagath*	Estd.: 1983 Tel.: 6637547 6635737 Fax: 6637547	Agents : K.L. Koh Enterprises Pvt. Ltd., Singapore M. Rawji Brothers Bombay, Nishant Aromas, Bombay Balaji Chemicals, Bombay

Name & Address	Phone/Fax Telex Nos.	Business Activities
Kohinoor Aroma Enterprises 20-A Block, Balaji Complex 125, Sultanpet Bangalore-560 053 *Chief: P.K. Sitaram*	Estd.: 1974 Tel.: 2877512 622703	Manufacturers : Aromatic Chemicals Natural Essentia Oils & Perfumes
Liya Aromatics 40/396, Azad Road, Kaloor Cochin-682 017 *Chief: P.A. George*	Estd.: 1985 Tel.: 348599 348782 Tlx.: 885-5023 LIYA IN Fax: 348782	Manufacturers & Traders : Natural Essential Oils Sandalwood Oil
Lux Flavours 2, Dutalraj Street Balavanthangal Madras-600 014 *Chief: V. Neelakantan* *Alternate: V. Anantharamkrishnan*	Estd.: 1981 Tel.: 2343818 4826345 Fax: 2344112	Manufacturers : Flavouring Essences
Mas Enterprises 13/1, 1st Floor, 7th Cross Setwen 3rd & 4th Main Chamarajpet Bangalore-560 018 *Chief: Madhav Bhagwat*	Estd.: 1993 Tel.: 6618933 Fax: 6612749	Agents : S.H. Kelkar & Co. Ltd. For Perfumes, Flavours and Aroma Chemicals
M.M. Abdul Hameed & Sons Post Box No. 12 Alwaye-683 101 *Chief: M.a. Mohammed* *Alternate: Ameen Mohammed*	Estd.: 1970 Tel.: 24014/24314 Tlx.: 0882-210 MMAH IN Fax.: 25127/24013	Traders & Merchant Exporters : Lemongrass Oil, Vetivert Oil, Citronelia Oil, Citrodora Oil Chaulmoogra Oil & Palmarosa Oil
Madras Aromatic Co. 48, Ellis Road Post Box No. 374 Mount Road Madras-600 002 *Chief: S.A. Rahim*	Estd.: 1974 Tel.: 840556 Fax: 833770	Manufacturers : Perfumes & Allied Products

Name & Address	*Phone/Fax Telex Nos.*	*Business Activities*
Mahalakshmi Trading Co. 107, Nyniappa Naick Street Madras-600 003 *Chief: K.U. Raghu* *Alternate: K.R. Hareesh*	Est.: 1947 Tel.: 563602	Traders : Aromatic Chemicals Raw Bathi and Agarbathi
Manju Chemicals No. 50, Kumaraswamy Nagar Villiwakkam Madras-600 049 *Chief: V.M.Yoosuf*	Estd.: 1984 Tel.: Off.: 626 1246 Fac.: 626 9354	Manufactuerers : Flavouring Essences & Food Colour Preparations
Maschmeijer Aromatics (India) Ltd. P.B. No.3, G.S.T. Road Chromepet Madras-600 044 *Chief: S.A. Md. Shareef*	Estd.: 1960 Tel.: 2368788 2368789 2368790 Tlx.: 041-26150 MAIL IN Fax: 2366828 2341375	Manufacturers : Musk Ambrette Musk Xylol, Musk Ketone; Perfumery Compounds and Aromatic Esters
Mattupalli Sambamurthy 2/4, Brodipet Guntur-522 002 (AP) *Chief: Mattupalli Gopala Krishnamurthy*	Estd.: 1990 Tel.: 235821	Manufacturers : Perfume Compounds Indenting Agents for Aromatic Chemicals
Mercantile Corporation 105, Mount Road Madras-600 002 *Chief: V.K. Eashwar*	Estd.: 1948 Tel.: 849324 4937412 Fax: 4937412 Tlx.: 41-6517 TRUE IN	Dealers : Perfumery Raw Essential Oils and Aroma Chemicals
Mysore Y.G. Agarbatti Works Metro Mansion Purani Haveli Road Hyderabad-500 002	Estd.: 1960 Tel.: 522864 521307	Manufacturers : Perfumery Compounds and Perfumed Agarbathies
N.K.M. Subburama Iyer & Sons 77, South Avani Moola St. Madurai-625 001 *Chief: N.S. Pandari Nathan*	Estd.:1926 Tel.: 24194	Dealers : Aromatic Chemicals Natual Ess. Oils Flavouring Compounds

Name & Address	*Phone/Fax Telex Nos.*	*Business Activities*
Naresh Trading Co. 36, K.V. Temple Street Bangalore-560 053 *Chief: Naresh Khakhar* *Alternate: Manoj Khakhar*	Estd.: 1969 Tel.: 2871800 Fax.: 2871800	Traders : Aromatic Chemicals Ntural Essential Oils Resinoids, Perfumery Compounds
Nasir & Bros. 1101 Akbar Road Mandi Mohalla Mysore-570 021	Estd.: 1985 Tel.: 31677 Fax: 37540	Dealers : Agarbatti Raw Aromatic Chemicals Perfumery Compounds and Natural & Synthetic Ess. Oils
Nat-Con No. 490 (L) IV Phase Peenya Industrial Area Bangalore-560 058 *Chief: Sujit Mukund*	Estd.: 1987 Tel.: 8396545 Fax: 8392986	Manufacturers : Spice Oils, Spice Oleoresins, Herbals Extract, Dry Fruit Extracts & Natural Products
The National Tading Co. (Madras) 57, Velachery Road Madras-600 032 *Chief: J.R. Shah* *Alternate: P.J. Shah*	Estd.: 1948 Tel.: 2352317 2350771 Fax: 2352317	Manufacturers : Perfumes & Cosmetics Agents : Fobile Daniled Ltd. U.K
Natural & Essential Oils Pvt. Ltd. No. 224, 8th Cross Gokulam III Stage Mysore-570 002 *Chief: M.R. Tyagarajan* *Alternate: T. Gowrishankar*	Estd.: 1979 Tel.: Off.: 512021 Fac.: 77738/ 77857 Fax.: 512021	Manufacturers : Jasmine Concrete Jasmine Absolute Tuberose Concrete Tuberose Absolute Sambac Concrete Sambac Absolute Champaka Concrete Champaka Absolute & Davana Oil
Navrat Fragrances Pvt. Ltd. J.P. Tower, 8th Floor 7/2 Nungambakkam High Road Madras-600 034 *Chief: N. Pater Penanayagam*	Estd.: 1984 Tel.: 8260134 Fax: 8270346	Manufacturers : Tuberose Concrete & Absolute Jasmine Grandiflorum Concrete & Absolute, Jasmine Sambac Concrete & Absolute

Name & Address	*Phone/Fax Telex Nos.*	*Business Activities*
Nesstate Flora No. 4, Veerapandi Coimbatore-641 019 *Chief: K. Longanathan* *Alternate: T. Gowishankar*	Estd.: 1984 Tel.: 892587 Fax: 892286	Manufacturers : Jasmine Concrete Jasmine Sambac Concrete, Tuberose Concrete
Nikhil Products 14/2, II Cross, SSI Area V Block, Rajajinagar Bangalore-560 010 *Chief: Hitesh. C. Nathvani* *Alternate: Nikhil C. Nathvani*	Estd.: 1986 Tel.: 3350752 Fax.: 3351115	Manufacturers : Aromatic Chemical & Natural Essential Oil
Odochem Industries C-71, II Stage Peenya Industrial Estate Bangalore-560 058 *Chief: P. Annaputnaiah* *Alternate: M.S. Raikar*	Estd.: 1989 Tel.: Fac: 8392229 Fax: 8392229	Manufacturers : Aldehyde C16, Rectified Clove Leaf Oil, Eugenol Propenyl Guethol, Geraniot Ex-Palmrosa
People's Chemical Agency Post Box No. 7562 38, Arcot Srinivasachar Street Bangalore-560 053 *Chief: B.L. Kishore* *Alternate: B.L. Kiran*	Estd.: 1853 Tel.: 2870470 2877485 Tlx.: 0845-2527 Fax: 2256089	Traders & Agents : Dyes, Chemicals & Allied Products
Perfumery Industries PKCCI Buidlings, K.G. Road Bangalore-560 009 *Chief: S.V. Raghavan* *Alternate: s. Vasudevan*	Estd.: 1962 Tel.: 2268498	Manufacturers : Perfumery Compounds
Plant Lipids Pvt. Ltd. Kadayiruppu Kolechery-682 311 Cochin, Kerala *Chief C.J. George* *Alternate: Dr. A.G. Mathew*	Estd.: 1979 Tel.: (04853)- 60395 60497 Tlx.: 8856598 LIPID IN Fax: (04853)- 60689 (0484) 370981	Manufacturers & Exporters : Spice Oils, Oleoresins Natural Food Colours Flavour Concentrates etc.

Name & Address	*Phone/Fax Telex Nos.*	*Business Activities*
The Punjab Aromatics A.G. Road Calicut-673 032 *Chief: Bharat Bhusan Agarwal*	Estd.: 1981 Tel.: 54042 51987 Tlx.: 804308 TPA IN Fax: 0495-51760	Manufacturers : Sandalwood Oil
Purandas Ranchhoddas & Sons No. 22-6-786, Gulzar Houz East Paneshah, Guruvannagalli Hyderabad-500 002 *Chief: Madanlal* *Alternate: Kantilal*	Estd.: 1895 Tel.: 520343 522203 Fax.: 565009	Manufacturers : Flavoured Chewing Tobacco (Quiwam & Zardal) Cosmetics and Perfumery Compounds
Radhas Perfumery Enterprises Convent Road Kollam-6591 001 *Chief: Dr. B.A. Rajakrishnan*	Estd.: 1974 Tel.: 79010 79511 Tlx: 886-296 Fax: 0474-740610	Manufacturers : Radhas Ayurvedic Soap
Reliable Industrial Syndicate 85-B, Industrial Suburb II Stage, Yeshwanthpur Bangalore-560 022 *Chief: Ramesh Puri* *Alternate: Ajay Puri*	Estd.: 1960 Tel.: 3373952 3377608 Tlx.: 0845-2104 RIS IN Fax: 3378304	Manufacturers : Natural Essential Oils Aromatic Chemicals
Robin Chemicals Pvt. Ltd. 103, Nelson Manickam Road Aminjikarai Madras-600 029 *Chief: Mukund R. Shah* *Alternate: Surendra N. Shah*	Estd.: 1972 Tel.: 422806 4837514 Fax: 422220	Manufacturers : Flavouring Essences, Food Colours, etc.
S.V. Rangaswamy & Co. Ltd. 2, 3rd Cross, Kalasipalayam New Extension, P.B. No. 6539 Bangalore-560 002 *Chief: S.V. Rangswamy*	Estd.: 1964 Tel.: 2222301 (4 lines) Fax: 2224497 Tlx: 0845-2267 SVR IN	Agents : Haarmann & Reimer GmbH Hozminden Germany, Indian Organic Chemical Ltd. Bombay

Name & Address	*Phone/Fax Telex Nos.*	*Business Activities*
S. Chandanmull Mutha No. 2, Nyniappa Naick Street Madras-600 003 *Chief: P. Chandanmull* *Alternate: J. Vasant Kumar*	Estd.: 1948 Tel.: 563529 560999 565609	Traders : Aromatic Chemicals and Commission Agents
Saibaba Sugandh Bhandar P.B. 7905 53, Santhusapet Bangalore-560 053 *Chief: M.D. Khasnis* *Alternate: Ajit Khasnis*	Estd.: 1959 Tel.: 2879762 2874802	Dealers : Perfumery Compounds and Chemicals
Sathyanarayana & Co. 61, Mamulpet Bangalore-560 053 *Chief: T.N. Seetharamaiah* *Alternate: T.S. Sathyakumar*	Estd.: 1962 Tel.: 7870125 2874326 Fax: 6601141	Manufacturers : Representative of Aromatic Chemicals, Natural Ess. Oils Resinoids & Perfumery Compounds
Sathyanarayana Traders 62, Mamulpet Bangalore-560 053 *Chief: S. Jayaprakash* *Alternate: J.G. Mohan*	Estd.: 1969 Tel.: 2259819 6652801	Manufacturers : Aromatic Chemicals Perfumery Compounds
Shanbhag Aromatics 794, Khanapur Rd. Belgaum-590 006 *Chief: Dr. Mohan R. Shanbhag*	Estd.: 1980 Tel.: Off.: 28540 Fac.: 23120 Fax: 429430	Manufacturers : Aromatic & Fine Chemicals
Shilpa Aromatics K.C. Rani Road Gadag-582 101 *Chief: Kashinath Patwardhan*	Estd.: 1979 Tel.: 8658	Manufacturers : Perfumery Compounds Aromatic Chemicals and Agarbathies
Shri-Aroma Agencies No. 961, 24th Main 4-T Block, Jayanagar Bangalore-560 041 *Chief: S.H. Rizvi* *Alternate: Saquib A. Rizvi*	Estd.: 1984 Tel.: 6633822 6634768 Tlx.: 0845-2277 SHRI IN Fax: 6634765	Indenting Agents : Cavallier Freres S.A. Grasse, France, for Natural Essential Oils Resinoids Absolutes etc.

Name & Address	Phone/Fax Telex Nos.	Business Activities
Shri Rathod Trading Company 532, Mount Road Madras-600 018 *Chief: Chandrakant Tolia*	Estd.: 1935 Tel.: 4349757	Traders : Perfumery Compounds
Sita Traders 1595/8, Vinivilas Road Mysore-570 004 *Chief: S. Jayaprakash* *Alternate: J.G. Mohan*	Estd.: 1975 Tel.: 36261	Dealers : Perfumery Raw Materials
Sonarome Chemicals Pvt. Ltd. C-136, Peenya Industrial Area II State Bangalore-560 058 *Chief: Mrs. R. Gulhati*	Estd.: 7980 Tel.: Off.: 8394804 Fac.: 8395595 Tlx.: 845-8848 Fax: 3334802	Manufacturers : Flavours & Fragrances
South East Enterprises 91/13, S.S.I. Area, 4th Cross V Block Rajajinagar Bangalore-560 010 *Chief: Sanjay Mehta* *Alternate: Anup Chand Mehta*	Estd.: 1989 Tel.: 33550311 Fax.: 3300245	Traders & Agents : Perfumery Compounds & Aromatic Chemicals
Sri Murugan & Co. 124, Nyniappa Narchen Street, Park Town Madras-600 003 *Chief: M. Suresh Kumar*	Estd.: 1980 Tel.: 567662 560387	Traders : Aromatic Chemicals
Srivasta Industries 45/12, Gubbanna Industrial Estate, VI Block, Rajajinagar Bangalore-560 010 *Chief: V.P. Mani*	Estd.: 1976 Tel.: 3306023 3385320	Manufacturers : Aroma Chemicals & Natural Essential Oils
Sudarshana Enterprises 91-2, K.V. Temple Street Bangalore-560 053	Estd.: 1961 Tel.: 2875295 Fax: 2875295	Agents : Satish Rosin & Terpentine Works and Sumesh & Terpene Industries, Hoshiarpur for Perfumery Raw Materials

Name & Address	*Phone/Fax Telex Nos.*	*Business Activities*
Sundar Agency No. 66, 3rd Road Seshadripuram Bangalore-560 020 *Chief: A.G. Sundarvardan*	Estd.: 1983 Tel.: 3348390 3348739	Agents : D.G. Gore, Bombay Shree Chemical Industries Privi (P) Ltd. U.K. Aromatic & Chemicals
Sunrise Chemical Industries 66, bazullah Rd., T. Nagar Madras-600 017 *Chief: N.M. Venkatesh*	Estd.: 1984 Tel.: Off.: 8252516 Fac.: 8282219 Tlx.: 41-7558 PCO IN WDT260 Fax: 8256971	Manufacturers : Concentrated Perfumery Compounds for Industrial purpose
Suresh Chemicals 298/2, N.S. Palya Bannerghatta Rd. Bangalore-560 076 *Chief: K.S. Suresh Babu*	Estd.: 1986 Tel.: Fac.: 6634118 Fax: 628912	Manufacturers : Hydroxy Citronellal & Perfumery Compounds
Swastik Eucalyptus Oil Co. 166, Main Bazar ootacamund-643 001 Bangalore-560 010 *Chief: Shantilal B. Mehta*	Estd.: 1954 Tel.: Off.: 42527 Fac.: 43489	Manufacturers : Eucalyptus Oil, Geranium Oil, Lemongrass Oil Citronella oil, Cittriodora oil and Vertivert Oil
Synat Aromatix Pvt. Ltd. P.O. Box 793 40-3-4, Krishna Nagar Vijayawada-520 010 *Chief: N.V. Rama Rao*	Estd.: 1990 Tel.: 471184 Tlx.:0475-239 PCO IN Fax: 473433	Manufacturers : Perfumes & Flavours Drug Intermediates Fine Organic Chemicals
Syed Attars 'Syedna' Ground Floor Masjid lane, S.R.M. Road Ernakulam Cochin-682 018 *Chief: S.M. Malik Mohamed*	Estd.: 1976 Tel.: 341783	Manufacturers : Perfumery Compounds

Name & Address	*Phone/Fax Telex Nos.*	*Business Activities*
Synthite Industrial Chemicals Ltd. Ajay Vihar, M.G. Road Cochin-682 016 *Chief: C.V. Jacob* *Alternate: George Paul*	Estd.: 1972 Tel.: Off.: 355794 360698 Fac.: 04853 60285 Tlx.: 0885-6328 SYN IN Fax: 370405	Manufactures : Spice oleoresins Essential oils, Resinoids, Floral concentrates, Natural food colours, Dry Flowers, Seasonings etc.
T.M.V. Aromatic (P) Ltd. Mahakavi Bharathiyar Rd. Emakulam Kochi-682 035 *Chief: T.V. Rajesh Shenoi* *Alternate: T.M.V. Shenoi*	Estd.: 1991 Tel.: Off.: 373121 361330 Fac.: 855340 Tlx.: 0885-6612 TMV IN Fax: 373121	Manufacturers : Aromatic Chemicals Essential Oils and Perfumes
T.M.V. Shenoi Mahakavi, Bharathiyar Road Ernakulam Kochi-682 035 *Chief: T.M.V. Shenoi* *Alternate: T.V. Rajesh Shenoi*	Estd.: 1958 Tel.: 361330 373121 Tlx: 885-6612 TMV IN Fax: 373121	Manufacturers : Aromatic Chemicals Essential Oils Perfumes for Agarbathies, Washing and Toilet Soaps
Technagi Laboratories 53, 3rd Cross, MICO Layout Bangalore-560 076 *Chief: Dr. K.R. Lakshminarayanan*	Estd.: 1983 Tel.: Off.: 6636165 Fac.: 646486 Fax: 6636165	Manufacturers : Aromatic Chemicals Resinoids and Perfumery
Trade India Exports (Regd.) 209E, Missionary Hill P.B.No. 13 Ootachmund-643 002 *Chief: V. Narayanan* *Alternate: V.N. Ranjith*	Estd.: 1981 Tel.:42553 41413 Tlx.: 8504-204 PCO IN Fax: 41413	Manufacturers : Natural Geranuum Oil Wintergreen Oil and Java Vitronella Oil

Name & Address	*Phone/Fax Telex Nos.*	*Business Activities*
Universal Oleoresins VIII/946, Navaratna House Jawahar Road Cochin-632 002 *Chief: Chetan Shah* *Alternate: Dipak Shah*	Estd.: 1981 Tel.: Off.: 223671 226673 225029 Tlx.: 8857002 BREW IN Fax: 226542	Manufacturers: Spice Oils & Oleoresins Natural Colours, 'Spice Drops' Instant Spice Extracts
V.V. Southern Aromatics Pvt. Ltd. 7, Venkatachala Mudali St. Park Town Madras-600 003	Estd.: 1977 Tel.: 581841	Manufacturers : Perfumery Compounds for Soaps, Toiletries Cosmetics, Tobacco & Agarbathi
Venkateswara Essences and Chemicals Pvt. Ltd. 145/2, Benniganahalli Old Madras Road Bangalore-560 016 *Chief: M.G. Joseph*	Estd.: 1988 Tel.: 5283753 Fax: 5283753	Manufactures : Soft Drink Concentrate & Flavours
Vin Enterprises **'Anugrah'** Near Govt. Girls High School Tripunithura-682 301 *Chief: Dr. Mohan S. Venkastesh*	Estd.: 1993 Tel.: 0484-	Agents : Indenting Agent for Aroma Chemicals, Spice Oils & Oleoresins Essential Oils Menthol & Allied Products
Vina Fragrances 459, Ashoka Pillar Road Jayanagar Bangalore-560 011 *Chief: K.L. Negendra*	Estd.: 1994 Tel.: 6639344 Fac.: 64272 Fax.: 6650338	Manufacturers : Perfumery & Flavour Compouds for Soaps Shampoos Agarbathi Aerosol Room Spray and Tobacco/Zarda
Vinarom Limited 1101, Bartor Centre M.G. Road Bangalore-560 001 *Chief: Ajit Pal* *Alternate: V. Nandakumat*	Estd.: 1985 Tel.: Off.: 5091104 5091105 Fac.: 425343 Fax: 425344	Manufacturers and Exporters : Industrial Perfumery Compounds

Name & Address	Phone/Fax Telex Nos.	Business Activities
Vinod Kumar Rekesh & Company 'Gyanmalaya' 32 Mount Plesant Road Coonoor-643 102 *Chief: P. Vinod Kumar* *Alternate: P. Rakesh*	Estd.: 1958 Tel.: 20868 Fac.: 21767 Fax: 04264-20868	Manufacturers : Eucalyptus oil I.P. & B.P.
Vinod Perfumers NO. 49, M.B.T. Street Nagarthpet Cross Bangalore-560 002 *Chief: G.V.R. Prasad*	Estd.: 1993 Tel.: 2234109	Dealers : Perfumery Raw Materials & Aroma Chemicals
Vivek Trading Company 10/3, 1st. Floor, 5th Cross Victona Layout Bangalore-560 047 *Chief: Vimal M. Mashru*	Estd.: 1988 Tel.: 568028 Tlx.: 0845-2199 (SUB-21) Fax.: 5576384	Traders & Agents : Nirmal Colorants & Chemicals Mfg. Co. Atlas Fine Chemicals Pvt. Ltd. Dealers : Aromatics Chemicals Natural Essential Oils
Yash & Company 157, B.V.K. Iyengar Road Bangalore-560 053	Estd.: 1961 Tel.: 2268350	Agents : Ambernath Chemical Industries, Bombay Alcheme Laboratories Bombay Dearlers: Aroma Chemicals, perfumes & Flavours
Dubey Perfumers 19-2-422, Chandulal Baradari Colony Hyderabad-500 264 *Chief: Devesh Dubey* *Alternate: Nisheeth Dubey*	Estd.: 1991 Tel.: 523350 Fax: 524083	Manufacturers : Natural Essential Oils & Perfumes
S.V.P. Chemicals (P) Ltd. B.C. 85, Lytton Road, Camp Belgaum-590 001 *Chief: Vinayak Pattanshetti* *Alternate: Basawaraj Pattanshetti*	Estd.: 1983 Tel.: 421585 423585 Fax: 428298	Manufacturers : Di-Ethyl Phthalate

Name & Address	*Phone/Fax Telex Nos.*	*Business Activities*
Associate Members		
Cigma Essence & Aromatics Pvt. Ltd. 910/1 Thimmampalayam Karamadai-641 104 Coimbatore (Dt.) T.N. *Chief: S.R. Varadharajan*	Estd.: 1994 Tel.: 04267 72001 72480 Fax: 04267--	Manufacturers : Jasmine, Tuberose Jasmine Sambac, Mimosa Marigold Concretes & Absolutes
Dragoco India Ltd. 144, 1st Street Seevaram Village Perungudi Madras-600 096 *Chief: C. Venkat* *Alternate: S. Balasubramanian*	Estd.: 1994 Tel.: 1926172 4926539 4927325 Fax: 4925773	Dealers : Fragrances and Flavours
I.T.C. Limited ITC Tobacco Technology Centre Peenya Bangalore-560 058 *Chief: Dr. P.P. Singh* *Alternate: Ashok Madbhavi*	Estd.: 1973 Tel.: 8394351 Tlx.: 845-5050 ITCR-IN Fax: 8394352	Manufacturers : Tobacco Flavours
J.N.T.U. Oil Technological Research Institute Ananntapur-515 004 Andrapradesh	Estd.: 1948 Tel.: 20376	R & D : Research activities on Essential Oils, perfumery Products Spices & Oleoresines
The Karnataka State Agarbatti Manufacturer's Co-operative Society Ltd. No. 18/3, 1st Main Road Sampangiram Nagar Bangalore-560 027	Estd.: 1961 Tel.: 2221468	Traders : Supplying raw materials required for the manufacture of Agarbattis in Karnataka
Reckitt & Colman of India Limited 176, SIPCOT Indl. Complex, Hosur-635 126 Hosur-635 126 T.N. *Chief: Dr. B.B. Singh*	Estd.: 1981 Tel.: 6661, 6766 Fac.: 6756 Tlx.: 0458-210 RCI IN Fax: 04344-6662	Manufacturers : Bulk Drugs Aromatic Chemicals Insecticides etc.

Name & Address	*Phone/Fax Telex Nos.*	*Business Activities*
Adarsh Sugandh Bhandar Katra Purohitji Johri Bazar Jaipur-302 003 *Chief: Desraj Taneja* *Alternate: Anurag Pamami*	Estd.: 1950 Tel.: 564872	Dealers : Perfumery Chemicals Essences, Food Colour Petroleum Jelly, White Oils etc.
Alka Chemi-Cosmetics 1578 Lallu Ramji's Vanda Opp. Jansatta Bldg. Mirzapur Ahmedabad-380 001 *Chief: Mahendrabhai C. Saraiya* *Alternate: Rameshbhai C. Saraiya*	Estd.: 1966 Tel: 5505183 5351150 5351022	Manufactures : Perfumery Compounds Flavours, Agarbathies Dealing in Aromatic Chemicals
Ambica Agencies 26, Professor Colony. Opp. Memnagar Fine St. Near Vijay Char Rasta Navrangpura Ahmedabad-380 009	Estd.: 1979 Tel.: 491403	Agents : Bush Boake Allen (I) Ltd. for Perfumery Compounds and Flavouring Compounds
Anant Agarbatti Works 1761, Gautam Chamber Gandhi Road, Nr. Bala Hanuman Ahmedabad-380 001 *Chief: Kamleshu C. Shah* *Alternate: Mukesh C. Shah*	Estd.:1985 Tel.: Off.: 334255 Fac.: 2740520 2741484 *Fax: 2743689*	Manufacturers : Agarbatti and Synthetic Essential Oil & Aroma Compounds
Armate Trading Corporation 9, Mihir Apartments Near Opera Society Dhumketu Marg, Paldi Ahmedabad-380 007 *Chief: Milan V. Mehta*	Estd.: 1990 Tel.: 418999 Fax: 418999	Agents : Synthie Industrial Chemicals Ltd. & Drachem Speciality Chemicals Ltd. Dealing in Aromatic Chemicals, Synthetic Musks, Spice Oil & Oleoresins
Arochem Industries 454 Rambag Ratlam-457 001 *Chief: Mohanbhai B. Patel*	Estd.: 1969 Tel.: 31026	Manufacturers : Aromatic Fine Chemicals, Perfumery Compounds & Agarbatties

Name & Address	*Phone/Fax Telex Nos.*	*Business Activities*
Arochem Industries 780 GIDC Estate Makarpura Baroda-390 010 *Chief: Dr. Rajnikant R. Shah*	Estd.: 1980 Tel.: 443214	Manufacturers : Benzyl Acetate, Benzyl Alcohol, Alpha Amyl Cinnamic Aldehyde, Rose Crystals
Bharti Perfumers 9, Pragati Industrial Estate Gujarat Bottling Road Opp. Dena Bank, Rakhial Ahmedabad-380 023 *Chief: Panchabhai B. Sukhadia* *Alt.: Kint Panchabhai Sukhadia*	Estd: 1983 Tel.: Off.: 2744691 (F) 2744586	Manufacturers : Perfumes
Boyce Pharma 1, Rameshwar Chambers Opp. Paface Talkies Bunder Road Bhavnagar-364 001 *Chief: H.K. Patel* *Alternate: M.C. Patel*	Estd.: 1985 Tel.: Off.: 25456 22617 Fac.: (02846)-22361	Manufacturers : Aromatics Chemicals Fine Chemicals and Essential Oils
Chinubhai Motilal Saraiya 3101, Three Gates Ahmedabad-380 001 *Chief: Mahendrabhai C. Samajya* *Alternate: Rameshbhai C. Sariya*	Estd.: 1933 Tel.: Off.: 5351150 5351022	Traders : Agarbatti, Perfumes Flavours & Aromatic Chemicals Fac.: 5505183
Dayal Chemical Works 41 Jail Road Indore (MP)	Estd.: 1960 Tel: Off.: 534307 531962 Fac.: 420515	Manufacturers : Essence & Food Colours
Dayalal Velji & Sons Ranjit Road Jamnagar-361 001 *Chief: Harilal D. Nagrecha*	Estd.: 1947 Tel.: 551092 78396	Manufacturers : Flavouring Essence Dealers : Perfumes and Agarbathies
G. Aromas 2, Jyotikapark Society Shahbag Road Ahmedabad-380 004 *Chief: Udayam G. Shah* *Alternate: Kiran G. Shah*	Estd.: 1991 Tel.: 2112877 Fax: 2112878	Manufacturers : Industrial Perfumes

Name & Address	Phone/Fax Telex Nos.	Business Activities
Gujarat Aromatic 416, Sugandh Ghar Jethabhai's Pole, Khadia Ahmedabad-380 001 *Chief: Nikunj H. Dyer*	Estd.: 1967 Tel.: (O) 2148949 (F) 7459754	Manufacturers : Synthetic Industrial Perfumes
Gujarat Organic Chemicals 32, Vithal Udyognagar Anand Sojitra Road Distt. Kaira Gujarat-388 121 *Chief: Navinbhai S. Patel*	Estd.: 1975 Tel.: (02692)- 46205 Fax: 46446	Manufacturers : Benzyl, Benzoate, Benzyl Alcohol Silver Sulpha Diazine USP
Hams Trading Corporation 4, Shanti Sadan Estate Opp. Dinbhai Tower Lal Darwaja Ahmedabad-380 001 *Chief: D.C. Shah*	Estd.: 1970 Tel.: 5353153 5354085 Fax: 5354085	Agents : Saiba Industries P. Ltd. Bombay
Iscon Research Laboratories Pvt. Ltd. 16-B (II) Heavy Indl. Area Jodhpur-342 003 *Chief: M.L. Jain* *Alternate: C.S. Bhandari*	Estd.: 1984 Tel.: Off.: 42582 40418 Fac.: 40468 Fax: 0291-41193	Manufacturers : Benzyl Acetate Benzyl Alcohol Benzyl Benzoate Di-Benzyhl Ether etc.
J.B. Shah & Co. Pankaj Soceity Ahmedabad-380 007 *Chief: Shashin V. Sheth* *Alternate: Jatin V. Sheth*	Estd.: 1954 Tel.: 6620072 Fax: 6620202	Manufacturers : Aroma Compounds and Perfumery Compounds
K.V. Arochem Ltd. 170-175 GIDC Indl. Estate Vipi-396 195 *Chief: S.V. Vaze*	Estd.: 1978 Tel.: (02638) 30699 Tlx: 011-71960	Manufacturers : Organic Chemicals Benzyl Alcohol, and Esters, Phenyl ethyl Alcohol and esters Phenyl ethyl methyl ether etc.

Name & Address	*Phone/Fax Telex Nos.*	*Business Activities*
M.L. Rathod & Co. 7/8 Galaxy commercial Centre 1st Floor, Jawahar Raod Post Box No. 224 Rajkot-360 001 *Chief: Manshinhji L. Rathod*	Estd.: 1955 Tel.: Off.: 55903 Fac.: 43905	Manufacturers : Perfumery Compounds
M.M. Khambhatwala Akashethkl 'a's' Pole Raipur Ahmedabad-380 001 *Chief: K.R. Khambhatwala* *Alternate: S.G. Khambhatwala*	Estd.: 1924 Tel.: Off.: 2146400 2146500 Fac.: 5324148 5326918	Manufacturers : Perfumed Hair Oil Agarbattis, Dhoop Masala for preparing Hair Oil, Perfumes etc.
Nangrani Industries Post Box 150 Bhavnagar-364 001 Gujarat	Estd.:1977 Tel.: (0278) 5311 5010	Manufacturers : Flavouring Compounds
Natwarlal Nathalal & Co. 49, Balahanuman Gandhi Road Ahmedabad-380 001 *Chief: Mahendrabhai N. Shah* *Alternate: Niren G. Shah*	Estd.: Tel.: 2140147 Fax: 2144807	Dealers : Food Colour Aromatic Chemicals Fragrances
NIcon Traders Chokshi Bazar Mahatma Gandhi Road Vadodara-390 001 Gujarat *Chief: Ashwindbhai M. Chokshi*	Estd.: 1980 Tel.: 551844 66205	Dealers : Aromatic Compounds Flavours, Food Colours Natural Essential Oil
Nidaan Chemicals P. Ltd. Plot No. 84 GIDC Phase 1, Vatwa Ahmedabad-382 445 *Chief: B.B Shah* *Alternate: B.P. Shah*	Estd.: 1987 Tel.: 831709 831816 832997	Manufacturers : Aromatic Chemicals
Nirmesh 42, Jaota Compound Mittal Chamber 2nd Floor Indore-452 001 (MP) *Chief: Nirmal Bagree*	Estd.: 1976 Tel.: 464121 to 464124 Fax: 731-4611963 Tlx.: 735402 GMBN IN	Agents : Chemicals Pharmaceuticals Raw Materials Bulk Drug Drug Intermediate Solvents Pigments etc.

Name & Address	Phone/Fax Telex Nos.	Business Activities
Opal Aromatics 35-A/4, Indl. Estate Fort Indore-462 006 (MP) *Chief: J.K. Shetty*	Estd.: 1980 Tel.: 410177	Manufacturers : Aromatic Chemicals Industrial Perfumes
P.C. Lalani & Co. Chauta Bazar, Kelapith Surat-395 001 *Chief: Sunil A. Lalaru*	Estd.: 1940 Tel.: 423280	Manufacturers : Perfumery Agarbatti Raw OIl etc.
P.M. Rathod & Co. 10/11, Empre Tower Nt. Petrol Pump Panchwali, C.G. Road Ahmedabad-380 009 *Chief: Ashsin C. Patel* *Alternate: Bipin C. Patel*	Estd.: 1981 Tel.: Off.: 6420261 466846 Fac.: 7470821 7474557 Fax: 6420261	Manufacturers : Perfumes & Aroma Chemicals
Parasmani Products 1st B. Road, Sardarpura Jodhpur-342 001 *Chief: R.K. Parekh*	Estd.: 1976 Tel.: 34283 37378 Fax: 0291-34896	Manufacturers : Industrial Perfumes
Parnami Perfumery Works Adarsh Nagar Jaipur-302 004 *Chief: Praveen Pamami* *Alternate: Alok Pamami*	Estd.: 1980 Tel.: 620131 48633 605751	Manufacturers : Perfumes Agarbatties
Pioma Industries 8th Floor, Rasna House Panchwati Ahmedabad-380 006 *Chief: Areez Khambatta*	Estd.: 1984 Tel.: 6427774 6423338 Fax: 9179- 466574 Tlx.: 1216460	Dealers : Essence, Food Colours Saccharin Flavours & Perfumery Chemicals
R.D. Agencies 7, Raghuvir Park Shnji Complex Dhebar Road Rajkot-360 001 *Chief: Pryush Kotak*	Estd.: 1990 Tel.: 22272	Dealers : Aromatic Chemicals & Perfumery Compounds Agent : Privi Organics Pvt. Ltd. Bombay

Name & Address	*Phone/Fax Telex Nos.*	*Business Activities*
R.R. Gondalwala & Co. Tower Road Surendranagar-363 001 *Chief: R.R. Gondalwala*	Estd.: 1970 Tel.: 20032 23640	Dealers : Flavours, Food Colour Perfumes and other Food Chemicals
Rupangi Impex Ltd. 4th Floor, Agarwal Complex Near Muncipal Market C.G. Road, Navarangpura Ahmedabad-380 009 *Chief: Radheshyam Kabra* *Alternate: C.D. Patel*	Estd.: 1989 Tel.: Off.: 401170 6420223 4011533 Fac.: 2870105 2874358 Fax: 2872255	Manufacturers : Natural Menthol & Peppermint Oil
S.M; Associates 1, Bapudas Apts Nar Vijay Restaurant Ahmedabad-380 009 *Chief: Vijay Podar*	Estd.: 1992 Tel.: 402708 Fax: 6420819	Agents : For Food Colours Flavours Soft Drink Concentrate and Aromatic Compounds
Sabari Chemicals P. Ltd. A/2/236 G.I.D.C. Estate Nandesari-391 340 Distt. Baroda *Chief: Ravi Nair* *Alternate: Mohan Nair*	Estd.: 1984 Tel.: Off.: 23081 338334 Fac.: 840429 840143 Fax: 481265 840890	Manufacturers : Benzyl Alochol Benzyl Acetate Benzyl Benzoate Benzyl Chloride Phenyl Acetic Acid Sodium Benzoate etc.
Sanghi Organics & Phytochem Ltd. 144, Piplia Rao Agra Bombay Road Indore-452 001 *Chief: Rajeev Sanghi* *Alternate: K.K. Jain*	Estd.: 1979 Tel.: Off.: 62651 65830 67308 Fac.: 07292 47239 47360 Fax: 474392 Tlx.: 0735-412	Manufacturers : Phenyl Ethyl Alcohol Phenyl Ethyl Methyl Ether Phenyl Ethyl Acetate, Phenyl Ethyl Formate Sulphamide etc.

Name & Address	*Phone/Fax Telex Nos.*	*Business Activities*
Sanjay Chemicals 3, Sanjay Society No. 2 Shahibag Ahmedabad-380 004 *Chief: Dinesh M. Shah* *Alternate: Jatin G. Shah*	Estd.: 1973 Tel.: Off.: 386458 2140147 Fac.: 813025 Fax: 2144807	Manufacturers : Synthetic Essential Aroma Compounds Speciality Agarbatti Compounds
Sapan Chemicals Moti Nagar Sagar (MP)-470 002 *Chief: Ramanbhai Patel* *Alternate: Ramashankar Dhagat*	Estd.: 1982 Tel.: 22478 25278	Agent : Daurala Sugar works New Delhi Bush Boake Allen (India) Ltd. Calcutta Arochem Industries Baroda
Saraiya Brothers 3101/1 Three Gates Ahmedabad-380 001 *Chief: B.K. Saraiya*	Estd.: 1938 Tel.: 5351561	Dealers : Perfumes, Essence Chemicals Agarbatties
Saraiya Ramlal Maganlal & Sons 3106, Three Gates Ahmedabad-380 001 *Chief: Jogen G. Saraiya* *Alternate: Gopal G. Saraiya*	Estd.: 1944 Tel.: 5351640	Dealers : Perfumery Compounds Flavours, Essential Oils
Shah Agency 1574/1 Kalupur Road Opp. Jain Upashray Ahmedabad-380 001 *Chief: Chandrakant Shah* *Alternate: Harshad R. Shah*	Estd.: 1978 Tel.: 337974 334695	Dealers : Agarbatti Tobacco Snuff. Perfume & Aromatic Chemicals
Varia Sunderji Virji Near Railway Crossing Main Road Surendranagar-363 001 *Chief: Chaitanya Vana* *Alternate: Suvidhi Vana*	Estd.: 1962 Tel.: Off.: 21524 31206 Fac.: 23142 25142	Manufacturers : Flavours, Fragrances Flavouring Emulsions Soft Drink Concentrates

Name & Address	*Phone/Fax Telex Nos.*	*Business Activities*
Varia Sunderji Virji & Co. Natakshala Road Jamnagar-361 001 *Chief: Arvind S. Varia*	Estd.: 1940 Tel.: Off.: 77277 551071 Fac.: 40311 Fax: 553121	Traders: Perfumery Compounds Aerated Water requisites Flavouring Essences and Edible Colours Manufactures : Carbondioxide
Vijay Industries E-4, Patel Industrial Estate Pratap Nagar Baroda-390 004 *Chief: Mahesh Nagrecha* *Alternate: Bhaumik Nagrecha*	Estd.: 1974 Tel.: Off.: 554439 Fac.: 460495	Manufacturers : Flavouring Essences Food Colours etc.
Vikalpa Rasayan P. Ltd. 3F, P.K. House Near M.J. L:ibrary, Ellisbridge Ahmedabad-380 006 *Chie: R.J. Gandhi* *Alternate: P.J. Gandhi*	Estd.: 1983 Tel.: 467157 467716	Dealers : Natural Essential Oils and Aromatic Chemicals
Vikram Enterprise 202, Classic Avenue 2nd Floor, Opp. Sales India Ashram Road Ahmedabad-380 009 *Chief: B.K. Patel* *Alternate: D.K. Patel*	Estd.: 1985 Tel.: 6569269 403745 Fax: 409562	Manufacturers : Diphenyl Oxide
Vin Flavors 1, Krishna Society Haribhakti Ext.Old Padra Road Baroda-390 015 *Chief: P.C. Vin*	Estd.: 1978 Tel.: Off.: 322048 fac.: 461496 Fax: 461936	Manufactures : Flavouring materials Food & Phamaceutical Companies
Wala & Company Nanbhawadi, Kalanala Bhavnagar-364 002 *Chief: Pratapsing M. Wala* *Alternate: Prakash P.Wala*	Estd.:1950 Tel.: 24628	Manufacturers : Perfumery Compounds

Name & Address	*Phone/Fax Telex Nos.*	*Business Activities*
Silversons 110, Narayan Chamber Nehru Bridge Corner Ashram Road Ahmedabad *Chief: D.K. Patel*	Estd.: 1993 Tel.: 4579314	Manufacturers : Di-Phenyl Oxide
A.L. Chaudhary & Co. 1, Waston Street Calcutta-700 013 *Chief: R.K. Chaudhary* *Alternate: M.M. Chaudhry*	Estd.: 1952 Tel.: 263989 271277	Agents : M/s. Daurala Sugar Works, New Delhi Dealers : Benzaldehyde, Benzyl Alcohol, Benzyl Benzoate Cinnamic Aldehyde etc.
B. Kamdar & Co. 1, Sun Yat Sen Street Calcutta-700 012 *Chief: B. Kamdar* *Alternate: Ilesh Kamdar*	Estd.: 1964 Tel.: 27-0643	Dealers : Fragrances, Flavours Natural & Synthetic Essential Oils
Basha Perfumery House 8, Ezra Street Calcutta-700 001 *Chief: Ismail Basha* *Alt: E.M. Khaja Kamal Basha*	Estd.: 1959 Tel.: 225-4347	Manufacturers : Perfumery Compounds Aromatic Chemicals Essential Oil cartons etc.
Bosco Laboratory 63, Radha Bazar Street Calcutta-700 001 *Chief: S.L. Bose* *Alternate: H.L. Bose*	Estd.: 1958 Tel.: Off.: 242-0186	Manufacturers : Raw Materials for Perfumery i.e. Synthetic Essential Oils & Perfumery Compounds
Breeze Fragrances 63, Ratan Sirkar Garden Street Calcutta-700 007 *Chief: Pradip Kumar Prasad*	Estd.: 1990 Tel.: 231-1348	Traders : Aromatic Chemicals & Perfumery Compounds Agents : Beeta Chemicals, Bombay Amish Aromatics Calcutta

Directory of Perfumes and Flavours–Manufacturers/
Distributors/Suppliers/Traders/Exporters/Importers

Name & Address	Phone/Fax Telex Nos.	Business Activities
C. Prabhudas & Co. 1, Bonfield Lane, 1st Floor Calcutta-700 001 *Chief: Anil Kumar Hemani* *Alternte: Manharlal Hemani*	Estd.: 1974 Tel.: Off.: 242-8091 2426315 Fac.: 25-6856 25-5636 Fax: 2423617	Manufacturers : Perfumery Compounds & Synthetic Ess. Oil
Calcutta Essence Supply Co. 41, Ezra Street Calcutta-700 001 *Chief: Kanubhai Kothan*	Estd.: 1951 Tel.: 254298	Dealers : Fragrances, Flavours and Perfumery Raw Materials
Chunilal Prabhudas & Co. (Calcutta) P. Ltd. 1, Bonfield Lane, 1st Floor Calcutta-700 001 *Chief: Viraj Hemani* *Alternate: Surendra R. Shah*	Estd.: 1930 Tel.: 242-8091 2426315 Fax: 2423617	Dealers : Aromatic Chemicals Perfumery Compounds Resinoids, Flavouring Essence, Food Colours etc.
D. Jayantilal & Company 33, B.R.B. Basu Road (Canning Street) Calcutta-700 001 *Chief: Lalit Kumar Shah* *Alternate: Mahendra Shah*	Estd.: 1950 Tel.: 2428167 2424282 Fax: 242-1960	Dealers : Essential Oils, Food Colours and Pharmaceutical Raw Materials
Dabur (Dr. S.K. Burman) P. Ltd. P.O. Narendrapur-743 508 Distt-24 Parganas West Bengal	Estd.: 1884 Tel.: 4779324 4779325	Manufacturers : Ayurvedic and Patent Medicines and Pharmaceuticals
Desai Chemical Co. Pvt. Ltd. 11, Ezra Street Calcutta-700 001 *Chief: Pratp H Desai* *Alternate: Jatin P. Desai*	Tel.: 247-9541 247-1759 Fax: 2479738 2407173	Dealers : Aromatic Chemicals Essential Oils Perfumery Compounds Fragrances & Flavours
Du Croco Fragrances (India) 23A, Netaji Subhas Road 5th Floor Calcutta-700 001 *Chief: Asit Baran Bhattacharya*	Estd.: 1972 Tel.: 2201121	Manufacturers : Perfumery Compounds

Name & Address	*Phone/Fax Telex Nos.*	*Business Activities*
East India Aromatic Traders 44, Ezra Street, 2nd Floor Calcutta-700 001 *Chief: Dhirajlal Kamdar* *Alternate: Bharat Kamdar*	Estd: 1965 Tel.: 256834 259511	Agents : for S.H. Kelkar & Co. Ltd., K.V. Arochem Ltd.
F.C. Aromatics 22, Rabindra Sarani Calcutta-700 073 *Chief: F.C. Dhingra* *Alternate: Satyen Dhingra*	Estd.: 1970 Tel.: 270845 272864	Manufacturers : Soap Compound Detergent Compound Agarbatti Compounds etc.
Fine O Chem Industries 13/D Palit Street Calcutta-700 019 *Chief: Vasant K. Shanghvi* *Alt.: Mahendra K. Shanghvi*	Estd.: 1972 Tel.: Off.: 4751250 Fac.: 3503692	Manufacturers : Cinnamic Aldehyde Cinnamic Alcohol Indole, Bromostyrol and Alpha Amyhl Cinnamic Aldehyde
Florasynth Armatics 44, Ezra Street Post Box No. 2066 Calcutta-700 001	Estd.: 1976 Tel.: 268011 262095 Tlx.: 021-5293 NAIK IN	Manufacturers : Industrial Perfumery Compounds and Synthetic Essential oils
Jamnadas & Brothers Pvt. Ltd. 1, Bonfield Lane, 1st Floor Calcutta-700 001 *Chief: Arun Khanderia* *Alternate: Ranjen Hemani*	Estd.: 1929 Tel.: 2426121 2426576 Fax.: 2433582	Indenting Agents : Dealing in Aromatic Chemicals Natural Ess. Oils and Perfumery Compounds
Jayesh & Company 8-C Suhasini Ganguli Lane Calcutta-700 025 *Chief: Jayesh Shah*	Estd.: 1976 Tel.: 483668	Dealers : Aromatic Chemicals Natural Ess. oils, Solvents, and Resinoids
K. Kar 32E, Jackson Lane Calcutta-700 001 *Chief: Nital Kar* *Alternate: S. Kar*	Estd.: 1939 Tel.: 2427839 Fax.: 2422573 Tlx.: 214080 KARK IN	Dealers : Aromatic Indgredients Distributors for Givaudan-Roure

Name & Address	*Phone/Fax Telex Nos.*	*Business Activities*
Keshavlal Khanderia & Co. 167, Old China Bazar Street Calcutta-700 001 *Chief: Shashikant Khanderia* *Alternate: Chhanda Kar*	Estd.: 1961 Tel.: 2422334	Agents : Distributors of Aromatic Chemicals Flavours, Food Colours and Perfumery Compounds
Lakshmi Bottle Stores 17, Ezra Street Post Box No. 450 Calcutta-700 001 *Chief: Vijay Sanganeria*	Estd.: 1940 Tel.: 253706	Dealers : Aromatic Chemicals Industrial Fragrances Essences, Colours and Commission Agents
Latin Flavourosynthesis Co. 161/1 Mahatma Gandhi Road 2nd Floor, Bangur Bldg. Calcutta-7000 007 *Chief: Sanjive Mehrotra* *Alternate: Kuldeep Mehrotra*	Estd.: 1986 Tel.: 2382243	Manufacturers : Essential Oils and Oriental Perfumes
Madan Lal Burnwal Munshi Bazar Asansol-713 301 (Burdwan) *Chief: Madanlal Burnwal*	Estd.: 1885 Tel.: 203455	Manufacturers : Perfumery Compounds
Makhuylal Ayodhya Prasad and Grandsons 4B, Madan Mohan Burman Street Calcutta-700 007 *Chief: Sanjeev Kumar Gupta* *Alternate: Harishu Chandra Gupta*	Estd.: 1976 Tel.: 2393340 2390447	Manufacturers : Indian Attars Perfumery Compounds Agents : Sanjeev Perfumery works
Mansukhlal & Brothers 1, Bonfield Lane 1st Floor Calcutta-700 001 *Chief: Manharlal Hemani* *Alternate: Pankaj Hemani*	Estd.: 1966 Tel.: 2428091 25-5636 25-6856 Fax.: 2423617	Dealers : Aromatic Chemicals Perfumery Compounds Resinoids, Flavouring Essence, Food Colours etc.

Name & Address	*Phone/Fax Telex Nos.*	*Business Activities*
Moolraj & Co. 33, Braboume Road 2nd Floor Calcutta-700 001 *Chief: Bharat Kumar Kampani*	Estd.: 1955 Tel.: 2426622 749457	Dealers : Aromatic Chemicals Natural Ess. Oils Resinoids etc.
Mukti Agencies (P) Ltd. 23A, Netaji Subhas Road 11th Floor Calcutta-700 001 *Chief: Ashim Kumar Das* *Alternate: Ashis Kumar Das*	Estd.: 1963 Tel.: 220-8595	Dealers : Aromatic Chemicals Perfumery Compounds Resinoids Agents : Industrial Perfumes Ltd. Bombay
N.H. Enterprises 82, Purani Godown Road Gaya-823 001 *Chief: Nurul Haque Khan*	Estd.: 1990 Tel.: 21765	Dealers : Aromatic Chemicals Perfumery Compounds Natural Ess. Oils Heavy Chemicals etc.
National Perfumery House 44, Ezra Street Post Box 328 Calcutta700 001 *Chief: Subhash K. Naik* *Alternate: Mrinal S. Naik*	Estd.: 1949 Tel.: 25-8144 25-5547 25--6426 Fax: 250617	Dealers : Aromatic Chemicals Natural Ess. Oils Resinoids, Industrial Perfumery Compounds
Neshat Perfumery House 21, Parsee Church Street Calcutta-700 001 *Chief: S.M. Asiam*	Estd.: 1940 Tel.: 25-4859 277985	Dealers : Industrial Perfumery Compounds, Flavours and allied-Products Essential Oils Aromatic Chemicals etc.
North Eastern Mercantiles Ltd. Jainarayan Road Fancy Bazar Gauhati-781 001 *Chief: S.K. Jain*	Tel.: 1986 Tel.: 545503 521613 Fax.: 522037 Tlx.: 0235-2291 GALVA IN	Dealers : Citronella Oil, Lemon Lemon Grass Oil Palma Rosa Oil etc.

Name & Address	*Phone/Fax Telex Nos.*	*Business Activities*
O.T. Kader Basha Sahib 17, Ezra Street Calcutta-700 001 *Chief: Saleem* *Alternate: Basha*	Estd.: 1930 Tel.: 257970 Fax: 2254402	Dealers : Aromatic Chemicals Perfumery Compounds Essential Oils etc.
Orient Perfumery House 7, Parsee Church Street Calcutta-700 001 *Chief: Nawab Mushtaque Ahmed*	Estd.: 1961 Tel.: 259594 Fax: 266863	Dealers : Perfumery Raw Materials
Paul & Son 18 Ezra Street G.P.O. Box No. 902 Calcutta-700 001 *Chief: G.P. Jhunjhunwalla* *Alternate: Anadn Jhunjhunwaalla*	Estd.: 1946 Tel.: 253023 2250234 Fax: 2259832	Dealers : Aromatic Chemicals Natural & Synthetic Essential Oils, Resinoids, Fragrance & Flavours
Quality Perfumery Centre 5/5 Clive Row, 5th Floor Calcutta-700 001	Estd.: 1972 Tel.: 2209057 Fax: 2429834	Dealers : Agarbathi Materials and Soap Compounds
Raj Aromatics 14/2 Old China Bazar Street 3rd Floor, Room No. 193 Calcutta-700 001 *Chief: Nikesh Sheth* *Alternate: Ajay Sheth*	Estd.: 1966 Tel.: 2423606 2422564 Fax: 2421615	Manufacturers : Perfumery Compounds for Agarbathies Cosmetics, Soaps and Toiletnes
Reprocess 103B, Dhan Devi Khanna Road Calcutta-700 054 *Chief: J.P. Sarkar*	Estd.: 1987 Tel.: 346314 34-7278	Traders : Industrial Perfumes
Royson 34, Chitaranjan Avenue 2nd Floor, Room No. 4 Calcutta-700 012 *Chief: A.M. Roy*	Estd.: 1986 Tel.: 27-7546 27-4858 Fax: 2252434	Manufacturers : Petroleum Jelly Agarbathi Oil Cosmetic Oil White Oil L.L.P.
S.D. Bose 63, Radha Bazar Street Calcutta-700 001 *Chief: S.L. Bose* *Alternate: H.L. Bose*	Estd.: 1946 Tel.: Off.: 2422110 2420186 Fac.: 74-2987	Manufacturers : Raw Materials for perfumery & Blended Perfumery Compounds

Name & Address	*Phone/Fax Telex Nos.*	*Business Activities*
Seth Brothers (Perfumers) Pvt. Ltd. 11, Rabindra Sarani 1st Floor Calcutta-700 073 *Chief: A.K. Shukla* *Alternate: R.P. Shukla*	Estd.: 1949 Tel.: 225-0792	Manufacturers : Industrial Fragrance & Flavours, Essential Oils etc.
Soni Aromatics 70 Canning Street Calcutta-700 001 matic *Chief: Pravin Soni* *Alternate: Haresh Soni*	Estd.: 1990 Tel.: 258580 258931	Manufacturers : Perfumery Compounds and Dealing in Aro- Chemicals, Natural Essential Oils Rosinoids etc.
Swastik Industries 32, Ezra Street Room No. 321 & 322 3rd Floor Calcutta-700 001 *Chief: Chandrakant Kothan* *Alternate: Rishabh Kothari*	Estd.: 1977 Tel.: 25-0306 250207 Fax: 25-0207	Manufacturers : Industrial Perfumery Compounds
Synthodor Company Meghdoot Garden Udairajpur Madhyamgram, 24 Parganas (N) Pin-743 275 WB *Chief: Susanta Kar*	Estd.: 1966 Tel.: 5523218 Fax: 5524121	Manufacturers : Syntjhetic Ess. Oils Mixture of Odoriferous Substances
Synthroma Laboratories 3A Pollock Street 1st Floor, Unit 30 & 31 Calcutta-700 001 *Chief: V.r. Shah* *Alternate: Dhimant Mehta*	Estd.: 1987 Tel.: 261411 257226 258459 Fac.: 665-3858 Fax: 258618	Manufacturers : Aromatic Chemicals & Essential Oils
Tulsi Fragrances 17, Ezra Street G.P.O. Box 2491 Calcutta-700 001 *Chief: V.N. Jhunjhunwalla*	Estd.: 1989 Tel.: Off.: 25-2939 256098 Fac.: 40-9442 Fax: 40-9599	Manufacturers : Fragrances

16

Manufacturers of Standardized Herbal Extracts, Phytochemicals and Essential Oils in India

S.No.	Name of Address	Main Products
1.	Amsar Private Limited 47, Laxmibai Nagar Indl. Estate	Extract Phytochemicals Fort, Indore452006 Essential Oils
2.	Ansar Drugs Laboratories Salabbatpura Moti Begumwadi Surat395002	Extracts
3.	Alchem International Pvt. Ltd. 240, Jhandewalan Extension New Delhi110055	Phytochemicals
4.	Alembic Chemical Works Baroda	Extracts
5.	Alkaloids Corpn. 8, Bentick Street Calcutta-700001	Phytochemicals
6.	Auro Impex Pvt. Ltd. 8, C14 936, Dehgam Road Industries Township Vapi-396195	Phytochemicals
7.	Bengal Chemicals & Pharmaceuticals Ltd. 153, Dharmatala Street Calcutta700013	Extracts
8.	Biological Evans Ltd. C-1-4936, Dehgam Road Industies Township Vapi--396195	Phytochemicals
9.	Bengal Chemicals & Pharmaceuticals Ltd. 164, Maniktala Main Road Calcutta-700054	Extracts

10.	Bhavnagar Oil & Chemicals Industries Pvt. Ltd. 141, Dalamal Tower Nariman Point Mumbai-400021	Castor Oil
11.	Bicon India Pvt. Ltd. 20th K.M. Hosour Road Hebbagodi562158 Bangalore Distt.	Papain
12.	Bombay Extractions Pvt. Ltd. Daya Mandir, 1st Floor 123-25, Mumbadevi Road Mumbai-400003	Castor Oil
13.	Chemical, Industrial & Pharmaceuticals Laboratories Ltd. Vikhorli Mumbai400079	Phytochemicals
14.	CIPLA Research Centre & Factory Vigonagar P & T Office Bangalore	Phytochemicals
15.	CIBA–Giegy of India Ltd. Bhandup Mumbai-400078	Phytochemicals
16.	Central Institute of Medicinal & Aromatic Plants Post Bag No. 1 Ram Sagar Misra Nagar Lucknow--226016	Essential Oils
17.	Chemiloids 4045, 10B, Brindavan Colony Labbipet Vijayawada510010	Extracts Phytochemicals Essential Oils
18.	Drug Research Laboratory (Farm and Factories J&K) Jammu-Tawi-180001	Extracts Phytochemicals
19.	Enzo Chem. Laboratories Pvt. Ltd. Ybola-423401 Maharashtra	Papain
20.	Govt. Opium and Alkaloid Works Ghazipur (UP)	Opium Alkaloids
21.	Govt. Quinine Factory Mungpoo	Quinine Salts

22.	Govt. Quinine Factory Anamallais, Tamil Nadu	Quinine Salts
23.	Glaxo Laboratories (P) Ltd. Dr. Annie besant Road Worli, Mumbai-400018	Phytochemicals
24.	Herbochem 38, Technocrats Idustrial Estate Balanagar, Hyderabad-500037	Extracts
25.	Indo German Alkoloids Mahakali Caves Road Andheri (East), Mumbai-400093	Phytochemicals
26.	Jayant Oil Mills 13, Sitalwadi, Mazgaon, Mumbai	Castor Oil
27.	Kothari Phytochemicals International 766, Anna Nagar Madurai625020	Phytochemicals
28.	Kisalaya Pharmaceuticals Pvt. Ltd. Plot No. 548, Secotor-III Industrial Area, Pithampur Distt. Dhar (M.P.)	Tannic Acid
29.	Kulu Aromatics Shamshi175126 Distt. Kullu (HP)	Essential Oils
30.	Kumaon Chemical Products Village Shivalalpur P.O. Ramnagar-244715 Nainital	Pytochemicals Ginger Oil
31.	Liberty Oil Mills Pvt. Ltd. 302, Dalamal House 206, Nariman Point Mumbai-400021	Castor Oil
32.	Mehta Pharmaceuticals Pvt. Ltd. G.T. Road, Chheharta Amritsar-143105	Brucine Sulphate N.F. Berberine Hydro- chloride Podophyllum Resin BP/USP Santonin I.P./J.P. Strychnine Calcium sennosides A+B Xanthotoxin (USP) Mathoxsalen Valerian Extract Herbal Extract

33.	New India Agro Chemical Industries 4013, Yawai Road, Bhusawal	Phytochemicals
34.	Organokem Laboratories Near Janata Vidyalaya Yeola Distt., Nasik	Phytochemicals
35.	Polybond Chemicals 4, Bhaktinagar Station Plot Rajkot-360002	Papain
36.	Rathi Papains Pvt. Ltd. 75-76-A Mittal Court Nariman Point, Bombay-400021	Papain
37.	Regional Research Laboratory Jammu Tawi	Phytochemicals Essential Oils
38.	Sandoz India Ltd. Sandoz House, Dr. A.B. Road Worli, Mumbai-400018	Phytochemicals
39.	Smith Stanistreet Pharmaceuticals Ltd. 18, Convent Road Calcutta-700014	Phytochemicals
40.	Shashi Phytochemicals Industry 1, Old Industrial Area, Alwar	Phytochemicals
41.	Sheeba Laboratories Pvt. Ltd. B-151, Avas Vikas Colony Delhi Road, Saharanpur-247001	Phytochemicals
42.	Standard Essential Oil Distillers 84/113, Carvalongar Kanpur-208003	Essential Oils
43.	True Food Corporation 17, Kamer Building 38, Cawaji Patel Street Mumbai-400 023	Papain
44.	Uma Ayurved Bhawan Pvt. Ltd. Kasganj-207123 (UP)	Kupipakva Rasayans Parpati Bhasma & Pishtees Kharaliya Rasayan & Gutika Guggul Loh & Mandur Others

17

Ayurvedic Colleges in India

S.No.	Name of Address	Courses Offered
1.	ALN Rao Memorial Ayurved Medical College, Koppa-577126 Distt. Chickmagalore (Karnataka)	Under Graduate
2.	Anantha Laxmi Govt. Ayurved College Station Road WArangal-506002 (AP)	Under Graduate
3.	Aryakanya Shuddha Ayurved Mahavidyalaya, Kareli Bagh Vadodara-390018 (Gujarat)	Under Graduate
4.	Ashtang Ayurved Mahavidyalaya 2062, Sadashiv Peth Vijayanagar Colony Pune-411030 (Maharashtra)	Under Graduate & Post Graduate
5.	AV Samiti's Ayurved Maha Vidaylaya Bijapur586101 (Karnataka)	Under Graduate & Post Graduate
6.	Ayurved Mahavidyalaya Gaya-823991 (Bihar)	Under Graduate
7.	Ayurved & Unani Tibbia College Ajmal Khan Road, Karol Bagh New Delhi-1100055	Under Graduate
8	Ayurved Mahavidyalaya Heggerio Extension Old Hubli-580024 (Karnataka)	Under Graduate
9.	Ayurved Mahavidyalaya Near Sion Railway Station Sion Mumbai-400022 (Maharashtra)	Under Graduate & Post Graduate
10.	Ayurved Mahavidyalaya Ganeshwadi, Panchavati Nasik-422003 (Maharashtra)	Under Graduate & Post Graduate

11.	Ayurved Mahavidyalaya (Shri Shivaji Nagar) Tal, Rahuri, Rahuri Factory413796 Distt. Ahmednagar (Maharashtra)	Under Graduate
12.	Ayurved College Pathanjali Puri, Thadgam (via) Coimbatore-641108 (Tamil Nadu)	Under Graduate
13.	Bundelkhand Govt. Ayurved College Jhansi-294001 (Uttar Pradesh)	Under Graduate
14.	Chaitanya Ayurved Mahavidyalaya Sakegaon Bhausawal-425201 (Maharashtra)	Under Graduate
15.	Dayanand Ayurved Medical College & Hospital Siwan-841221 (Bihar)	Under Graduate
16.	Dayanand Ayurved College Mahatma Hansraj Marg Jalandhar City-144088 (Punjab)	Under Graduate
17.	DMM Ayurved Mahavidyalaya Aarni Road, Shivaji Nagar Yeotmal-445001 (Maharashtra)	Under Graduate & Post Graduate
18.	Dr. BRKR Govt. Ayurvedic College S.R. Nagar, Erragadda Hyderabad-500038 (A.P.)	Under Graduate & Post Graduate
19.	Dr. NR Sastry Govt. Ayurved College Bandar Road Vijayawada-520002 (A.P.)	Under Graduate
20.	Ganga Educational Society's Ayurved Medical College Kolhapur-416012 (Maharashtra)	
21.	Gaur Brahaman Ayurved College Rohtak-124001 (Haryana)	Under Graduate
22.	Gopabandhu Ayurved Mahavidyalaya Puri-752002 (Orissa)	Under Graduate & Post Graduate
23.	Govt. Ayurved College Herbala Road, Ulubari Guwahati-781001 (Assam)	Under Graduate
24.	Govt. Ayurved College Kadam Kuan Patna-800003 (Bihar)	Under Graduate & Post Graduate

25.	Government Dharam Samaj Sanskrit Mahavidyalaya Muzaffarpur (Bihar)	Under Graduate
26.	Govt. Akhandanand Ayurved College Opp. Victoria Garden Bhadra Ahmedabad-380001 (Gujarat)	Under Graduate & Post Graduate
27.	Govt. Ayurved College Ajwa Road Baroda-390001 (Gujarat)	Under Graduate
28.	Govt. Ayurved College Sadar Bagh Junagarh-362001 (Gujarat)	Under Graudate
29.	Govt. College of Indian Medicine & Hospital Vishweshwariah Circle Sayu Rao Road Mysore-570021 (Karnataka).	Under Graduate & Post Graduate
30.	Govt. College of Indian Medicine Dhanvantari Road Bangalore-560009 (Karnataka)	Under Graduate & Post Graduate
31.	Govt. Taranath Ayurved College Anantapur Road Bellary-583101 (Karnataka)	Under Graduate
32.	Govt. Ayurveda College Dhanwantari Nagar Tripunithura-682301 Distt. Ernakulam (Kerala)	Under Graduate
33.	Govt. Ayurveda College MG Road Thiruvananthapuram-695001 (Kerala)	Under Graduate & Post Graduate
34.	Govt. Ayurvedic College Raipur-492001 (MP)	Under Graduate & Post Graduate
35.	Govt. Ayurvedic College Gwalior-473001 (MP)	Under Graduate & Post Graduate
36.	Govt. Ayurvedic College Gorakhpur Jabalpur-482001 (MP)	Under Graduate
37.	Govt. Dhanwantri Ayurved College Mangalnath Road Ujjain-456001 (MP)	Under Graduate

38.	Govt. Ashtang Ayurved Mahavidyalaya & Hospital Lok Manya Nagar Indore-420009 (M.P.)	Under Graduate
39.	Govt. Ayurved College Rewa486001 (MP)	Under Graduate
40.	Govt. Ayurved College Wazirabad Nanded431601 (Maharashtra)	Under Graduate & Post Graduate
41.	Govt. Ayurvedic College Tuijapur Road, Madhban Osmanabad-413501 (Maharashtra)	Under Graduate
42.	Govt. Ayurved Mahavidyalaya Raje Raghuji Nagar Nagapur440001 (Maharashtra)	Under Graduate & Post Graduate
43.	Govt. Ayurved College & Hospital Balangir-76701 (Orissa)	Under Graduate
44.	Govt. Ayurved College Patiala--147001 (Punjab)	Under Graduate & Post Graduate
45.	Govt. Rishikul Ayurved College Haridwar-249401 (Uttar Pradesh)	Under Graduate Post Graduate
46.	Govt. Gurukul Ayurved College Gurkul Kangari Haridwar-249401 (UP)	Under Graduate
47.	Govt. Ayurved College Atarra-210201 Distt. Banda (Uttar Pradesh)	Under Graduate
48.	Hanuman Shikshan Prasark Mandal's Ayurved Mahavidyalaya Peth Vadagaon, Tq. Hatkanacgala Distt. Kolhapur (Maharashtra)	Under Graduate
49.	J.S. Ayurved Mahavidyalaya College Road Nadiad-387001 (Gujarat)	Under Graduate
50.	Karmavir Vyankatrao Tanaji Randhir Ayurved College Boradi-401701 Tal. Shirpur (Maharashtra)	Under Graduater
51.	Karnataka Liberal Education Society Shri BM Kankanwadi Ayurved Mahavidyalaya, Shajapur Belgaum-590003 (Karnataka)	Under Graduate

52.	Kaviraj Ananta Tripathy Sarma Ayurved College Ankushpur-761100, Ganjam (Orissa)	Under Graduate
53.	Lal Bahadur Shastri Govt. Ayurved Mahavidyalaya Handia-221503 (Allahabad) (Uttar Pradesh)	Under Graduate
54.	Maharashtra Arogya Mandal Hadapsar-411028 Pune (Maharashtra)	Under Graduate
55.	M.M.M. Govt. Ayurved Mahavidyalaya Udaipur-313001 (Rajasthan)	Under Graduate & Post Graduate
56.	Mohta Ayurved Mahavidyalaya Sadulpur-331023 Distt. Churu (Rajasthan)	Under Graduate
57.	National Institute of Ayurved Madhav Vilas Palace, Amer Road Jaipur-302002 (Rajasthan)	Under Graduate & Post Graduate
58.	Nitishwar Bhartiya Chikitsha Vigyan Sansthan & Hospital Mukherjee Seminar Campus Harisabha Chowk, Ramna Muzaffarpur-842002 (Bihar)	Under Graduate
59.	Parsurampuriya Ayurved College Sikar-332001 (Rajasthan)	Under Graduate
60.	PBN Institute of Indian Medical Sciences Ranti Road Madhubani-847211 (Bihar)	Under Graduate
61.	RA Podar Medical College (Ayurved) Worli, Mumbai-400018 (Maharashtra)	Under Graduate & Post Graduate
62.	Rajkiya Ayurved Mahavidalaya Paprola176115 Distt. Kangar (HP)	Under Graduate
63.	Rajkiya Ayodhya Shivkumari Ayurved Mahavidayala Begusarai-850101 (Bihar)	Under Graduate
64.	Rajkiya Lalit Hari Ayurved College Pilibhit-262001 (Uttar Pradesh)	Under Graduate & Post Graduate
65.	Rajkiya Maharani Rameshwari Bhatriya Chikitsa Vigyan Sansthan Mohanpur-846007 (Darbhang) (Bihar)	Under Graduate

66.	Ravindernath Mukherji Ayurved Mahavidyalaya Distt. Champaran Motihari-845401 (Bihar)	Under Graduate
67.	Sangam Sewabhavi Trust's Ayurved Mahavidyalaya S/o Sanjivan Hospital Nasik Poona Road Sangamner-422605 (Maharashtra)	Under Graduate
68.	Seth Chandanmal Mutha Aryangla Vaidyak Mahavidyalaya Cendamal Satara-415001 (Maharashtra)	Under Graduate & Post Graduate
69.	Seth Govindji Raoji Ayurved Mahavidyalaya 21/A/13, Budhwar Peth Samarat Chowk Sholapur-413002 (Maharashtra)	Under Graduate
70.	Seth JP Govt. Ayurved Mahavidyalaya Opp. Sardar Bagh Bhadra Bhavnagar--3640o01 (Gujarat)	Under Graduate
71.	Sh. DM College of Ayurveda Udupi-576101 (karnataka)	Under Graduate
72.	Sh. Gangadhar Shasti Gune Ayurved Vishrambag Ahmednagar-414001 (Maharashtra)	Under Graduate
73.	Shri Ayurved Mahavidyalaya Dhanwantri Marg, Hanuman Nagar Nagpur-440009 (Maharashtra)	Under Graduate & Post Graduate
74.	Shri Balahanuman Ayurved Mahavidyalaya At & Post Lodhra--382835 Distt. Mehsana (North Gujarat)	Under Gradaute
75.	Shri Bhanwar Lal Dugar Ayurved Vishwabharati (Gandhi Vidya Mandir Sardar Shehar--331403 Distt. Churu (Rajasthan)	Under Graduate
76.	Shri Dhanwantry Ayurved College & Pandit Kedarnath Memorial Ayurved Hospital, Secto 46-B Chandigarh-160017 (Punjab)	Under Grduate

77.	Shri Dhanwantri Ayurved Mahavidyalaya Ahiroli, Buxar Bhojpur-802101	Under Graduate
78.	Shri Gulab Kunverba Ayurved Mahavidyalaya Dhanwantri Mandir Jamnagar-361008 (Gujarat)	Under Graduate
79.	Shri Gurudev Ayurved Mahavidyalaya Gurukunj Ashram (Mozari) Amrawati-444601 (Maharashtra)	Under Graduate & Post Graduate
80.	Shri Krishna Govt. Ayurved College Kurukshetra-132118 (Haryana)	Under Graduate
81.	Shri Laxminarayan Ayurved College Sant Tulsidas Marg Amritsar-143001 (Punjab)	Under Graduate
82.	Shri Maru Singh Memorial Mahila Ayurved Degree College Kanya Gurukul Khanpur Kalan-124301 (Sonepat) Haryana	Under Graduate
83.	Shri Mastnath Ayurved College Ashal Bohar Rohtak124001 (Haryana)	Under Graduate
84.	Shri Moti Singh jageshwari Ayurved Mahavidyalaya Chhapra-841301 (Bihar)	Under Gradaute
85.	Shri Nursinghanath Ayurved College & Research Institute Nrisinghnath P.O., Paikmal Distt. SDmbalpur-768029 (Orissa)	Under Graduate
86.	Shri OH Nazar Ayurved College Near Railway Station Shri Swami Atmanand Saraswati Road Surat-395003 (Gujarat)	Under Graduate
87.	Shri Radha Krishna Toshniwal Ayurved Mahavidyalaya Station Road Akola-444001 (Maharashtra)	Under Graduate & Post Graduate
88.	Shri Venkataramana Ayurved College 144, Kutchery Road, Mylapore Madras-600004 (Tamilnadu)	Under Graduate

89.	Smt. KG Mittal Punarvasu Ayurved College Netaji Subash Road Mumbai-400002 (Maharashtra)	Under Graduate & Post Graduate
90.	Sri Yastindra Narayan Ashtang Bhagalpur-812006 (Bihar)	Under Graduate
91.	SRM Govt. Ayurved College Baeilly-243001 (Uttar Pradesh)	Under Graduate
92.	S.S.M.D. Ayurved College & Hospital G.T. Road Moga-142001 (Punjab)	Under Graduate
93.	State Ayurved College Tulsidas Marg Lucknow--226004 (UP)	Under Graduate & Post Graduate
94.	S.V. Ayuved College T.T. Devasthanams Tirupati-517501 (AP)	Uder Graduage
95.	Swami Kalyandev Govt. Ayurved College Rampur Muzaffar Nagar (UP)	Under Graduate
96.	Swami Raghavandracharya Ayurved Mahavidyalaya Karjara Station P.O., Manjholi Gaya-823001 (Bihar)	Under Graduate
97.	Tilak Ayurved Mahavidyalaya 583/2, Rasta Peth Pune-411011 (Mahrashtra)	Under Graduate & Post Graduate
98.	Vaidyaratnam Ayurveda College Ollur-Thikkattussery Tirchur-680322 (Kerala)	Under Graduate
99.	Vasant Dada Patil Ayurved Medical College South Shivaji Nagar Sangli-416416 (Maharashtra)	Under Graduate
100.	Vasant Kusum's Rural Yog & Ayurved Sandhodhan Paratishthanam's Sidh Kalan Ayurved Mahavidyalaya Nehru Chowk Sangamner-422605 Distt. Ahmednagar (Maharashtra)	Under Graduate

101.	Vidarbha Ayurved Mahavidyalaya Hanuman Nagar Amrawati-444605 (Maharashtra)	Under Graduate & Post Graduate
102.	VPS Varier Ayurveda College Kottakkal, Edarikode P.O.-676501 Malappuram Distt. (Kerala)	Under Graduate
103.	Yashwant Shikshan Prasark Mandal's Sri Yashwant Ayurved College At & Post Kdeali-416114 Tal. Panhala Distt. Kohapur (Maharashtra)	Under Graduate
104.	Verala Medical Trust & Research Centre's Ayurved Medical College Mumbai-400012 (Maharashtra)	Under Graduate

18

Institute of Unani Medicine

1. Central Research Institute of Unani Medicine
   Opposite E.S.I. Hospital
   A.G. Colony Road, Erragadda
   Hyderabad-500838 (Andhra Pradesh)
2. Regional Research Institute of Unani Medicine
   1, West Mada Church Street, Royapuram
   Chennai-600001 (Tamil Nadu)
3. Regional Research Institute of Unani Medicine
   Bhadrak-756100 (Orissa)
4. Regional Research Institute of Unani Medicine
   Nawab Manzil, Guzri
   Patna-800008 (Bihar)
5. Regional Research Institute of Unani Medicine
   163-164, Terhi Pulia, Kursi Road
   P.O. Batha Saboli, Aliganj
   Lucknow226997 (Uttar Pradesh)
6. Regional Research Institute of Unani Medicine
   A.K. Tibbiya College Hospital (New Block)
   Al;igarh Mulsim University
   Aligarh-202002 (Uttar Pradesh)
7. Regional Research Institute of Unani Medicine
   J.J. Hospital Compound
   behind Eye Bank, Byculla
   Mumbai-400008 (Maharashtra)
8. Regional Research Institute of Unani Medicine
   University of Kashmir, Hazrat Bal
   Srinagar-190006 (Jammu & Kashmir)
9. Regional Research Institute of Unani Medicine
   79-B, 1st Floor, Chittaranjan Avenue
   Calcutta-700073 (West Bengal)
10. Clinical Research Unit
    Ayurvedic & Unani Tibbiya College
    Karol Bagh, New Delhi-110005

11. Clinical Research Unit
Community Centre, Neb Sarai
P.O. Mehrauli
New Delhi--110068
12. Clinical Research Unit
Unani Medical College
Himmat Ganj
Allahabad-211016 (Uttar Pradesh)
13. Clinical Research Unit
Civil Hospital, Masjid Road
Krimganj-788710 (Assam)
14. Clinical Research Unit
40-23, Park Road
Kurnool-518001 (Andhra Pradesh)
15. Clinical Research Unit
Sri Jayachamarajender Institute of Indian Medicine
Bangalore-560009 9Karnataka)
16. Clinical Research Unit
Department of Pharmacology
Gandhi Medical College
Bhopal-462001 (Madhya Pradesh)
17. Clinical Research Unit
368, Kothi Atanas, Meerut-250002 (Uttar Pradesh)
18. Clinical Research Unit
Kurupatil Nina Memorial MEs Orphanage
Edathala-683564
Distt. Alwaye (Kerala)
19. Clinical Research Unit
S.H. Unani Tibbiya College
Ganpati Naka
Burhanpur-450331 (Madhya Pradesh)
20. Clinical Research Unit
Unani Medical College & Hospital
Anglo-Urdu School Campus
New Modi Khana, K.B. HIdayatullah Road
Pune-411001 (Maharashtra)
21. Drug Standardisation Research Unit
Jamia Hamdard, Hamdard Nagar
New Delhi-1100062
22. Drug Standardisation Research Unit
Regional Research Institute of Unani Medicine
163-164, Terhi Pulia, Kursi Road
P.O. Batha Saboli, Aliganj
Lucknow-226007 (Uttar Pradesh)

23. Drug Standardisation Research Unit
Department of Chemistry, New College
P.B. NO. 684, P.Ol Rayapatta, 87 Peters Road
Chennai-600014 (Tamil Nadu)
24. Drug Standardisation Research Unit
Central Research Institute of Unani Medicine
Opposite E.S.I. Hospital
AG Colony Road, Erragadda
Hyderabad--500838 (Andrha Pradesh)
25. Drug Standardisation Research Unit
Department of Chemistry, Central College
Bangalore-560001 (Karnataka)
26. Chemical Research Unit
Department of Research in Unani Medicine
Near Office of Dean, Faculty of Science
Aligarh Mulsim University
Aligarh-202002 (Uttar Pradesh)
27. Central Herb Garden & Museum
Regional Research Insitute of Unani Medicine
163-164, Terhi Pulia
Kursi Road, P.O. Batha Sboli, Aliganj
Lucknow-226007 (Uttar Pradesh)
28. Literary Research Institute of Unani Medicine
Jamia Hamdard, Hamdard Nagar
New Delhi-110062
29. Family Welfare Research Unit
Government Nizamiah Tibbiya College
Hydrabad-500 002 (Andhra Pradesh)
30. Family Welfare Research Unit
Regional Research Institute of Unani Medicine
J.J. Hospital Compound
Behind Eye Bank, Byculla
Mumbai-400008 (Maharashtra)
31. Pilot Project on Clinical Research
222, Kaila Road, Near Junir High School
Ghaziabad (Uttar Pradesh)
32. Information Centre
Central Council for Research in Unani Medicine
61-65, Istitutional Area
Pankha Road, Janakpuri
New Delhi-110058

19

Colleges of Unani Medicine in India

Name of Address of the College	*Affiliated to*
Andhra Pradesh	
1. Government Nizamiah Tibbi College Charminar, Hyderabad-500001	Andhra Pradesh University of Health Sciences, Vijayawada
2. Dr. Abdul Hq Unani Medical College & Hospital Park Road, Kurnool-518001	-do-
Bihar	
3. Unani Medical College and Hopsital Muzaffarpur Kadam Kuan, Patna-800003	Bihar University
4. Zalfequar Haider Unani Medical College & Hospital P.O Box No. 12, Nawalpur Siwan-841226	-do--
5. Salfia Unani Medical College laheria Saria, Darbhanga-846001	-do-
6. Nizamia Unani Medical College & Hospital Bari Raod, Gaya-823001	-do-
Delhi	
7. Hamdard Tibbia College Hamdard Nagar New Delhi-110062	Jamia Hamdard, New Delhi
8. Ayurvedic and Unani Tibbia College Karol Bagh, New Delhi-110005	University of Delhi, Delhi

Karnatakla

9.	Goverment Unani Medical College No. 26, 1st Floor, Indian Red Cross Society Building Mahadeva Nagar, Race Course Road Bangalore-560039	Bangalore University Bangalore

Madhya Pradesh

10.	Saifia Hamidia Unani Tibbia College Burhanpur-450331 Distt Khandwa	Hari Singh Gaur Vishwavidyalya, Sagar

Maharashtra

11.	A.K.I. Tibbia College and Hospital Nagpad, Hasrat Mohani Chowk Mumbai-400001	Bombay University, Mumbai
12.	Mohammedia Tibbia College and Assayer Hospital P.O. Box No. 128, Mansoora Malegaon--423203, Distt. Nasik	Poona University, Pune
13.	Unani Medical College & Hospital Ango-Urdu School Campus New Modi Khana K.B. Hidayatullah Road Pune-411001	-do-
14.	Taj Tibbia College Jamia Arabias, Rasheed Nagar Nagpur-440002	Nagpur University, Nagpur
15.	Unani Medical College and Hospital Gulshan-e-Masoom Azam Colony Dargah Road, Parbhani-431401	Dr. Babasaheb Ambedkar University Aurangabad

Rajasthan

16.	Rajputana Unani Tibbia College Khander ka Rasta, Near Char Darwaza Jaipur-302002	University of Rajasthan Jaipur
17.	Rajasthan Unan Tibbia College 11/4636, Handipura chawkri Ram Chandra ji Jaipur-302002	-do-

Tamil Nadu

18.	Government Unani Medical College Arignar Anna Government Hospital of Indian Medicine Chennai-600106	Dr. MGR Medical University, Chennai

Uttar Pradesh

19.	Ajmal Khan Tibbia College Aligarh University Aligarh-202002	Aligarh Muslim University, Aligarh
20.	Takmil ut-Tibb College Jhawai Tola, Hakim Abdul Aziz Road Lucknow-226003	Kanpur University
21.	Unani Medical College Himmatganj, Allahabad-211001	-do-
22.	Jamia Tibbia, Deoband-247554 Distt. Sahranpur	Affiliation in process
23.	Deoband Unani Medical College Naya Bans, Near Talhavi Chungi Deoband-247554 Distt. Saharanpur	-do-
24.	Ibn-e-Sina Tibbia College Binapara, Distt. Azamgarh	-do-

West Bengal

25.	Calcutta Unani Medical College Maulvi Abdul Haleem Lane Calcutta-700016	-do-

20

World Importers of Natural Medicines

BELGIUM

PARC Scientifique
Rue Du Bosquet 7
B-1348 Louvain-La-Neuve, Balgium
Tel.: 0032-10-455.257
Fax: 0032-10456.076 or 454.934

Codidex Pharma S.P.R.L.
Rue Josse Impens
1030 Brussels, Belgium
Telephone: (32) (02) 2415324
Fax: 21662933

Du Pont De Nemours (Belgium)
100, Rue De La Fusee, B-1130
Bruxelles, Belgium
Telephone: (32) 2724 2611
Telex: 62788, Fax: (32) 7210460

Hybritech Europe S.A.
12, All. Des Noisetierrs, S.A.
B-4900 Angleur, Belgium
Telephone: (32) 416770000
Telex: 42208, Fax: (32) 676210

Sofarex N.V.
Van Varenberghstraat 49
B-2600 Berchem

Introplant Tropenpflanzen
Trottstrasse 16, D-3500 Kassel, Germany
Telephone: (49) (0561) 300001-3
Telex: 992511 Breks

Pfannenschmidt
P.O. Box 20224, D-2000
Hamburg 54, Germany
Antwerp, Belgium
Telephone: (32) 32189032
Telex: 71710, Fax: (32) 2189955

Somejant Sa
Rue De Boetendael 147
B-1180 Bruxelles, Belgium
Fax: (32) 23453806

Thissen S.A. Laboratories
4-6, Rue e La Papyree
B1420 Briane L'aleud, Belgium
Telephone: (32) 23861211
Telex: 61254, Fax: (32) 3851782

FRANCE

Docks Des Alcools SA
57 Rue De Villiers, F-9200
Neuilly Sur Seine, France
Telephone: (33) 147572420
Telex: 620048 F

GERMANY

Homviora Arznei Hagedorn Gmbh
Arabellastrasse 5, D-8000
Munchen 81, Germany
Telephone: (49) (089) 92322800

POLAND

Rolimpex, P.O. Box 364
PL-00950 Warszawa, Poland
Telephone: (48) 301000/300636
Telex: 814341 RLX PL
Fax: (48) 301867
Telephone: (49) 0405531057
Fax: (49) 0405536414

Verhaelen GMBH
Muelheimmer Str. 176, W-4100
Duisburg 1, Germany
Telephone: (49) 0203355005
Fax: (49) 0203355006

GREECE

Vioergex, V. Salateas Sons Ltd.
35 Deligiorgi St., GR-10437
Athens, Greece
Telephone: 30/1/5237484, 524271
Telex: 219482

ITALY

Ely Lilly Italia SPA
Via Gramsci, 733
I-50019 Sesto Florentino (Fi), Italy
Telephone: (39) 55421130

Istituto Gentili SPA
Via Mazzini, 11
I-56100 Pisa, Italy
Telephone: (39) 50501980

Sclavo SPA
Via Fiorentina, 1
I-53100 Siena, Italy
Telephone: (39) 577293111

Laboratio de applicationes
Calle Lope de ruedo 46
E30220 Madrid Spain
Telephone: (34) (1) 57440342
Fax: (34) (1) 5736537

SWEDEN

Kemila-Preparat AB, Box 609
S-19126 Solentuna, Sweden
Telephone: (46) 08359040
Telex: 15396 KEMILABS
Fax: (46) 08250545

PORTUGAL

Aquario Commercio De Electonica
Rua de Alegria 93-A
4000 Porto Portugal
Telephone: 02323381, 318817
Telex: 2082746
Fax: 02-2001379

RUSSIA

Medexport, Import Dept.
31, Korp., 2, UI Kakhovka
Moscow 113461, Russia
Telephone: (7) 121-0154, Telex: 411247

SPAIN

Borrasosa S.L.
C/Locom., 5 Cabezo de Torres
E-30110 Murcia, Spain
Telephone (34) (5) 4359669

Industrias La Locomotora S.L.
C/Locom., 5 Cabezo De Torres
E-30110 Murcia, Spain
Telephone: (34) 68831025
Fax: (34) 68832017

Mr. A.A. Spencer
69 Pine Grove Brookmans Park
GB-Hatfiedl AL 9 7BL, England
Telephone: (44) 707/553354
Telex: 296369
Fax: (44) 1/4009928

BAHARAIN

Baharain Pharmacy & Gen. Store
P.O. Box 56, Manama, Baharain
Telephone: (973) 253491

SWITZERLAND

Equilibriumn S.A.
8, Route De Buchillon, Ch-1162
Saint Prex, Switzerland
Telephone: (41) 0221/8062245
Fax: (41) 021/8062109

UNITED KINGDOM

Andard Mount Ltd.
West Africa House, Ashbource R
GB-London W 5 3QP, England
Telephone: (44) 819915150
Fax: (44) 819915001

Bush Beach Ltd.
Stanely Green Ltd.
GB-Cheadle Hu.,
Cheadle SK8 6RN, England
Telephone: (44) 61/4858231
Telex: 669583
Fax: (44) 61/485-6445

Mootah Medical Co.
P.O. Box 17561
Jeddah 21494, Saudi Arabia
Telephone: 966-026400196/6400918

SYRIA

Bechara Yordan Obegi
P.O. Box 343, Damascus, Syria
Telephone: 17693
Telex: 11360 SY

CANADA

Flora Distributors Ltd.
7400 Fraser Park Drive, Burnaby
BC V5J 5B9, Canada
Telephone: (697) 436-6000
Fax: (604) 436-6060

Wing Hing Co. Ltd.
8823 E. Cordova St., Vancouver
BC V6A 1M5, Canada
Telex: 04-352848

Gulf Delta Corp.
P.O. ox 252, Safat 13003, Kuwait
Telephone: (965) 4814499
Fax: (965) 4837817

OMAN

United National Commercial Co.
P.O. Box 4428, Ruwi, Oman
Telephone: 706670/796701
Telex: 3441 UNCC ON

SAUDI ARABIA

Bafarat Spices and Herbs Shops
P.O. Box 11652
Jeddha 21463, Saudi Arabia
Telephone: (966) 6421058
Fax: (966) 6433379

Mobarak H Al Dosari
P.O. Box No. 59462
Riyadh-11532, Saudi Arabia
Fax: 2332585

F.H. Taussing Inc.,
111 Brook St. Scardale,
NY 10583, U.S.A.
Telephone: (914) 472-6464
Telex: 13-1481
Fax: (914) 472-1846

Foreign-Domestic Chemicals
95 Chestnut Ridge Road, Montvale
NJ 07645, U.S.A.
Telephone: (201) 307-3333
Telex: 423-659
Fax: (201) 307-3398

G.D. Searle
5200 Old Orchard Rd.
Skokie, IL 60077, U.S.A.
Telephone: (708) 470-3028
Fax: (708) 967-2099

Golombeck, Morris J. Inc.
960 Fanklin Ave., Brooklyn
Ny 11225, U.S.A.
Telephone: (718) 284-3505
Fax: (718) 693_1941

U.S.A.

Botanicals International
2550 El Presidio Street
Long Beach, CA 90810, U.S.A.
Telephone: (310) 637-9566
Fax: (310) 637--3644

Cyclo Product, Inc.
P.O. Box 01557, Los Angeles
CA 90001, U.S.A.
Telephone: (213) 582-6411
Fax: (213) 582-8038

Maway Corporation
1338 Cypress St., Mandela Pkwy.
Oakland, CA 94607, U.S.A.
Telephone: (510) 208-3113
Telex: 3716659
Fax: (510) 208-3069

Olfactory Corporation
P.O. Box 21620, Ornard
CA 93034, U.S.A.
Telephone: (805) 644-8965

Sunrider International
3111 Lomita BL Vd.
Torrance, CA 90505, U.S.A.
Telephone: (310) 534--4786

The Lebermuth Co.
P.O. Box 4103, South Bend
IN 46634, U.S.A.
Telephone: (219)259-7000
Telex: 276424
Fax: (219) 258-7450

Whole Herb Co.
P.O. Box 1085, Mill Valley
CA 94942, U.S.A.
Employees : 4
Telephone: (415) 383-6485
Fax: (415) 383--1747

ARGENTINA

Michans Y Roy Ltd.
Hauser Chemical Research Inc.
4750 Nautilus Court S.
Boulder, Co 80301, U.S.A.
Telephone: (303) 530-4750
Fax: (303) 530-7083

Herbarium Inc.
11016 151nd Ave
kenosha, WI 53142, U.S.A.
Telephone: (414) 857-2373
Telex: 264-445
Fax: (414) 857-9501

CHILE

Laboratorio Vitafarma Ltd.
P.O. Box 51130, Santiago, Chile
Telephone: (56) 2/2742332
Telex: 242162 RTTR
Fax: (56) 2/2742407

Reutter Ltd.
P.O. Box 51130, Santiago, Chile
Telephone: 56-2/2742332, 2742482
Telex: 242162 RTTR
Fax: (56) 2/2742407

AUSTRALIA

Herbimex
GPO Box 1514, Brisbane QLD 4001
Australia
Telephone: (61) (07) 3\2854454

JAPAN

Alps Pharmaceutical Ind. Co. Ltd.
TSUJI-Koraibashi Bldg., 4-7
Koraibashi 2-Chome, Osaka 541, Japan
Telephone: (81) 06-201-4561
Telex: 5228763 ALPSOS J
Fax: (81) 06-223--0376

Crew Corp.
10-9-606, Uehommachi, 6-Chome
Tennoji-Ku, Osaka 543, Japan
Florida 734, Piso 1, Off
1005 beunos Aires, Argentina
Telephone: (54) (1) 322-1322
Telex: 23560 MACREN AR

Dainan Boeki Kaisha, Ltd.
3-3, Minami-Kyuhoji-Machi
3-Chome, Chuo-Ku, Osaka 541, Japan
Telephone: (81) 06-251-1191
Telex: J64519 DAINANBO
Fax: (81) 06-251-1192

Fukunda Ryu Co. Ltd.
5-11, Nishitemma 1-Chome
Kita-Ku, Osaka 530, Japan
Telephone: (81) 06-364-5861
Fax: (81) 06-364-6562

Hino Pharmaceutical Co. Ltd.
3-15, Doshomachi 2-Chome
Chuo-Ku, Osaka 541, Japan
Telephone: (81) 06-231-5847
Telex: J64490 HINO
Fax: (81) 06-231-7309

Hip Shing Tai Co. (Japan) Ltd.
P.O. Box 620, Kobe Port
Kobe 650, Japan
Telephone: (81) 078 (391) 2191
Telex: HST JAPAN J78654

Ichimaru Co. Ltd.
J Bldg. 3-7, Fushimimachi, 2-Chome
Chuo-Ku, Osaka 541, Japan
Telephone: (81) 06-201-0612
Telex: J63412 QUAPRO
Fax: (81) 06-201-0617

Koshiro Co. Ltd.
5-8, Doshomachi 2-Chome
Chuo-Ku, Osaka 541, Japan
Telephone: (81) 06-231-1803
Telex: KOSHIRO J64859
Fax: (81) 06-227-0187

UHA Marketing (M) Sdn. Bhd.
8 JL. Mega Mend. 5/M Old Kland
58200 Kuala Lumpur, Malaysia
Telephone: (81) 06-773-2118
Telex: J63023 CREW CORP
Fax: (81) 06--773-1813

Koyaku Company Limited
13-1, Shimosone Shimachi
Kokuram-Ku, Kitakyushu 800-02 Japan
Telephone: (81) 093-47-1981
Telex: 712815 Pharmk J
Fax: (81) 471-1862

Manage Develop. Fukunaga Co. Ltd.
457-8 Tonohara
Chikushino City, 818, Japan
Telephone: (81) (092) 922-2028
Fax: (81) (092) 924-4710

Morishita Jintan Co. Ltd.
1-30, Tamatsukuri 1-Chome
Chuo-Ku, Osaka 540, Japan
Telephone: (81) 06-761-1133
Telex:5278973 Jintan J
Fax: (81) 06-768-1661

MALAYSIA

Heron Product (M) Sdn. Bhd.
10-A JL. Jejaka 7, T. Mal. Cheras
55100 Kuala Lumpur, Malaysia
Telephone: (60) 3/9858552
Fax: (60) 3/9858366

Nature's Sunshine Products
95A Jalan Jejaka Sembilan
55100 Kuala Lumpur, Malaysia
Telephone: (60) (03) 9852722
Fax: (60) (03) 9856231

Natures Herbs Sdn. Bhd.
62, 1/F, Jalan SS 2/66, 47300 Petaling
Jaya, Selangor, Malaysia
Telephone: (60) 3/7765887
Fax: (60) 3/7745142

TAIWAN

Chang Sen Tang Co.
Telephone: (60) 3/7839536
Fax: (60) 3/7817353
Voon Ng Tong Trading Co. Bhd
489 Jalan Sungei Rambai
14000 Bukti Mertajam, Malaysia
Telephone: (60) (04) 51153
Telex: MA 40848 TECKAN

Weng Aun Thye
258 Lebuh Pantai
10300 Penang, Malaysia
Telephone: 60-04-612310/622200
Telex: MA 40506 PGWAT

PHILLIPPINES

Pharma Industries Inc.
P.O. Box 604, Manila, Philippines
Telephone: (63) 885-311

SOUTH KOREA

Dooley International Corp.
C.P.O. Box 10696
Seoul, South Korea
Telephone: 82022520741, 2355713
Telex: Y.B. KIM K26634
Fax: (82) (02) 236-0040

Pharmaton-Korea Co. Ltd.
C.P.O. Box 2533, Seoul, South Korea
Telephone: (82) (02) 755378
Telex: WYPARK K28589
Fax: (82) (02) 754-6732

General Medicine Sup Ctr. Ltd.
P.O. Box 792, Taipei City, Taiwan
Telephone: 886-02/5510031
Fax: (886) (02) 5377392

Giant Medical Corporation
P.O. Box 101-53, Taipei City, Taiwan
Telephone: (886) (02) 7151651-4
Telex: 11735 GRERICH
Fax: (886) (02) 7170521
9F, 2, Hsi Sheng S Rd, Sec. 2
Ta-An Dist, Taipei City, Tawian
Telephone: (886) 02/3225516
Fax: (886) (02) 3225518

Chia Shin Trading Co. Ltd.
P.O. Box 22841, Taipei City, Taiwan
Telephone: (886) (02) 5641700
Telex: 10495 SANDEERS
Fax: (886) (02) 5426694

Chii Yea Trading Co. Ltd.
10, Alley 19, Lane 50, Wu Hsing
Sungshan Dist, Taipei City, Taiwan
Telephoe: 886-02-7389005
Telex: 19559 Chiiyea
Fax: (886) (02) 7363028

Chinese-Cheer Trading Co. Ltd.
2F, 2, Lane 107, San Ho Rd, Sec 3
Sanchung City, Taipei Hsein, Twiwan
Telephone: (886) (02) 9731121-3
Fax: (886) (02) 9753516

Chun Che Trading Co. Ltd.
55, Ku Shan 1 Rd, Kushan Dist,
Kaohsiung City, Taiwan
Telephone: (886) (02) 5513700
Fax: (886) (02) 7717022

Edwin Trading Co. Ltd.
7F-1, 337, Hsin Yi Rd, Sec 4
Ta-An Dist, Taipei City, Taiwan
Telephone: (886) (02) 7003861-2
Fax: (886) (02) 7086820

Hyades Trading Co. Ltd.
4F-1, 142, Cheng An E Rd, Sec. 2
Chungshan Dist, Taipei City, Taiwan
Telephone: (886) (02) 7712755
Fax: (886) (02) 7762397

I Chang Trading Co. Ltd.
66, Ho Chuan St. Kushan Dist.
Kaohsiung City, Taiwan
Telephone: (886) (02) 5311177-8
Fax: (886) (02) 5317688

Great Eurasia Corp
9F, 101, Fu Hsin N Rd, Chungshan Dist
Taipei City, Taiwan
Telephone: (886) (02) 7131155
Telex: 10262 GECTPE
Fax: (886) (02) 7169656

Great Wealth Intern'l Corp.
P.O. Box 55-134, Taipei City, Taiwan
Telephone: (886) (02) 5814027
Telex: 14003 AJLC
Fax: (886) (02) 5614824

Hiap Ho Trading Co. Ltd.
2, Al 17, Ln 46, Ti Hua St, sec. 1
Yenping Dist, Taipei City, Taiwan
Telephone: (886) (02) 5315258
Telex: 27627 TEKHO
Fax: (886) (02) 5623643

Hsiangou Trading Co. Ltd.
P.O. Box 634, Taipei City, Taiwan
Telephone: (886) (02) 3411969
Telex: 15324 KINGCESS
Fax: (886) (02) 3971895

New Great Asia Tradingg Co. Ltd.
P.O. Box 3191, Taipei City, Taiwan
Telephone: (886) (02) 5061247
Telex: 26609 YENHAI
Fax: (886) (02) 5069309

Oranon Taiwan Ltd.
P.O. Box 39558, Taipei City, Taiwan
Telephone:(886) (02) 3121267-8
Telex: 10587 ORGTPE
Fax: (86) (02) 3121269

Seng Yuang Trading Co. Ltd.
3/F, 14, Lane 185, Nanking W Rd.
Yenping Dist., Taipei City, Taiwan
Telephone: (886) (02) 5316157
Telex: 25179 Sengyuan
Fax: (886) (02) 5366046

Shin Ho Shing Company Ltd.
P.O. Box 1566, Taipei, City, Taiwan
ICC Trading (Taiwan) Ltd.
P.O. Box 1369, Taipei City, Taiwan
Telephone: (886) (02) 5627131
Telex: 114261 ICCTRADE
Fax: (886) (02) 5511455

Jin Jin Enterprise Co. Ltd.
P.O. Box 3717, Taipei City, Taiwan
Telephone: (886) (02) 7475090-1
Telex: 17491 JWJIN
Fax: (886) (02) 7475092

Kaisers Pharm & Medical Corp.
P.O. Box 3717
Taipei City Taiwan
Telephone: (886) (02) 5641681
Telex: 11654 KAISERS
Fax: (886) (02) 5236690

Lucid Import & Medical Corp.
283, Ming Shen W Rd
yenning Dist., taipei City, Taiwan
Telephone: (886) (02) 5419139
Telex: (260921 LUCID
Fax: (886) (02) 5362307

Sun Tsuang Enterprise Co. Ltd.
1F, 29, The Ho Rd
Yungho City, Taipei Shien, Taiwan
Telephone: (886) (02) 9213410
Fax: (886) (02) 9229666

Swechen Co. Ltd.
P.O. Box 59269, Taipei City, Taiwan
Telephone: (886) (02) 5110453

Swegian Company
P.O. Box 59269
Taipei City, Taiwan
Telephone: (886) (02) 5110453

Taiwan Excelsior Inc
5F, 141, Jen Ai Rd, Sec 3
Ta-An Dist, Taipei City, Taiwan
Telephone: (886) (02) 7713121
Telex: 11739 TWATCEL
Fax: (886) (02) 7310299
Telephone: (886) (02) 3115517--9
Fax: (886) (02) 3754148

Shing Yu Trading Co. Ltd.
4F-1, 42, Chang An E Rd, Sec 2
Chungshan Dist, Taipei City, Taiwan
Telephone: (886) (02) 7718333
Fax: (886) (02) 7762397

Shuang Lung Trading Co., Ltd.
2F, 112, Ti Hua St, Sec 1
Yenping Dist, Taipei City, Taiwan
Telephone: 886-02-5224787
Fax: (886) (02) 5515028

Union Medical Ent. Co. Ltd.
P.O. Box 26-784, Taipei City, Taiwan
Telephone: (886) (02) 7365657
Telex: 10177 FUERLOOK

Weiming Union Trading Co. Ltd.
4F, 11, Lane 125, I Tung St
Chungshan Dist, Taipei City, Taiwan
Telephone: (886) (02) 5061916

Yuen Fung Trading Co. Ltd.
P.O. Box 1-52, Kaohsiung City, Taiwan
Telephone: (886) (07) 5510399
Telex: 73209 YUENFUNG
Fax: (886) (07) 5315234

EGYPT

Ankram Company
30, Abdel Raheim Sabri Street
Dokki, Cairo, Egypt
Telephone: (20) 709093
Telex: 92598 UN

N.I. Ibrahim Company (Flavogypt)
8, Falaki Street, Alexandria, Egypt
Telephone: (20) 3 4825064
Fax: (20) 4833923

The Yuh Trading Co. Ltd.
P.O. Box 68-280, Taipei City, Taiwan
Telephone: (886) (02) 5017217
Telex: 23819 TEHYUHCO
Fax: (886) (02) 5007019

Tow Star Trading Co. Ltd.
P.O. Box 58052, Taipei City, Taiwan
Telephone: 886) (02) 3625275
Telex: 20110 Honchang
Fax: (886) (02) 3628308

Tzu Sheng Company, Ltd.
P.O. Box 71, Taipei City, Taiwan
Telephone: (886) (02) 2222016
Fax: (886) (02) 2213081

- Automatic Bread Plant
- Automatic Papad Plant
- Automatic Toffee & Candy
- Baby Cereal Food
- Baby Health Care Food & Milk
- Bakery Industries
- Baking Powder
- Banana & Its By Products
- Banana Powder
- Banana Puree
- Banana Waffers
- Basmati Rice Trading
- Beer & Wine
- Beer Industry
- Beer Plant (5000 Bottle/Day)
- Besan Plant
- Biscuits Making Plant
- Bottling Plant (Alcoholic & Non Alcoholic)
- Bottling Plant Country Liquor
- Brandy
- Buffalow Meat Processing
- Candy Hard Boiled
- Canning And Preservation
- Cashew Feni
- Cashew Kernels (Dried & Fried)
- Cashew Nut (Dried & Fried)
- Casine From Milk
- Cattel Feed
- Cattle & Poultry Feed
- Cattle Feed From Molasses & Bagasse
- Cattle Feed From Tapioca
- Chewing Gum & Bubble Gum
- Chewing Tobacco (Khaine) In Pounch Pack
- Chicken Meat Processing & Packaging
- Chicken/Mutton (Sheep Meat) Processing
- Chilli Oil
- Chilli Powder
- Chocklate
- Cocoa Butter And Cocoa Powder
- Coconut And Cashew Feni
- Coconut Oil From Copra
- Coconut Oil In Containers (Filteration & Airtight Packaging)
- Coconut Powder
- Coconut Processing Complex Unit
- Coconut Sqush Jam & Cream
- Coconut Water
- Coffee Processing & Packaging
- Cold Drink
- Confectionery Products (Toffee & Candy)
- Country Liquor
- Curry Powder
- Custard Powder
- Dairy Product &Milk Packaging In Pouch (Ghee, Casein, Butter
- Dairy Products
- Dall/Pulse Mill
- Dehydrated Garlic Flakes & Granulated Powder
- Dehydrated Onion & Onion Powder
- Dehydrated Vegetables
- Dehydration & Pickling Oyster Paddy Straw Mushroom
- Dehydration Of Fruit & Vegetable Juice
- Dehydration Of Fruits & Vegetable
- Dehydration Of Vegetables & Tropical Fruit/Drying/Crystallisation
- Dog Food
- Drum Stick Powder
- Dry Ginger From Green Ginger
- Drying Of Red Chillies
- Edible Oil Product Start From Grind Raw Material To Fiber
- Edible Oil Refind Oil
- Edible Plasticizer For Ragi Papad
- Edible Vegetable Oil
- Egg Powder
- Fish & Poultry Food
- Fish Canning In Tin (Pouching) (Dehydration Of Fish)
- Fish Meal
- Fish Processing
- Flour Mill (Atta & Besan)
- Food Colour (Naturla & Synthetic)
- Freezing Of Fresh Vegetable For Export
- French Fries & Allied Potato Products
- Fresh Processed Frozen Vegetable Puree & Sauce 100% Eou
- Frozen Food (Fruit & Vegetables
- Fruit Drink In Tetra Pack
- Fruit Juice & Allied Products
- Fruit Juice (Mango) In Tetrapack
- Fruit Juice Bottling Plant
- Fruit Juice In Plastic Cups
- Fruit Juice Manufacturing
- Fruit Juice Powder
- Fruit Juice, Jam, Jellies And Allied Products
- Fruit Processing
- Fruit Pulp & Juices
- Fruit Pulp & Squashes
- Garlic Oil
- Garlic Paste
- Garlic Powder
- Ginger Glazing & Preservation
- Ginger Powder
- Ginger Processing (Peeling, Drying, Grinding & Blending
- Gluten
- Gram Dall & Flour Mill With Modern Automatic Plant
- Gram Dall And Flour Mill
- Gur From Cane (Export Quality)
- Hing (Asafetida)
- Honey Processing & Packaging
- Honey Roasted Peanut
- I.M.F.L. (Indian Made Foreign Liquors)
- Ice Cream Manufacturing
- Ice Cream Of Different Flavours
- Ice Cube Plant
- Ice Making Plant
- Instant Foods (Idli Mix, Vada Mix, Gulabjamun Mix, Sambar Mix
- Instant Noodles
- Instant Tea
- Instant Tea & Coffee (Premixed With Sugar & Milk)
- Iodised Salt Free Flowing Form Sea Water
- Iodized Salt (Ordinary & Moistureless Free Flowing)
- Iodized Salt Free Flowing
- Jam Jally (Chutny, Pickels & Squash Etc.)
- Katha
- Katha And Cutch (Chuna)
- Khaine (Chewing Tobacco)
- Khandsari Sugar
- Lacithin (Soyabased)
- Lichi Juice
- Locally Made Foreign Liquor
- Macaroni Manufacturing
- Macaroni Spaghetti Vermicelli & Noodles
- Maize & Its By Product
- Maize & Its Products
- Maize Processing For Glucose
- Makhana Processing Unit
- Malting Plant
- Mango Juice
- Mango Pappad (Aam Pappad)
- Mango Powder
- Mango Processing
- Mango Pulp
- Mango Pulp & Slices
- Masala (Spices) [Eou]
- Milk Paneer
- Milk Plant With Pouch Packing
- Milk Powder And Ghee
- Milk Product Cheese
- Mineral Water
- Mineral Water In Pouches
- Mini Flour Mill (Disk Type)
- Mini Sugar Plant
- Modern Basmati Rice
- Modern Bread & Buns (Bakery Unit)
- Modern Chilly Powder
- Mushroom Processing And.Canning
- Musturd Oil Mill
- Namkeen (Dalmoth, Bhujia, Chanachoor Etc.)
- Oleoresin From Chilly
- Onion & Potato Powder
- Onion Powder
- Pan Masala In Pouch & Tin Pack Sada, Meetha, Zarda
- Pan Masala In Pouch Pack
- Pan Masala, Gutka & Pouch Making Plant
- Paneer From Soya Milk
- Papad & Bari
- Papad Plant (Imported/Automatic)
- Parboiled Rice Mill
- Pectin From Mango Peel
- Pickles (Vegetarian & Non Vegetarian)
- Pickles Murabbas (Veg. & Non Veg.)
- Pickles, Morabas, Sauces & Squashes
- Pig Meat Processing (800 Pig/Day)
- Piggery Meat Processing
- Piggery/Meat/Chicken Processing
- Pine Apple Slice Canning
- Pineapple Juice Manufacturing & Canning
- Poha (Chiwra)
- Pork Products
- Potato And Onion Flakes
- Potato Chips
- Potato Chips (Imported M/C.)
- Potato Granules
- Potato Powder (Automatic)
- Potato Starch
- Potato Waffers (Imported Plant)
- Poultry Feed
- Poultry Processing (Processed Meat)
- Processed Fruits And Vegetable
- Processing Of Food Grain/Pulse And Retail Packaging
- Refining Of Edible Oil
- Rice & Corn Flakes
- Rice Noodles
- Roasted & Fried Dry Fruits, Grain, Grams, Peas Etc.(In Pouch)

- Roasted/Salted/Coated Cashewnut, Peanuts, Almonds
- Roller Flour Mill (Mini Flour Mill)
- Salted Cashewnut Processing
- Sattu Manufacturing
- Semi Automatic Plant For Toffee Etc.,
- Silver Coated Sugar Balls
- Skimmed Milk Powder
- Snack Food (Crax Type) Roll & Ball Type
- Soft Drink (Carbonated)
- Softy Ice Cream Cones (Automatic/Imported Plant)
- Sounf Supari (Elaichi Flavour)
- Soya Been Milk From Soya
- Soya Products
- Soyabean Bariyan (Automatic)
- Soyabean Meat
- Soyabean Product (Soyabean Oil Soya Paneer, Soya Extract)
- Soyabean Products
- Spice & Allied Product
- Spice Oleoresin (Ginger)
- Spices (EOU)
- Starch & Allied Product From Maize
- Starch (A & B)
- Starch From Maize
- Starch From Tapioca
- Sugar Candy (Bombay Mishri Type)
- Sugar Candy (Pearl Type)
- Sugar Cane Juice Preservation
- Sugar Cubes
- Sugar Pellets
- Sugar Plant
- Sun Flower Seed Oil
- Sweet Scented Supari
- Tamarind Juice Concentrates
- Tamarind Kernel Powder
- Tea Bag
- Tea Bag (Dip-Dip Type)
- Tea Processing
- Tea Processing & Packaging
- Tomato Paste (Tomato Concentrate)
- Tomato Powder
- Tomato Product In Pouch (Souce Ketchup Etc.)
- Tomato Product Manufacturing
- Trading Business (Rice,Salt,Dry Fruits, Etc.)
- Turmeric Powder
- Tuty Fruity From Papaya
- Upgrading Of Salt
- Vanaspathi Ghee (Hydrogenated Vegetable Oil)
- Vegetable Oil (Refined)
- Vermicelli
- Vodka From Potatoes
- Wheat Puff
- Wine, Brandy, Whisky & Champagne
- Yogurt In Plastic Cups
- Zarda Kimam Tobacco
- Zarda Of Various Grades

Biochemicals & Biotechnology

- Absolute Alcohol From Molasses
- Acetic Acid From Molasess
- Alcohol From Potatoes
- Aqua Culture Shrimp Farming
- Aquaculture Prawn Farming
- Bio Fertilizer
- Bio-Fertiliser (Organic Fertilisers) From Garbage
- Bio-Fertilisers From Cowdung & Other Wastes
- Bio-Fertilizer (Organic Manure)
- Bio-Fertilizer Frim Birds Excreata
- Bio-Stimulant And Fertilizer Suppliment
- Button Mushroom Cultivation, Processing & Canning
- Citric Acid From Molasses
- Compressed Yeast From Molasses
- Cut Flower Rose [Floriculture]
- Dehydration And Pickling Of Oyster Paddy Straw Mushroom
- Enzymes
- Ethyl Alcohol From Molasses
- Floriculture With Green House (Cut Flower Rose)
- Hybrid Seed Production
- Industrial Enzymes
- Insecticides From Neem Seeds Neemoil & Leaves
- Mini Fertilizer Plant (Urea)
- Municipal Garbage Treatment
- Mushroom (Oyster & Paddy) Cultivation, Processing, Dehydration
- Mushroom Cultivation & Processing
- Mushroom Cultivation & Processing With Air Conditioning
- Mushroom Processing And Canning
- Organic Fertiliser
- Papain [Ip/Bp Grade]
- Papain Manufacturing
- Prawn Fish Farming
- Shiitake Mushroom
- Tissue Cultures (100 Eou)
- Vermi Compost
- Vermiculture

Chemical & Allied Industries

- 2-4, Dichlorophenoxy Acetatic Acid
- 2-Chloroethyl Phosphate Acid 39% Emulsifying Concentrate
- 4,4, Diamino Stilbene 2-2-Dis-Sulphonic Acid
- Acetic Acid (Glacial)
- Acetic Acid From Molasess
- Acetic Acid From Natural Gas
- Acetic Anhydride
- Acetone
- Acetylene Gas
- Acetylene Gas & Oxygen Gas
- Acid Slurry (From Linear Alkyl Benzene)
- Acid/Spirit Proof Caramel
- Activated Bleaching Fuller Earth
- Activated Carbon & Sodium Silicate From Rice/Paddy Husk
- Activated Carbon From Cashewnut Shell
- Activated Carbon From Coconut Shell
- Activated Carbon From Fuller Earth Slum
- Activated Carbon From Rice Husk
- Activated Carbon From Rice Husk Coconut Shell
- Activated Carbon From Saw Dust, Rice Husk And Coconut Shells
- Activated Carbon From Wood
- Activated Carbon Powder & Granulated
- Activated Charcoal
- Air Freshners (Odonil Type)
- Alcohol From Potato
- Alcohol From Rice (Grains)
- Alcohol From Rice Straw
- Alkyd Resin
- Alkyd Resin (Soyabeen Oil And Lineseed Oil)
- Alum (Ferric & Non Ferric)
- Alum For Paper Industries
- Aluminium Hydroxide (I.P.)
- Aluminium Hydrcxide Gel
- Aluminium Silicate
- Aluminium Slug (Used For Collapsible Tube Containers)
- Amino Acid
- Ammonium Nitrate
- Ammonium Nitrate From Fertilizer
- Ammonium Sulphate
- Amonium Chloride
- Amyl Acetate
- Anhydrous Ferric Chlolride
- Antimony Trioxide
- Assaying Gold
- Barium Carbonate
- Barium Compounds
- Basic Chromium Sulphate
- Basic Chromium Sulphate From Waste Sulfurdioxide
- Beneficiation Of Maganese Ore
- Benzoic Acid
- Benzyl Alcohol
- Benzyl Benzoate
- Bleaching Powder
- Boric Acid
- Buffing & Polishing Compound
- Cable Jelly Compound
- Cable Jelly Filled Compound
- Caffeine From Tea Waste
- Calcining Of Magnesite & Dead Burnt Mangnese Oxide
- Calcium Carbide
- Calcium Carbonate (Activated)
- Calcium Carbonate (Precipitated & Activated)
- Calcium Carbonate From Lime Stone
- Calcium Carbonate From Marble Chips
- Calcium Chloride
- Calcium Gluconate
- Calcium Hypochloride
- Calcium Nitrate
- Calcium Oxide (Lime Stone Powder)
- Camphor Tablet
- Carbon Black From Dry Cell Batteries
- Carbon Black From Fertilizer's Waste
- Carbon Dioxide (Co2)
- Carbon Dioxide From Boiler Exhaust Gases
- Carboxy Methyl Cellulose (Cmc)
- Cationic Softner
- Caustic Soda
- Cellulose Acetate
- Cellulose Powder & Microcrystalline Cellulose Powder
- Chelated Zinc (Zn-Edta)
- Chemical Etching Of Stainless Steel
- China Clay Washing/ Purification
- Chlorinated Paraffin Wax (Cpw)

- Chromic Acid
- Coalchar From Activated Carbon
- Cobalt Octoate
- Construction Chemicals
- Coolent Engines
- Copper Sulphate
- Copper Sulphate From Copper Ash
- Corrosion Controlling Chemicals (Pipe Lines)
- D.O.P. (Dioctyle Phthalate)
- Dehydrated Lime
- Dhop (Loban) Benzion
- Di Calcium Phosphate From Rock Phosphate Haifa Process
- Di-Butyl Phthalate (Dbp)
- Di-Calcium Phosphate From Rock Phosphate
- Diethyle Phathilate (D.E.P.)
- Dough Moulding Compound (Dmc)
- D-Phenyl Glycine
- Dry Ice By Breaking Of Air
- Dye Fixing Agent (By Cold Process)
- Emulsifiers For Cutting Oil
- Etching Process
- Ethyl Acetate
- Ethyl Alcohol From Molasses
- Ethylene Diamine
- Extraction Of Gold Silver & Copper From The Alloy By Chemical Process
- Extraction Of Lead From Lead Waste
- Extraction Of Silver From Hypo Solution (Chemical Process)
- Fatty Acid
- Ferric Alum
- Ferric Chloride (Anhydrous)
- Ferric Oxide
- Ferric Sulphate
- Ferro Alloy
- Ferro Manganese
- Ferro Silicon
- Ferrous Silicate
- Ferrous Sulphate
- Fire Works
- Fluorine Chemical (Hydro Fluoic Acid)
- Foaming Agent
- Formaldehydeformic Acid
- Furfural From Rice Husk/ Hull
- Gasket Shellec Compound
- Gelatin (Edible, Pharmaceutical & Photography Grade)
- Glycerine
- Gold Salt
- Ground Calcium Carbonate
- Heat & Uv Stabilizers For Pvc & Other Engineering Plastics
- Heat And Water Proof Compound For Construction
- Hexachloroethane
- Hexachloroethane From Ethylene Dichloride
- Hexamine From Formaldehyde
- High Concentrated Formalin
- Hydrated Lime From Sea Shell
- Hydrochloric Acid
- Hydrogen Peroxide
- Hydrogen Peroxide (By Auto Oxidation Process)
- Hydrogen Peroxide By Ethyle Anthraquinine Catalytic
- Hydroxide (Naoh)- Caustic Soda
- Hydroxy Amine Sulphate
- Hydroxylamine Sulphate
- Industrial Gases
- Insoluble Sulphur
- Iron Oxide For Making Ferrites
- Isoephthalic Acid
- L A B (Linear Alkyl Benzene)
- Laboratory Chemical Unit
- Lactic Acid
- Lead Extraction From Scrap Batteries
- Lead Oxide
- Lead Oxide (Mono Red And Gray)
- Lead Oxide (Mono-Oxide, Red Lead Tetranickel)
- Lead Recovery From Scrap Battery
- Lead Stearate
- Leather Chemicals (Hydrated Lime, Chromium Sulphate, Borax)
- Lecithin From Sunflower Oil
- Light Magnesium Oxide
- Lime Stone Powder
- Liquid Oxygen Botteling Plant
- M - Dinitrobenzene
- Magnesium From Sea Water
- Magnesium Hydroxide
- Magnesium Hydroxide Powder
- Magnesium Powder (Light)
- Magnesium Sulfate As Fertilizer Grade
- Magnesium Sulphate
- Maleic Anhydride
- Managnese Sulphate
- Melamine Formaldehyde Powder
- Menthyl Methacrylate
- M e t a - D i n i t r o Benzaldehyde
- Metal Naphathenates
- Metal-Pre-Treatment Chemicals
- Methy Ethyl Ketone Oxime (Mek Oxime)
- Methyl Ethyl Ketone Peroxide
- Methyl Salicylate
- Metol
- Micro Nutrients Mixture Solid
- Moisquito Coil
- Mono Ethylene Glycol
- Mono Sodium Glutamate
- N-Acetyl Glucosamin Through Chitin Biotechnically
- N-Butyl Acetate
- Nickel Catalyst For Hydrogenation Of Vegetable Oil
- Nitro Cellulose
- Nitrous Oxide
- Non Formal Dye Fixing Agent (Natural)
- Non Formaldehyde Fixing Agent
- Non-Ferric Alum
- N-Paraffin
- Ortho-Toluene Solvent
- Ossein From Bones
- Oxalic Acid From Molasses
- Oxalic Acid From Paddy Husk
- Oxalic Acid From Saw Dust
- Oxalic Acid From Vegetable Waste
- Oxygen And Nitrogen Gas Plant
- Oxygen Gas Collection And Bottling Plant
- Oxygen Gas Plant
- Oxygen Gas Plant (Air Seperation Method)
- Oxygen Liquid Plant
- P.V.C. Stabiliser (Lead Stearate & Calcium Stearate)
- Pectin From Citrus, Lemon & Oranges
- Pectin From Orange Lime Peels
- Pectin From Raw Papaya
- Phenyl
- Phenyl (Black And White)
- Phenyl (Pine Oil Disinfectant)
- Phenyl Brown & White
- Phosphoric Acid (Purification) From Crude
- Photo-Emulsion For Rotary Screen Printing
- Phthalic Anhydride
- Phthalocyanine Blue & Green
- Plaster Of Paris
- Poly Acetal Unit
- Poly Corbonate (Dry Process)
- Poly Vinyl Alcohol
- Polyester Resin
- Polyvinyl Acetate
- Potassium Chloride
- Potassium Cyanide (Silver & Gold)
- Potassium Iodate
- Potassium Nitrate
- P o t a s s i u m Permanganate (Kmno4) In Solution Form
- Potassium Silicate
- Potassium Silicate Using Autoclave
- Pottasium Iodide
- Precipitated Calcium Carbonate
- Precipitated Silica
- Precipitated Silica From Rice Husk Ash
- Reclamation Of Nickel From Spent Catalyst Of Vanaspati Industry
- Recovery Of Silver From Waste Fixer Bleach Obtained From Photo Colour Lab By Sulphide Process
- Recovery Of Zinc Metal From Zinc Ash
- Ringer's Lactate Solution
- Roofing Compound & Water Proffing Compound
- Saccharine
- Silica Jel
- Silica Sand Benefication (50 Ton Per Hour)
- Silicone
- Silicone Carbide
- Silicone Emulsion
- Silicone From Rice Husk
- Silver Extraction From Waste Hypo Solution (Chem. Process)
- Silver Extraction From Waste Hypo Solution (X-Ray/Cinema Film
- Silver Extraction From Waste X-Ray & Cinema Film
- Silver Extrusion From Waste Fibre Bleach And From Photo Film
- Silver Nitrate
- Single Super Phasphate & Mix Npk Fertilisers (Ssp & Npk)
- Single Super Phasphate (S.S.P.)
- Single Super Phasphate (S.S.P.) & Sulphuric Acid
- Soda Ash
- Sodium Aluminates
- Sodium Aluminium Sulphate

- Sodium Benzoate
- Sodium Bicarbonate From Soda Ash
- Sodium Carboxy Methyl Cellulose
- Sodium Hexa Meta Phosphate
- Sodium Hypo Chlorite From Waste Chlorine Gas
- Sodium Hypochloride (Bleaching Powder)
- Sodium Meta Bi Sulphite
- Sodium Meta-Silicate
- Sodium Silicate From Rice/Paddy Husk
- Sodium Silicate From Silica And Soda Ash
- Sodium Sulphate (Anhydrous)
- Sodium Sulphide From Barium Compound
- Sodium Sulphide From Sulfur Caustic Soda
- Sodium Sulphite
- Sodium Tripoly Phosphate
- Softner (Cationic, Anionic & Nomiric)
- Solder Fluxes
- Solid Fuel Cake
- Solvent Extraction & Refining Plant
- Solvent Extraction And Refining Of Soyabeen Plant
- Solvent Extraction Plant
- Stearic Acid
- Strontium Carbonate
- Sulphur Milling Plant
- Sulphuric Acid
- Super Phosphate & Mixed Fertiliser (Npk)
- Synthetic Iron Oxide (Yellow)
- Tartaric Acid From Maleic An-Hydride
- Tartaric Acid From Tamarind
- Tartaric Acid From Tarmind Powder
- Tartaric Acid, Food Colour, Crude Pectine, Tamarind Oil
- Titanium Dioxide
- Tri Basic Lead Sulphate
- Ultra Marine Blue (5 Mt/Day)
- Urea Formaldehyde
- Urea Formeldehyde Resin
- Water Proofing Compound (Liquid & Powder)
- Water Proofing Compound (Liquid & Solid)
- Water Treatment Chemicals
- X-Ray Photography Developers & Fixer
- Zeolite - A
- Zinc & Copper Sulphate From Brass Ash
- Zinc Brightner
- Zinc Chloride
- Zinc Oxide
- Zinc Oxide (Chemical Process)
- Zinc Phosphate
- Zinc Stearate
- Zinc Sulfate 21% Agricultural Grade From Waste Ash
- Zinc Sulphate
- Zinc Sulphate Micro Nutrients Or Fertilizer
- Zinc Sulphate Micro-Nutrient Mixture
- Zinc-Metal From Zinc Ash
- Zircon

Computer Products

- Call Centre (Domestic)
- Call Centre (International)
- Compact Disc
- Computer Assembly (Hardware)
- Computer Education Institute
- Computer Monitor (Monochrome Monitor)
- Computer Ribbon (For Printer)
- Computer Ribbon Refilling/Reinking
- Computer Software (EOU)
- Cybercafe
- E-Commerce
- Floppy Disks
- Internet Servicd Provider(Isp)
- Laptop Computers
- Medical Transcription Centre
- Online Shopping Mall Portal
- Plastic Flopy Storage Box
- Portal

Cosmetics, Perfumes, Flavours & Essential Oils

- Aerosol Spray [Rose Flavour , Night Qeen, Jasmin]
- After Shave Lotion
- Agar Oil From Black Agar Wood
- Agarbatti Synthetic Perfumery Compound
- Air Freshner & Purifiers
- Air Freshners (Odonil Type)
- Aromatic Perfumery Compounds
- Bindi
- Bindiya (Shilpa Type)
- Car Shampoo
- Cosmetic Industries
- Detol Type Antiseptic Lotion
- Dhoop Batti Sticks
- Essences For Biscuit, Confectionery Items (Non-Essential Flavour)
- Essential Oil From Flowers
- Essential Oils From Jawa Citronella Oil
- Essentical Oil Form Lily, Mogra, Nishigandha
- Eucalyptus Oil
- Extraction Of Essential Oil & Packaging
- Extraction Of Oil (Jeera, Ajowon, Ginger,Cardamom Oil Etc.)
- Formulation Of Flavours
- Fractional Distillation Of Essencial Oil And Medicinal Plant
- Garlic Oilginger Oil
- Ginger Oil (Super Critical Co2 Process)
- Hair Dye (Godrej Type)
- Hair Dye Powder
- Hair Shampoo
- Herbal Cosmatic
- Herbal Hair Oil (Banphool Type)
- Herbal Natural Essential Oil
- Herbal Natural Essential Oil (Steam Distillation Process)
- Lamon Grass Oil
- Lily Essence
- Menthol Crystal Bold From Menthol Oil
- Menthol Crystals
- Menthol Crystals & Menthol Oil menthol Oil
- Nail Polish
- Non-Alcoholic Flavours
- Oleo-Resin & Capsisin Product Extraction Plant
- Oleoresin & Essential Oil Mfg
- Palmrosa Grass Oil
- Peppermint Oil
- Perfumery Chemicals Synthetic And Natural
- Red (Lal) Tooth Powder
- Rose Oil (Essential Oil From Flowers)
- Rose Plantation & Rose Oil Extraction (Rose Essential Oil)
- Sandal Wood Oil & Powder
- Scent & Perfumes
- Shampoo & Creams
- Shampoo & Creams (Cold Cream, All Purpose Cream & Varnishing Cream) Shaving Cream
- Shaving Cream & Shaving Soap
- Spice Oil Or Oleoresins (Extraction Of Essential Oil From Spices)
- Synthetic Purfumery Compound
- Talcum Powder (Face & Toilet Powder)
- Tejpatta Oil From Tejpatta
- Telcum Powder
- Tobacco Based Tooth Powder
- Tooth Paste
- Tooth Paste (Gel Type)
- Yara Yara (Perfumes For Soap, Detergent & Agarbatti Etc.)

Dyes & Dye Intermediates

- Acetonaphthone
- Azo Die Stuffs
- Beta Napthol (100 Eou)
- Coumarin
- Dye Fixing Agent (By Cold Process)
- Dye Intermediates
- Dye Intermediates - Indigo Blue
- Dyes & Dye Intermediates
- Fast Colour Base
- Leather Auxiliaries
- Metal Naphthenates
- Naphthalene Balls
- Naphthnol Astr
- Natural Coloured Oil (Turmeric Colour & Oil)
- Phthalo Cyanine Blue And Green
- Re-Active Dyes (Red,Orange,Yellow Colour) Used B-Napthol
- Textile Dyeing Auxiliaries
- Textile Printing Pigment Binder
- Ultra Marine Blue

Electrical & Electronic Industries

- Air Conditioner (A/C) Car & Room Servicing
- Air Conditioners (Window Type)
- All Aluminium Alloy Conductor (Aaac)
- Alternator (1 To 75 Kva)
- Aluminium Power Cables
- Aluminium/Copper Cable Lugs
- Arial Bunched Cable
- Armoured Cables
- Audio Cassette Assembling & Recording Unit
- Audio Cassette Manufacturing & Recording
- Audio Cassettes Manufacturing
- Audio Magnetic Tape
- Audio Stereo Cassette

Recorder Players
- Audio Video Assembling Unit
- Audio Video Cassette Assembling
- Auto Bulb/Lamp
- Auto Lamps (Auto Tail Lights)
- Battery (Ups, Invertor, Solar System, & Automobile Battery)
- Battery Plates & Assembly
- Button Cell (Miniature Watch Battry)
- Cable Creeping Lungs, Socket & Cable Creeping Tools
- Calculator, Torch & Alarm Capacitors
- Cardless Telephone
- Cassette Tape Recorder
- Ceiling Fan
- Chocke And Patti For Fluorescent Tube
- Choke & Starter For Fluorescent Tube
- Clay Plate For Electric Heater
- Colour Television (T.V.)
- Commutators
- Compact Disc Rom (Cd-Rom)
- Compact Disk Player
- Compact Fluorescent Lamps
- Compressor For Ac (Hermetic)
- Computerised Washing Machine
- Cooling Coils (For Airconditioners)
- Copper Clad Laminated Sheet Used For Making P.C.B.
- Ct/Pt Epoxy Casting Transformers
- Diesel Generator (20-200 Kva) Dg Set
- Dish Antenna And Satellite Network Equipment
- Distribution Transformer (250kva) Repairing
- Distribution Transformers
- Domestic Refrigeration
- Dry Cell Battery Manufacturing Unit
- Dry Cell Manufacturing
- Dry Cells, Rechargeable Cells
- Electric & Ordinary Detonators(Used In Explosive For Hard Rock Cutting & Blasting
- Electric Bulb (Gls Bulb)
- Electric Energy Meters
- Electric Fan
- Electric Fluorescent Tube
- Electric Gyser
- Electric Mixer
- Electric Motor
- Electric Motor Pumps
- Electric Panel Board (Switch Boards)
- Electric Steam Iron
- Electric Water Heater
- Electrical Accessories (Plugs, Switches, Sockets Etc.)
- Electrical Lamp
- Electrical Panel (Switch Board)
- Electronic Calculator
- Electronic Choke (Ballast)
- Electronic Cut Out For Automobiles
- Electronic Digital Weighing Machine
- Electronic Energy Meter
- Electronic Service Centre
- Electronic Toys
- Emergency Light
- Epabx/Epax System
- Exhaust Fans (Cooler Fan)
- F.H.P. Motors
- Ferrite Magnets
- Fluorescent Tube Starter
- G.L.S. Bulbs/Lamps
- Gas Based Power Project (600 Mv)
- Halogen Lamps
- House Wiring Cables
- Ht & Mv Industrial Cubic Switch Boards
- Hydro Based Power Plant (15mw)
- Immersion Heater
- Information Moving Display (Lead Type)
- Invertors
- Jelly Filled Cables
- Lamp Shades & Chandliers
- Light Emitting Diodes
- M.C.B. (Miniature Circuit Breaker)
- Maintenance Free Re-Chargable Battery
- Micro Oven
- Miniature Transformer
- Multilayer Printed Circuit Board
- Musical Door Bell
- Neon Sign Board Manufacturing
- Optical Fibre Cable
- Optical Pickup Unit
- P.V.C. Stablizers
- P.V.C. Wire & Cables
- Pcb Manufacturing (Flexible)
- Pcb Manufacturing (Multilayer)
- Pcb Manufacturing (Totally Automatic Plant)
- Plastic Coolar Body (Symphony Type)
- Polyurethene Battery Separator
- Portable Television (B & W)
- Portal
- Power Capacitor
- Power Generating Unit From Agricultural Waste Heat Energy
- Power Plant (5 Mw/Hr) By Agro Waste
- Power Plant (Hydro Based) Cap: 10 Mw
- Power Project (100% Foreign Funded)
- Power Supply (Linear Switch Mode)
- Power Transformer
- Printed Cricuit Board
- Pvc Battery Separator
- Pvc Electric Wires & Cables
- Rechargeable Battery - Maintenance Free (Sealed Lead Acid)
- Re-Conditionig Of Fluorescent Tube
- Refrigeration & Mini Refrigeration
- Rewinding Of Burnt Electric Motor
- Rosin Cored Soft Soldering Wire
- Sattelite Receiver
- Soft & Hard Ferrites
- Solar Cooker
- Solar Electrical Cell & Heating Pannel
- Solar Energy Water Heater
- Solar Photo Voltaic System
- Solar Power Plant
- Switch Mode Power Supply
- Tape Recorder's Pinch Roller, Rubber, Drive, Belt Flat
- Telephone (Push Button Type)
- Terminal Connectors
- Transformer/Servomotor/Relay
- Un-Intrupted Power Supply (Ups)
- Variable Frequency, Variable Voltage A.C. Voltage
- Video Cassette
- Video Compact Disc (V.C.D.)
- Voltage Stablizer (Solid State)
- Voltage Stablizer Using Ic Timer
- Washing Machine
- Washing Machine & Geyser
- Wind Energy Power Project
- Winding Wires Pvc Insulated For Submersible Motors
- Xlpe Cables

Electroplating Industries

- Aluminium Anodizing Plant
- Aluminium Hard-Anodizing Unit
- Chrome Plating
- Electro Polishing Of Steel
- Electroplating Of Gold & Their Chemical Treatment In Golden Colour
- Electroplating Of Plastic
- Electroplating Of Various Metal
- Gold Electroplating On Cheaper Ornaments (Without Using Gold)
- Gold Plated Silver Jewellery
- Gold Plated Silver Jewellery & Cutlery
- Hard Chromium Plating
- Silver & Gold Plating On Pvc And Nylon-6
- Watch Case Buffing

Glass & Cement Industries

- Acrylic Mirror
- Ceramic (Porcelain) Insulator
- Ceramic Hotel Ware Bone China
- Ceramic Thread Guide
- Ceramic Unit
- Glass Ampoules (Distilled Water)
- Glass Bangles & Glass Pressed Wares
- Glass Bottle
- Glass Marble
- Glass Sheet
- Glass Sheet (Automatic Plant)
- Glazed Ceramic Tiles
- Granite Slab & Tiles
- High Alumina Ceramic
- Laminated Safety Glass
- Mirror Colouring (Pink, Black,Golden, Silver)
- Mirrors (Silver, Golden, Pink Black And Yellow Colour)
- Non Glazed Ceramic Tiles
- Optical Glass
- Optical Lenses Manufacture
- Safety Glass
- Watch Glass

Gums & Adhesives

- Acrylic Adhesive
- Adhesive (Fevicol Type)
- Adhesive Based Polyurethanes
- Adhesive Content Pvc Resin & Dop Paste Grade

- Disposable Needles For Syringes
- Drip Irrigation System
- Drum & Berrels (35 To 200 Ltr)
- E.R.W.Steel Conduit Pipes
- Earth Moving Equipment
- Electrical Stamping
- Electronic Horn For Automobile
- Fasteners (Nut,Bolt,Rivet Etc.)
- Fasteners (Nuts Bolts Rivets & Washers
- Ferrite Magnets
- Filter (Micro Filter Inserts For Automobile)
- Filter For All Vehicles
- Fire Extinguisher
- Fire Fighting Equipments
- Flush Doors
- Forging Unit
- Forging Unit (General)
- Foundry Sand (Non Ferrous Metal)
- G.I. Wire From H.B. Wire
- Galvanised Iron Strips
- Galvanising Of Zinc (Electrical Process)
- Galvanising Of Zinc (Hot-Dip Process)
- Galvanising Plant
- Galvenising Cans For Gardening
- Garden Tools & Fencing Accessories
- Gas Welding Torch & Nozzles
- Gold & Platinum Jewellery Manufacturing With Die-Casting
- Graphite Carbon Plate
- Graphite Crucibles
- Graphite Electrode For Arc Furnace
- Grinding Media Ball
- Hand Pump Mark-Ii Unit
- Hand Tools (E.O.U.)
- Handle For Bucket
- Helmet
- Hot Dip Galvanizing
- Hydraulically Regulated Doors Closer (Everest Type)
- Hydroulic And Pneumatic Items
- Industrial Valve
- Investment Casting
- Iron Powder (Cost)
- Iron Powder From Mill Scale Scrap
- Jali For Fan [Fan Gaurd][Metalic] Automatic Plant
- Kitchen Sinks (Stainless Steel
- Kudali, Fawra, Gaiti, Belcha Manufacturing
- L.P.G. Cylinder
- L.P.G. Cylinder & Regulator
- L.P.G. Cylinders
- L.P.G. Regulators (Domestic Purpose)
- Laminated Tube (Multilayer)
- Lead Metal From Lead Ore
- Link Chain
- Locks (Aligarh Type)
- Lpg Regulators (For Domestic Purpose)
- M.S. Binding Wires
- M.S. Hinges
- M.S. Ingots (Mini Steel Plant) 5 Mt Induction Furnace
- M.S. Pipe From Strips
- M.S. Winding Wire & Anealing
- Magnet
- Material Handling Equipments
- Measuring Tapes
- Mechanical Toys
- Metal Container For Packaging
- Metal Drums & Barrels 25 To 200 Litres
- Metal Hardening
- Metallic Drum (Used For Oil Storage)
- Micro Filters For Automobile
- Micro Irrigation System
- Mini Steel Plant (25-T V H F Electric Arc Furnace &Int Rolling Mill)
- Non Stick Cookwares
- Non-Stick Kitchen Ware
- Nut & Bolts (Cold Formed Steel Fastners)
- Nut And Bolts (Mild Steel)
- Oil Seals
- Open Top Sanitary Cans For Food, Pesticides, Paint
- P.P. Caps (Aluminium)
- Packaging Printing Tin Container & Other Metals
- Pad Locks/Door Locks
- Pig Iron
- Pilfer Proof Caps
- Pilfer Proof Crown Caps
- Pig Iron
- Piston Assembly (Aluminium Alloy)
- Piston-Rings For Ic Engines (Cost Iron)
- Plant Protection Equipment
- Plastic Cladded Aluminium Squeeze Tube
- Press Steel Doors & Window
- Pressure Die-Casting
- Printed (Multi Colour) Tin Container (Air Tight) Packing
- Printed Tin Containers
- Railway Air Break
- Refrigeration Strand Various Model
- Rerolling Mill For Sariya & Twisting Rod
- Re-Rolling Mill For Tor Steel
- Resin Cored Soldring Wire
- Rice Huller
- Rock Drill Bits
- Rolling Mill With Furnish Plant
- Rolling, Bearing & Forging Of Outer/Inner Rings
- Rubber Auto Parts
- S.G. Iron Casting & Melleable Iron Casting
- S.S. Alloy Steel Casting
- S.S. Bright Bars & Wire Mfg.(Cold Drawn Process)
- S.S. Cutlery
- Safety Helmate
- Safety Pin, Paper Pin, Gem Clips
- Sandwiched Bottom (Al-Alloy & S.S.) Utensils
- Seemless M.S. Tube & Pipes
- Selenium Coated Aluminium Drum Used In Plain Paper Copier
- Self Taping Steel Screws
- Sewing Needles (For Use With Domestic/Indl. Sewing M/C.)
- Silencer For Auto Vehicles
- Silencer For Two And Three Wheelers
- Silicone Metal (Cap. 25 Mt/A)
- Sintered Bearing
- Sintered Bushes
- Sintered Metal Auto Components
- Sponge Iron
- Sponge Iron With Captive Power Plant (Agro Based)
- Spring Washers
- Stainless Steel Cutlery
- Stainless Steel Tube
- Stainless Steel Utensile
- Stainless Steel Wire Drawing
- Steel Balls For Ball Point Pen
- Steel Casting For Railways
- Steel Drums And Barrels
- Steel Fabrication (Fabrication Unit)
- Steel Forging For Automobile Parts
- Steel Furniture
- Steel Ingot (Furnace)
- Steel Plant (Blast Furnace)
- Steel Re-Rolling Mill (Steel Roof & Coil From Scrap)
- Steel Rolling Mill
- Steel Safty Pins
- Steel Shot/Steel Grits
- Steel Wool
- Structural Steel
- Submerged Arc Welded Pipes
- Submersible Pump Manufacture
- Super Enameled Copper Wire
- Surgical Suture
- Taper Roller Bearing Manufacturing
- Thermocole
- Three Wheelers Manufacturing
- Torch & Tri-Light Unit (Integrated Plant)
- Carbon Brush, Brush Holder Slipring
- Tripod Stands, Tables & Chairs (100% E.O.U.)
- U Bolt & Centre Bolt For Autoleaf Springs
- Vacuum Metalising Process
- Vacuum Thermoflask
- Valve Guide
- Washerless Faucet (Taps)
- Watch Straps/Chains/Belt
- Watch Case Manufacturing Unit
- Watch Strraps/Chains/Bracelets /Belt (Brass & Steel)
- Welding Brass Rod
- Welding Electrodes
- Welding Fluxes
- Wick Stoves
- Wick Stoves Stainless Steel
- Wind Mill
- Wind Screen Cleaner
- Wire Mesh (Hexagonal Square)
- Wire Nail
- Wire Nail/Wire Drawing
- Zinc Amd Aluminium Anode Foundry Marine & Oil Industry

Miscellaneous Products

- Advertising Agency
- Agarbatti (Sticks)
- Air Taxi (12 Seater)
- Amusement Park
- Amusement Park Cum Water Park
- Artificial Marble Tiles
- Artificial Flowers (Paper & Cloth)
- Asphlatic Roofing Sheet
- Auto Workshop/Garage & Service Station

- Bamboo Chips For Paper Mill
- Bamboo Sticks Used For Agarbatti
- Bank (Private Sector)
- Banquet Hall
- Bentonite (Quarrying, Processing & Exporting)
- Bone Crushing Plant
- Buttons From Cattle Houses
- Buttons From Hoves & Horns
- Canvas Shoes
- Car-Leasing & Finance
- Cigarettes Unit
- Cinema Hall
- Coal Washing Unit
- Coir Handicraft
- Cold Storage
- Cold Storage & Ice Plant
- Combine Coke
- Community Hall
- Compozite Carbon Fiber
- Cricket Ball, Bat Manufacturing
- Daily Need Stores
- Departmental Stores
- Diagnostic Centre
- Diamond & Gem Cutting & Processing Unit
- Diamond Cutting & Export
- Dispensary
- Disposable Cigarete Gas Lighter
- Dry Cleaners
- Dry Cleaning And Laundry Unit
- Dry Flowers
- Engineering College
- Expansion Joint Filler
- Eye Hospital
- Fast Food Corner
- Fire Fighting Equipment,Chemicals & Refilling
- Fire Works
- Five Star Hotel (Delux)
- Five Star Hotel Industry
- Flush Door, Chip Board, Hard Board, Insulating Board
- Flush Door, Clip Board & Hardboard
- Games Parlour
- Gas Filling Of L.P.G. Cylinder
- Gems Manufacturing (Original)
- Gold & Silver Jewellery
- Gold Jewellery (100% Eou)
- Handicrafts (Can & Bamboo)
- Hard Board From Saw Dust
- Hawan Samgri
- Health Club & Beauty Parlour
- Health Club Cum Beauty Parlour Cum Hair Saloon
- Heat Chamber Painting
- Holiday Resorts
- Holiday Resorts Cum Ent. Club 4 Star Hotel
- Holiday Village Resort
- Hospital
- Hospital (20 Beds)
- Hospital 300 Beds To 700 Beds Teaching Facility
- Hospital Bed
- Hotel
- Hotel Industries 5 Star, 3 Star Holiday Resorts
- Hotel Unit (Three Star)
- Hotel/Small Motel
- L.P.G. Cylinder Retesting Uint
- L.P.G. Cylinder Testing Centre
- Laminated Partical Board
- Laundry
- Leasing Hire Purchase A/C
- Local Area Bank
- Mfg. Of Coloured Joint Filler Used For Jointing Tiles
- Marketing Arrangement And Distribution Strategy Of Wd-40
- Marketing Of Gram Shilpa
- Match Box Plant (Automatic)
- Medical College
- Medical College Hospital & Research Institute
- Melamine Crockery
- Mineral Fillers For Application Paint, Paper, Rubber, Plastic
- Mineral Wool
- Motel/Small Hotel With Banquet Hall, Restaurant & Catering
- Multistoryed Commercial Complex
- Natural Care Centre
- Nursing Home
- Paeditric Hospital 25 Beds
- Paint Brush
- Particle Board & Block Board With Sanding And Laminating
- Petrol Pump
- Photo Lab. Cum Studio (100% Computerised)
- Plaster Of Paris Bandages
- Plywood
- Plywood & Plyboard
- Plywood (Phenol Bonded)
- Pvc Joint Fillings
- Q.S.S. Colour Lab.
- Quering Of Lime Stone
- Recreation And Health Club
- Residential Appartments
- Restaurant
- Restaurant/Fast Food Parlour
- Rubber Wood Processing Plant
- Saw Mill
- School
- Shellac Manufacturing
- Shoe Uppers
- Slaughter House Beef Processing
- Slimming Centre & Health Club
- Snake Park
- Sport Shoe (Automatic Imported Plant
- Sterilize Bone Meal
- Straw Board
- Stuff Toys
- Sunmica
- Super Market (Commercial Market)
- Synthetic Floating To Fishing Industry
- Synthetic Rubyand Sapphire
- Tennis Ball
- Timber (Wood) Seasoning
- Trading Business (With Packaging Rice, Salt, Pulses, Etc)
- Travelling Agency
- Venetian Blind
- Video Film Studio
- Ware House
- Water Park
- Wind Mill
- Wooden Furniture
- Wonder Fuel (Gel Type)
- Wood Wool Industry
- Wooden Chips For Supplying To Paper Mills
- Wooden Doors Windows Sheets Tv Cabinet
- Wooden Furniture
- Wooden Furniture With Mediocre Automation
- Wooden Furniture With Seasoning Plant
- Wooden Needles For Tooth & Wooden Spoon For Ice Cream
- Wooden Tooth Pick
- Work Shop For Telco Truck

Oils & Fats

- Castor Oil (Batch Process)
- Castor Oil (Extraction & Refining)
- Castor Oil (Refining & Extraction)
- Castor Oil Derivative Oleo Resin
- Coconut Oil From Copra
- Coconut Oil In Containers (Filteration & Airtight Packaging)
- Corn Oil (Maize Oil)
- Cotton Seed Oil
- Cotton Seed Oil (Extraction & Refined)
- Extraction Of Sesame, Rice Bran & Palm Oil
- Extraction Of Oil From Neem Seed
- Extraction Of Oil From Soyabean & Cotton Seed
- Fat Liquor (Sulfated Oil)
- Hydrogenation Of Non-Edible Oil
- Maize Oil
- Margarine/Fat
- Neem Oil From Seeds
- Non-Formal Dye Fixing Oil
- Palm Oil
- Poppy Seed Oil By Expeller Process
- Poppy Seed Oil By Solvent Extraction Process
- Rainbow Colours On Metal
- Refined Oil (Cotton Seed Ground Nut Oil & Sunflower Oil
- Refined, Bleached, Palm Oil From Crude Palm Oil
- Rice Bran Extraction & Refining
- Rice Bran Oil
- Rubber Processing Oil
- Shesham Oil From Shesham Seed
- Shortening & Liquid Palm (Olien)
- Sun Flower Seed Oil
- Turpentine Oil And Rosin

Paints, Pigments, Enamels & Varnishes

- Aluminium Paint
- Anti-Corrosive Thinner & Paint
- Automobile Paints For Car
- Cement Paint
- Chrome Pigments
- Cement Paint
- Clear Transparent Lacquer For Coating On Brass
- Dry Distemper And Cement Paint
- Emulsion Paint (Road Marking & Airodrome Runways -Water Base)
- Insulating Varnish
- Insulating Varnishes & Wire Enamels
- Latex Paints For Roof
- Lead Chrom Pigment From Lead Scrap (97%)
- Lithopone Pigment
- Red Oxide Pigments From Ferrous Sulphate
- N.C. Thinners Used In Auto Parts
- Naphtha Base Thinner

- Newsprint Paper
- Nitro Cellulose (Lacquers)
- Paint And Varnish
- Paint Industries
- Ultra Violet Varnish
- Pigments
- Poster Colour
- Powder Coating
- Powder Coating (Chamber Type)
- Red Oxide Paint
- Solvent & Thinner
- Stoving Paint
- Synthetic Iron Oxide (Red, Yellow, Green, Blue Etc)
- Thinner/Solvent & Its Allied Product
- Thinners
- Titanium Dioxide
- Colour Cem (Snowcem)
- Ultra Violet Varnish
- Vacuum Metalizing Lacquers

Paper & Allied Products

- Absorbent Kraft Paper
- Amonia Paper
- Card Board Boxes & Cartoons Of Paper
- Card/Gray Board From Pulp & Waste Paper
- Coated Paper & Board Art & Chrom
- Corrugated Board Box Plant (Printed & Laminated)
- Corrugated Sheet Board & Boxes
- Craft Paper & Special Paper
- Paper Bags For White Cement Bags
- Emery Sand Paper
- Exercise Note Book & Register
- Flute Paper From Waste Paper
- Hand Made Paper
- Hard Board From Baggase
- Kraft Paper & Mill Board From Waste Cartoon Boxes
- Kraft Paper From Waste Cartoon Boxes
- Manufacturing Of Recycled Paper Products
- Mini Paper Plant
- Mini Paper Plant By Waste Paper
- Mini Paper Plant From Eucalyptus Wood
- Mini Paper Plant From Jute Sticks & Wheat Husk Rice Husk
- Paper & Paper Products
- Paper (E.C.G. & E.E.G.)
- Paper And Paper Board From Jute Sticks
- Paper Bags For General Use
- Paper Board Manufacturing Unit
- Paper Cones & Tubes
- Paper Cones & Tubes (Automatic Plant)
- Paper Cups For Ice Cream
- Paper Envelopes
- Paper From Bagasse
- Paper From Bamboo
- Paper From Rice Husk & Wheat Husk
- Paper From Waste Paper, Bamboo Chips Rice & Wheat Husk
- Paper From Wood Pulp Bamboo Etc.,
- Paper Napkin, Facial Paper & Toilet Roll From Tissue Paper
- Paper Napkins & Air Mail Paper
- Paper Plates
- Paper Shopping Bag· Poly Coated Paper
- Printed Paper Shopping Bags
- Pulp From Bamboo Wood
- Self Sealing Paper Envelopes
- Silicon Release Paper
- Silicone Coated Paper
- Straw Board (Automatic Plant)From Rice Husk & Bagasse
- Sundried Board From Waste Paper & Pulp
- Tissue Paper
- Tissue Paper, Toilet Paper & Air Mail Paper Roll
- Tracing Paper
- Wall Paper
- Writing & Printing Paper

Pesticides, Insecticides & Allied Products

- Aerosol Insecticide Spray
- Ayurvedic Gamaxane (Using Red Moing)
- Bagon Spray
- Boot Polish
- Copper Oxychloride
- D.D.T. Powder
- Grease Manufacturing Unit
- Mosquito Coil And Mats
- Mosquito Coils
- Mosquito Mats And Liquids
- Mosquito Repellant Candle
- Mosquito Repellant Liquidator
- Mosquito Repellant Oil
- Mosquito Repellant Mats
- Mosquito Repellant Agarbatti
- Pesticide Formulation
- Pesticides
- Phenyl (Black & White)
- Phenyl Pine Oil Disinfectants

Petroleum, Waxes & Allied Products

- Anti-Static Lubricating Oil Used For Polyster Fibre Spinning
- Automatic Candle Making Plant
- Bees Wax
- Bituminous Felts For Water Proofing And Damp Proofing
- Brake Fluids [Dot-3 Type)
- Brake Oil, Coolant & Packaging Of Lubricant Oil & Grease
- Break Oil
- Calcined Petroleum Coke
- Candle Making Plant (Semi Automatic)
- Candle Making Unit (Automatic)
- Chlorinated Paraffin Wax (Cpw)
- Coaltar Distillation
- Coloured Flamed Candles (Red, Blue & Green)
- Coloured Flamed & Perfumed Candles
- Compound Wax From Residual Oil
- Coolant & Brake Oil
- Cutting Oil
- Feldspar
- Furnace Oil
- Grease & Lube Oil From Used Engine Oil
- Grease Manufacturing
- Grease Manufacturing (Calcium, Lithium & Sodium)
- Grease Used For Chasis
- Jute Batching Oil
- Liquid Shoe Polish
- Lube Oil From Cnsl Reduce Friction
- Lubricating Oil & Greases
- Lubricating Oils & Grease (Blending Of Lubricating Oil & Manufacture Of Greases
- Microcrystaline Wax From Sludge Of Petrolium
- Microcrystalline Wax From Sludge Of Petrochemical Refinery
- Mobile Oil (Lube) & Grease
- Poly Ethylene Wax
- Polyester Polyol Air Foam Mfg.By Using Petroleum Base As Raw Material
- Reclaimation Of Wax Sludge For Mfg. Of Microcrystaline Wax
- Reclamation Of Transformer Oil
- Reclamation Of Used Engine Oil
- Refining Of Used Lubricating Oil
- Re-Refining Of Used Lubricating Oils
- Road Emulsion Bitumen Or Modified Bitumen
- Shoe Polish
- Transformer Oil
- Turkey Red Oil
- Wax Floor Polish
- Wetting Oil (Textile Yarn Wetting Agent)
- White Oil From Kerosene Oil
- Wire Drawing Lubricants
- Wood Polish

Pharmaceuitcal Drugs & Fine Chemicals

- Acyclovir
- Adhesive Tape For Hospital Use
- Aloevera Gel
- Amoxycillin
- Ampicillin
- Aspirin
- Ayurvedic Churan & Tablets
- Ayurvedic Pain Balm Onintment
- Ayurvedic Pharmacy (Capsules, Liquid, Oral Ointment, Powder)
- Ayurvedic/Herbal Pharmacy
- Baby Health Care Food & Milk
- Bulk Drugs
- Camphor Tablets
- Ciprofloxacin
- Cloxacillin
- Cotton Buds/Swab
- Dettol Like Antiseptic Lotion
- Dextrose (Monohydrous)
- Dextrose 5%
- Dextrose Powder From Potatoes
- Dextrose Saline 5% 10% 25% Solution
- Dextrose Saline Solution In Plastic Bottles
- Disposable Baby Diaper
- Disposable Needles For Syringes
- Disposable Plastic Syringes & Needles Tube Plant
- Distilled Water
- Empty Gelatine Capsules
- Gelatine From Bones
- Glucose Saline
- Herbal Concentrate In The Mfg.Of Herbal Drugs & Concentrate
- Herbal Extract

- Herbal Formulation (Herbal Plant)
- Homeopathic Sugar Giobules
- Homoeopathic Medicines
- I.V. Bottle (F.F.S. Technology)
- I.V. Fluid In Plastic Bottles
- I.V. Fluids
- Ibuprofen
- Injectables For Pharmaceutical
- Isobgol Husk
- L-Ascorbic Acid (Vitamin C) From Lemons
- Liquid Glucose From Maize And Maize Oil
- Liquid Glucose From Potatoes
- Medicinal Plant Extract
- Mother Tincture & Bio Chemic Medicines
- Paracetamol
- Pentaerythritol
- Pharmaceutical Unit
- Pharmaceutical Unit (Tablet, Syrup, Capsules)
- Salicylic Acid/Aspirin
- Saline And Injection Water
- Sanitary Napkins & Baby Diaper
- Starch Liquid Glucose Dextrose Sorbitol
- Sulfamethoxazoline
- Surgical Suture
- Tablet Capsules Syrup & Lotion
- Tooth Brush & Tooth Powder/Paste
- Tooth Paste & Tooth Powder
- Trimetheprime
- Veternary Medicines (Powder, Tablets & Capsules)

Plantation

- Amla Plantation
- Aromatic Plants Cultivation & Processing
- Banana Plantation & Its By Products
- Cardamom Cultivation
- Coconut Plantation
- Coffee Plantation
- Eucalyptus Tree Plantation
- Ginger Cultivation & Storage
- Herbal Medicinal Plant & Processing
- Herbal Plantation (Medicinal)
- Maize Cultivation & Its By Products
- Mango Plantation
- Mustered Seed Cultivation
- Neem Plantation
- Palm Tree Plantation
- Papaya Cultivation
- Papaya Cultivation & Papain Manufacturing
- Plantation Of Medicinal Plant & Herbs
- Poplar Plantation
- Rose Plantation & Rose Oil Extraction (Rose Esential Oil)
- Rubber Plantation
- Saffron Cultivation
- Shisham Plantations
- Tea Plantation
- Teak Plantation
- Teak Plantation By Tissue Culture
- Turmeric Plantation

Plantation/ Agro Based

- Aloevera Juice, Gel And Powder
- Aquaculture/ Shrimp Farming
- Asparagus Cultivation And Processing
- Banana & Its By Products
- Banana Powder
- Bee Keeping & Honey Processing
- Bee Keeping, Honey Processing And Packaging
- Bio-Coal Briquetts From Agri.Cellulosic Waste
- Cashew Nut Kernal Extraction From Cashew Nut Fruits
- Cashew Nut Shell Liquid & Kernel Processing
- Cashew Nut Shell Liquide (Cnsl)
- Cashewnut Kernel Extraction From Cashewnut Shell
- Cattle Farm (Cap. 500 Cow)
- Cattle Breeding
- Cattle Breeding & Dairy Farm To Produce Milk
- Cattle Feed With Molasses
- Cement From Fly Ash & Lime
- Cement From Rice Husk
- Charcoal From Baggasse
- Charcoal From Coconut Shell
- Chicken Meat Processing & Packaging
- Coconut Fibre Unit
- Coconut Processing Unit (Complex)
- Coconut Shell Powder
- Coffee Processing & Packaging
- Coir Industry
- Coir Pith
- Dairy Agro Farm (Cow, Goat, Broiler) Farming
- Dairy Farm To Produce Milk
- Dairy Farm To Produce Milk In Poly Pack
- Dairy Farming & Dairy Products
- Dairy Farming To Produce Milk For Co-Operative Society
- Dairy Products
- De-Carbonised (Smokeless Coke/Soft Coke)
- Dehulling Of Sesam Seeds
- Dehydrated Onion & Onion Powder
- Desiccated Coconut Powder From Coconuts
- Dry Ginger From Green Ginger
- Fish Farming
- Fish Farming (Prawn & Others) & Marine Products
- Fruit Pulp And Juice Concentrate
- Fuel Briquetts From Agro Waste
- Ginger Processing (Peeling Drying, Grinding, Bleaching
- Goat And Sheep Farming
- Goat Farming
- Gram Dall & Flour Mill With Modern Automatic Plant
- Gram Dall And Flour Mill
- Green House (Micro Plant Propagation)
- Hard Board For Rice Husk
- Hard Board From Bagasse
- Hard Board From Coir Dust
- Hard Board From Saw Dust
- Herbs Cultivation & Processing
- Honey Processing & Packaging
- Liquid Glucose From Potatoes
- Medicinal / Herbal Plants
- Mini Sugar Plant
- Modren Rice Mill
- Mushroom Cultivation & Processing With Air Conditioning
- Nursery Farms
- Nursury For Producing Tree - Sapling
- Onion & Potato Powder
- Onion Storage
- Papaya Cultivation & Papain Manufacturing
- Particle Board From Cotton Stem
- Particle Board From Rick Husk
- Particle Board From Saw Dust
- Pig Farming
- Pig Farming With Pork Processing
- Pig Meat Processing (800 Pig/Day)
- Poultry & Poultry Farm With Hatchery
- Poultry And Broiler Farming
- Poultry Farm (Cap. 5000 Fowls/Annum)
- Poultry Farm (Cap: 100000 Birds/Annum)
- Poultry Feed
- Poultry Processing Plant
- Rabbit Farming
- Seed Grading/Processing
- Soft Board & Hard Board From Coir Dust
- Soyabean Products
- Sugarcane Juice Preservation
- Tamarind Kerenel Powder
- Tamarind Seed Decoradicating & Powder Starch Making
- Tea Packaging Industry
- Tea Plantation & Processing
- Tea Processing & Packaging
- Tobacco Creamy Snuff
- Trading Business (Rice,Salt,Dry Fruits, Etc.)

Printing & Publishing

- Aluminium Printing Plates For Offset Printing Machine
- Aluminium Ps (Pre-Sensitised) Plates
- Automatic Book Binding Unit
- Ceramic Transfers (For Printing On Ceramics)
- Computer Farms & Security Printing Press
- Dtp Cum Offset Printing
- Dtp, E-Mail, Internet & Leased Access For Commercial Purpose
- Flexographic & Rotogravure Printing
- Flexographic Printing On Polyethylene
- Graphic Art Conversion & Packing
- Gravure Printing Cylinders
- Heat Transfer Label For Rubber
- Letter Press Printing Unit
- Modern Advertisement Agency With Dtp & Film Studio
- Multi Colour 8 Page Offset Unit
- News Paper Publishing Unit
- Offset Printing [Mini]

Above mentioned Project Reports are Readily available with "National Institute of Industrial Research"
106-E, Kamla Nagar, Delhi - 110 007. Ph: 23843955, 23845886, 23845654 Fax: 91-11-23841561

k

- Offset Printing Press Single Colour
- Offset Printing Press-4 Colour
- Photo Polymer Coating For Plate & Block Making
- Pre-Sensitised (Ps) Plates Of Aluminium For Offset Printing
- Printing On Cartoon
- Screen Printing

Rubber & Plastic Industries

- 100% Polyster Wadding
- Abs Granules
- Acrylic Sheet & Moulded Products
- Acrylic Sheet From Acrylic Waste
- Acrylic Tiles (Extruded)
- Acrylic Yarn
- Air Bubble Packaging
- Armoured Cables
- Auto Tubes
- Automobile Tyre For Bus,Truck,Trolly
- Automobile Tyre Tube & Flaps
- B.O.P.P. Film
- Bakelight Electrical Accesseries
- Bakelite Moulded Products
- Bakelite Powder For Electric Goods & Pressure Cooker
- Bakelite Sheet (Phenolic Sheet)
- Bicycle Tubes
- Bicycle Tyres 4000 Pcs./ 8 Hr.
- Blood Bags
- Blow Moulding (Plastic Containers)
- Bopp Pressure Sensetive Self Adhesive Tape
- Coir Foam (Rubberised Coir)
- Colour Master Batches For Various Plastic
- Conveyor Belting
- Cycle Tyres & Tubes
- Disposable Plastic Cup, Glasses
- Disposable Plastic Syringes
- Epoxy Resin
- Eva (Ethylene Vinyl Acetate Sheet & Sole)
- Expanded Polystyrene
- Expanded Polystyrene Board
- F.R.P. Boat Building
- F.R.P. Product (Fiber Rainforced Plastic Products)
- Fibre Glass
- Fibre Reinforced Plastic Pipes
- Flexible Office Furniture Systems
- Flexible Polyurethane Foam
- Foam & Its Products As Mattresses,Cushion, Pillows
- Frp Auto Scooter Roofs/ Celling
- Frp Sheet & Product
- H.D.P.E. Bags (Stitching)
- H.D.P.E. Film & Sheets
- H.D.P.E. Tarpaulins
- H.D.P.E. Woven Sacks/ Stitching
- Hard Rubber Battery Container
- Hawai Chappal
- Hawai Chappal & Micro Cellular Sheet Manufacturing
- Hdpe Container (1 To 5 Ltr)
- Hdpe Container (All Purpose)
- Hdpe Plastic Tank (Cap.1000 L)
- Hdpe Twine & Rope
- Hdpe/Pp Box Strapings
- Hoses (Air-Based-Welding Hoses & Pesicides Spray Pipe)
- I.V. Cannula
- Injection Moulded Plastic Components
- Injection Moulded Plastic Products
- Intra Venous (I.V.) Sets
- Latex Foam (Rubber) Products
- Latex Rubber Condoms
- Liquid Storage Tank
- Lpg Gas Pipe
- Lpg Rubbr Tube (Pipe) Flexible
- Manufacturing Of Hdpe & Ldpe Pipes & Fittings
- Medical X-Ray Film Slitting And Repacking
- Moulded Luggage
- Moulded Shoe & Hawai Chappal Mfg.
- Multi-Layer 3-Layer Film Printing & Lamination
- Multi-Layer Co-Extrusion, 3-Layer Film With Lamination & Printing
- Neon Sign Board Manufacturing
- Nylon Fish Net
- Nylon Polyester & Polypropylene Rope Making
- Nylone Zip Fasteners
- Optical Fibre
- P V C Bottles
- P.U. Foam (Polyurethane Foams)
- P.V.C. Coating On G.I.Wire
- P.V.C. Conduit Pipe
- P.V.C. Conduit Pipe (Electrical)
- P.V.C. Film
- P.V.C. Granules, Film & Bag (Printed)
- P.V.C. Hand Gloves
- P.V.C. Lining For Metal Crown Caps
- P.V.C. Pipe & Fitting
- P.V.C. Wire & Cables
- P.V.C. Wires And Cables (Flexible)
- Patches Tube Repairing Material
- Pet Bottle
- Pet Bottles From Pre-Form Pet
- Pet Bottles/ Containers
- Pet Pre-Form From Pet Resin
- Plastic Buckets, Bottles & Doli
- Plastic Buttons From Polyester Sheet & Rod
- Plastic Card Mfg. Smart Card, Credit Card, Discount Card
- Plastic Cards (Smart Cards)
- Plastic Cards (Smart Cards) Utilised Credit Cards
- Plastic Collapsible Tube For Tooth Paste & Cream
- Plastic Collopsible Tubes & Printing
- Plastic Corrogated Sheet & Box
- Plastic Fan Guard (Automatic Plant)
- Plastic Felt
- Plastic Films & Sheet With Printing (Flexo & Roto)
- Plastic Granules From Scraps/Waste
- Plastic I. V. Bottles
- Plastic Mats Extruding & Weaving
- Plastic Moulded Furniture
- Plastic Moulded Furniture (Chairs)
- Plastic Moulded Toys
- Plastic Office Products
- Plastic Processing Moulds
- Plastic Sequince
- Plastic Spectacle Frame
- Plastic Sutli
- Plastic Toys
- Plastic Water Storage Tank (H.D.P.E.)(Syntex Type)
- Poly Propylene Measuring Cup
- Polyester Film
- Polyester Polyol Air Foam Mfg.By Using Petroleum Base As Raw Material
- Polyester Resin
- Polyster Film
- Polythene Bags
- Polythene Bags And Automatic Prinitng
- Polythene Pouches For Ghee, Butter, Milk And Oil
- Polythene Printed Bags
- Polythene Printed Bags (Pp & Hm)
- Polyurethane
- Polyurethane Foam & Its Products
- Polyurethane Product (Rigid & Moulded)
- Polyurethane Foam (Flexible)
- Polyurethane Pipe Section,Slab Panels, Rigid Foam, Moulding
- Pvc (Hdpe) Water Storage Tank
- Pvc Bottles For Mineral Water
- Pvc Compound From Pvc Resin
- Pvc Compounding
- Pvc Conduit Pipes
- Pvc Felexible Pipe
- Pvc Footwear
- Pvc From Ethanols
- Pvc Granules & Rigid Pipes
- Pvc Hoses (For Irrigation Purposes)
- Pvc Pipe & Fittings
- Pvc Profiles (Door, Window And Chairs) Decorative Accessories
- Pvc Rexine Cloth
- Pvc Section Hoses
- Pvc Section Pipe
- Pvc Soles
- Pvc Tube
- Rubber (Floor Mat) For Automobile
- Rubber Auto Parts
- Rubber Ball For Childrens
- Rubber Band
- Rubber Band (Disco Type)
- Rubber Baskets
- Rubber Belting (V - Belt)
- Rubber Compound For Automobiles
- Rubber Floor Mat
- Rubber Linning & F.R.P. Linning
- Rubber Powder From Waste Tyres
- Rubber Reclamation Industry
- Rubber Roller & Ebonite Roller
- Rubber Roller For Printing M\C
- Rubber Roller For Rice Mill
- Rubber Rollers
- Rubber Sheet For